Essential Clinical
Global Health

D1341649

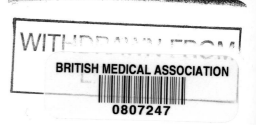

Essential Clinical Global Health

Edited by

Brett D. Nelson
MD, MPH, DTM&H
Director of Pediatric and Newborn Programs
Division of Global Health and Human Rights, Department of Emergency Medicine
Division of Global Health, Department of Pediatrics
Massachusetts General Hospital

Assistant Professor
Harvard Medical School
Boston, Massachusetts
USA

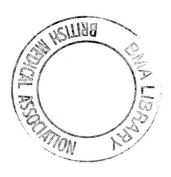

WILEY Blackwell

Registered Office
John Wiley & Sons Ltd, The Atrium, Southern Gate, Chichester, West Sussex, PO19 8SQ, UK

Editorial Offices
350 Main Street, Malden, MA 02148-5020, USA
9600 Garsington Road, Oxford, OX4 2DQ, UK
The Atrium, Southern Gate, Chichester, West Sussex, PO19 8SQ, UK

For details of our global editorial offices, for customer services, and for information about how to
apply for permission to reuse the copyright material in this book please see our website at
www.wiley.com/wiley-blackwell.

Library of Congress Cataloging-in-Publication Data

Essential clinical global health / edited by Brett D. Nelson.
     p. ; cm.
  Includes bibliographical references and index.
  ISBN 978-1-118-63844-6 (pbk.)
  I. Nelson, Brett D., editor.
  [DNLM: 1. Clinical Medicine. 2. Evidence-Based Practice. 3. World Health. WB 102]
  RC46
  616–dc23

                                                    2014032272

A catalogue record for this book is available from the British Library.

Cover image: Reproduced from Tara Clark Photography © Tara Clark Photography

Set in 10/12 pt AGaramondPro by Toppan Best-set Premedia Limited
Printed and bound in Singapore by Markono Print Media Pte Ltd

1   2015

Contents

Editor and Editorial Board

Contributors

Adam M. Ackerman MD
Resident in Surgery
Department of Surgery
Maine Medical Center
Portland, ME, USA

Hans C. Ackerman MD, DPhil, MSc
Assistant Clinical Investigator
Laboratory of Malaria and Vector Research
National Institute of Allergy and Infectious Diseases
Rockville, MD, USA

Asya Agulnik MD, MPH
Fellow in Pediatric Critical Care
Boston Children's Hospital
Boston, MA, USA

Roy Ahn MPH, ScD
Associate Director
Division of Global Health and Human Rights
Department of Emergency Medicine
Massachusetts General Hospital
Instructor in Surgery
Harvard Medical School
Boston, MA, USA

Melanie Anspacher MD
Pediatric Hospitalist
Children's National Medical Center
Assistant Professor of Pediatrics
George Washington University
Washington, DC, USA

Natasha M. Archer MD, MPH
Instructor Pediatrics
Dana-Farber/Boston Children's Cancer and
Blood Disorders Center
Harvard Medical School
Boston, MA, USA

Peter S. Azzopardi MB, BS, MEpi, FRACP
Centre for Adolescent Health
Royal Children's Hospital
Murdoch Childrens Research Institute
Department of Paediatrics
University of Melbourne
Melbourne, Australia
Wardliparingga Aboriginal Research Unit
South Australian Health and Medical Research Institute
Adelaide, Australia

Marouen Ben Guebila
Chairperson of Education
International Pharmaceutical Students' Federation
The Hague, The Netherlands

Dalia Brahmi MD, MPH
Senior Clinical Advisor
Ipas
Chapel Hill, NC, USA

Helen Brotherton MBChB, MRCPCH, DTM (RCSI)
Paediatric Registrar
Royal Hospital for Sick Children
Edinburgh, Scotland, UK

Thomas F. Burke MD, FACEP
Chief, Division of Global Health and Human Rights
Department of Emergency Medicine
Massachusetts General Hospital
Assistant Professor of Surgery
Harvard Medical School
Boston, MA, USA

Alejandro J. Candelario MD
Resident in Pediatrics
Seattle Children's Hospital
University of Washington
Seattle, WA, USA

Ryan W. Carroll MD, MPH
Instructor in Pediatrics
Program Director
Global Health Collaborative
MUST, Uganda
Center for Global Health
Division of Pediatric Critical Care Medicine
Department of Pediatrics
Massachusetts General Hospital
Harvard Medical School
Boston, MA, USA

Mohammod Jobayer Chisti MBBS, MMed Pediatrics
Clinical Lead, Intensive Care Unit and Scientist
Centre for Nutrition and Food Security
International Centre for Diarrhoeal Disease and Research
Dhaka, Bangladesh

David C. Christiani MD, MPH, MS
Professor of Medicine, Professor of Occupational Medicine
and Epidemiology
Massachusetts General Hospital
Harvard Medical School
Harvard School of Public Health
Boston, MA, USA

Cordelia E.M. Coltart MBBS, BSc, MPH, MRCP
Academic Clinical Fellow
London School of Hygiene and Tropical Medicine
The Hospital for Tropical Diseases
University College London Hospitals
London, UK

Peter B. Cooch MD
Resident in Pediatrics
Department of Pediatrics
University of California
San Francisco
San Francisco, CA, USA

Carrie M. Cox MD
Assistant Professor Internal Medicine and Pediatrics
Loyola University Chicago
Stritch School of Medicine
Maywood, IL, USA

Mick B. Creati MBBS, MPH, FRACP
Adolescent Physician
Centre for Adolescent Health
Royal Children's Hospital
Victoria, Australia

Susan Cu-Uvin MD
Professor, Obstetrics and Gynecology and Medicine
Division of Infectious Diseases
Director, Brown Global Health Initiative
Brown University
Providence, RI, USA

Patricia A. Daoust RN, MSN
Associate Director of Nursing, Center for Global Health
Chief Nursing Officer
Seed Global Health
Massachusetts General Hospital
Boston, MA, USA

Ranu S. Dhillon MD
Brigham and Women's Hospital
Harvard Medical School
Boston, MA, USA
Earth Institute and School of International and Public
Affairs
Columbia University
New York, NY, USA

Nathalie Dhont MD, PhD
Gynaecologist
The Walking Egg Foundation
Ziekenhuis Oost-Limburg Hospitals
Genk, Belgium

Sahera Dirajlal-Fargo MS, DO
Instructor of Pediatrics
Case Western Reserve University
Rainbow Babies and Children's Hospital
Cleveland, OH, USA

Paul K. Drain MD, MPH
Massachusetts General Hospital
Harvard Medical School
Boston, MA, USA

Melody Eckardt MD, MPH
Director of Maternal Health
Division of Global Health and Human Rights
Department of Emergency Medicine
Massachusetts General Hospital
Instructor in Obstetrics and Gynecology
Director of Global and Refugee Health
Department of Obstetrics and Gynecology
Boston University School of Medicine
Boston, MA, USA

Claire W. Fung MD, MPH
Clinical Instructor
Department of Family Medicine
University of Washington
Seattle, WA, USA
The Everett Clinic
Everett, WA, USA

Diane L. Gal BSPharm, MPH
Formerly with the International Pharmaceutical Federation
(FIP) Education Initiative
The Hague, The Netherlands

Michael B. Hadley MPH
MD candidate
Harvard Medical School
Boston, MA, USA

Jason B. Harris MD, MPH, FAAP, FIDSA
Associate Professor
Division of Infectious Diseases
Department of Pediatrics
Massachusetts General Hospital
Harvard Medical School
Boston, MA, USA

Tabish Hazir MBBS, DCH, MCPS, FCPS
Professor and Head of Pediatrics
Children's Hospital
Pakistan Institute of Medical Sciences
Islamabad, Pakistan

Caroline S. Hesko MD, MPH
Pediatric Resident
Case Western Reserve University
Rainbow Babies and Children's Hospital
Cleveland, OH, USA

Nadi Kaonga MHS
Division of Global Health and Human Rights
Department of Emergency Medicine
Massachusetts General Hospital
Tufts University School of Medicine
Boston, MA, USA

Jennifer Kasper MD, MPH
Assistant Pediatrician
Division of Global Health
MassGeneral Hospital for Children
Instructor and Chair
Harvard Medical School
Boston, MA, USA

Johannes Kataraihya MD, MMED, DIC
Principal Consultant Physician and Cardiologist
Bugando Medical Centre
Associate Professor of Medicine
Weill Bugando School of Medicine
Catholic University of Health and Allied Sciences
Mwanza, Tanzania

Francine R. Kaufman MD
Chief Medical Officer and Vice President
Medtronic Diabetes
Emeritus Professor of Pediatrics and Communications
University of Southern California
The Center for Diabetes, Endocrinology, and Metabolism
Children's Hospital Los Angeles
Los Angeles, CA, USA

Elissa C. Kennedy MBBS, MPH
Principal for Maternal and Child Health
Centre for International Health
Burnet Institute
Adjunct Senior Lecturer, School of Public Health and
Preventive Medicine
Monash University
Melbourne, Victoria, Australia

Suwat Kusakul MD
Director, Nakhon Phanom Hospital
Nakhon Phanom, Thailand

Joy E. Lawn B MedSci, MB BS, MRCP (Paeds), MPH, PhD
Director, MARCH
Professor, London School of Hygiene and Tropical Medicine
London, UK
Saving Newborn Lives/Save the Children
Cape Town, South Africa

Anne C.C. Lee MD, MPH
Instructor in Pediatrics
Department of Newborn Medicine
Brigham and Women's Hospital
Harvard Medical School
Boston, MA, USA

Lois K. Lee MD, MPH
Attending Physician
Division of Emergency Medicine
Boston Children's Hospital
Assistant Professor of Pediatrics
Harvard Medical School
Boston, MA, USA

Els M.M. Leye MSc, PhD
Postdoctoral Researcher
International Centre for Reproductive Health
Ghent University
Ghent, Belgium

Susan C. Lipsett MD
Clinical Fellow in Pediatric Emergency Medicine
Boston Children's Hospital
Boston, MA, USA

Hillary Mabeya MBChB, MMed
Lecturer, Obstetrics and Gynecology
Chairman, Division of Reproductive Health
Moi University and Moi Teaching and Referral Hospital
Eldoret, Kenya

Alice G. Mark MD, MSc
Senior Clinical Advisor
Ipas
Chapel Hill, NC, USA

Lloyd K. Matowe BPharm (Hons), MSc, PhD
Director, Pharmaceutical Systems Africa
University of Liberia
Monrovia, Liberia

Alishya Mayfield MD
Brigham and Women's Hospital
Boston Children's Hospital
Harvard Medical School
Boston, MA, USA

Sarah E. Messmer
MD Candidate
Harvard Medical School
Boston, MA, USA

Danny A. Milner Jr MD, MSc
Associate Professor
Pathology and Assistant Medical Director (Microbiology)
Brigham and Women's Hospital
Harvard Medical School
Harvard School of Public Health
Boston, MA, USA

Radoslaw Mitura MD, MSc
President
International Pharmaceutical Students' Federation
The Hague, The Netherlands

Katharine E. Morley MD, MPH
Clinical Instructor in Medicine
Massachusetts General Hospital
Harvard Medical School
Boston, MA, USA

Michael G. Morley MD, MHCM
Ophthalmic Consultants of Boston
Assistant Clinical Professor of Ophthalmology
Harvard Medical School
Boston, MA, USA

Peter P. Moschovis MD, MPH
Clinical Research Fellow, Pulmonary and Critical Care
Medicine
Research Fellow, Pediatric Global Health
Massachusetts General Hospital
Harvard Medical School
Boston, MA, USA

Marisa Nádas MD, MPH
Assistant Professor
Department of Obstetrics & Gynecology and
Women's Health
Albert Einstein College of Medicine
Bronx, NY, USA

Brett D. Nelson MD, MPH, DTM&H
Director of Pediatric and Newborn Programs
Division of Global Health and Human Rights
Department of Emergency Medicine
Division of Global Health, Department of Pediatrics
Massachusetts General Hospital
Assistant Professor
Harvard Medical School
Boston, MA, USA

Michelle L. Niescierenko MD
Attending Physician
Division of Emergency Medicine
Boston Children's Hospital
Instructor of Pediatrics
Harvard Medical School
Boston, MA, USA

Elizabeth Nowak
MD candidate
Ben-Gurion University
Columbia University Medical Center
Be'er Sheva, Israel

Karen Olness MD
Professor of Pediatrics
Global Health and Diseases
Case Western Reserve University
Rainbow Babies and Children's Hospital
Cleveland, OH, USA

Suzinne Pak-Gorstein MD, MPH, PhD
Assistant Professor
Department of Pediatrics
University of Washington
Harborview Medical Center
Seattle Children's Hospital
Seattle, WA, USA

Judith Palfrey MD
Professor of Pediatrics
Harvard Medical School
Boston, MA, USA

Kinjan Parikh
MD candidate
Harvard Medical School
Boston, MA, USA

Shreya Patel MD, MPH
Resident, Global Primary Care Program
Massachusetts General Hospital
Harvard Medical School
Boston, MA, USA

Elizabeth Peacock-Chambers MD
Attending Pediatrician
Boston University School of Medicine
Boston, MA, USA

Robert N. Peck MD, DTM&H
Assistant Professor of Medicine and Pediatrics
Weill Cornell Medical College
New York, NY, USA
Senior Lecturer
Catholic University of Health and Allied Sciences
Weill Bugando School of Medicine
Consultant Physician
Bugando Medical Centre
Mwanza, Tanzania

Ronald E. Pust MD
Director
Office of Global and Border Health
Co-Director
Global Health Distinction Track
Professor of Family and Community Medicine
Professor of Public Health
College of Medicine, University of Arizona
Tucson, AZ, USA

Shamim A. Qazi MBBS, MSc, MD
Department of Maternal, Newborn, Child and
Adolescent Health
World Health Organization
Geneva, Switzerland

Nancy E. Ringel MD
Lecturer in Global Health
Harvard Medical School
Boston, MA, USA

Kirsti Rinne RN, MSN
Nurse Practitioner
University of Utah Medical Center
Salt Lake City, UT, USA

Lauren C. Riney DO
Pediatric Resident
Case Western Reserve University
Rainbow Babies and Children's Hospital
Cleveland, OH, USA

Sara Ritchie MBChB, MRCGP, DFFP, DTM&H, MPH,
Dip Derm
Honorary Clinical Fellow in Dermatology
University College London Hospitals
London, UK

Jeff A. Robison MD
Assistant Professor of Pediatrics
University of Utah
Salt Lake City, UT, USA

Carlos Rodriguez-Galindo MD
Associate Professor of Pediatrics
Dana-Farber/Boston Children's Cancer and
Blood Disorders Center
Harvard Medical School
Boston, MA, USA

Sylvia V. Romm MD, MPH
Clinical Teaching Staff
Boston University School of Medicine
Massachusetts General Hospital
Boston, MA, USA

Christopher Sanford MD, MPH, DTM&H
Associate Professor, Department of Family Medicine
Associate Professor, Department of Global Health
Director
University of Washington Neighborhood
Northgate Travel Clinic
Director
University of Washington Department of Family Medicine
Global Health Fellowship
University of Washington
Seattle, WA, USA

Thuss Sanguansak MD
Assistant Professor of Ophthalmology
Khon Kaen University
Khon Kaen, Thailand

Susan M. Sawyer MBBS, MD, FRACP
Director, Centre for Adolescent Health
Murdoch Childrens Research Institute
Royal Children's Hospital and Department of Paediatics
University of Melbourne
Professor of Adolescent Health
The University of Melbourne
Melbourne, Australia

Sandra K. Schumacher MD, MPH, CTropMed
Instructor of Pediatrics
Boston Children's Hospital
Harvard Medical School
Boston, MA, USA

Brittany A. Seymour DDS, MPH
Assistant Professor
Department of Oral Health and Epidemiology
Harvard School of Dental Medicine
Harvard Global Health Institute
Boston, MA, USA

Lisa E. Simon DMD
Resident
Department of Oral Health Policy and Epidemiology
Harvard School of Dental Medicine
Cambridge Health Alliance
Boston, MA, USA

Luke R. Smart MD
Global Health Fellow
Department of Medicine
Weill Cornell Medical College
New York, NY, USA
Lecturer
Catholic University of Health and Allied Sciences
Mwanza, Tanzania

Aliyah R. Sohani MD
Medical Director
Hematology Core Laboratory
Massachusetts General Hospital
Assistant Professor of Pathology
Harvard Medical School
Boston, MA, USA

Diane Stafford MD
Training Program Director
Division of Endocrinology
Boston Children's Hospital
Harvard Medical School
Boston, MA, USA

Sara N. Stulac MD, MPH
Deputy Chief Medical Officer
Partners In Health
Department of Global Health and Social Medicine
Harvard Medical School
Division of Global Health Equity
Brigham and Women's Hospital
Department of Global Health
Boston Children's Hospital
Boston, MA, USA

Mark Tomlinson PhD
Professor of Psychology
Alan J. Flisher Centre for Public Mental Health
Department of Psychology
Stellenbosch University
Stellenbosch, South Africa

Lynda A. Tyer-Viola RNC, PhD, FAAN
Assistant Clinical Professor
Baylor College of Medicine
Director of Nursing
Pavilion for Women
Texas Children's Hospital
Houston, TX, USA

Patience Ugwi MBBS, MPH
University of Benin, Nigeria
PhD candidate
Health Services and Policy
University of Iowa
Iowa City, IA, USA

Amelia van der Merwe PhD
Post-doctoral fellow
Alan J. Flisher Centre for Public Mental Health
Department of Psychology
Stellenbosch University
Stellenbosch, South Africa

Francisco Vega-Lopez MD, MSc, PhD, FFTM, RCPSG, FRCP
Honorary Professor and Consultant Dermatologist
National Medical Center
Universidad Nacional Autónoma de México
Mexico City, Mexico
University of London, London School of Hygiene and Tropical Medicine
University College London Hospitals NHS Trust
London, UK

Julia E. von Oettingen MD
Clinical Fellow in Endocrinology
Boston Children's Hospital
Harvard Medical School
Boston, MA, USA

Ariel Wagner
MD/MMSc candidate
Harvard Medical School
Boston, MA, USA

Ana A. Weil MD, MPH
Clinical Fellow in Infectious Diseases
Division of Infectious Diseases
Massachusetts General Hospital
Harvard Medical School
Boston, MA, USA

Christopher J.M. Whitty DSc, FRCP, FFPH, FMedSci
Professor of International Health
London School of Hygiene and Tropical Medicine
The Hospital for Tropical Diseases
University College London Hospitals
London, UK

Susanna E. Winston MD
Fellow in Pediatric Infectious Diseases
Warren Alpert Medical School at Brown University
Hasbro Children's Hospital
Providence, RI, USA

Traci A. Wolbrink MD, MPH
Associate in Critical Care Medicine
Boston Children's Hospital
Instructor in Anesthesia
Harvard Medical School
Boston, MA, USA

Elizabeth R. Wolf MD, MPH
Acting Instructor, Senior Fellow
Department of Pediatrics
Seattle Children's Hospital
University of Washington
Seattle, WA, USA

Tana Wuliji BPharm, PhD
Senior Improvement Advisor
Quality and Performance Institute
University Research Co., LLC
Bethesda, MA, USA

Faiza Yasin MHS
Division of Global Health and Human Rights
Department of Emergency Medicine
Massachusetts General Hospital
Boston University School of Medicine
Boston, MA, USA

About the Editor

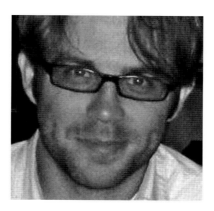

Brett D. Nelson, MD, MPH, DTM&H
Harvard Medical School
Massachusetts General Hospital
Boston, Massachusetts
USA

Dr Nelson is an attending pediatrician and global health faculty member at Harvard Medical School and Massachusetts General Hospital (Boston, Massachusetts, USA). His interests are healthcare provision, development, research, and advocacy for vulnerable populations, particularly newborns and children in settings affected by poverty, conflict, or disaster. Dr Nelson received advanced degrees in medicine and public health from Johns Hopkins and a diploma degree in tropical medicine from the London School of Hygiene and Tropical Medicine. He has been involved in clinical care, academic research, program management, and global health consultancy in dozens of resource-limited areas while working for organizations such as the Centers for Disease Control, Médecins Sans Frontières, International Rescue Committee, UNICEF, International Red Cross and Red Crescent, Johns Hopkins University, and Harvard University. Dr Nelson helped establish the United States' first Pediatric Global Health Fellowship at Massachusetts General Hospital and was its first fellow. Recently in Liberia, he served as the country's Senior Pediatrician and as the Interim Chair of the Department of Pediatrics and Newborn Medicine for Liberia's sole teaching hospital. He currently leads newborn and child health programs in several countries in East and West Africa. Dr Nelson works clinically as a newborn hospitalist, he is the Director of Pediatric and Newborn Programs at the Massachusetts General Hospital Division of Global Health and Human Rights, and he co-directs a popular course at Harvard Medical School on global health and tropical medicine.

Preface

Welcome to *Essential Clinical Global Health!*

There has never been a more exciting and opportune time to be involved in global health, with more health care students and providers than ever before working clinically abroad. And for very good reasons. Health care needs are significant in low- and middle-income countries, and when done thoughtfully, clinicians and clinicians-in-training can contribute considerably to addressing gaps in health services and to building local capacity. Meanwhile, being engaged in these global health experiences can also be incredibly rewarding to those serving – with clinicians typically receiving far more (in terms of experiences, knowledge, and friendships) than they ever give.

Essential Clinical Global Health is a first-of-its-kind clinically focused textbook for students, trainees, and clinicians interested in global health. Our goal with this textbook is to provide readers with the knowledge and skills essential for rewarding and effective global health experiences in resource-limited settings.

This textbook represents the collective experience and dedication of nearly 100 leading global health experts from around the world. Contributors include seasoned clinicians and topic leaders who have had decades of experience living and working in low- and middle-income settings. The textbook also integrates the valuable perspectives of students and clinical trainees as they participate in global health experiences. The common thread amongst all of the contributors is that we find clinical work in global health incredibly important and rewarding, as we suspect you do as well, and we are excited to share this book with you.

We have organized *Essential Clinical Global Health* into six parts. Within the Introduction, we discuss approaches to working successfully within resource-limited settings. We provide an orientation to health care systems and the development and evaluation of clinical programs in these settings. We also include a chapter with critical guidance on preparing for travel and remaining safe while working abroad. Part 2, Newborn and Child Health, begins with an overview of childhood health, followed by chapters on addressing the leading causes of under-five mortality, specifically, newborn causes, acute respiratory infections, diarrheal illnesses, malaria, measles, and malnutrition. After this child health section, we move on in Part 3 to address health in the next stage of life, including issues related to Adolescent, Reproductive, and Maternal Health. Important global Infectious Diseases are discussed in Part 4, with particular emphasis on HIV/AIDS and tuberculosis. We also examine in this section the large number of important but often neglected tropical diseases, which may not be commonly seen in high-income countries but which have a significant impact on health in many low- and middle-income countries. In Part 5, Non-communicable Diseases, we recognize the growing burden of chronic and non-infectious diseases worldwide and discuss the setting-appropriate diagnosis, management, and prevention of conditions such as cardiovascular disease, chronic respiratory disease, endocrine conditions, cancer, trauma, emergency care, critical care, mental health, skin conditions, dental disease, and eye disease. Lastly, Part 6 of the textbook involves chapters on Other Global Health Topics crucial to working successfully in global health, including essential laboratory, nursing, and pharmacy skills and special chapters on humanitarian assistance, technology in global health, illness in returning travelers, and development of global health careers.

Each chapter is filled with key learning objectives, evidence-based clinical guidelines, practical clinical skills, real-world experiences from practitioners in the field, and a list of core readings. We hope you will also find useful the supplementary resources, videos, and self-assessment questions and answers provided in the textbook's electronic supplement. The companion Wiley E-Text version of the textbook may be particularly valuable for carrying abroad for reference on a laptop, tablet, or mobile device.

It is our sincere goal that this textbook is as useful to you and other readers as possible. Therefore, we very much welcome your thoughts and suggestions. Please feel free to send any recommendations and corrections to the editor at medicalstudent@wiley.co.uk.

Whether you are a student preparing for your first global health experience or an established clinician interested in expanding your understanding of the management of illnesses in low- and middle-income countries, we hope *Essential Clinical Global Health* helps make your global health experiences even more rewarding and effective.

- brett
Brett D. Nelson, MD, MPH, DTM&H
Boston, Massachusetts, USA

How to Use Your Textbook

Features contained within your textbook

Every chapter begins with an **abstract, list of key words and learning objectives**.

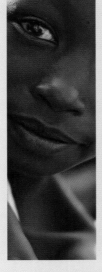

Key learning objectives

Discuss the similarities and differences among clinical roles in resource-rich countries and resource-limited settings.

Review the evidence-based rationale for relying on patient demographics, history, and physical examination in any clinical setting, whether or not resource-constrained.

Cite additional resources for acquiring the skills and knowledge for working effectively in resource-limited settings, including books, websites, and courses emanating from and/or designed for low- and middle-income countries.

Abstract

Learning to provide quality medical care in a resource-limited setting can be both challenging and rewarding if the clinician is prepared with global health knowledge, problem-solving skills, and cultural humility. Although clinical resources may be limited in global health practice, the underlying bases of diagnosis and therapy are not fundamentally altered by resource level. However, the application of those principles in a resource-limited setting differs significantly from typical practice in resource-rich countries, where patient demography, cultural contexts, disease epidemiology, and cost-effectiveness may be viewed differently by clinicians. This chapter concentrates on these differences and the similarities in underlying clinical principles, illustrating several implications for a clinician's role in resource-limited settings. It concludes with an extensive list of resources, including international clinical reference books that can facilitate practice in sustainable, equitable partnerships with host-nation clinicians and mentors.

Key words: global health, international health, cross-cultural, advocacy, evidence-based medicine, syndromic diagnosis, resource-limited settings, cost-containment, clinical decision-making, medical ethics, case studies, bibliographies

Red flag boxes highlight important points.

🚩 Red flag

Patients with severe malnutrition require an alternate approach to rehydration because of the serious risk of fluid overload and electrolyte imbalances.

Clinical experience boxes gives real-life experiences from students and clinicians working in resource-limited settings.

Clinical experience

"During a cholera outbreak, I worked with nurses to register patients as they arrived in a treatment center. A child was carried in who could not open her eyes, and she was vomiting more than five times per hour. She had only been sick with diarrhea for one day, but her skin looked dull and stiff. She would not even cry. Healthcare workers felt no pulse and placed two intravenous catheters in her arm veins before she was even out of her father's arms. After receiving intravenous fluids for an hour, she was awake. A few hours later, after more treatment, she was smiling brightly and eating a banana. I was amazed that this small child arrived completely lifeless and, in a few hours with one simple treatment, seemed like a healthy child."

Kayla, working in Haiti

Clinical pearl boxes provide further insight into topics.

Clinical pearl

For patients with acute diarrhea who are able to feed (e.g., breast milk, formula, or foods), never withhold feeding and give zinc supplementation.

The anytime, anywhere textbook

Wiley E-Text

For the first time, your textbook comes with free access to a **Wiley E-Text: Powered by VitalSource** version – a digital, interactive version of this textbook which you own as soon as you download it.

Your **Wiley E-Text** allows you to:

Search: Save time by finding terms and topics instantly in your book, your notes, even your whole library (once you've downloaded more textbooks)

Note and Highlight: Color code, highlight, and make digital notes right in the text so you can find them quickly and easily

Organize: Keep books, notes, and class materials organized in folders inside the application

Share: Exchange notes and highlights with friends, classmates, and study groups

Upgrade: Your textbook can be transferred when you need to change or upgrade computers

Link: Link directly from the page of your interactive textbook to all of the material contained on the companion website

The **Wiley E-Text** version will also allow you to copy and paste any photograph or illustration into assignments, presentations, and your own notes.

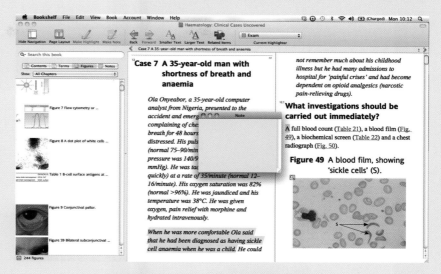

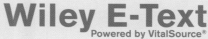

To access your Wiley E-Text:

- Find the redemption code on the inside front cover of this book and carefully scratch away the top coating of the label. Visit **www.vitalsource.com/software/bookshelf/downloads** to download the Bookshelf application to your computer, laptop, tablet or mobile device.
- If you have purchased this title as an e-book, access to your **Wiley E-Text** is available with proof of purchase within 90 days. Visit **http://support.wiley.com** to request a redemption code via the 'Live Chat' or 'Ask A Question' tabs.
- Open the Bookshelf application on your computer and register for an account.
- Follow the registration process and enter your redemption code to download your digital book.
- For full access instructions, visit **www.wileyessential.com/globalhealth**.

The VitalSource Bookshelf can now be used to view your Wiley E-Text on iOS, Android and Kindle Fire!

- **For iOS:** Visit the app store to download the VitalSource Bookshelf: **http://bit.ly/17ib3XS**
- **For Android and Kindle Fire:** Visit the Google Play Market to download the VitalSource Bookshelf: **http://bit.ly/BSAAGP**

You can now sign in with the email address and password you used when you created your VitalSource Bookshelf Account.

Full E-Text support for mobile devices is available at: **http://support.vitalsource.com**

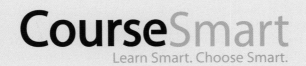

CourseSmart

CourseSmart gives you instant access (via computer or mobile device) to this Wiley-Blackwell e-book and its extra electronic functionality, at 40% off the recommended retail print price. See all the benefits at **www.coursesmart.com/students**.

Instructors ... receive your own digital desk copies!

CourseSmart also offers instructors an immediate, efficient, and environmentally-friendly way to review this textbook for your course.

For more information visit **www.coursesmart.com/instructors**.

With **CourseSmart**, you can create lecture notes quickly with copy and paste, and share pages and notes with your students. Access your **CourseSmart** digital textbook from your computer or mobile device instantly for evaluation, class preparation, and as a teaching tool in the classroom.

Simply sign in at **http://instructors.coursesmart.com/bookshelf** to download your Bookshelf and get started. To request your desk copy, hit 'Request Online Copy' on your search results or book product page.

CourseSmart
Learn Smart. Choose Smart.

We hope you enjoy using your new textbook. Good luck with your studies!

About the Companion Website

Don't forget to visit the companion website for this book:

 www.wileyessential.com/globalhealth

There you will find additional resources, videos, and multiple choice questions (MCQs) to test your knowledge. Scan this QR code to visit the companion website:

Acknowledgments

Dr Nelson, the editorial board, and the contributors would like to sincerely thank all who assisted in making this textbook possible. In particular, we would like to thank for their expertise and valuable input Carrie Cox, Sahera Dirajlal, Christine Griffin, Patricia Hibberd, Christopher Huston, Elizabeth Hutton, Ronald Kleinman, Patrick Lee, Alishya Mayfield, Kinjan Parikh, Jeff Robison, Mairead Shaw, Sara Stulac, Christina Wojewoda, the International Pharmaceutical Federation's Education Initiative Steering Committee, and leaders from the Consortium of Universities for Global Health and the former Global Health Education Consortium.

We are also deeply grateful to the many students and clinicians-in-training who contributed to this textbook, including Maren Blonk, Jim Carr, Elizabeth Crow, Camille Gérin, Rachel Fraser, Luise Gram, Elina Harju, Geneviève Lavallée, Carolyn McLellan, Cory Nelson, Helen Noh, Lucy Philpott, Christopher Wiley, and the student volunteers in the International Pharmaceutical Students' Federation. We send a special thanks to Elizabeth Nowak and the many students who contributed 'Clinical experiences' to the textbook: Elisabeth Berger, Jesse Berry, Sam Enumah, Mathias Essman, Shiv Gaglani, Brandi Harless, Elizabeth Majzoub, Maayan Melamed, Jonah Mink, Martha Tesfalul, Richard Vinroot, and others. Dr Nelson would also like to thank the many medical students over the years who have participated in our global health course at Harvard and who first inspired this textbook.

Additionally, we appreciate the outstanding support of the team at Wiley-Blackwell publishers and its affiliates, including Elizabeth Johnston, Elizabeth Norton, Jolyon Phillips, Katrina Rimmer, and Kathy Syplywczak.

Lastly, and most importantly, we thank our many healthcare colleagues in low- and middle-income countries who inspire us daily and who have taught us so much.

Part 1
Introduction

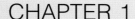

CHAPTER 1

Working Clinically in Resource-Limited Settings

Ronald Pust[1], Peter S. Azzopardi[2,3], and Shreya Patel[4]
[1]University of Arizona, Tucson, AZ, USA
[2]Royal Children's Hospital, Murdoch Children's Research Institute, and University of Melbourne, Melbourne, Australia
[3]Wardliparingga Aboriginal Research Unit, South Australian Health and Medical Research Institute, Adelaide, Australia
[4]Massachusetts General Hospital, and Harvard Medical School, Boston, MA, USA

Key learning objectives

- Discuss the similarities and differences among clinical roles in resource-rich countries and resource-limited settings.

- Review the evidence-based rationale for relying on patient demographics, history, and physical examination in any clinical setting, whether or not resource-constrained.

- Cite additional resources for acquiring the skills and knowledge for working effectively in resource-limited settings, including books, websites, and courses emanating from and/or designed for low- and middle-income countries.

Abstract

Learning to provide quality medical care in a resource-limited setting can be both challenging and rewarding if the clinician is prepared with global health knowledge, problem-solving skills, and cultural humility. Although clinical resources may be limited in global health practice, the underlying bases of diagnosis and therapy are not fundamentally altered by resource level. However, the application of those principles in a resource-limited setting differs significantly from typical practice in resource-rich countries, where patient demography, cultural contexts, disease epidemiology, and cost-effectiveness may be viewed differently by clinicians. This chapter concentrates on these differences and the similarities in underlying clinical principles, illustrating several implications for a clinician's role in resource-limited settings. It concludes with an extensive list of resources, including international clinical reference books that can facilitate practice in sustainable, equitable partnerships with host-nation clinicians and mentors.

Key words: global health, international health, cross-cultural, advocacy, evidence-based medicine, syndromic diagnosis, resource-limited settings, cost-containment, clinical decision-making, medical ethics, case studies, bibliographies

Essential Clinical Global Health, First Edition. Edited by Brett D. Nelson.
© 2015 John Wiley & Sons, Ltd. Published 2015 by John Wiley & Sons, Ltd.
Companion website: www.essentialseries.com/globalhealth

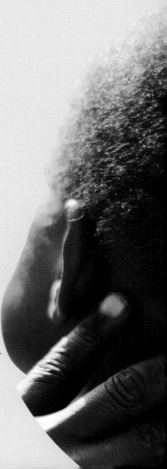

Introduction

Working as a healthcare professional in resource-limited settings is both a rewarding and an enriching experience (Pust, 1984a; Azzopardi & Gray, 2010). Professionally, providing clinical care in the context of limited resources nurtures development of clinical diagnostic and therapeutic skills, which are widely valued in any setting (Palfrey, 2011). Working in diverse sociocultural settings promotes the development of communication skills, confidence, flexibility, adaptability, and resilience (Parker *et al.*, 2011). Global health also fosters a more sound understanding of health, well-being, and their complex determinants (Ventres & Wilson, 1995).

A goal of healthcare professionals working in a resource-limited setting is to promote attitudes and approaches that foster respectful and collaborative relationships within each uniquely diverse culture, community, and health system (Nelson *et al.*, 2012). This chapter begins by considering the role and responsibilities of visiting health professionals and the importance of understanding local context, capacity, and priorities. We introduce broad concepts of providing cross-cultural clinical care to build on a foundation of existing clinical skills. The underlying premise is that an accurate medical history and physical examination, judicious use of investigations, coupled with knowledge of local prevalence of diseases and health resources, will enable clinicians to provide good clinical care. We illustrate syndromic approaches to diagnosis using a case study of a child with fever. The chapter concludes with a comprehensive list of books and websites that may serve as additional resources.

Orientating to the health system

Resource-limited settings are largely characterized by high burdens of disease and injury, economic disadvantage, political turmoil, natural disaster, racial and gender-based discrimination, or marked socioeconomic disparity. "Developing country" is an alternate term; however, it sometimes implies a Western concept of development, viewed as derogatory by some. The World Bank utilizes terminology based on gross per-capita income level (e.g., low- or middle-income country, or LMIC). Over the past 15 years, the term "international health" has increasingly become "global health," the latter term encompassing an interdisciplinary cooperative approach to health and its determinants (Koplan *et al.*, 2009).

Perhaps what these terms do not reflect is the great heterogeneity both within and across these settings; consequently, experience in one setting may not necessarily translate to another. Most importantly, communities that have limited material resources are likely to be wealthy in terms of cultural, communal, and environmental resources (Marsh *et al.*, 2004).

The determinants of health and well-being are complex, and many health-related programs in resource-limited settings focus on health outcomes or disease, often distinct from promoting health and wellness. Focusing on disease is a pragmatic response to the combination of overwhelming disease burden and limited resources (Jamison *et al.*, 2006). However, the opportunity that each clinical interaction provides to address broader health and well-being should be maximized whenever possible, especially as people living in resource-limited settings often experience significant barriers in accessing healthcare. Initiatives such as the Integrated Management of Childhood Illness (IMCI) include this strategy of making the most of each clinical encounter.

Health systems, as described in Chapter 2, include organizations, policies, resources, and people whose primary purpose is to improve health (WHO, 2010). Global health systems are growing increasingly complex. Every country, as well as different global health stakeholders, may have differing interests and influences (Frenk & Moon, 2013). While working in resource-limited settings, understanding the health system is paramount. Figure 1.1 highlights the major tiers of health service, using the example of the World Health Organization (WHO) program for Integrated Management of Adolescent and Adult Illness (IMAI). While community-based health centers usually provide the majority of initial primary care for patients, district and regional hospitals provide referral services and commonly host visiting healthcare clinicians.

Clinicians should not feel overly daunted at the prospect of working in a resource-limited setting. The language of medicine is universal, and basic scientific and clinical methods remain relatively unaltered by resource level. Increasing globalization and urbanization may result in your host country not feeling as "foreign." Additionally, you may be surprised with the familiarity of the health conditions you encounter: while communicable or infectious diseases have traditionally been more common in LMICs, non-communicable diseases (e.g., mental disorder, cardiovascular disease, diabetes, chronic respiratory disease and cancer) have increasingly "gone global" and now account for more premature death and disability than infectious diseases in nearly every nation. There are, however, some important considerations that can help clinicians prepare for working in resource-limited settings, outlined in Table 1.1. It is these considerations that form the focus of the remainder of this chapter.

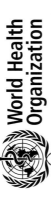

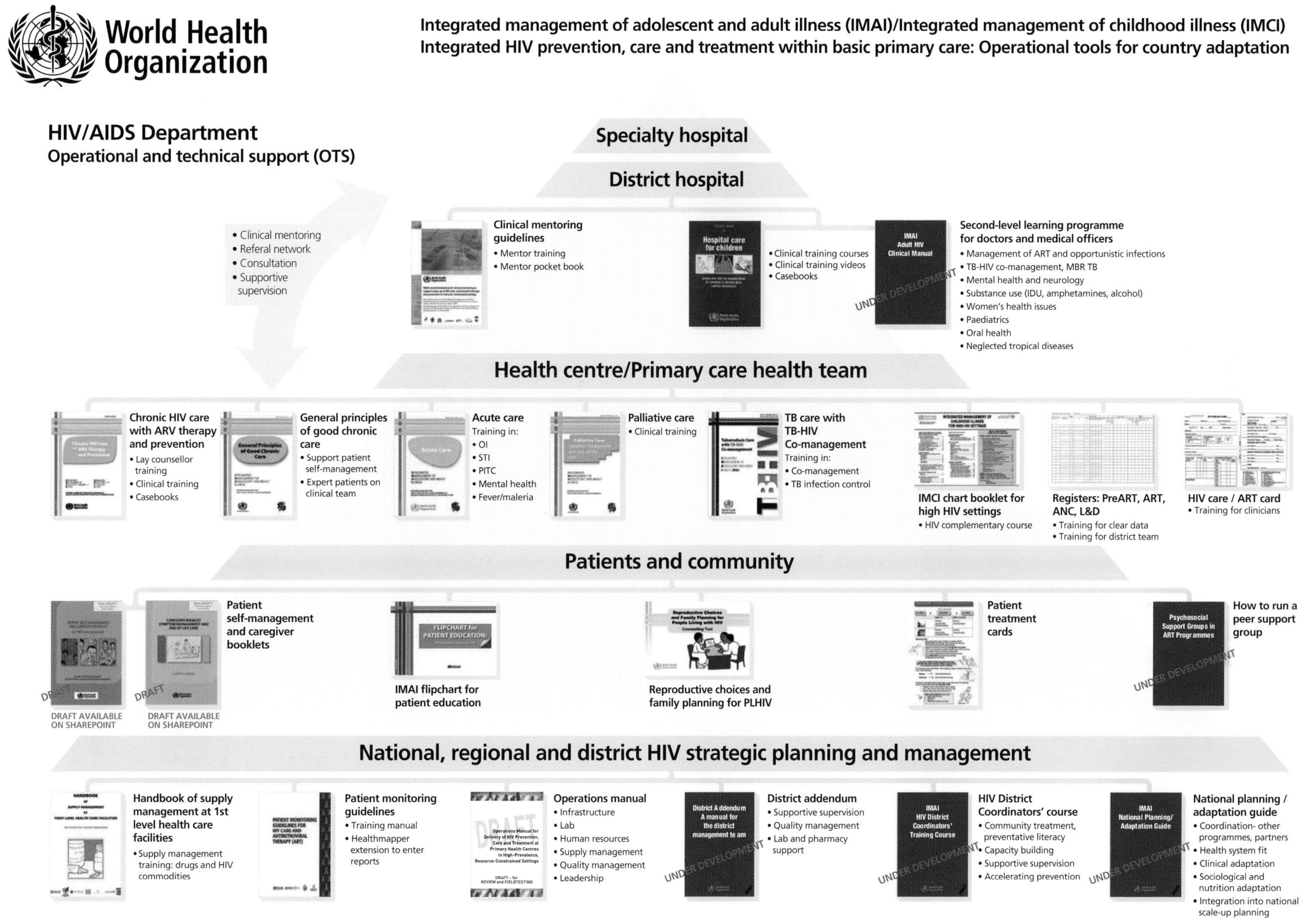

Figure 1.1 Tiers of the typical healthcare system, with the corresponding WHO guidelines for each level of care. The district hospital plays a key role in terms of clinical mentoring, supporting a referral network, consultations, and supportive supervision. *Source:* World Health Organization. Reproduced with permission of the World Health Organization.

Table 1.1 Some key considerations relating to clinical practice in resource-limited settings.

Clinical care

- With fewer resources, clinicians and patients often have fewer options, and even these limited options may not be available with the immediacy expected or required.
- Clinical encounters will include both the familiar and esoteric with regard to diseases, treatment modalities, and medications. For example, Chagas disease or tuberculosis may be extremely common, zinc might be included as treatment of diarrhea, and salbutamol tablets may be used rather than inhalers.

Patient populations

- Culturally, clinicians will find differences in language, family, and social norms. For example, elders are often highly regarded, and sometimes families will shelter them from devastating diagnoses. Or, it may be inappropriate for male healthcare providers to treat female patients.
- LMICs are often at different stages along the demographic transition with some still experiencing high birth and death rates, resulting in a young mobile population.
- Even within a given setting, there may be major differences in health and health resources depending on wealth or class, especially in urbanized settings, leading to vast disparities in outcomes.
- There are often differing expectations of health and wellness; patients may be incredibly trusting and unquestioning of decisions from healthcare professionals.
- The role of spirituality and health are often interrelated, with traditional healers playing key, revered roles in the community.
- Patients may have had little prior contact with the healthcare system. Barriers to healthcare access may be complex; geographic isolation, personal financial resources, health illiteracy, competing commitments, permission, and fear are common.

Laws and regulations

- In some settings, for example, it may be illegal to provide termination of pregnancy. While personal views among clinicians may differ, remember that as a guest, breaching local laws is likely to result in greater harm than good for the patient, the health service, colleagues, and oneself.

National systems and resources

- Healthcare systems may be structured differently, and perhaps more or less equitably, than in high-income countries. Often the costs covered by the patient or system will be very different than in resource-rich countries. For example, in LMICs, the government may provide all antiretroviral therapy (ART), but a patient may have to pay out of pocket for an intravenous kit and fluids.
- Health services may be delivered by a myriad of health and social service agencies – government, non-governmental, and faith-based organizations – with differing levels of integration.
- "Task-shifting/-sharing" is increasingly employed to address health-workforce shortages and involves training individuals to provide specialized healthcare usually outside their typical role. For example, in a setting where doctors are limited, the ministry of health may train and support nurses to staff primary care clinics or to prescribe and dispense ARTs. Community health workers, who are usually community members with basic health training, are another key player in resource-limited settings; they can facilitate health service access, provide care, and serve as links between health services and the community.

The clinician's role working in a resource-limited setting

Given the heterogeneity of resource-limited settings and diversity of clinical roles, it is impossible to provide comprehensive guidance to working in these settings. However, the principles that follow may assist the clinician in developing a clinical approach that is most effective.

Understanding your clinical role, capacity, privilege, and limitations

Having the host clearly define your clinical role will help delineate how best to contribute and learn. Ideally, the role should be defined by the host before you commence and be continuously reviewed and refined during your stay.

Working in a resource-limited setting will invariably require stepping outside comfort zones, both within and beyond one's specialty. However, it is essential to practice within your skills and training: "If you wouldn't back home, don't do it abroad" (Crump & Sugarman, 2010; Parker *et al.*, 2011). It is critical to be honest with oneself, colleagues and patients regarding clinical skills, capabilities, and limitations. Expect to not have all the answers, and be prepared that outcomes of clinical care may not always be good, even if it is an area of expertise. Identify a mentor, distinguish personal and professional limits, and recognize when and how to take care of yourself (see Chapter 4).

As a visiting clinician, one will likely be treated with a great deal of respect by the host institution. The visiting clinician's opinions may be accepted over those of local, more experienced clinicians, so facilitating and respecting the input of local clinicians is paramount. Local staff may be reluctant to question one's decisions or behavior. In general, open inquiring communication is best for patients and the healthcare team. Additionally, it is also important to consider personal behaviors outside the clinical environment, to be respectful of local cultures and norms, and to preserve a professional reputation and collegial relationships.

Role as an educator

Health knowledge is an important determinant of health outcomes for populations in resource-limited settings. It follows that knowledge exchange is an important component of working in global health. Every stage of medicine involves the opportunity to both teach and learn from patients and colleagues, and this exchange is often enriched in new settings. Evidence, guidelines, and approaches that are effective in the home setting may not be appropriate for the resource-limited working environment (Davey, 2001). Consult local clinicians and professionals about their professional development needs and how you might help address those needs.

Flexibility in teaching style becomes particularly important in the diverse settings of resource-limited settings. For example, busy crowded wards may or may not be the appropriate place for bedside teaching based on both logistics and cultural norms. However, case discussions conducted in a non-threatening and supportive environment can provide a powerful vehicle for education and professional development. Providing a discharge summary to the nurse at the clinic and to the admitting officer can improve patient care and follow-up and can also be educational.

In addition to opportunities to teach, working in a resource-limited setting provides an opportunity to learn (Ventres & Wilson, 1995). Professional development, however, should not be at the expense of local staff and patients (Parker *et al.*, 2011).

Role as an advocate

Medical work in LMICs can frequently be witness to human injustice (Foege, 1998), which may include discrimination and abuse, political turmoil in conflict situations, or famine and extreme poverty. Clinicians have an opportunity to bear witness (or *témoignage*, as described by Médecins Sans Frontières) and to raise awareness around important health injustices. Open discussions with the hosts and patients are vital in pursuing advocacy. Yet it is essential not to impose one's own values and expectations. Be realistic around what can be achieved, and consider the implications of advocacy, both in its success and failure.

Role as a clinician

The role as a clinician is to provide healthcare, and this may seem like second nature to experienced clinicians. However, there are some important considerations in working in a cross-cultural setting. Working closely with an interpreter, community health worker, or local colleague can help one translate both language and culture. For example, there may be specific protocols for addressing community elders or greeting patients (e.g., shaking hands may be impolite). It may be disrespectful in some cultures to ask about deceased children, "bad luck" to ask in detail about pregnancy, or improper to take a sexual health history from a patient of the opposite gender. Remember, many patients in resource-limited settings have had limited contact with the Western healthcare system and may be unfamiliar or overwhelmed by what might be considered a "routine" question. In Sara's case for example (Boxes 1.1–1.3), there may be important reasons why her first contact with the health systems was delayed for two days. Reasons may include financial, alternate care seeking (Hill *et al.*, 2003), or fear of the health system. Perhaps there is no reason at all, and detailed questioning may be misinterpreted as placing blame. Indeed, many of the determinants of health and health-seeking behavior in resource-limited settings are shaped by complex factors, and many are beyond the patient's control.

There may also be important considerations in conducting a physical examination, especially in patients of the opposite gender. Importantly, if a sociocultural protocol is breached, be gracious, apologetic, and never defensive (Shah & Wu, 2008).

Understand local context, priorities, capacity, and opportunities

Orienting to the country in which one will be working is fundamental to providing healthcare that is effective and efficient. Key contextual factors include the structure of the health system; local diseases (Lim *et al.*, 2013) and treatment patterns; basic cultural and historical facts; and health indicators for that country, such as the infant mortality rate and maternal mortality ratio (which are indicative of the country's overall level of health and stage of epidemiological and demographic transition). In Sara's case, an understanding of the local epidemiology and seasonal prevalence of malaria, for example, is critical to appreciating the potential causes of her fever.

There are some aspects of working in resource-limited settings that can be particularly discomforting or overwhelming for clinicians. Health services can be significantly over-stretched by both volume of patients and severity of disease. Common therapies, such as oxygen, may be either very limited or unavailable. Oftentimes, clinicians may need to decide which patients are most needing of this precious resource. These decisions are difficult and should involve local staff. A pragmatic approach is to focus on what can be done (Pust, 1984b) and

---

Box 1.1 Case study: Sara from Kenya – health center to district hospital

This actual case of "Sara" from Kenya (for whom we are using a pseudonym and a non-patient photo [Figure 1.2]) is divided into three stages in her care. At the end of each stage, discuss how Sara's care should be managed, based on the principles in this chapter.

Sara is a 3-year-old girl from a remote district of Kenya at an elevation of 1680 m (5500 feet). Because of 2 days of fever and malaise, her parents took her to the local health center. Her WHO "Road to Health" card documented full immunization and steady growth tracking the 50th percentile. The nurse at the health center found Sara to have fever and "hard breathing." A malaria blood smear was performed and reported "positive." Therefore, the nurse gave Sara antimalarials, and she was taken home. Later that day, her breathing became deep, rapid, and somewhat labored, so her father took her to the district hospital, 30 km from home.

   At the hospital, Sara was assessed by the clinical officer, who found her very unwell with decreased consciousness and fast breathing. Her vital signs showed tachycardia (154 beats per minute), tachypnea (72 breaths per minute), and fever (39°C).

What are the possible causes of Sara's presentation? Does the season and elevation contribute to the initial assessment (pre-test probability)? What should be done next?

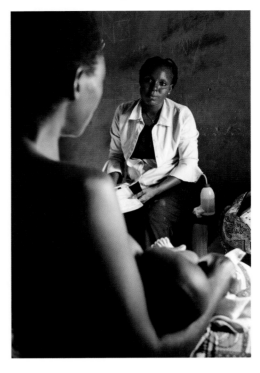

Figure 1.2 "Sara" is brought by her parents to the local health center, where she is found to be febrile and breathing fast. *Source:* Science Photo Library.

Box 1.2 Case study: clinical assessment of Sara at the district hospital

Sara's blood smear was reported as "3+ *P. falciparum* malaria." Her hemoglobin was 6.1 g/dL, and her blood glucose was normal (5 mmol/L = 90 mg/dL). The clinical officer made two diagnoses: (1) complicated malaria and (2) severe pneumonia. Sara was admitted and given oxygen plus intravenous quinine (for malaria), ampicillin, and gentamicin. On evening ward rounds, Sara was reviewed by the doctor, who confirmed these vital signs but found Sara unresponsive. Her neck was not stiff. Her palms and tongue were slightly pale. She had no cough or chest retraction, despite her respiratory rate of 72. Her abdominal examination was normal, other than a barely palpable liver and spleen. Her last urine output was approximately 8 hours earlier.

What is your assessment at this point? How many diseases does Sara have?

What if the assessment is incorrect (false-positive or false-negative diagnosis)? What small device might help differentiate between malaria and pneumonia? Should treatment for both malaria and pneumonia be continued? Are more treatment(s) necessary? If so, for what other diagnoses?

---

do that well. Some patients will present with diseases that, unfortunately, cannot be treated with local resources (e.g., a newborn with spina bifida). However, there is still likely much that can be done to improve health outcome. Explaining the disease to the parents or the fact that this condition has been seen before can help foster acceptance (in some cultures, congenital disease is associated with an evil curse or shame). Palliation may involve dressings and antibiotics for infection. There is also an opportunity for education and health promotion for future pregnancies.

Box 1.3 Case study: management of Sara's complex illness

The doctor's assessment was severe *P. falciparum* malaria. The two complications appeared to be cerebral malaria and metabolic acidosis, both of which are common in children with falciparum malaria, the predominant species in Africa.

The doctor continued treatment for severe malaria with intravenous quinine (first-line treatment with intravenous artesunate was not available). Special attention was paid to monitoring and preventing hypoglycemia (which would be undetectable in an unconscious child like Sara), fluid overload, and hyponatremia.

The doctor was not convinced that Sara had pneumonia; she assessed the respiratory rate and depth to be due to compensatory respiratory alkalosis in response to the severe metabolic acidosis brought about by complicated malaria.

Nevertheless, she did not stop the intravenous ampicillin and gentamicin or oxygen therapy. This was for two reasons.

1. In some cases it can be very difficult to clinically distinguish pneumonia from severe malaria.
2. Sara was by now comatose, presumably from cerebral malaria. However, there is some chance that her altered mental status (Area 4 in Figure 1.5) could be due to concurrent meningitis. No lumbar puncture had been done in the outpatient department prior to starting ampicillin and gentamicin; therefore, it would now be difficult to completely exclude bacterial meningitis, a rapidly devastating disease.

Should a lumbar puncture have been performed on Sara? What are the potential outcomes of "missing" meningitis (a false negative)? What about treating with effective drugs (ampicillin and gentamicin) without first having evidence of meningitis (a potentially false-positive diagnosis)? Does it make any difference?

The next day, Sara's vital signs became normal, but she was still unconscious and her malaria smear remained 2+ positive. The same treatment continued. By day three, Sara was clinically normal, sitting up, and eating well.

What can be learned from Sara's case? What can be learned about working clinically in a resource-limited setting? In what ways is it different from working in a resource-rich setting? How is it similar?

It is important not to focus on the deficits. Instead, take a strengths-based approach (Marsh *et al.*, 2004; Pust, 2007). You may well be surprised to learn the diversity of resources and skills available within your health service. Local health staff in a resource-limited setting are often very skilled at providing care across specialties, such as anesthesia, obstetrics, minor surgery, and neonatal care. There may also be other services within the health system that can complement what the health facility can provide.

Understanding referral pathways, which may be quite complex and/or costly for a patient, can assist in providing more comprehensive healthcare. This is especially critical in resource-limited settings as many patients will have had limited contact with the health system, and each clinical encounter provides the opportunity for health education, promotion, and prevention.

Clinical diagnosis and case management in resource-limited settings

The scientific bases (Sackett, 1992; Straus *et al.*, 2005; Herrle *et al.*, 2011) and goals of clinical care remain largely unchanged by resource level. Common principles of good clinical care anywhere include efficient (Palfrey, 2011; Dhaliwal & Detsky, 2013) and evidence-based stewardship in the allocation of resources (McGee, 2012). In practice, resources are limited or constrained in almost all settings. However, it is often when clinicians from resource-rich settings practice in resource-limited settings that they truly learn the value and effectiveness of the science underlying diagnosis and treatment. To illustrate this, consider the questions in the case of Sara (Boxes 1.1–1.3).

Diagnosis on the basis of your patient's demographics, symptoms, and signs

Patient demographics and the presence or absence of findings on history and physical examination are just as much "tests" as laboratory investigations (Straus *et al.*, 2005; McGee, 2012). In the case example, Sara's history of fever and malaise are **sensitive** tests for a host of diseases. However, neither fever nor malaise is **specific** for any disease; if based on these findings alone, the diagnosis will likely be imprecise or incorrect. Figure 1.3 reinforces the need for other findings – those with higher specificity and predictive value – if we are to have higher diagnostic accuracy.

Three principles can be used to increase the diagnostic accuracy of clinical findings:

1. interpreting clinical findings in the context of the local epidemiology;
2. considering "clusters" of clinical findings or syndromes;
3. using laboratory investigations judiciously.

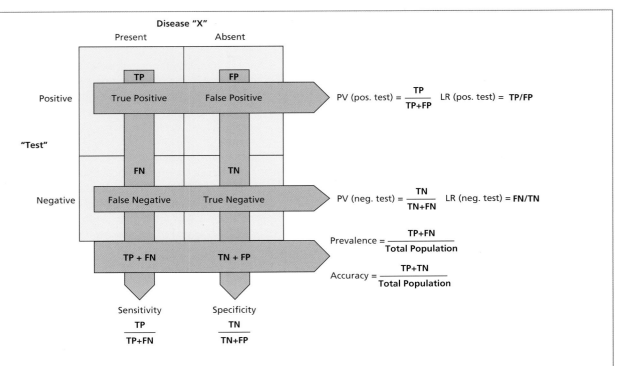

Figure 1.3 Two-by-two table on the relationship between test and disease: the basic concepts of clinical diagnosis in all settings. TP, true positive; TN, true negative; FP, false positive; FN, false negative; PV, predictive value. Likelihood ratio (LR) can also be computed from any such two-way table: LR of a positive test or finding = TP/FP; LR of a negative test = FN/TN. A positive high-specificity test tends to "rule in" the suspected diagnosis (remembered as SpIn+). A negative high-sensitivity test tends to "rule out" the suspected diagnosis (remembered as SnOut−).

Interpreting clinical findings in the context of the local epidemiology

The classic triad of time, place, and person (i.e., patient demographics) determine to a great extent the relative prevalence of disease. The fact that Sara was a child and from a malaria-prevalent area increased the risk that she had clinical malaria (Taylor *et al.*, 2010). These epidemiological findings must be considered when estimating her pre-test probability of any specific disease, such as malaria (Richardson, 1999). Additional diagnostic tools are then used to generate a **likelihood ratio**, which is the ratio of true positives to false positives of any clinical finding ("test") for the disease being considered, in this case malaria. The Fagan nomogram (Figure 1.4), or the equivalent in hand-held software, can be used to calculate the post-test probability of that disease. The red and green lines in Figure 1.4 demonstrate these concepts. While experienced clinicians are not formally completing this analysis with each patient test, the foundation of their veteran decision-making is often based on this thoughtful, data-driven approach.

In the context of a high post-test probability for malaria, most clinicians would advise treatment (Davey, 2001; Simoes *et al.*, 2003). However, the implications of a false-positive diagnosis, leading to inappropriate treatment, must also be considered (Chandler *et al.*, 2008). In the case of Sara, this would unnecessarily expose Sara to the risks of antimalarial medications and, more importantly, delay the diagnosis and treatment of her actual disease.

Any individual physical finding may not have significant sensitivity or specificity for clinical malaria (Bisoffi & Buonfrate, 2013). Splenomegaly, for example, may be absent (falsely negative) in a child's first few attacks of malaria, and these are the cases most likely to be fatal. Since many children (often 50%) in endemic communities have enlarged spleens from prior malaria episodes, there is little correlation between splenomegaly and **current** clinical malaria, thereby lowering the likelihood ratio of splenomegaly for the diagnosis of current clinical malaria (Hackett, 1944; WHO, 2012). Therefore, in the example in Figure 1.4, if the positive likelihood ratio of splenomegaly for current clinical malaria is approximately 2, the post-test probability is raised only modestly, to 67% (red line).

Considering "clusters" of clinical findings or syndromes

Since any one given physical finding may not yield a high likelihood ratio for a specific disease, a skilled clinician will use a combination of findings in the patient's history and physical examination to quickly limit the differential diagnosis. When

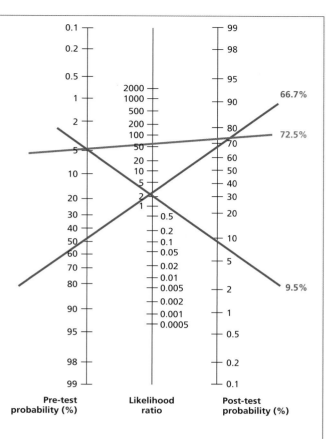

Pre-test probability (%)   Likelihood ratio   Post-test probability (%)

Figure 1.4 Fagan nomogram demonstrating the relationship between pre-test probability, likelihood ratio, and post-test probability (see Figure 1.3 for the definition of likelihood ratio). Many diagnostic calculations, including those in this chapter, are available on several smartphone apps, including MedCalc (www.medcalc.com/bayes.html). Alternately, in the field, one can use the Fagan nomogram and a straight edge. This nomogram, often used for laboratory tests, can also be used to conceptualize clinical decision-making. The red and green lines represent two individual patients who each present with a single clinical finding suggestive of a particular disease. The likelihood ratio is arbitrarily 2 in these examples. However, it is only the patient who comes from a setting where this disease is prevalent (high pre-test probability, red line) that is likely to have that disease. The blue line demonstrates that the presence of multiple or convincing clinical findings for a particular disease (arbitrarily, here, a likelihood ratio of 50) greatly increases the post-test probability of that disease, even in the context of low pre-test probability.

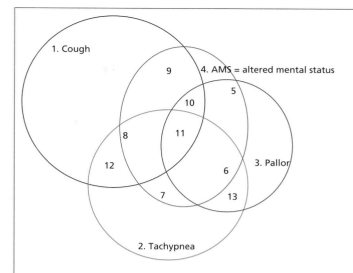

Figure 1.5 Syndromic diagnosis: a Venn diagram of acutely febrile children in sub-Saharan Africa. Total area of rectangle indicates all acutely febrile children in sub-Saharan Africa. Area of colored circles indicates prevalence of each of four clinical signs: cough (black), tachypnea (green), pallor (blue), and altered mental status (red).

dromes" and can suggest specific diagnoses, of which the following are examples.

• Cough (black circle 1) plus tachypnea (green circle 2) suggests pneumonia. If the child has only these two findings (area 12), this is potentially pneumonia, which is much more likely if there is also chest retraction. However, if the child has additional symptoms or combinations (areas 6, 7, 8, and/or 11), the child has complicated pneumonia and/or additional disease(s).
• Palmar pallor (blue circle 3) in the febrile child suggests malaria. If the patient also has altered mental status (area 5) and/or tachypnea (area 6), complicated malaria is likely.
• Altered mental status (red circle 4) in the febrile child suggests meningitis; lumbar puncture is recommended, regardless of other finding, and especially if there are no other findings. In resource-limited settings, where comprehensive work-ups are usually not available, syndromic management becomes increasingly important.

combined with epidemiologic assessment of pre-test probabilities of diseases, this very efficient clinical approach considers the likelihood of a combination of findings in order to make a "syndromic diagnosis" (English *et al.*, 2003), as illustrated by the Venn diagram in Figure 1.5. The areas on the diagram are approximate and will vary by time, place, and person. Combinations of findings, or areas of numbered overlaps, are "syn-

In general, the greater the number of combined findings or elements of a syndrome present, the more likely and specific is the diagnosis of the suspected disease. Palmar pallor (Muhe *et al.*, 2000) could indicate anemia (Montresor *et al.*, 2003; Calis *et al.*, 2008) from a variety of causes. However, the likelihood of malaria is raised if palmar pallor is part of a syndrome of findings consistent with malaria (Taylor & Molyneux, 2003).

As the case of Sara showed us, pneumonia (Shann *et al.*, 1983) and malaria can present with clinical similarities, and both are common among children in this setting (Margolis & Gadomski, 1998; Principi & Esposito, 2011). In The Gambia, for example, among children presenting with overlapping clinical findings in the rainy season, 33% had pneumonia and 38% had malaria (O'Dempsey *et al.*, 1993). In the dry season, 48% had pneumonia and only 6% had malaria. As Sara became seriously ill and comatose, additional or alternative diagnoses must be considered, including tuberculosis meningitis (Wright *et al.*, 1993; Berkley *et al.*, 2001; Weber *et al.*, 2002; Green *et al.*, 2003; Azzopardi & Graham, 2008; Best & Hughes, 2008).

Many health professionals who have trained in resource-rich countries have been taught the concept of "Occam's razor" or diagnostic parsimony. This is an attempt by clinicians to identify a single disease that accounts for nearly all the patient's findings. While this principle is usually also true in resource-limited settings, comorbidity is both common and difficult to exclude without highly sensitive and specific laboratory tests. Broader management may therefore be necessary.

Using laboratory investigations judiciously

Laboratory tests and imaging should serve to increase diagnostic certitude primarily, and perhaps only, when the results will change patient management. The potential harm of investigations should also be considered and weighed against potential benefits. In the case of Sara, for example, the risk of performing a lumbar puncture in a comatose child (who is treated with antibiotics regardless) far outweighs the benefits. Harm may also come from cost and delays in therapy. If treatment for a specific disease (e.g., acromegaly or thalassemia) is unavailable, unaffordable, or culturally unacceptable, use of additional resources to pursue that diagnosis might be injudicious (Pust, 1984b). As mentioned previously, the clinician's role in such a setting may be to advocate for the relevant resources, if consonant with other competing priorities.

Conversely, laboratory confirmation of even a fairly likely diagnosis may be indicated if there are significant implications of a false-positive diagnosis. For example, in the context of increasing resistance to antimalarial drugs, the WHO now recommends laboratory confirmation of malaria before treatment is commenced (d'Acremont *et al.*, 2010; WHO, 2012).

In Sara's case, does a diagnosis of malaria indicate that antibiotic therapy should be ceased (Newton, 2004)? Returning to Figure 1.3, the 2 × 2 table helps conceptualize the potential outcomes of "incorrect" (false-positive or false-negative) diagnoses. Given the comorbidities of serious diseases and the paucity of investigations having high accuracy in resource-limited settings, it is usually better to err on the side of treatment of serious disease (i.e., when a falsely negative diagnosis may be fatal). In Sara's case the physician did not discontinue these antibiotics, which are effective in most cases of bacterial meningitis and pneumonia. The extended case of Sara demonstrates some universal principles of clinical care as applied in resource-limited settings.

In this chapter, diagnosis based chiefly on clinical findings has been emphasized. However, because several simple diagnostic aids are portable and affordable, many clinicians routinely carry these in a pocket or bag. Table 1.2 highlights some diagnostic tools a clinician may consider bringing (and leaving), after consulting with the host institution about their appropriateness.

Implications of diagnosis and treatment

Consider the costs of healthcare in resource-limited settings

In resource-limited settings, it is essential to know the costs of diagnostic and treatment resources. Tests and imaging are costly to health facilities and patients. Even when affordable, many diagnostic modalities in resource-limited settings may not have regular quality control or calibration. Radiographers may not be available to interpret imaging. Many investigations have a long turn-around time, especially those processed elsewhere, thus delaying your patient's care. Non-essential treatments may be prohibitively expensive, resulting in displacement of funds from purchasing other essential items.

Consider the cultural context of clinical care

Diagnosis can be associated with significant stigma. For example, in many cultures there remains great discrimination against people living with HIV. Implications of certain diagnoses should be considered and planned for before any investigations are performed.

Additionally, before prescribing treatment in resource-limited settings (as in any setting), consider its impact on the patient, family, and staff (Hill *et al.*, 2003). Inpatient hospital care may be preferred when resources at home are limited. For example, there may be no clean water to prepare oral rehydration solution for a child with diarrhea. However, hospitalization also can co-opt relatives or friends who have other important commitments (e.g., employment, caring for other family members). Patients may travel great distances at significant cost to reach health services, so consider the need and options for continuing care carefully.

Expatriates, by definition, are guests "working in someone else's country" (Stark, 2011; Pust, 2012). With continued welcome, a short rotation may grow into a longer stay, which may transform into a lifelong relationship. Yet regardless of the length of the experience, a visiting clinician should always have the sincere humility of a guest, a strong mutual respect with the hosts, an eagerness to learn from them, and a shared determination to help build a better future. As Senegalese novelist Cheikh Hamadou Kane explained: "We have not had the same past, you and ourselves. But we shall have the same future. The era of separate destinies has run its course."

Table 1.2 Small diagnostic tools you may consider taking to a resource-limited setting (in addition to these diagnostic tools, see Chapter 4 for a general list of items to pack when traveling abroad).

Clinical items to consider taking when relevant

- Items specifically requested by your host
- Portable pulse oximeter: can be very useful at bedside or outpatient triage in distinguishing, for example, "difficult breathing" of malaria (normal oxygenation) versus pneumonia (low oxygenation) (see case study in this chapter)
- Peak expiratory flow meter: low-cost meters are now available and can provide reliable lung function test results. A less precise but even lower-cost alternative is the Snider match blowing test, in which a patient's ability to blow out a match at 15 cm (6 inches) is approximately correlated with FEV_1 and PEFR
- Tape measures, including those for mid-upper arm circumference (MUAC) (see Chapter 12)
- Pocket visual acuity cards that are independent of culture and literacy
- Tuning fork(s) (256/512 Hz) for Weber and Rinne hearing tests
- 10-g filament to test for protective foot sensation (diabetes and leprosy)
- Extra thermometer(s) for spot checks of patient temperature
- Pen-lights
- Extra batteries for any battery-operated device
- Blood pressure cuff with stethoscope
- Glucose or Hemoglobin A1C meter and testing strips
- Low-tech hemoglobin card test
- Rapid diagnostic test (RDT) cards (e.g., for pregnancy, malaria, HIV, syphilis, typhoid)
- Fecal occult blood test cards and developer
- Urinalysis test strips
- Nitrazine pH paper (e.g., when testing for the presence of amniotic fluid in suspected rupture of membranes)
- Portable ultrasound: now available at a much lower cost and may help avoid (or facilitate) procedures
- Vacuum extractor (VE), for those properly trained in its use. While many resource-limited settings have VEs, they are often underutilized in favor of cesarean section, even when VE is indicated. One small, affordable, lightweight example is the KiwiVac

Clinical items that should *not* be taken

- Anything that the hosts do not support
- Medications that are not on the WHO or the country's Essential Drug List (with some exceptions, if requested by your host)
- Equipment that is difficult or expensive to maintain (especially if it detracts from methods already in use that are appropriate, cost-efficient, and sustainable)
- New, packaged equipment that may require import duties (unless you are prepared to cover these)

Additional resources

This section includes some of the general resources we have found most useful while working clinically in resource-limited settings. For additional topic-specific resources, please also refer to the resources listed in their respective chapters.

Clinical care

- Local clinical guidelines. Before or on your arrival at your destination, seek copies of the locally approved clinical guidelines, which are often adapted from international sources, such as the WHO. These local guidelines may be available on the Ministry of Health website, from your host institution, or from other local partners/NGOs.
- World Health Organization (2013) *Pocket Book of Hospital Care for Children*, 2nd edn. Available at http://www.who.int/ maternal_child_adolescent/documents/child_hospital_care/ en/index.html

- World Health Organization (2011) *Integrated Management of Adolescent and Adult Illness (IMAI) District Clinician Manual: Hospital Care for Adolescents and Adults*, Vols 1 and 2. Available at http://www.who.int/hiv/pub/imai/imai2011/en/
- World Health Organization (2003) *Surgical Care at the District Hospital*. Available at http://www.who.int/surgery/ publications/scdh_manual/en/
- Davidson R, Brent A, Seale A (2014) *Oxford Handbook of Tropical Medicine*, 4th edn. Oxford: Oxford University Press.
- Beeching N, Gill GV (eds) (2014) *Lecture Notes: Tropical Medicine*, 7th edn. Oxford: Wiley-Blackwell.
- Farrar J, Hotez PJ, Junghanss T, Kang G, Lalloo D, White N (eds) (2013) *Manson's Tropical Diseases*, 23rd edn. Philadelphia: Saunders Elsevier.
- Davies AM (2002) *The WHO Manual of Diagnostic Imaging*. Geneva: WHO.
- Guerrant RL, Walker DH, Weller PF (eds) (2011) *Essentials of Tropical Infectious Diseases: Principles, Pathogens and Practice*, 3rd edn. Philadelphia: Saunders Elsevier.

- King M, Bewes P, Cairns J, Thornton J (eds) (2009) *Primary Surgery. Vol. 1, Non-trauma; Vol. 2, Trauma; Vol. 3, Primary anesthesiology.* Oxford: Oxford University Press. Available at http://www.primary-surgery.org/start.html
- Magill AJ, Ryan ET, Hill DR, Solomon T (eds) (2013) *Hunter's Tropical Medicine and Emerging Infectious Diseases*, 9th edn. Philadelphia: Saunders Elsevier.
- Schull CR (2010) *Common Medical Problems in the Tropics*, 3rd edn. Oxford: Macmillan.
- Shah SP, Price DD (eds) (2011) *The Partners in Health Manual of Ultrasound for Resource-limited Settings.* Boston, MA: Partners in Health. Available at http://parthealth.3cdn.net/3ad982b2456f524cf8_kxvm6qpr9.pdf
- Watters DAK, Wilson IH, Leaver RJ, Bagshawe A (eds) (2004) *Care of the Critically Ill Patient in the Tropics*, 2nd edn. Oxford: Macmillan.
- Werner D, Thuman C, Maxwell J (2011) *Where There Is No Doctor: A Village Health Care Handbook.* Berkeley, CA: Hesperian Foundation.

Modern methods in clinical diagnosis and treatment decisions

- McGee S (2012) *Evidence-based Physical Diagnosis*, 3rd edn. Philadelphia: Saunders Elsevier.
- Straus SE, Richardson WS, Glasziou P, Haynes RB (2011) *Evidence-based Medicine*, 4th edn. Edinburgh: Churchill Livingstone.

Sources for setting-appropriate resources and guidelines

- World Health Organization. WHO guidelines approved by the Guidelines Review Committee. Available at http://www.who.int/publications/guidelines/en/
- Médecins Sans Frontières/Doctors Without Borders. Several clinical reference manuals. Available at http://www.refbooks.msf.org
- World Health Organization. Blue trunk libraries: a collection of books for the health district. Available at http://www.who.int/ghl/mobile_libraries/bluetrunk/en/print.html
- Teaching Aids at Low Cost (TALC). TALC selects the most practical books from various publishers and distributes them in LMICs and online at subsidized prices. Available at http://www.talcuk.org
- Hesperian Foundation. Non-profit organization that develops setting-appropriate educational materials, including the series, *Where There Is No Doctor.* http://www.hesperian.org
- African Medical and Research Foundation (AMREF). http://www.amref.org.

Global health courses and curricula

- American Society of Tropical Medicine and Hygiene. Diploma Courses in Clinical Tropical Medicine and Travelers' Health. http://www.astmh.org/certification/certificate.cfm
- Consortium of Universities for Global Health (CUGH), formerly Global Health Education Consortium. Many online clinical modules. Available at http://www.cugh.org/
- University of Arizona. Global health: Clinical and community care. An annual, open, 3-week course since 1982. Described at http://www.globalhealth.arizona.edu/description
- Harvard Medical School. Clinical topics in global health: A practical introduction for preclinical medical students. Available in part at www.mededportal.org/publication/9471. For further details see Nelson BD, Saltzman A, Lee PT. Bridging the global health training gap: design and evaluation of a new clinical global health course at Harvard Medical School. *Medical Teacher* 2012;34:45–51.
- USAID. Global Health eLearning Center. Available at http://globalhealthlearning.org
- Ethical challenges in short-term global health training. A case-based training course in global health ethics. Available at http://www.ethicsandglobalhealth.org

Websites and reports

- World Health Organization's annual World Health Report. Available at http://www.who.int/whr/en/
- UNICEF's annual report on the State of the World's Children. Available at http://www.unicef.org/sowc/
- Measure DHS. Latest Demographic and Health Survey (DHS) data by country. Available at http://www.measuredhs.com/
- Multiple Indicator Cluster Survey. Child health data by country. Available at http://www.childinfo.org/
- CDC Travelers' Health information on vaccination, prophylaxis, and diseases. Available at http://wwwn.cdc.gov/travel/default.aspx
- *The Lancet* global health series, including "Child survival series" (June–July 2003, Vols 361–362); "Neonatal survival series" (March 2005, Vol. 365); "Maternal survival series" (September 2006, Vol. 368); "International child development series" (January 2007, Vol. 369); "Chronic diseases series" (December 2007, Vol. 370); "Neglected tropical diseases series" (January 2010, Vol. 375); "Tuberculosis series" (May 2010, Vol. 375); "Stillbirths" (April–May 2011, Vol. 377).

REFERENCES

Azzopardi P, Graham S (2008) What are the most useful clinical indicators of tuberculosis in childhood? International Child Health Review Collaboration, March 2008. Available at http://www.ichrc.org/sites/www.ichrc.org/files/clinicaltb.pdf

Azzopardi P, Gray N (2010) Developing country health in a developed country: personal perspectives. *J Paediatr Child Health* 46:549–51.

Berkley JA, Mwangi I, Ngetsa CJ *et al.* (2001) Diagnosis of acute bacterial meningitis in children at a district hospital in sub-Saharan Africa. *Lancet* 357:1753–7.

Best J, Hughes S (2008) Evidence behind the WHO Guidelines: Hospital care for children: what are the useful clinical features of bacterial meningitis found in infants and children? *J Trop Pediatr* 54:83–6.

Bisoffi Z, Buonfrate D (2013) When fever is not malaria. *Lancet Global Health* 1:e11–12.

Calis JCJ, Phiri KS, Faragher EB *et al.* (2008) Severe anemia in Malawian children. *N Engl J Med* 358:888–99.

Chandler CIR, Jones C, Boniface G, Juma K, Reyburn H, Whitty CJM (2008) Guidelines and mindlines: why do clinical staff over-diagnose malaria in Tanzania? *Malaria J* 7:3.

Crump JA, Sugarman J (2010) Ethics and best practice guidelines for training experiences in global health. *Am J Trop Med Hyg* 83:1178–82.

d'Acremont V, Malila A, Swai N *et al.* (2010) Withholding antimalarials in febrile children who have a negative result for a rapid diagnostic test. *Clin Infect Dis* 51:506–11.

Davey G (2001) Adapting international protocols to local settings. *Trop Doct* 31:65.

Dhaliwal G, Detsky AS (2013) The evolution of the master diagnostician. *JAMA* 310:579–80.

English M, Berkley J, Mwangi I *et al.* (2003) Hypothetical performance of syndrome-based management of acute paediatric admissions of children aged more than 60 days in a Kenyan district hospital. *Bull WHO* 81:166–73.

Foege WF (1998) Global public health: targeting inequities. *JAMA* 279:1931–2.

Frenk J, Moon S (2013) Governance challenges in global health. *N Engl J Med* 368:936–42.

Green DA, Ansari BM, Davis S, Cameron D (2003) Reagent strip testing of cerebrospinal fluid. *Trop Doct* 33:31–2.

Hackett LW (1944) Spleen measurement in malaria. *J Natl Malaria Soc* 3:121–33.

Herrle SR, Corbett EC, Fagan MJ, Moore CG, Elnicki DM (2011) Bayes' theorem and the physical examination: probability assessment and diagnostic decision making. *Acad Med* 86:618–27.

Hill Z, Kendall C, Arthur P, Kirkwood B, Adjei E (2003) Recognizing childhood illnesses and their traditional explanations: exploring options for care-seeking interventions in the context of the IMCI strategy in rural Ghana. *Trop Med Int Health* 8:668–76.

Jamison DT, Breman JG, Measham AR *et al.* (eds) (2006) *Disease Control Priorities Project*, 2nd edn. Washington, DC: Disease Control Priorities Project. Available at http://www.dcp2.org/pubs/DCP

Koplan JP, Bond TC, Merson MH *et al.* (2009) Towards a common definition of global health. *Lancet* 373:1993–5.

Lim SS, Vos T, Flaxman AD *et al.* (2013) A comparative risk assessment of burden of disease and injury attributable to 67 risk factors and risk factor clusters in 21 regions, 1990–2010: a systematic analysis for the Global Burden of Disease Study 2010. *Lancet* 380:2224–60.

Margolis P, Gadomski A (1998) Does this infant have pneumonia? *JAMA* 279:308–13.

Marsh DR, Schroeder DG, Dearden KA, Sternin J (2004) The power of positive deviance. *BMJ* 329:1177–9.

McGee S (2012) *Evidence-based Physical Diagnosis*, 3rd edn. Philadelphia: Saunders Elsevier.

Montresor A, Ramsan M, Khalfan N *et al.* (2003) Performance of the Haemoglobin Colour Scale in diagnosing severe and very severe anaemia. *Trop Med Int Health* 8:619–24.

Muhe L, Oljira B, Degefu H, Jaffar S, Weber MW (2000) Evaluation of clinical pallor in the identification and treatment of children with moderate and severe anaemia. *Trop Med Int Health* 5:805–10.

Nelson BD, Kasper J, Hibberd PL, Thea DM, Herlihy JM (2012) Developing a career in global health: considerations for physicians-in-training and academic mentors. *J Grad Med Educ* 4:301–6.

Newton CRJC (2004) Management of severe falciparum malaria in African children. *Trop Doct* 34:65.

O'Dempsey TJD, McArdle TF, Laurence BE, Lamont AC, Todd JE, , Greenwood BM (1993) Overlap in the clinical features of pneumonia and malaria in African children. *Trans R Soc Trop Med Hyg* 87:662–5.

Palfrey S (2011) Daring to practice low-cost medicine in a high-tech era. *N Engl J Med* 364:e21.

Parker J, Mitchell R, Mansfield S *et al.* (2011) A guide to working abroad for Australian medical students and junior doctors. *Med J Aust eSupplement* 194(12): 1–95.

Principi N, Esposito S (2011) Management of severe community-acquired pneumonia of children in developing and developed countries. *Thorax* 66:815–22.

Pust RE (1984a) US abundance of physicians and international health. *JAMA* 252:385–8.

Pust RE (1984b) Clinical practice roles for the doctor in developing countries. *Ariz Med* 41:327–32.

Pust RE (2007) Balance of trade: export–import in family medicine. *Fam Med* 39:746–8.

Pust RE (2012) Indication. *Ann Fam Med* 10:75–8.

Richardson WS (1999) Where do pretest probabilities come from? *Evid Based Med* 4:68–9.

Sackett DL (1992) A primer on the precision and accuracy of the clinical examination. *JAMA* 267:2638–44.

Shah S, Wu T (2008) The medical student global health experience: professionalism and ethical implications. *J Med Ethics* 34:375–8.

Shann F, Hart K, Thomas D (1983) Acute lower respiratory tract infections in children: possible criteria for selection of patients for antibiotic therapy and hospital admission. *Bull WHO* 62:749–53.

Simoes EA, Peterson S, Gamatie Y *et al.* (2003) Management of severely ill children at first-level health facilities in sub-Saharan Africa when referral is difficult. *Bull WHO* 81:522–31.

Stark R (2011) *How to Work in Someone Else's Country.* Seattle, WA: University of Washington Press.

Straus SE, Richardson WS, Glasziou P, Haynes RB (2005) *Evidence-based Medicine*, 3rd edn. Edinburgh: Churchill Livingstone.

Taylor SM, Molyneux ME, Simel DL, Meshnick SR, Juliano JJ (2010) Does this patient have malaria? *JAMA* 304:2048–56.

Taylor TE, Molyneux M (2003) Clinical features of malaria in children. In: Warrell DA, Gilles HM (eds) *Essential Malariology*, 4th edn. London: BookPower, chapter 8.

Ventres WB, Wilson CL (1995) Teaching (and learning) family medicine internationally: a cultural survival guide. *Fam Pract* 12:324–7.

Weber MW, Herman J, Jaffar S *et al.* (2002) Clinical predictors of bacterial meningitis in infants and young children in The Gambia. *Trop Med Int Health* 7:722–31.

WHO (2010) *Monitoring The Building Blocks Of Health Systems: A Handbook of Indicators and their Measurement Strategies.* Geneva: World Health Organization.

WHO (2012) *Management of Severe Malaria*, 3rd edn. Geneva: World Health Organization.

Wright PW, Avery WG, Ardill WD, McLarty JW (1993) Initial clinical assessment of the comatose patient: cerebral malaria vs. meningitis. *Pediatr Infect Dis J* 12:37–41.

CHAPTER 2
Healthcare Systems

Jennifer Kasper[1,2], Patience Ugwi[3], and Nancy E. Ringel[2]
[1]MassGeneral Hospital for Children, Boston, MA, USA
[2]Harvard Medical School, Boston, MA, USA
[3]University of Iowa, Iowa City, IA, USA

Key learning objectives

- Learn the definition and key functions of a healthcare system.
- Understand the challenges facing healthcare systems in resource-limited settings.
- Understand the critical roles of the leading organizations and funders involved in improving healthcare systems and delivery in these settings.

Abstract

Healthcare systems represent an interface of many different governmental and non-governmental organizations (NGOs) and stakeholders working together with the goal of improving the health of the populations they serve. Healthcare systems are incredibly complex and vary widely from one country to another. As a clinician working in global health, it is important to understand a country's health system, how it functions, and its strengths and challenges in order to tailor health services to meet the needs of the population. In this chapter, we provide an overview of the components that constitute a health system, discuss some of the challenges of implementing system interventions in low- and middle-income countries (LMICs), and describe different models of healthcare delivery. We also discuss the role of healthcare systems in meeting the Millennium Development Goals. We highlight a number of LMICs that have successfully implemented universal health coverage.

Key words: healthcare systems, health systems strengthening, health policy, health financing, health resources, human resources for health, IMCI, Millennium Development Goals, post-2015 development agenda, universal health coverage

Essential Clinical Global Health, First Edition. Edited by Brett D. Nelson.
© 2015 John Wiley & Sons, Ltd. Published 2015 by John Wiley & Sons, Ltd.
Companion website: www.essentialseries.com/globalhealth

Introduction

A functioning healthcare system is essential for combating various diseases and promoting health for all people. According to the World Health Organization (WHO), a healthcare system consists of "all institutions, organizations, and resources whose primary goals are to improve health, provide financial risk protection to its users, and be responsive to population expectations" (WHO, 2000). Healthcare systems exist in every country, but the structure of these systems varies. Integrated health systems – those that provide both preventive and curative services to the population across different levels of the healthcare system – are associated with more successful public health interventions and better health outcomes (WHO, 2008a; Ahmed *et al.*, 2010; Atun *et al.*, 2010).

For anyone working in global health, it is critical to understand the components of the local healthcare system, where they are situated and how they function, and the challenges facing healthcare workers in providing optimal care to patients. The key functions of a healthcare system and the benchmarks by which its performance is measured are listed in Table 2.1 (WHO, 2000; Mills *et al.*, 2004). We will discuss each of these functions separately.

Table 2.1 Key functions of a healthcare system.

1. Stewardship: leadership, policy, and system regulation
2. Financing: raising and pooling funds to pay for health services
3. Resource generation: personnel and materials used in healthcare delivery (e.g., medical supplies, diagnostic equipment, medications, information systems)
4. Service provision: healthcare providers and ancillary staff in clinical settings, private and public, formal and informal

Stewardship

Stewardship and governance of the healthcare system play a crucial role in achieving its goals. Stewardship is the responsibility of a country's department or ministry of health (MOH). These responsibilities include the following (WHO, 2000):

- *Policy-making and implementation.* The MOH's national health policy statement defines the roles of stakeholders and partners. In low-income countries, where external assistance from donors is often an important part of the healthcare system, the MOH employs a sector-wide approach to coordinate the large range of stakeholders.
- *Regulation.* The MOH oversees the activities of all stakeholders (e.g., public and private sector, NGOs) to ensure they abide by the guidelines set in the national health policy statement.
- *Information gathering.* Data collection is important for understanding and prioritizing the population's health needs and those of potentially vulnerable groups (e.g., women, disabled, HIV-positive); identifying the focus and activities of NGOs and who within the population is served by them; coordinating the efforts of NGOs within the country's overall implementation plan; writing policies to guide activi-

ties; and monitoring and evaluating the effectiveness of health programs.

One aspect of healthcare system strengthening is enhanced leadership development for ministers of health and others in low-income countries (Omaswa & Boufford, 2010). One example is the World Bank's "Flagship Program on Health Sector Reform and Sustainable Financing" that delivers short-term training to policy-makers, managers, and administrators involved in national health systems (Shaw & Samaha, 2009).

Financing

Financing for a healthcare system, primarily the responsibility of the country's ministry of finance, is imperative for conducting operations. The structure of this financing greatly influences the size, function, and population covered by the healthcare system. Oftentimes, there are distinct differences in healthcare financing between LMICs and high-income countries.

On average, wealthier countries spend up to twice as much of their gross domestic product (GDP) on health compared with low-income countries (Figure 2.1). As a result, low-income countries are often reliant on external sources, which account for 17–60% of their healthcare funding (WHO, 2011). Key external funders include the United States Agency for International Development (USAID), the Bill and Melinda Gates Foundation, the World Bank, the UK's Department for International Development (DFID), and the European Union (EU). In low-income countries, citizens generally contribute a high percentage (40–50%) to healthcare financing through personal out-of-pocket spending. The remainder of funding comes from government tax funds (40–60%) and social insurance (10–15%) (Roberts *et al.*, 2008). The private health sector provides a significant portion of healthcare services in low-income countries, with patients paying for services at the point of care (Tangcharoensathien *et al.*, 2008). Patients in these

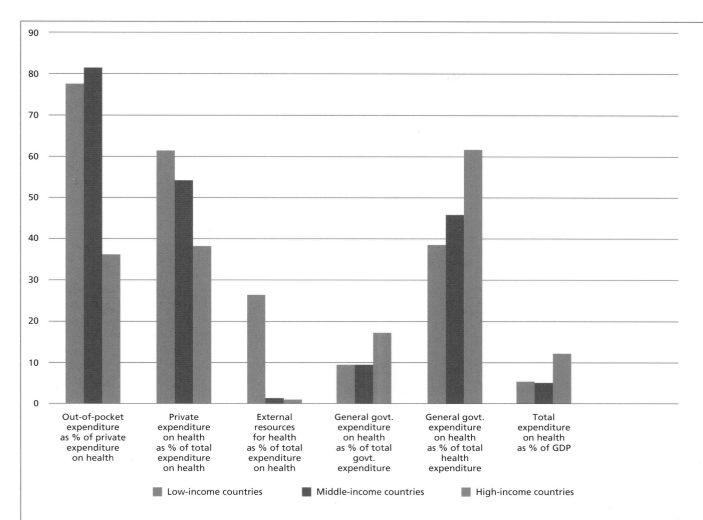

Figure 2.1 Comparing health expenditure ratios in low-income, middle-income, and high-income countries. *Source*: WHO Health Statistics 2013. Adapted from WHO (2013a).

countries, many of whom already live below the poverty line, carry a higher financial burden and are at greater risk of catastrophic healthcare expenditure, defined as a household expenditure on health that exceeds 40% of the household income after subsistence needs have been met (Xu *et al.*, 2003). They may forgo care and treatment, leading to worsening health outcomes that require even greater out-of-pocket spending. This can lead to a vicious cycle of poor health and inability to pay for healthcare. In contrast, the majority of healthcare financing in high-income countries comes from general taxation or mandatory social health insurance plans (Roberts *et al.*, 2008). Hence, the financial risk of caring for patients is distributed among the citizens as a result of greater risk pooling. In this system, people are less likely to become destitute by paying for healthcare.

Resource generation

Resource generation refers to the acquisition of the materials (e.g., medical and surgical supplies, diagnostic equipment, medications, and health information systems) and various types of human resources (e.g., doctor, nurse, midwife, community health worker) needed to provide healthcare to the population.

Physical resources

Diagnostic and therapeutic supplies in all sectors of a healthcare system are critical to provide timely and appropriate management of patients in primary, secondary, and tertiary care centers and to minimize morbidity and mortality.

Medical products, such as essential medicines, vaccines, diagnostics, and health technologies, constitute the second largest component of most countries' healthcare budgets and the largest component of private health expenditure in low-income countries (WHO, 2000). Well-functioning health sectors also have systems to support appropriate use of these products, which include diagnostic and treatment protocols, supply and distribution systems, price monitoring, and safety protocols (WHO, 2000).

WHO (2013b) defines essential medicines as

those that satisfy the priority healthcare needs of the population. They are selected based on public health relevance, evidence of efficacy and safety, and comparative cost-effectiveness. These medicines should be available within the context of functioning healthcare systems at all times, in adequate amounts, in appropriate dosage forms, with assured quality, and at a price the individual and community can afford.

WHO publishes an Essential Medicines List and an Essential Medicines List for Children that are updated every 2 years (http://www.who.int/medicines/publications/essential medicines/en/).

In some low-income countries, medication stock-outs, even of essential medications, are a common occurrence. The WHO estimates that the median availability of essential medications in public health facilities in low-income countries is approximately 40% (WHO, 2013c). Insufficient supplies may occur for any of the following reasons: medication price, inadequate financing, low priority setting by policy-makers, inappropriate drug selection and prescription, limited distribution to remote areas, development of medication resistance, and poor storage facilities and fragile supply chains (Department for International Development, 2004).

Additional challenges affect the availability of essential medicines for children in low-income countries. First, pediatric-specific formulations of medications are often unavailable, so children are administered fractions of adult medications that may not be appropriately dosed. Additionally, scales for weighing children are in many cases broken or unavailable, so healthcare providers can only estimate the necessary milligram per kilogram dose. These challenges lead to inaccuracies that may result in drug resistance or toxicity (Qazi & Hill, 2010).

Chapter 33 further discusses issues related to medications in low-resource settings.

Health information systems

A health information system is a tool for collecting, storing, and managing data to understand and address the health status and needs of a population. Health information data are important for effective clinical management, strategic planning, and policy development at all levels of the healthcare system. The WHO divides health information data sources into population-based and health facility-based (WHO, 2013d).

The main population-based sources of health information are national census and national household surveys, including demographic and health surveys (IFC International, 2013). Key health facility-related data sources include public health surveillance (e.g., community outreach by community health workers), health services data (sometimes referred to as health management or routine health information systems, such as birth registers, death registers, inpatient and outpatient data), and health system monitoring data (e.g., human resources, health infrastructure, financing).

Major challenges exist in health data documentation. In low-income countries, documentation is usually paper-based, which may be incomplete, illegible, misfiled, damaged, or completely absent. Governments and NGOs working in low-income countries have begun to use computer-based and cell-phone-based data collection tools that may overcome the challenges of a paper-based system. However, these have their own challenges, such as user training, equipment maintenance, and power outages. The demands of donor organizations for additional data and the competing interests of different stakeholders may lead to fragmentation and often duplication of data collection systems. If the needs of the population are not known to policy-makers, then the lack of rigorous data collection makes planning and evaluation of policies and programs difficult. Figure 2.2 illustrates the different types of tools employed to collect socio-demographic and health data at different levels of the healthcare system (AbouZhar & Boerma, 2005).

Human resources for health

Healthcare providers who deliver public health, clinical, and environmental services are key for healthcare delivery (WHO, 2000; Narasimhan *et al.*, 2004). Many low-income countries have an insufficient supply of healthcare workers (HCWs) to meet their health system needs. The WHO recommends a ratio of 23 HCWs (doctors, nurses and midwives) per 10,000 population, and many low-income countries fall far short of this ratio. The WHO estimates that 57 countries worldwide have a critical shortage of health workers, and 36 of those countries are in sub-Saharan Africa. Of note, sub-Saharan Africa contains 11% of the world's population and 25% of the global disease burden, but only 3% of the global health workforce (Anyangwe & Mtonga, 2007; Kasper & Banujirwe, 2012). Figure 2.3 illustrates the relative paucity of a number of types of health personnel in LMICs compared with high-income countries.

The reasons for this human-resource shortage are complex. One contributing factor is the unequal distribution of HCWs: the majority of HCWs are located in urban areas while a majority of the population may live in rural areas. Another factor is the migration of HCWs externally to high-income countries, which offer HCWs better professional opportunities and often better lifestyles. Similarly, migration of HCWs internally from the public sector to higher-paying NGO or

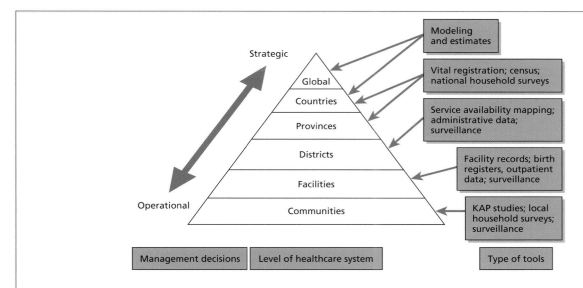

Figure 2.2 Data needs and sources at different levels of the healthcare system. *Source*: AbouZhar & Boerma (2005), figure 1, p. 580. Reproduced with permission of the World Health Organization.

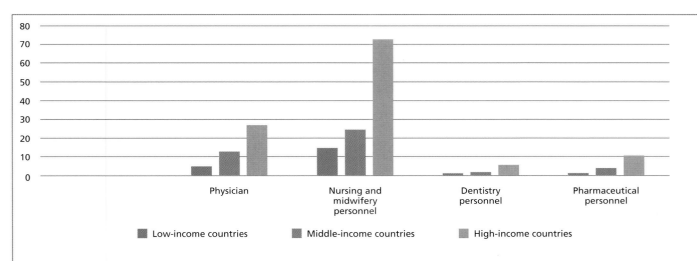

Figure 2.3 Health workforce density per 10,000 population. *Source*: WHO Health Statistics 2013. Adapted from WHO (2013a).

private-sector positions also contributes to the shortage. Lastly, a limited number of training facilities and teaching faculty mean that countries train inadequate numbers of HCWs to begin with. Tackling the problem will require a multifaceted approach (Kasper & Banujirwe, 2012; Sherr *et al.*, 2012).

Governments, the WHO, and other organizations are working to increase the number of HCWs in low-income countries. Meanwhile, task-shifting – the use of trained, less specialized workers – will continue to be an important aspect of healthcare delivery (WHO, 2007; May *et al.*, 2013; Omaswa, 2006). Community health workers, in particular, have been shown to contribute significantly to the decline in maternal, child, and infant mortality in several low-income countries (Perez *et al.*, 2009; Nelson *et al.*, 2012; Frontline Health Workers Coalition, 2013).

Models for health program implementation

A large number of stakeholders are involved in implementing programs to improve care in low-income countries. There is wide variation in the approaches used in integrating health programs into the healthcare system (Atun *et al.*, 2009);

however, implementation often falls along a spectrum among "vertical," "horizontal," and more recent "diagonal" models.

Vertical model

The vertical model of program implementation often targets specific diseases or interventions and may have varying degrees of integration within the local healthcare system. Vertical implementation may be useful for achieving specific health outcomes rapidly in target populations that are difficult to reach in countries with weak healthcare systems (Atun *et al.*, 2008). External donors and NGOs typically employ this model (Sridhar & Tamashiro, 2009; Patel *et al.*, 2012). Examples of largely vertical initiatives include the US President's Emergency Plan for AIDS Relief (PEPFAR), Direct Observed Treatment Strategy (DOTS) for tuberculosis, the Global Access to Vaccine Initiative's (GAVI) Hib vaccine program, and polio eradication programs.

Some advantages of the vertical model include faster implementation of highly specialized healthcare, achieving faster targeted health outcomes, and easier program evaluations. Disadvantages of this model include typically poor integration into the existing healthcare system and competing interests in donor and government priorities. Vertical programs may overburden a limited workforce to engage in activities that take them away from usual clinical duties. Vertical implementation may also cause inequities in access and health outcomes, as this approach characteristically is often short term and may focus on only a select portion of the population.

Horizontal model

The horizontal model of program implementation involves strengthening the existing healthcare infrastructure with a goal of providing improved comprehensive preventive and curative health services (Atun *et al.*, 2009). It delivers health services through a public-funded healthcare system and focuses on long-term healthcare system strengthening, across multiple sectors, particularly at the primary care level (Msuya, 2003; Sridhar & Tamashiro, 2009). Examples of horizontal programs include the Integrated Management of Childhood Illness (IMCI) (Box 2.1), India's Integrated Child Development Services (ICDS), and Bangladeshi Rural Advancement Committees' (BRAC) health programs.

Advantages of the horizontal model include increased likelihood of long-term sustainability and increased access to a broader range of services, which is especially beneficial to those who cannot afford private services. It has also been shown to be the most effective way to deliver services that require an integrated and comprehensive delivery method, such as HIV care (Msuya, 2003). A disadvantage of the horizontal approach is that it depends on the existing health system to deliver care. In countries with weak health systems, these programs can be difficult to manage. It can also be difficult to evaluate the impact of specific projects as the interventions and health outcomes are usually long term, impacted by other concurrent

> ## Box 2.1 IMCI: a case example
>
> Integrated Management of Childhood Illness (IMCI), developed jointly by the WHO and UNICEF in the 1990s, is a system-wide initiative implemented in low-income countries to reduce childhood deaths from preventable causes. A disproportionate number of under-five deaths occur in low-income countries, and five countries account for half of the deaths. About three-quarters of these deaths are due to preventable causes, including neonatal conditions, pneumonia, diarrhea, malaria, and measles, and can be avoided by well-known and relatively uncomplicated interventions (WHO, 2013e). IMCI replaces or complements a number of "vertical" child health programs aimed at specific groups of conditions, including control of diarrheal diseases, acute respiratory infections, and the Expanded Program on Immunization (WHO/UNICEF, 2005).
>
> IMCI aims to reduce child mortality and improve child health and development with these three components: improvement of case-management skills of health staff through the provision of locally adapted guidelines; improvement of health systems; and improvement of household and community practices (Angus, 2009).
>
> Implementation of IMCI has been associated with improved health outcomes and improvement in the quality of healthcare delivery, including appropriate antibiotic prescriptions, early recognition of danger signs, and appropriate referrals to higher-level medical centers alongside cost savings in some countries (Ahmed *et al.*, 2010).

programs, and affected by political will (Msuya, 2003; Atun *et al.*, 2009).

Diagonal model

For many years, the public health community debated the merits of vertical versus horizontal programming and financing of health services. In 2006, the concept of an integrated "diagonal" approach was introduced for health systems strengthening in resource-limited settings (Sepúlveda *et al.*, 2006). Frenk and Sepúlveda describe the diagonal approach as a

> strategy in which we use explicit intervention priorities [such as diagnosis and treatment of HIV] to drive the required improvements into the health system, dealing with such generic issues as human resource development, financing, facility planning, drug supply, rational prescription, and quality assurance (Frenk, 2006).

In effect, the diagonal model advocates for use of vertical interventions (e.g., vaccines for children or care and treatment

Clinical experience

"I worked with Doctors Without Borders at an HIV clinic in a slum of Nairobi, Kenya following the post-election violence in 2008. Within the clinic, I oversaw a TB treatment program, which cared for hundreds of patients with TB and multi-drug resistant TB. My clinic would receive patients in advanced stages of TB and HIV, as well as those co-infected with both diseases. One of the biggest challenges we faced was providing patients with access to care – although patients who received care improved quickly and dramatically. We found that the HIV clinic became an access-point not only for the treatment of TB and HIV, but for many of the other health issues that affected the community. While HIV and TB care should remain a global healthcare priority, we can also think of ways to use these programs to extend access to primary care within communities."

Richard, physician working in Kenya

of HIV-positive people) to strengthen all aspects of a healthcare system (e.g., human and material resources, financing, training, planning) (see Clinical experience box). This integrated approach is now widely recognized as the most effective approach for improving healthcare systems in resource-poor settings.

Other challenges for healthcare systems in low-income countries

Low-income countries face numerous financial, material, human, and structural challenges. They also face both a high burden of communicable diseases and a growing burden of non-communicable diseases (NCDs). The emergence of NCDs such as cancer, cardiovascular disease, chronic respiratory disease, and diabetes is a major cause of morbidity and mortality in low-income countries (WHO, 2013f). The WHO projects that, by 2030, NCDs will be the leading cause of mortality in all low-income countries. NCDs require a different approach to health service delivery, including sustainable health services, patient education and community involvement, reliable medication supplies, and other therapies (Robinson & Hort, 2011; WHO, 2012).

Conflicting interests among stakeholders and governments can limit the successful implementation of health programs. A high burden of historic loan debt further cripples many countries' ability to adequately fund healthcare. Today, 36 countries (30 of them in Africa) qualify for the International Monetary Fund's debt reduction packages through the Heavily Indebted Poor Country Initiative. Logistical challenges, such as disrupted supply lines, problems with the cold chain for vaccine storage, and insufficient and/or unpredictable electricity, have negative impact on appropriate healthcare provision. Finally,

in many of these countries, armed conflicts, civil unrest, and natural disasters can disable and destroy already fragile health systems.

Millennium Development Goals

The Millennium Development Goals (MDGs), a set of eight international goals, was one major global response to the health and socioeconomic challenges faced by many low-income countries. The aim of the MDGs was "to create an environment – at the national and global levels alike – conducive to development and the elimination of poverty." These goals were adopted by all the member nations of the United Nations, following the United Nations Millennium Summit in 2000 (World Bank, 2013). Using baseline data from 1990, the eight MDGs aimed to achieve the following by the year 2015 (World Bank, 2013).

1. Reduce by half the number of people living in absolute poverty.
2. Ensure access to primary education for all children.
3. Promote gender equality and empower women.
4. Reduce by two-thirds the number of children that die before their fifth birthday.
5. Reduce by three-quarters the number of women that die in childbirth.
6. Combat HIV/AIDS, malaria, and other diseases.
7. Reverse environmental degradation by ensuring countries originate and implement "green strategies."
8. Develop a global partnership for development.

Although progress has been made towards achieving the MDGs (United Nations Development Programme, 2013), significant work still remains, and strong comprehensive health systems play an important role.

With the passing of 2015, the next generation of MDGs will focus on sustainable development, transforming economies, building peace, and forging a new global partnership (Figure 2.4) (United Nations, 2013). One of the proposed goals includes universal health coverage (UHC). To reach this goal, and many of the others, health systems worldwide will need to be highly functioning and responsive to the population.

Primary care and universal health coverage

Primary care and universal health coverage are priorities in low-income countries. Many interventions from donors and other stakeholders can be integrated into a strong primary care system to ensure equitable distribution of health services.

UHC is defined as

ensuring that all people having access to needed promotional, preventive, curative, and rehabilitative health services, of sufficient quality to be effective, while also ensuring that people

ILLUSTRATIVE GOALS AND TARGETS

 1. End Poverty

 2. Empower Girls and Women and Achieve Gender Equality

 3. Provide Quality Education and Lifelong Learning

 4. Ensure Healthy Lives

 5. Ensure Food Security and Good Nutrition

 6. Achieve Universal Access to Water and Sanitation

 7. Secure Sustainable Energy

 8. Create Jobs, Sustainable Livelihoods, and Equitable Growth

 9. Manage Natural Resource Assets Sustainably

 10. Ensure Good Governance and Effective Institutions

 11. Ensure Stable and Peaceful Societies

 12. Create a Global Enabling Environment and Catalyse Long-Term Finance

Figure 2.4 Goals of the post-2015 development agenda. *Source*: United Nations (2013).

Table 2.2 Services that may be in a basic or essential health package.

1. Family health: antenatal care, delivery and newborn care, postnatal care, family planning, child health, child growth monitoring, essential nutrition, immunization, and adolescent reproductive health
2. Treatment and surveillance for communicable diseases: tuberculosis, leprosy, HIV/AIDS and sexually transmitted infections, epidemic diseases (including malaria), and rabies
3. Basic curative care and treatment of major chronic conditions
4. Hygiene and environmental health
5. Health education and communication

Source: adapted from WHO (2008b).

do not suffer financial hardship when paying for these services (WHO, 2010).

It is important to consider which people and what services will be covered by UHC. To make the most of available resources, many countries have designed a basic or essential health package of benefits available to all citizens. The contents of this package differ among countries since they are based on each country's economic, epidemiologic, and social conditions (WHO, 2008b). Table 2.2 details several services that may be in a basic or essential health package.

In order to achieve UHC, a healthcare system must extend coverage to the non-covered, reduce cost-sharing and patient fees, and include other services not covered (Figure 2.5). However, there are three fundamental challenges facing all countries trying to achieve UHC (WHO, 2010). These include having sufficient financial and human resources to finance UHC, providing protection of patients from financial hardships caused by out-of-pocket spending, and ensuring the efficient use of available resources.

Some LMICs, including Brazil, Chile, China, Mexico, Rwanda, Ghana, Thailand, and Taiwan, have successfully achieved or are very close to achieving full UHC for their populations (WHO, 2010). Rwanda and Ghana utilized health insurance programs that were largely initiated, and owned and operated, by the community. These programs provide insurance coverage for primary healthcare services and have been shown to be effective in achieving UHC even in the poorest settings (Soors *et al.*, 2010; Lu *et al.*, 2012).

Conclusion

Healthcare systems are complex and vary greatly between countries. Numerous low-income countries have healthcare systems that do not fully meet their population's health needs, and many factors contribute to the limitations of these systems. Much international attention is focused on improving healthcare systems, and addressing structural challenges must be an inherent part of strengthening health systems worldwide.

Additional resources

- World Health Organization (2000) *Health Systems: Improving Performance. World Health Report, 2000.* Geneva: WHO.
- Roberts MJ, Hsiao W, Berman P, Reich MR (2008) *Getting Health Reform Right.* New York: Oxford University Press.

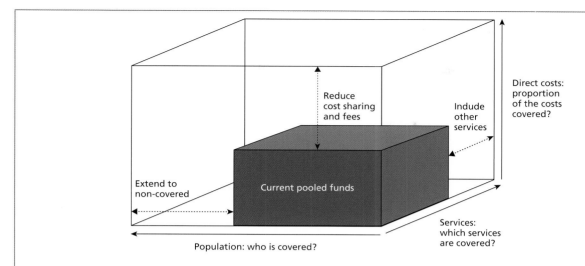

Figure 2.5 Three dimensions to consider when moving toward universal health coverage. *Source*: WHO (2010). Reproduced with permission of the World Health Organization.

- Mills A, Bennett S, Bloom G, *et al.* (ed.) (2004) *Strengthening Health Systems: The Role and Promise of Policy and Systems Research*. Geneva: Alliance for Health Policy and Systems Research.
- United Nations Development Program. The Millennium Development Goals Report, 2013. Available at http://www.undp.org/content/undp/en/home/librarypage/mdg/the-millennium-development-goals-report-2013/
- World Health Organization (2013) Health statistics and health information systems. Available at http://www.who.int/healthinfo/systems/en/

- World Health Organization (2008) World Health Report 2008: Primary health care (now more than ever). Available at http://www.who.int/whr/2008/en/
- World Health Organization (2007) Everybody's business. Strengthening health systems to improve health outcomes: WHO's framework for action. Available at http://www.who.int/healthsystems/strategy/everybodys_business.pdf

REFERENCES

AbouZhar C, Boerma T (2005) Health information system: the foundations of public health. *Bull WHO* 83:578–83.

Ahmed HM, Mitchell M, Hedt B (2010) National integration of Integrated Management of Childhood Illness (IMCI): policy constraints and strategies. *Health Policy (New York)* 96:128–33.

Angus N (2009) Integrated management of childhood illness in resource-poor countries: an initiative from the World Health Organization. *Trans R Soc Trop Med Hyg* 94:9–11.

Anyangwe S, Mtonga C (2007). Inequities in the global health workforce: the greatest impediment to health in sub-Saharan Africa. *Int J Environ Res Public Health* 4:93–100.

Atun R, Bennett S, Duran A (2008) When do vertical (stand-alone) programmes have a place in health systems? Policy brief for World Health Organization and European Observatory on Health Systems and Policies. Copenhagen: World Health Organization.

Atun R, de Jongh T, Secci F, Ohiri K, Adevi O (2009) A systematic review of the evidence on integration of targeted health interventions into health systems. *Health Policy Plan* 25:1–14.

Atun R, Weil DE, Eang MT, Mwakyusa D (2010) Health-system strengthening and tuberculosis control. *Lancet* 375:2169–78.

Department for International Development (2004) Increasing access to essential medicines in the developing world: UK Government policy and plans.

June 2004. Available at http://hospicecare.com/uploads/2011/8/dfid_access_medicines.pdf

Frenk J (2006) Bridging the divide: comprehensive reform to improve health in Mexico. WHO Commission on Social Determinants of Health, Nairobi, June 29 2006. Available at http://www.who.int/social_determinants/resources/frenk.pdf

Frontline Health Workers Coalition (2013) Frontline Health Workers' lifesaving potential. Available at http://frontlinehealthworkers.org/

IFC International (2013) Demographic and Health Surveys 2013. Available at http://www.measuredhs.com

Kasper J, Banujirwe F (2012) Brain drain in sub-Saharan Africa: contributing factors, potential remedies and the role of academic medical centres. *Arch Dis Child* 97:973–9.

Lu C, Chin B, Lewandowski JL *et al.* (2012) Towards universal health coverage: an evaluation of Rwanda *Mutuelles* in its first eight years. *PLoS ONE* 7(6), e39282.

May S, Ingram M, Lofthouse HK, Montagu D (2013) What is the role of informal healthcare providers in developing countries? A systematic review. *PLoS ONE* 8(2):e54978.

Mills A, Bennett S, Bloom G, *et al.* (ed.) (2004) *Strengthening Health Systems: The Role and Promise of Policy and Systems Research*. Geneva: Alliance for Health Policy and Systems Research. Available at http://www.who.int/alliance-hpsr/resources/Strengthening_complet.pdf [accessed 11 July 2014]

Msuya J (2003) Horizontal and vertical delivery of health services: what are the trade-offs? Background Papers for the World Development Report 2004. Washington, DC: World Bank.

Narasimhan V, Brown H, Pablos-Mendez A *et al.* (2004) Responding to the global human resources crisis. *Lancet* 363:1469–72.

Nelson BD, Ahn R, Fehling M *et al.* (2012) Evaluation of a novel training package among frontline maternal, newborn, and child health workers in South Sudan. *Int J Gynaecol Obstet* 119:130–5.

Omaswa F (2006) Informal health workers: to be encouraged or condemned? *Bull WHO* 84:83. Available at http://www.who.int/bulletin/volumes/84/2/editorial20206html/en/

Omaswa F, Boufford JI (2010) Strong ministries for strong health systems. An overview of the study report: Supporting Ministerial Health Leadership: A Strategy for Health Systems Strengthening. Available at http://www.rockefellerfoundation.org/uploads/files/8819cca6-1738-4158-87fe-4d2c7b738932.pdf

Patel P, Hoyler M, Maine R Hughes CD, Hagander L, Meara JG (2012) An opportunity for diagonal development in global surgery: cleft lip and palate care in resource-limited settings. *Plast Surg Int* (2012), Article ID 892437.

Perez F, Ba H, Dastagire SG, Altmann M (2009) The role of community health workers in improving child health programmes in Mali. *BMC Int Health Hum Rights* 9:28.

Qazi S, Hill S (2010) What are the priority essential medicines for child survival? In: Priority Essential Medicines for Child Survival, UNICEF/WHO, Copenhagen, Denmark, 6–7 September 2010. Available at http://www.who.int/childmedicines/progress/Unicef_prioriry_meds_child_survival.pdf

Roberts MJ, Hsiao W, Berman P, Reich MR (2008) *Getting Health Reform Right*. New York: Oxford University Press.

Robinson HM, Hort K (2011) Non-communicable diseases and health systems reform in low- and middle-income countries. *Pac Health Dialog* 18:179–90.

Sepúlveda J, Bustreo F, Tapia R *et al.* (2006) Improvement of child survival in Mexico: the diagonal approach. *Lancet* 368:2017–27.

Shaw R, Samaha H (2009) *Building Capacity for Health System Strengthening: A Strategy That Works. The World Bank Institute's Flagship Program on Health Sector Reform and Sustainable Financing, 1997–2008*. Washington, DC: The World Bank Institute.

Sherr K, Mussa A, Chilundo B *et al.* (2012) Brain drain and health workforce distortions in Mozambique. *PLOS ONE* 7(4), e35840.

Soors W, Devadasan N, Durairaj V, Criel B (2010) Community health insurance and universal coverage: multiple paths, many rivers to cross. Background Paper, No. 48. Health Systems Financing: The Path to Universal Coverage. Geneva: World Health Organization. Available at http://www.who.int/healthsystems/topics/financing/healthreport/48_CHI.pdf

Sridhar D, Tamashiro T (2009) Vertical funds in the health sector: lessons for education from the Global Fund and GAVI. Paper commissioned for the EFA Global Monitoring Report 2010 Reaching the marginalized. Available at http://unesdoc.unesco.org/images/0018/001865/186565e.pdf

Tangcharoensathien V, Limwattananon S, Patcharanarumol W, Vasavid C, Prakongsai P, Pongutta S (2008) Regulation of health service delivery in private sector: challenges and opportunities. International Health Policy Program. Technical Partner Paper 8, June 2008. Available at http://healthmarketinnovations.org/sites/default/files/Regulation%20of%20Health%20Service%20Delivery%20in%20the%20Private%20Sector.pdf

United Nations (2013) A new global partnership: eradicate poverty and transform economies through sustainable development. New York: United Nations Publications.

Available at http://www.post2015hlp.org/wp-content/uploads/2013/05/UN-Report.pdf

United Nations Development Programme (2013) The Millennium Development Goals Report 2013. Available at http://www.undp.org/content/undp/en/home/librarypage/mdg/the-millennium-development-goals-report-2013/

WHO (2000) *World Health Report 2000. Health Systems: Improving Performance*. Geneva: World Health Organization.

WHO (2007) International action needed to increase health workforce. Available at http://www.who.int/mediacentre/news/releases/2007/pr05/en/

WHO (2008a) Integrated health services: what and why. Technical Brief No. 1. Available at http://www.who.int/healthsystems/service_delivery_techbrief1.pdf

WHO (2008b) Essential health packages: What are they for? What do they change? Available at http://www.who.int/healthsystems/topics/delivery/technical_brief_ehp.pdf

WHO (2010) World Health Report. Health systems financing: the path to universal coverage. Available at http://www.who.int/whr/2010/10_summary_en.pdf

WHO (2011) World Health Statistics 2011. Available at http://www.who.int/gho/publications/world_health_statistics/en/index.html

WHO (2012) *Prevention and Control of Non-Communicable Diseases: Guidelines for Primary Health Care in Low-Resource Settings*. Geneva: World Health Organization.

WHO (2013a) World Health Statistics 2013. Part III. Global health indicators. Available at http://www.who.int/gho/publications/world_health_statistics/EN_WHS2013_Part3.pdf

WHO (2013b) Essential medicines. Available at http://www.who.int/topics/essential_medicines/en/

WHO (2013c) Median availability of selected generic medicines. Available at http://www.who.int/gho/mdg/medicines/availability_text/en/index.html

WHO (2013d) Health statistics and information systems: country measurement and evaluation. Available at http://www.who.int/healthinfo/systems/en/

WHO (2013e) Child health epidemiology. Available at http://www.who.int/maternal_child_adolescent/epidemiology/child/en/

WHO (2013f) Non-communicable diseases. Available at http://www.who.int/mediacentre/factsheets/fs355/en/

WHO/UNICEF (2005) *Handbook IMCI Integrated Management of Childhood Illnesses*. Geneva: World Health Organization.

Xu K, Evans DB, Kawabata K, Zeramdini R, Klavus J, Murrat CJ. (2003) Household catastrophic health expenditure: a multi-country analysis. *Lancet* 362:111–17.

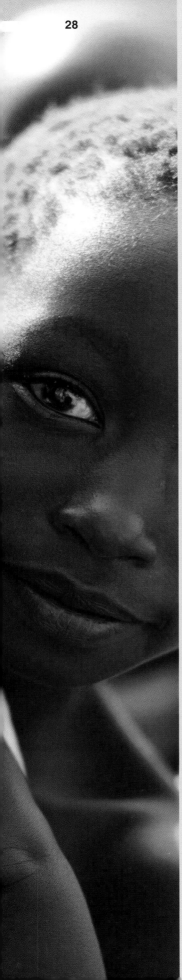

CHAPTER 3

Health Program Development and Evaluation

Alishya Mayfield[1,2,3], Kinjan Parikh[3], and Sara N. Stulac[1,2,3,4]

[1]Brigham and Women's Hospital, Boston, MA, USA
[2]Boston Children's Hospital, Boston, MA, USA
[3]Harvard Medical School, Boston, MA, USA
[4]Partners In Health, Boston, MA, USA

Key learning objectives

- Understand the importance of learning about culture and context when setting up local health programs.
- Learn about the key components of designing or revamping a health program at the level of a health center or hospital.
- Gain a basic understanding of how to design and conduct a needs assessment.
- Learn about basic tools for monitoring and evaluation and quality improvement.

Abstract

Clinicians working in resource-limited settings must address both individual patient care needs and programmatic and health systems challenges. Whether one's intended focus is program development or patient care, improved care will often require significant programmatic interventions, with their own unique set of challenges. This chapter describes key concepts in health program development, monitoring and evaluation, and quality improvement in resource-limited settings. It focuses on implementation at the level of a health center, hospital, or clinical program. It stresses the importance of understanding the politics, economy, geography, and epidemiology of a country and region, as well as forming meaningful connections with local and national leaders, prior to initiating programmatic changes. This chapter discusses issues to consider when forming partnerships with government officials and the community, staffing a program, and designing clinical programs. It provides clinicians with specific examples of tools they can use for conducting a needs assessment, implementing a monitoring and evaluation program, and designing quality improvement initiatives.

Key words: health program development, local context, needs assessment, social determinants of health, community health workers, objective-driven programmatic planning, monitoring and evaluation, quality improvement, fishbone diagram, cause-and-effect analysis, PDSA cycle

Essential Clinical Global Health, First Edition. Edited by Brett D. Nelson.
© 2015 John Wiley & Sons, Ltd. Published 2015 by John Wiley & Sons, Ltd.
Companion website: www.essentialseries.com/globalhealth

Introduction

Clinicians working at healthcare facilities in resource-limited settings are routinely faced with challenges beyond direct patient care. Whether one's intended focus is program development or patient care, improved care will often require significant programmatic interventions, with their own unique set of challenges. This chapter will provide readers with an explanation of key concepts in health program development, evaluation, and improvement in resource-limited settings at the level of a health center or hospital. It is meant to serve as an overview, rather than an exhaustive resource, for this broad topic. The chapter provides a basic orientation to key issues and available tools, and includes a list of more detailed resources available on each topic at the end of the chapter.

Table 3.1 Political questions to consider when developing a health program (Marmot & Wilkins, 2005).

What is the national, regional, and local political structure?

Which government departments or ministries will be important to the project, and who are the key contacts in those departments?

Which individuals have decision-making authority, and what is the chain of command?

How does healthcare spending compare with other social service expenditures and to overall government spending?

What laws exist for operating a non-governmental organization in this country?

Source: adapted from Partners In Health. Program Management Guide, 2011. Unit 1.

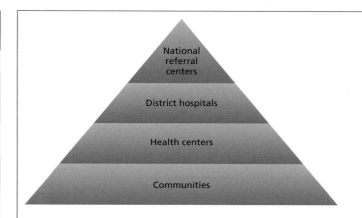

Figure 3.1 Local health systems pyramid.

Context and approach to health initiatives

Understanding local and regional culture, history, politics, economy, and geography

Developing a health program in a country with different cultural norms is a complex undertaking and can be particularly challenging in remote rural settings. Before embarking on such a journey, it is important to understand the country's history, geography, and political economy, and how each can impact a project on the local level. Seek out background information from the national government, non-governmental organizations (NGOs), journal articles, books, and online resources.

Getting to know local, regional, and national leaders can provide political context and information about local customs relevant to health program development. Engaging such individuals in meaningful discussions about projects in their area and building partnerships with them is critical to a project's success. Table 3.1 lists political questions to consider when developing a new health program in a country.

Approaching the community with genuine humility and respect, and establishing an environment of collaboration, will increase the chance of success when initiating programmatic changes. While certain local practices may be difficult to accept, it is important to consider the potential ramifications of challenging culturally ingrained practices.

Understanding regional health systems and epidemiology

Understanding the structure of national, regional, and local healthcare systems is a vital step in implementing or improving programs. Healthcare systems in resource-limited countries are often structured similarly to the example in Figure 3.1.

It is also helpful to develop a health profile of the most prevalent diseases in the region. Agencies such as the World Health Organization (WHO), the United Nations Children's Fund (UNICEF), and the United Nations Development Programme (UNDP) publish national health statistics for many countries. Other multinational organizations, including the United Nations Programme on HIV/AIDS (UNAIDS) and the Global Malaria Programme, publish disease-specific data for many countries (Marmot & Wilkins, 2005).

National ministries of health often publish data on the nationwide prevalence of disease and national protocols for the diagnosis and treatment of common illnesses. Government health officials can provide information on what data are routinely collected by healthcare facilities and how these data can be accessed. Finally, most hospitals and health centers keep patient registers with information about the local burden of disease. Even if incomplete, these data can help tailor healthcare services to the needs of a particular population.

Recognizing the social determinants of health

While healthcare has been identified as a human right in numerous international documents and forums, the extent to which the health of individuals and communities is impacted by social, economic, political, and cultural factors is often overlooked. A body of scholarly literature describes these factors as the social determinants of health (Marmot & Wilkins, 2005). In resource-limited settings, social and economic factors, including inadequate housing, drinking water, sanitation facilities, and nutrition, are often at the root of illness. Expanding a health program's objectives to address the social determinants of health can lead to improved health in a catchment area (Partners in Health, 2011a).

Identifying local partners and community engagement

Identifying local partners and engaging the community is another key step in initiating a health program. Solicit advice about the catchment area, community needs, established protocols, and previous programmatic successes and failures from local leaders. These leaders may include hospital administrators, clinicians, school principals, church officials, local government officials, tribal leaders, and representatives of community-based organizations. Community educational events, external relations activities, and community health worker (CHW) programs can also be used to engage the community in improving their own health.

Conducting a needs assessment

Whether designing a new healthcare facility or improving the services of an existing one, it is important to conduct a baseline needs assessment. A needs assessment provides a clear picture of a facility's strengths and weaknesses, identifies gaps in existing services, and facilitates the task of formulating a work plan. A wide array of existing assessment tools can be adapted for local use. The basic elements of an initial facility assessment (Table 3.2) can be expanded for a complex facility such as a referral hospital or condensed for a smaller health center. A link to a sample needs assessment can be found in the resources section.

Needs assessment tools are also useful when designing program-specific interventions or learning about community needs. These assessments share many basic elements with

Table 3.2 Components of a healthcare facility that need assessment.

Name and location of facility, year opened, and hours of operation

Contact information for key personnel

Size of catchment area and population served

Scope of inpatient wards, outpatient clinics, and mobile clinics, including range of activities (e.g., surgical services, malnutrition program, family planning, HIV testing and counseling)

Number of patients seen in hospital wards, outpatient clinics, and mobile clinics, and estimates on frequency of common clinical conditions

Information about medical and non-medical staff (e.g., number of physicians, nurses, and other clinicians, areas of expertise and level of training)

Assessment of pharmaceutical supply chain and distribution systems, as well as stock availability

Availability of laboratory equipment and supplies

List of existing medical equipment

Available imaging modalities

Existing infrastructure, including number of buildings and rooms, their function, area, and condition

Water source and availability

Modes of communication and transportation

Source and availability of electricity (e.g., municipal, generator, or solar power)

Warehouse and storage capacity

Availability of heating, cooling, and refrigeration

Security for personnel and materials

Sanitation facilities (e.g., hand washing, toilets, medical waste disposal)

Meals for staff and patients

Medical records systems

Staff housing

Waste disposal capacity and availability of an incinerator

Patient referral systems

Availability of non-medical supplies (e.g., sheets and blankets for patient beds)

facility-level assessments. For example, implementing an HIV treatment program requires clinical protocols, a pharmaceutical supply chain system, laboratory capacity, staff training, patient education, performance management, patient flow guidelines, and data management systems.

Implementing a baseline needs survey requires careful planning, trained staff, and systems for data entry and analysis. Tailor the survey to a particular facility or program. Obtain advance permission to conduct the survey from the appropriate officials. Create a schedule of assessment activities, including interviewing facility staff members, evaluating facilities, and observing activities. It is important to be sensitive to cultural norms and to the potential for disrupting employees' work when asking survey questions. Those conducting the survey should clearly explain its intent and provide reassurance that individuals will not be held responsible for gaps identified during the course of a needs assessment. Results of the survey should be analyzed and used to develop a work plan to address the needs identified.

Designing and developing healthcare facilities and programs

Mission statement, goals, and objective-driven programmatic planning

When designing a new healthcare program or improving upon an existing one, clearly outlined goals and objectives are important. Begin by collaboratively developing a mission statement and formulating a list of goals to fulfill that mission. Several guidelines for the development of a mission statement can be found online. Once goals have been identified, develop a series of objectives detailing how those goals will be accomplished. These objectives can then be translated into a work plan.

Utilizing objective-driven programmatic planning and an organized work plan can prevent the pitfall of pursuing projects unrelated to the core programmatic mission. The WHO Health System Framework Building Blocks (Figure 3.2) can be used as a guideline to help organize a work plan systematically.

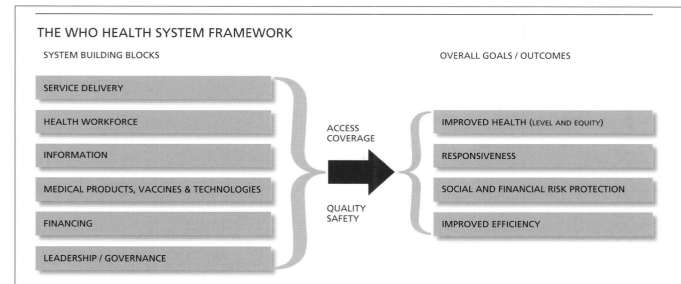

THE WHO HEALTH SYSTEM FRAMEWORK

SYSTEM BUILDING BLOCKS

- SERVICE DELIVERY
- HEALTH WORKFORCE
- INFORMATION
- MEDICAL PRODUCTS, VACCINES & TECHNOLOGIES
- FINANCING
- LEADERSHIP / GOVERNANCE

ACCESS COVERAGE

QUALITY SAFETY

OVERALL GOALS / OUTCOMES

- IMPROVED HEALTH (LEVEL AND EQUITY)
- RESPONSIVENESS
- SOCIAL AND FINANCIAL RISK PROTECTION
- IMPROVED EFFICIENCY

THE SIX BUILDING BLOCKS OF A HEALTH SYSTEM: AIMS AND DESIRABLE ATTRIBUTES

- Good health services are those which deliver effective, safe, quality personal and non-personal health interventions to those who need them, when and where needed, with minimum waste of resources.

- A well-performing health workforce is one which works in ways that are responsive, fair, and efficient to achieve the best health outcomes possible, given available resources and circumstances (i.e. there are sufficient numbers and mix of staff, fairly distributed; they are competent, responsive, and productive).

- A well-functioning health information sysytem is one that ensures the production, analysis, dissemination, and use of reliable and timely information on health determinants, health systems performance, and health status.

- A well-functioning health system ensures equitable access to essential medical products, vaccines, and technologies of assured quality, safety, efficacy, and cost-effectiveness, and their scientifically sound and cost-effective use.

- A good health financing system raises adequate funds for health, in ways that ensure people can use needed services, and are protected from financial catastrophe or impoverishment associated with having to pay for them.

- Leadership and governance involves ensuring strategic policy frameworks exist and are combined with effective oversight, coalition-building, the provision of appropriate regulations and incentives, attention to system-design, and accountability.

Figure 3.2 The WHO Health System Framework building blocks. *Source*: WHO (2007). Reproduced with permission of the World Health Organization.

Table 3.3 Example of a programmatic goal and corresponding objectives.

Goal

- To decrease mortality in children under 5 years of age

Objectives

- Increase the number of children under 5 years of age on antiretroviral therapy by 20% within the next 3 years
- Implement a protocol for identification and management of sepsis in children under 5 years of age within the next 4 months
- Vaccinate 1,000 children under the age of 5 in the next year

Table 3.4 Sample health facility budget.

Expense category	Approximate percentage of total expenditures
Pharmaceutical, laboratory, and other medical supplies	35
Staff salaries	30
Infrastructure and medical equipment	14
Communications and information technology	6
Transportation	6
Financial risk protection	4
Training and education	3
Medical records	2

Goals and objectives

Clearly defined goals and objectives are a necessary component of any program. Goals should be a broad statement of aims to accomplish over the duration of the project (American Red Cross and Catholic Relief Services, 2013). Objectives are narrower than goals and are specific statements about what should be accomplished through a given program or intervention. The mnemonic "SMART" can be helpful when formulating a list of objectives. Objectives should be *s*pecific, *m*easurable, *a*ttainable, *r*elevant, and *t*ime-bound (American Red Cross and Catholic Relief Services, 2013). Table 3.3 provides an example of a goal with several corresponding SMART objectives.

Budget and memorandum of understanding

Every work plan should have a corresponding budget that is closely aligned with the work plan's deliverables and long-term strategic goals. Table 3.4 provides an example of a health facility budget.

Creating a memorandum of understanding (MOU) is of critical importance when multiple parties are involved in a project. An MOU is a non-binding bilateral or multilateral document detailing the agreed-upon plan of action among multiple organizations. MOUs provide a concrete listing of mutual missions, goals, and responsibilities. If a project is jointly funded, both the budget and the MOU should delineate each parties' financial commitment to work plan deliverables. This helps avoid misunderstandings between organizations working together.

Staffing

Appropriate staffing is essential to the success of any healthcare program or facility and can be particularly challenging in resource-limited settings. While expatriate staff and volunteers can be useful for training and short-term implementation, their efforts should be focused on capacity-building and mentoring local staff to eventually carry out all functions.

Healthcare workers may be employed by governments, NGOs, for-profit organizations, or any combination thereof. When designing staff salary structures, NGOs can unintentionally destabilize existing public institutions by paying higher salaries than local rates. Adding a moderate bonus to the existing ministry of health salary is one approach that maintains the government as the primary stakeholder and protects the existing salary scale. Another approach is performance-based funding, through which staff salaries are adjusted based on the achievement of specific goals. Performance-based funding is used by organizations including The Global Fund To Fight AIDS, Tuberculosis and Malaria, the GAVI Alliance, the European Commission, and some ministries of health (The Global Fund To Fight AIDS, Tuberculosis, and Malaria, 2014).

Community health workers

Community health workers (CHWs) are an important component of a health system and play a crucial role on a healthcare team. Task-shifting of responsibilities to CHWs is becoming a widely recognized solution for the limited availability of nurses and doctors in low-income countries (WHO, 2008). CHWs are uniquely positioned to provide moral support, deliver community education, and identify socioeconomic needs. Health systems employing paid, accountable CHWs have been shown to have a significant impact on healthcare outcomes (Bhattacharyya *et al.*, 2001). In one model, CHWs deliver medications to patients with HIV and other chronic diseases, observe administration of medications, and report any adverse reactions or signs of infection to healthcare personnel. CHW-administered directly observed therapy for HIV and tuberculosis has led to high rates of adherence and retention (Rich *et al.*, 2012).

Another model is a population-based CHW program structure, whereby a CHW follows overall health indicators for a village, regularly visiting each household to collect information about illness, births, and deaths. Some CHWs provide clinical interventions, such as distributing insecticide-treated bednets, providing antimalarial medications, screening children for malnutrition, or serving as traditional birth attendants (Republic of Rwanda, Ministry of Health, 2008).

Important elements of any CHW program include training, clear job descriptions, supervision and reporting, integration with the clinical team, and data collection. Data collection may utilize household health charts (Partners in Health, 2013), patient medication administration sheets, and aggregate monthly reports. CHWs should be selected through transparent community-driven processes, and local leaders and healthcare personnel should participate in selecting respected community members to serve as CHWs.

Infrastructure

A thorough needs assessment should identify existing infrastructure gaps. Buildings may need to be modified or constructed, and new equipment will likely need to be purchased and maintained. Well-functioning laboratory and pharmaceutical supply chain systems are crucial components of any healthcare facility.

Pharmaceuticals, consumables, and laboratory equipment can use a large proportion of a facility's budget and should be carefully chosen based on programmatic goals and the catchment population's needs. The WHO Model List of Essential Medicines outlines medications commonly used in resource-limited settings and has been further refined to include country-specific lists (WHO, 2013). Médecins Sans Frontières (Doctors Without Borders) also publishes a handbook on essential medications for resource-limited settings (Médecins Sans Frontières, 2010). Such resources, in combination with local disease prevalence data, can be used to draft an appropriate formulary.

Depending on the availability of local information technology, medical records may be paper-based, electronic, or a combination thereof. An electronic medical record system requires the availability of hardware such as computers and servers, as well as the human capacity to maintain these systems.

Try to identify partners to assist with infrastructure needs. For example, The Global Fund has provided many healthcare facilities with improved diagnostic capacity by constructing and outfitting new laboratories (WHO, 2011).

Training and education

Appropriate and ongoing healthcare worker training and education in resource-limited settings is often a challenge and should be included in plans for any new program. Training initiatives should include all personnel – not just clinicians – and are most successful when they combine classroom-style didactics with hands-on practice and mentorship.

The Mentoring and Enhanced Supervision of Healthcare (MESH) model (Anatole *et al.*, 2012) developed in Rwanda has shown promise in strengthening provider capacity through on-site mentorship. The goal of MESH is to improve overall quality and efficacy of facility-based care through enhanced training and supervision of healthcare workers and integration of systems-based quality improvement (Doris Duke Charitable Foundation, 2012). This model includes interventions aimed at improving each of the WHO's six health systems building blocks at the health center level.

When developing programmatic systems, training manuals, or clinical protocols, utilize existing documents whenever possible and make sure they reflect national protocols and guidelines. Clinicians working in resource-limited settings commonly invest significant time into creating new clinical guidelines without realizing that such documents already exist.

The WHO has a wealth of publicly available protocols and training materials that can be adapted to specific locales, such as the *Integrated Management of Childhood Illness* (IMCI) and the *Integrated Management of Adult Illness* (IMAI) handbooks on the management of common pediatric and adult diseases. Many countries have nationally adapted IMCI training modules (UNICEF, 2005). In addition, most countries have national protocols for the diagnosis and treatment of diseases using diagnostic tests and medications available locally.

National trainings offered by the ministry of health can be useful, but these may remove staff from clinical duties for prolonged periods, so the utility of any off-site training should be carefully evaluated. On-site integrated training or educational events such as lectures, case conferences, educational games, and teaching rounds can provide appropriate education while keeping staff available for patient care. However, many countries require attendance at national clinical trainings.

Clinical systems

When designing clinical systems, consider patient flow and linkages between clinical services that reduce barriers to effective patient care. For example, when developing an HIV treatment program, consider creating mechanisms to provide multiple services within one clinical setting and/or to refer patients directly from one clinical service to the next. One approach is a system that seamlessly directs patients between pretest counseling, HIV testing, post-test counseling, and then to clinicians who prescribe antiretroviral (ARV) medications. When available and relevant, consider including reproductive health and social support services in this process. Mechanisms should also be in place to identify loss to follow-up and to reengage these patients in care.

Find out what kind of national or private health insurance systems are available and whether safety nets exist for individuals unable to pay for services. Try to obtain official descriptions of such systems as well as anecdotal accounts of people's experiences when utilizing these systems.

Monitoring and evaluation

Monitoring and evaluation basics

Monitoring and evaluation (often referred to as "M&E") is the process by which organizations assess how well programs are providing planned services, meeting service delivery targets, and achieving goals. Regular review of programmatic data provides supervisors with information on areas in which programs are succeeding and in which further strengthening or adaptation is needed. "A strong M&E system is a vital ingredient in your organization's accountability to stakeholders, who include patients, the community you are serving, donors, and national governments" (Partners in Health, 2011b). Consider sharing M&E results with the community and incorporating their feedback into future data collection efforts (American Red Cross and Catholic Relief Services, 2013).

The terms "monitoring" and "evaluation" are often used interchangeably but are two distinct concepts. Program monitoring refers to the "collection of routine data that measure progress toward achieving program objectives" (Frankel & Gage, 2007). Monitoring is an ongoing process that requires longitudinal data collection. Evaluation refers to systematic review of a program or project during specific time periods – at baseline, an interim point, or at the end of a project – to determine whether the intended goals are being achieved (American Red Cross and Catholic Relief Services, 2013). Baseline data are particularly important for documenting whether or not a change has occurred.

Monitoring without utilization of data is not a productive activity. When used together appropriately, monitoring and evaluation facilitate the production of reports showcasing a project's progress and its limitations. This information can then be transmitted across an organization to internal and external stakeholders. M&E data can also be used for accountability and can provide the basis for testing assumptions and improving on existing models.

Formulating an M&E matrix

An M&E matrix (also known as an indicator matrix or a performance indicator reference sheet) can be helpful when planning an M&E project. This is a chart outlining questions, indicators, resources needed, activities to be conducted, and reflections on the process of implementing a new program. As UNAIDS notes, "This matrix is important because it shows how data will be collected, where, when, and by whom, for each project you are monitoring and evaluating" (American Red Cross and Catholic Relief Services, 2013). Many guidelines for creating and utilizing M&E matrices exist, including the UNDP's Toolkit (American Red Cross and Catholic Relief Services, 2013) on M&E systems and the Monitoring and Evaluation Planning Guidelines and Tools published by the American Red Cross and Catholic Relief Services (Chaplowe, 2008). The M&E matrix can be incorporated into a Gantt chart (Figure 3.3), which provides a graphical display of program goals and objectives, a timeline for achieving them, and the person responsible for accomplishing them.

Staff require training and mentorship to develop skills in data collection, entry, quality assurance, and analysis (American Red Cross and Catholic Relief Services, 2013). There are an increasing number of good M&E resources available online, and there may also be in-country resources for M&E training.

Indicators and data quality

An indicator (often called a performance metric) is an objectively verifiable measurement used in monitoring and evaluation (Partners in Health, 2011). While indicators can be classified in various ways, they typically include programmatic inputs, outputs, and outcomes. One approach to indicators is outlined in Table 3.5.

Indicators for monitoring and evaluating a project are important for internal programmatic evaluation, as well as for reporting to national monitoring agencies. Many international agencies, governments, and other funders expect reports with standard indicators. Data collection and analysis can be time-consuming and costly, so indicators should be carefully chosen and not redundant with data already collected for another purpose or by another organization.

There are many tools available to help identify appropriate indicators for a range of program activities. The Global Fund, for example, publishes a toolkit that outlines a minimum set of indicators to be collected by all programs they support (The Global Fund to Fight AIDS, Tuberculosis and Malaria, 2011). In general, indicators should be valid, reliable, affordable, feasible, and relevant (American Red Cross and Catholic Relief Services, 2013), and the SMART mnemonic can also be applied to the selection of programmatic indicators (Langley *et al.*, 2009).

In order to minimize errors, data collection and recording systems should be simple and minimize time between data collection and entry. Written policies on data collection and mechanisms for ongoing training and supervision of data collection and entry contribute to consistency of data quality (American Red Cross and Catholic Relief Services, 2013).

Introduction to quality improvement methodology

Quality improvement (QI)

In program implementation, challenges frequently arise that limit the program's potential impact. This is often due to gaps in the system rather than problems with individual performance. The goal of QI is to address these gaps in a systematic manner. First, identify programmatic challenges that need to be addressed. Next, integrate performance measures into efforts to address the identified gaps. This QI work should utilize a team-based and systems-focused approach and should be

Objectives	Activities and Process Targets	2016												Person(s) Responsible	Notes
		Jan	Fab	Mar	Apr	May	Jun	Jul	Aug	Sep	Oct	Nov	Dec		
Improve education and training of clinical staff caring for patients with non-communicable diseases (NCDs)	Create a series of Powerpoint presentations on five most commonly seen NCDs (asthma, diabetes, hypertension, heart failure, and epilepsy)			■										Director of Training and Education	
	Conduct monthly lectures at noon conference covering major NCDs								■		■			Clinical Director	Asthma lecture given in June, hypertension in July, heart failure in August, epilepsy in September, and diabetes in October.
	Create protocols for treating each of the major diseases managed in NCD clinic (asthma, DM, HTN, CHF, epilepsy), and post in clinic						■							Clinical Director	
	Periodic one-on-one training and education in NCD clinic with all three clinicians												■	Clinical Director	Ongoing, but consists of Clinical Director working one on one in clinic with NCD clinicians at least one half day per month
	Create a website for clinical staff to access relevant protocols, presentations, and other educational materials													IT Director	
Ensure consistent staffing in NCD clinic with trained clinicians	Create and conduct full day training for three clinicians on NCD diagnosis and management						■							Clinical Director and clinical team	
	Create clinician schedule for NCD clinic					■								Clinical Director	
	Exam for clinicians on diagnosis and management of NCDs							■						Clinical Director	
	Additional training day for clinicians who score <70% on exam								■	■				Clinical Director	Only one NCD clinic physician needed this

Key: Yellow = in progress
Green = target completion date
Gray = actual completion date

Figure 3.3 Sample Gantt chart for improvements to a non-communicable disease (NCD) clinic.

Table 3.5 Types of indicators (Marmot & Wilkins, 2005; American Red Cross and Catholic Relief Services, 2013).

Inputs

Specific resources used in a program, such as supplies, staff, time invested, and financial outlays

Outputs

Short-term results of a program, such as number of home visits done or number of educational seminars conducted

Coverage

Proportion of a specific population receiving a service, such as percentage of adult men who have been tested for HIV

Performance

How well something is being done, such as number of patients reporting satisfaction with their clinical care or proportion getting correct treatment

Outcomes

Short-term results expected from program implementation, such as consistent recording of daily vital signs in the obstetrics ward during the month of July

Impact

Long-term effects or end results of a program, such as change in the incidence of tuberculosis in a particular district

Source: Adapted from Uganda Network of AIDS Service Organization (2005) and Partners in Health (2011b).

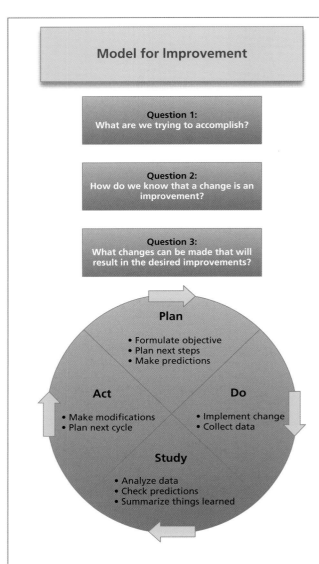

Figure 3.4 The Model for Improvement and PDSA cycle (Uganda Network of AIDS Service Organizations, 2005; WHO, 2007). Adapted from NHS Institute for Innovation and Improvement (2008a) and Langley *et al.* (2009).

supported by a multidisciplinary team drawn from clinicians, M&E staff, program leadership, and, ideally, consumers.

One of the most common approaches to QI is based on the Model for Improvement, which asks three key questions (Figure 3.4). This model uses small tests of change through the PDSA (Plan–Do–Study–Act) cycle, developed by Langley and colleagues in 1996 (Langley *et al.*, 2009). PDSA is shorthand for developing a plan to test a change in a program (Plan), carrying out the test (Do), observing and learning from the consequences (Study), and determining what program modifications should be made (Act) (NHS Institute for Innovation and Improvement, 2008a).

According to the United Kingdom's National Health Service (NHS) Institute for Innovation and Improvement (2008b):

You may not get the results you expect when making changes to your processes, so it is safer, and more effective to test out improvements on a small scale before implementing them across the board. Using PDSA cycles enables you to test out changes before wholesale implementation and gives stakeholders the opportunity to see if the proposed change will work …

By building on the learning from these test cycles in a structured way, you can put a new idea in place with greater chances of success.

This model allows evaluation of the impact of small programmatic changes and identification of potential problems before implementing changes on a larger scale.

Flow charts and cause-and-effect analysis

A flow chart provides a map of steps involved in the implementation of change. For example, if the guideline is that all pregnant women with HIV should receive antiretroviral drugs,

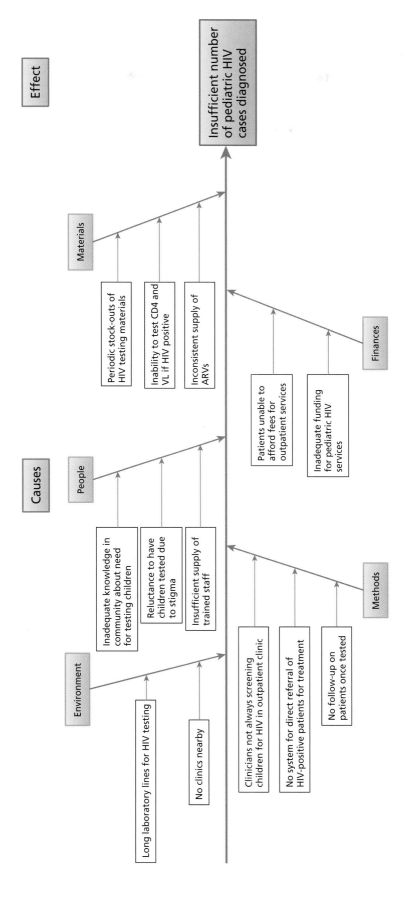

Figure 3.5 Fishbone diagram addressing the problem of insufficient number of pediatric HIV cases diagnosed.

a flow chart maps out the necessary steps to achieve this goal. This would include steps such as ensuring that all women are tested, linking HIV-positive women into clinical care, and the procurement of antiretroviral drugs. Once there is agreement on what ought to be happening, the next step is figuring out why it has not been happening.

Cause-and-effect analysis can facilitate a thorough examination of the various causes of a problem in order to effectively address them. A cause-and-effect diagram, also known as a fishbone or Ishikawa diagram, can assist with this process (Uganda Network of AIDS Service Organizations, 2005). In order to create a fishbone diagram, first identify the problem and then outline causes leading to it as shown in Figure 3.5.

The PDSA cycle and fishbone diagram are just two of many approaches to QI. Additional sources of information on QI can be found in the resource section of this chapter.

Additional resources

- WHO Commission on Social Determinants of Health (2008) Closing the gap in a generation: health equity through action on the social determinants of health. Commission on Social Determinants of Health final report. Geneva: World Health Organization. Available at http://www.who.int/social_determinants/thecommission/finalreport/en/index.html
- World Health Organization (2003) Health facility survey: tool to evaluate the quality of care delivered to sick children attending outpatient facilities Available at http://whqlibdoc.who.int/publications/2003/9241545860.pdf
- World Health Organization (2007) *Everybody's Business. Strengthening Health Systems to Improve Health Outcomes: WHO's Framework for Action.* Geneva: WHO. Available at http://www.who.int/healthsystems/strategy/everybodys_business.pdf
- Partners in Health (2013) Need to know: Malawi household chart. Available at http://www.pih.org/blog/malawi-health-data-collection
- US Department of Health and Human Services, Centers for Disease Control and Prevention (2011) Office of the Director, Office of Strategy and Innovation. Introduction to program evaluation for public health programs: a self-study guide. Atlanta, GA: Centers for Disease Control and Prevention. Available at http://www.cdc.gov/eval/guide/CDCEvalManual.pdf
- UNAIDS (2010) Basic terminology and frameworks for monitoring and evaluation. Available at http://www.unaids.org/en/media/unaids/contentassets/documents/document/2010/7_1-Basic-Terminology-and-Frameworks-MEF.pdf
- The Global Fund to Fight AIDS, Tuberculosis and Malaria (2011) *Monitoring and Evaluation Toolkit: HIV/AIDS, Tuberculosis and Malaria and Health Systems Strengthening*, 4th edn. Available at http://www.theglobalfund.org/en/me/documents/toolkit/
- National Quality Center. Quality improvement resources: Helpful tools to assist in your quality improvement efforts. Available at http://nationalqualitycenter.org/index.cfm/5852
- Institute for Healthcare Improvement (IHI). How to improve. Last modified December 4, 2012. Available at http://www.ihi.org/knowledge/Pages/HowtoImprove/default.aspx

REFERENCES

American Red Cross and Catholic Relief Services (2013) United Nations Development Group Toolkit. Available at http://toolkit.undg.org/overview

Anatole M, Magge H, Redditt V *et al.* (2012) Nurse mentorship to improve the quality of health care delivery in rural Rwanda. *Nurs Outlook* 61:137–44.

Bhattacharyya K, LeBan K, Winch P, Tien M (2001) Community health worker incentives and disincentives: how they affect motivation, retention, and sustainability. USAID, Basic Support for Institutionalizing Child Survival Project (BASICS II) for the United States Agency for International Development. Available at http://pdf.usaid.gov/pdf_docs/PNACQ722.pdf

Chaplowe SG (2008) Monitoring and evaluation planning: guidelines and tools. Washington, DC and Baltimore, MD: American Red Cross and Catholic Relief Services. Available at http://www.stoptb.org/assets/documents/countries/acsm/ME_Planning_CRS.pdf

Doris Duke Charitable Foundation (2012) Rwanda PHIT Partnership. Available at http://www.ddcf.org/Programs/African-Health-Initiative/Goals-and-Strategies/PHIT-Partnership-Grantees/Rwanda-PHIT-Partnership/

Frankel N, Gage A (2007) M&E Fundamentals: a self-guided minicourse. MEASURE Evaluation. Available at http://www.cpc.unc.edu/measure/publications/ms-07-20

Langley GJ, Moen RD, Nolan KM, Nolan TW, Norman CL, Provost LP (2009) *The Improvement Guide: A Practical Approach to Enhancing Organizational Performance*. San Francisco, CA: Jossey-Bass.

Marmot M, Wilkins RG (eds) (2005) *Social Determinants of Health*, 2nd edn. New York: Oxford University Press.

Médecins Sans Frontières (2010) Essential drugs: practical guidelines. Available at http://refbooks.msf.org/msf_docs/en/essential_drugs/ed_en.pdf

NHS Institute for Innovation and Improvement (2008a) Quality and service improvement tools: Plan, Do, Study, Act (PDSA). http://www.institute.nhs.uk/quality_andservice_improvement_tools/quality_and_service_improvement_tools/plan_do_study_act.html

NHS Institute for Innovation and Improvement (2008b) Quality and service improvement tools: cause and effect (Fishbone). http://www.institute.nhs.uk/quality_and_service_improvement_tools/quality_and_service_improvement_tools/cause_and_effect.html

Partners in Health (2011a) Program Management Guide. Unit 11: Addressing the social determinants of health. Available at http://www.pih.org/library/pih-program-management-guide/unit-11-addressing-the-social-determinants-of-health

Partners in Health (2011b) Program Management Guide. Unit 12: Using monitoring and evaluation for action. Available at http://www.pih.org/library/pih-program-management-guide/unit-12-using-monitoring-and-evaluation-for-action

Partners in Health (2013) Need to know: Malawi household chart. Available at http://www.pih.org/blog/malawi-health-data-collection

Republic of Rwanda, Ministry of Health (2008) National community health policy of Rwanda. Available at http://www.ipar-rwanda.org/index.php?option=com_docman&task

Rich M, Miller AC, Niyigena P *et al.* (2012) Excellent clinical outcomes and high retention in care among adults in a community-based HIV treatment program in rural Rwanda. *J Acquir Immune Defic Syndr* 59:e35–42.

The Global Fund to Fight AIDS, Tuberculosis and Malaria (2011) *Monitoring and Evaluation Toolkit: HIV/AIDS, Tuberculosis and Malaria and Health Systems Strengthening*, 4th edn. Available at http://www.theglobalfund.org/en/me/documents/toolkit/

The Global Fund To Fight AIDS, Tuberculosis, and Malaria (2014) Performance-based funding. Available at http://www.theglobalfund.org/en/about/grantmanagement/pbf/

Uganda Network of AIDS Service Organizations (2005) Monitoring and Evaluation: Participant Manual.

UNICEF (2005) *Handbook IMCI: Integrated Management of Childhood Illness*. Geneva: WHO. Available at http://whqlibdoc.who.int/publications/2005/9241546441.pdf

WHO (2007) Health services development: The WHO Health Systems Framework. Available at http://www.wpro.who.int/health_services/health_systems_framework/en/index.html

WHO (2008) Task shifting: rational redistribution of tasks among health workforce teams. Global recommendations and guidelines. Available at http://www.who.int/healthsystems/TTR-TaskShifting.pdf

WHO (2011) Increasing access to diagnostics through technology transfer and local production. Available at http://www.who.int/phi/publications/Increasing_Access_to_Diagnostics_Through_Technology_Transfer.pdf

WHO (2013) WHO model list of essential medicines. Available at www.who.int/selection_medicines/list/en/

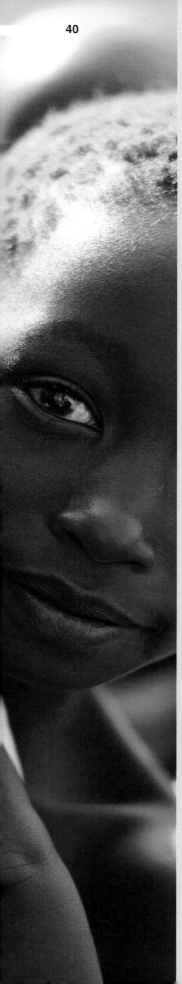

CHAPTER 4

Preparing for Travel and Staying Safe Abroad

Ariel Wagner[1] and Paul K. Drain[1,2]

[1]Harvard Medical School, Boston, MA, USA

[2]Massachusetts General Hospital, Boston, MA, USA

Key learning objectives

- To understand the preparations necessary prior to international travel.
- To understand how to avoid injury and illness while abroad.
- To understand the ethical issues of clinical practice in resource-limited settings.

Abstract

There are a number of important steps that trainees and clinicians should undertake in preparation for international work. This chapter provides an outline of these steps and suggests resources that may be helpful in the weeks and months prior to departure. The chapter also discusses ways for trainees and clinicians to stay safe and healthy during their time abroad. We also review ethical issues of providing direct medical care while abroad or while working in resource-limited settings.

Key words: international travel, preparation, trip planning, travel clinic, packing, health and safety, ethics, culture shock, insurance

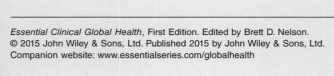

Essential Clinical Global Health, First Edition. Edited by Brett D. Nelson.
© 2015 John Wiley & Sons, Ltd. Published 2015 by John Wiley & Sons, Ltd.
Companion website: www.essentialseries.com/globalhealth

Introduction

International travel for clinical rotations, research, and volunteer opportunities can be a meaningful and even transformative experience. At the same time, travel abroad can be challenging and entail risks that may be different from those to which healthcare trainees and providers are accustomed at home. The topics in this chapter are therefore intended to help you prepare for your trip and to stay safe and healthy while abroad so that you can make the most of your international experience.

Box 4.1 Pre-departure checklist

- Visit a travel clinic to obtain prescriptions and immunizations
- Obtain passport and visas
- Obtain travel health insurance and medical evacuation insurance
- Provide contact information to your significant other, family, program or academic institution, and an emergency contact person
- Register your travel with your local embassy
- Research your destination
- Plan your research and/or clinical time at your destination
- Pack carefully

Table 4.1 Some commonly prescribed medications and common immunizations for travellers.

Medications
Malaria prophylaxis (see Table 4.2)
Antibiotics for traveler's diarrhea
Oseltamivir for influenza
Acetazolamide for altitude sickness

Immunizations[a]
Yellow fever
Typhoid
Hepatitis A and/or Hepatitis B
Meningitis
Rabies
Japanese encephalitis

[a] Specific immunizations provided will depend on one's destination (see CDC country-specific travel information: http://wwwn.cdc.gov/travel/destinationList.aspx).

Preparing for travel

See Box 4.1 for a quick-reference summary of the preparation required prior to traveling.

Travel clinic

Travelers should schedule a travel appointment with a healthcare provider at least 6 weeks prior to departure (Centers for Disease Control, 2014). This will allow time to obtain necessary medications and vaccinations (Table 4.1). Individuals should bring a copy of their immunization history to this appointment.

Passport and visa

Make sure you have a valid passport and any necessary visas. Many countries require one to two blank visa pages within the passport and may require a passport expiration date at least 6 months after your return flight. Some countries require you to obtain a visa prior to arrival, so check visa requirements for your destination countries well in advance of your trip as this process can take months. Travel and visa information can typically be found on your home country's consular department website.

Travel health insurance and medical evacuation insurance

Many domestic health insurance plans do not cover expenses related to illness or injury sustained abroad, nor do they typically cover the costs of emergency evacuation. Therefore, it is a good idea to purchase supplemental insurance to cover these services if needed. Travel health insurance, which covers such costs as doctor's visits abroad (often to specified providers), and medical evacuation insurance can be purchased together or separately from a number of different providers. Plans vary by company, making it important to research your available options. A comprehensive plan would include travel health insurance, medical evacuation, emergency medical expenses, and repatriation. As some organizations and institutions provide travel and/or evacuation insurance, especially for students, it is worth looking into this prior to purchasing insurance on one's own.

Contact information

Ensure that you have the contact information of key people at your destination and that others can contact you if needed.

Leave instructions for how to contact you while you are abroad (address, phone number, email address) with your family, significant other, program or academic institution, and at least one emergency contact person. Bring photocopies of your passport, visa, and other important documents with you should your wallet or purse be stolen or your documents lost or damaged. You may also want to leave photocopies of your passport, visa, and travel insurance card with a family member and/or responsible person from your program.

Register your travel

Register your travel with the local embassy of your home country so that they can contact you in case of an emergency. For US citizens, for example, this can be done through the US State Department website (https://travelregistration .state.gov/ibrs/ui/). Citizens of other countries should check with their state department or embassy for additional information. We recommend that you have the address and phone number for your local embassy or consulate office in case of emergency. Contact your bank and credit card companies to inform them of your travel plans in order to avoid accounts being frozen by your international transactions.

Research your site

It is strongly recommended that you familiarize yourself with the safety and security situation at your destination prior to your departure. Many governments publish up-to-date travel advisories and warnings by country, which can be easily accessed by citizens online. US citizens can sign up for automatic alerts from the US State Department to receive news or warnings within one's destination country (http:// travel.state.gov). Speaking with people who have traveled or worked at your destination can also be valuable. Country-specific health information is available online from the World Health Organization (http://www.who.int/countries/en/) and the US Centers for Disease Control (http://wwwn.cdc.gov/ travel/destinationList.aspx).

Once you have arrived in your country of destination, ask your hosts if there are certain neighborhoods or areas to avoid and when it might be safe to walk outside. Following the local news is a great way to keep yourself informed. You will also want to learn about the health situation at your destination. Learning about the local patterns of disease is often best achieved by speaking with local physicians, nurses, and other healthcare providers.

Plan your efforts at your site

For those who will be performing clinical work abroad, familiarizing yourself with clinical management protocols and drug availability in your host country ahead of time can help ease your transition. This may also help you avoid such pitfalls as prescribing medications or requesting diagnostic tests that are not locally available. Clinicians should also check the licensure requirements of the countries. Many countries will require foreign doctors to hold local licenses. The application process for these licenses can take several months and cost $200–400 on average. For students and trainees in particular, reading about common medical conditions at your destination site with which you may not be especially familiar (e.g., malaria) can also be helpful. Please refer to the other chapters in this textbook for more detailed information on a variety of relevant topics.

For those undertaking a research or public health project, reading about your topic prior to departure will enable you to make the most of your time at your site. For instance, an individual researching neonatal care at an urban hospital might prepare for her trip by reviewing her destination country's neonatal and infant mortality statistics and reading about evidence-based interventions to prevent neonatal mortality. For information about health conditions at your project destination, some helpful resources include the World Health Organization (www.who.int), UNICEF (www.unicef.org), and the United National Programme for HIV/AIDS (www.unaids.org). Demographic and Health Surveys are another excellent source of health statistics for many countries (www.measuredhs.com).

Packing

Knowing what to bring and what not to bring when traveling to a new place is always a challenge. In most cases, it is ideal to bring as little as possible, as this makes travel easier, and many items may be purchased on arrival. However, some items, such as contact lens solution and feminine hygiene products, can be difficult to purchase in some locations and would be best brought along. A packing list is included in Box 4.2, but be sure to check with your program or with people with experience at your destination for more specific recommendations.

For individuals working in a clinical setting, particularly a setting with limited resources, bringing basic medical supplies can be helpful. Check with your program regarding what items are best to bring. For those interested in donating items, it is essential to discuss these plans with your host institution ahead of time. This ensures that donated supplies are needed, are appropriate for the setting, and that the host organization is prepared to receive the items. Do not assume that all medications, supplies, or medical devices from your home institution will be of benefit to your host organization.

Large textbooks and other reading materials can take up significant space and weight and are usually best left at home. If you will have computer access at your destination, electronic copies of reference material are a great option. If you will be without electricity or computer access, some options include small portable medical reference books,

Box 4.2 Suggested packing list

General supplies
- Home prescriptions with adequate refills (in original containers)
- Over-the-counter medications (e.g., loperamide, diphenhydramine, hydrocortisone cream)
- Photocopies of important documents
- Headlamp or flashlight
- Electric plug adapter and converter (if needed)
- Insect repellant with DEET
- Battery- or solar-powered charger for electronics

Medical supplies
- White coat
- Stethoscope, oto-ophthalmoscope with tips
- N95 masks
- Specialty-specific tools (e.g., pregnancy wheel for an OB rotation)
- Pair of clinical scrubs
- Portable medicine or tropical medicine reference book
- Miscellaneous: latex gloves, suture supplies, hand sanitizer, etc.

(See Chapter 1, Table 1.2 for a list of diagnostic tools that may also be useful)

Other items to consider
- Mosquito net
- Rain gear

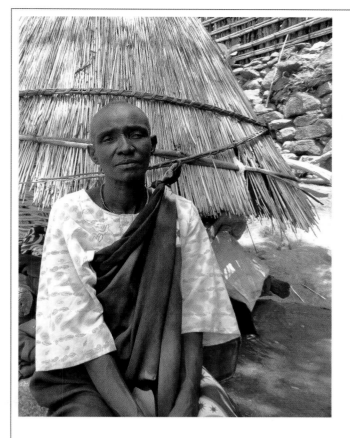

Figure 4.1 A traditional birth attendant serves her community in South Sudan. *Source*: B.D. Nelson, Harvard Medical School, Boston, Massachusetts, USA. Reproduced with permission of B.D. Nelson.

photocopies of relevant chapters, or a tablet/e-reader device that does not require frequent charging. Dozens of useful free clinical reference manuals are available (e.g., from WHO, UNICEF, international non-governmental organizations) and can be downloaded onto a tablet. If one will be carrying a smartphone, there are also numerous apps that can be helpful and are worth downloading onto your mobile device ahead of time, including Skype, a language translation app (e.g., Google Translate), a drug formulary app (e.g., Epocrates, Micromedex), and apps with other medical content (e.g., Medscape).

Understanding your local environment

Awareness, appreciation, and respect of the local culture at your destination are essential. This should be part of your trip planning, as understanding the local environment will help ease your transition into a new work and social context, improve your ability to work with your new colleagues, and help keep you safe. Begin by familiarizing yourself with the local history, political and economic system, cultural practices, attitudes and beliefs, and the artistic traditions of your destination country. Developing an understanding of the healthcare system and availability of resources can also be helpful. Many places also have an alternative healthcare system, such as traditional healers (Figure 4.1), and you should develop an understanding of their role in society. As before, speaking with individuals who have experience either working or living at your project site can be invaluable.

Dress

Acceptable dress can vary significantly from country to country, as well as within countries, depending on the region (rural versus urban), setting (clinical scrubs versus professional dress), and season of the year (rainy versus dry). Find out what types of clothing are appropriate ahead of time and pack accordingly. When in doubt, err on the side of dressing more conservatively and more professionally as a bad first impression at one's host hospital or community might be hard to overcome.

Clinical experience

"Anytime one travels to a new place to work, it's of course important to learn about and adjust to new cultural norms. While I was a second year medical student, I was part of a team providing eye care in a clinic in northern Thailand. Many of our patients were Buddhist monks who, as part of their vows, cannot touch women. When I first started working there I didn't know this! I walked up to our first monk patient and confidently offered my hand for a shake while introducing myself. He was so gracious and just bowed his head while our Thai guides quietly explained my gaffe. Nonetheless I went on to check his vision and get him into glasses without further missteps. Experiences like this are not uncommon, but it's great to try to learn as much as you can before working in a new community."

Jesse, physician working in Thailand

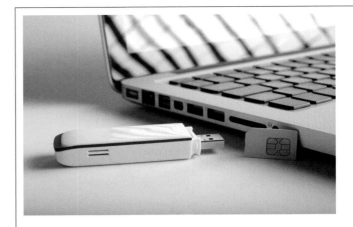

Figure 4.2 A local USB modem can provide internet access via the local cellular network. *Source*: iStock © Liens.

Language

Regardless of your destination, learning the local language can be an invaluable skill, and even speaking a few words often goes a long way. Bringing a pocket dictionary or phrase book to one's destination is advisable. Language materials for less widely spoken languages may be harder to find, but many programs can recommend helpful resources. In some settings, local language tutors are inexpensive and provide an excellent means by which to improve your language skills, learn about the local culture, and help support the local economy.

Resource availability

Electricity

The type of outlet and the voltage of the local power supply (e.g., 110 V vs. 220 V) differ from country to country. Using your electronic devices without converting the voltage can result in permanent damage to your device. Therefore, it is important to find out the standard voltage of electrical outlets in your country of destination in case an electrical adapter and a voltage converter or transformer is necessary. Even if your laptop computer has a built-in voltage converter, having the proper adapter will be important. In settings with minimal access to electricity, you may want to invest in solar- or battery-powered chargers for electronic equipment. A laptop or tablet with a long battery life, or having a second battery, can be helpful in these settings as well.

Currency and money

Withdrawing local currency at an ATM machine is generally the best way to obtain local currency without having to carry a lot of cash. However, ATM availability and acceptance of credit cards are often limited, especially outside of major cities,

and some banks charge transaction fees. Ask for recommendations from your program, but you may want to bring some cash in hard currency to exchange into the local currency on arrival. In addition, local counterparts may have recommendations about exchanging money as the rates, safety, and legality can vary significantly from country to country. For example, in some countries it is safe and recommended to exchange money in the informal sector, whereas in other countries these transactions are best made at a bank. In some countries, the exchange rate varies depending on the total amount of the transaction or the size of the bills exchanged. Older bills may not be accepted. In addition, credit cards are generally accepted for many formal purchases, such as at restaurants or hotels, but may incur a foreign exchange fee. However, many credit card companies now offer cards that do not charge foreign fees, and these may be worth acquiring before your departure. Visa is currently the most widely accepted credit card globally.

Internet and phone access

Internet availability and cellular phone service is expanding rapidly, but they are still absent in many settings. There is increasing availability of USB cellular modems that allow you to access the internet on your laptop across a local cell phone network (Figure 4.2). Local phone stores are available in major cities, and their staff can be helpful in understanding the local practice and options. A basic inexpensive phone and/or local SIM card can be purchased in most settings. International calls via an internet-based service, such as Skype, will generally be less expensive than cell phone calls. Purchasing international coverage through your home cell phone company is also an option but is often more costly than local options. Some phones may be "unlocked" for international use, enabling the use of a local SIM card with one's phone from home. For those without international coverage, or who are unsure of their plan details, it is prudent to turn your cellular data option off prior to departure from your home country as international charges are often astronomical.

Caring for yourself abroad

See Box 4.3 for a summary of how to stay safe when abroad.

Box 4.3 Being safe in a foreign environment

- Use common sense (e.g., avoid walking alone at night)
- Avoid wearing expensive clothing or displaying expensive items in public (leave important jewelry at home)
- Know your local environment (e.g., what neighborhoods have high crime?)
- Avoid dangerous activities and situations
  ○ Unprotected sex
  ○ Drugs and alcohol intoxication
  ○ Political gatherings, civil unrest
- Avoid unsafe transport, including mopeds and motorcycles. Motor vehicle accidents are the leading cause of death among foreign travelers! Always wear a seatbelt.

Food and water

Trying local foods can be a fun and delicious way to experience the local culture. However, it is important to keep in mind that the most common infections affecting international travelers are transmitted by contaminated food and water. Staying healthy does not require that you completely avoid local cuisine, but it does necessitate that you be more vigilant about hygiene and food safety than you might be at home.

- *Hand hygiene*: Soap and water, or hand sanitizer, are essential.
- *Fresh fruit and vegetables*: Words to live by: "Boil it, cook it, peel it, or forget it." Soak salad items for 20 min in water with a small amount of bleach (e.g., 1 teaspoon of 4% chlorine bleach per 1 L of water). Rinse with clean water prior to eating.
- *Water (and ice)*: Tap water may be safe in some countries. Where it is not, options include boiling for 10 minutes or treating your water. Bottled water is often an option but can get expensive. Many countries sell bags of water on the street and in stores. These are often safe, particularly the manufactured sealed brands, but it is a good idea to verify this with your host.

- *Dining out*: Avoid food that has been sitting out all day. Cooked foods that are still hot and dry items (e.g., cookies, bread) are typically safe to eat. Beverages in cans or sealed bottles are safe to drink.

Mosquito-borne illnesses

Several serious diseases are transmitted by mosquitoes, including malaria, dengue, and yellow fever. Malaria is transmitted by *Anopheles* mosquitoes, which typically bite from dusk to dawn. In contrast, dengue and yellow fever are transmitted by the *Aedes* mosquito, which bites during the day. For those traveling to areas where these diseases are endemic (Figures 4.3 and 4.4), minimizing the exposure of skin by wearing pants, long-sleeved shirts, and insect repellant with DEET during hours when mosquitoes are active will help avoid these illnesses. It is also important to sleep under an insecticide-treated mosquito bednet. If not provided for you, these are often available locally. Bednets can also be purchased before your trip from outdoor outfitters. In malaria-endemic regions, malarial prophylaxis is recommended (Table 4.2). Prophylactic options vary with regard to dosing frequency, duration of administration before and after travel, side-effect profiles, costs, and level of resistance at your destination.

Swimming

Schistosomiasis is a parasitic infection endemic in freshwater areas in certain parts of South America, the Caribbean, Africa, and Asia (Figure 4.5). Travelers should avoid swimming and wading in schistosomiasis-contaminated bodies of water (Figure 4.6).

Medical care

In case of an emergency, know where you should go for medical care and how your medical insurance works. If you need surgery, consider whether you can do this safely at the local hospital, whether you should be medically evacuated to a higher level of care, or whether the intervention can be delayed long enough for you to return home. Many local pharmacies will have antibiotics or other important treatments available. You should confirm with local colleagues which pharmacies have quality medications; some pharmacies carry knock-off drugs.

Safety in the medical environment

Tuberculosis exposure

For individuals working in clinical settings where they may experience prolonged exposure to tuberculosis, as well as for those spending an extended period of time in a country where tuberculosis is endemic, the CDC recommends pre- and post-exposure tuberculosis testing with either a two-step tuberculin skin test or a single interferon-gamma release assay (Centers

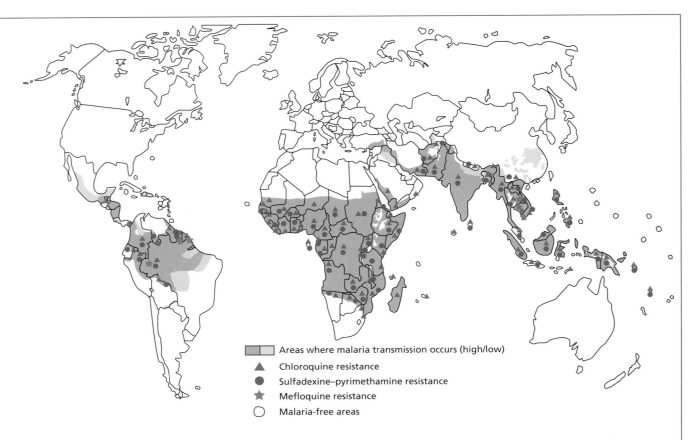

Figure 4.3 Global distribution of malaria, including areas of drug resistance to *Plasmodium falciparum* from studies in sentinel sites, up to 2004. *Source*: World Health Organization (2005). Reproduced with permission of the World Health Organization.

for Disease Control, 2013). The post-departure test should be performed 8–10 weeks after your return home. Healthcare trainees and providers who anticipate possible exposure to tuberculosis may want to bring N95 masks with them to prevent exposure, as these masks are unavailable in many high-risk settings.

Sharps injuries

It is estimated that 1000 healthcare workers globally are infected with HIV every year as a result of sharps injuries (Pruss-Ustun *et al.*, 2005). Risk of transmission varies widely with the nature of the exposure but is highest in individuals with a deep wound and exposure to a large volume of blood from a patient with known HIV and a high viral load. Table 4.3 provides a summary of the risk of transmission of HIV and hepatitis B and C from sources of known infection. In order to avoid exposure, providers should be vigilant and always follow universal precautions. For students and clinicians working in high-risk settings (e.g., an HIV or needle-exchange clinic), consideration should be given to bringing post-exposure prophylaxis in case of exposure (Box 4.4).

Culture shock

It is common and natural for travelers to experience a period of "culture shock" as they adapt to life in a new cultural setting. The trajectory of culture shock is depicted in Figure 4.7. On arrival, individuals typically experience a honeymoon period where everything is new and exciting. This is often followed by a low period of frustration and rejection, which eventually transitions into a period of adaptation and acceptance. These ups and downs are then frequently experienced again on return home.

In addition to culture shock, trainees and providers working in clinical settings often have to cope with additional stresses associated with their exposure to levels of suffering and death that they may not have encountered at their home institutions. It is therefore important to monitor your mental health while abroad and to find ways of releasing stress that are healthy and culturally sensitive, such as exercising, spending time with others, or keeping a private journal. While it is normal to experience culture shock and to struggle emotionally with many of the realities of providing healthcare in resource-poor settings, you should reach out to others if you start to feel

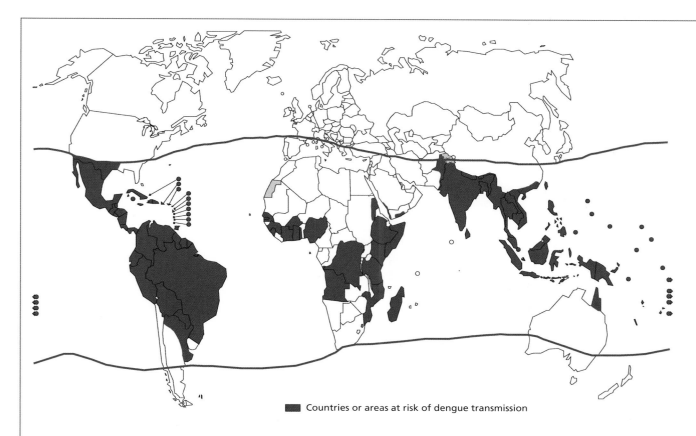

Figure 4.4 Global distribution of countries or areas at risk of dengue transmission, 2008. *Source*: World Health Organization (2010). Reproduced with permission of the World Health Organization.

overwhelmed. Friends, colleagues, and mentors can often provide needed support, as can counselors and other mental health professionals.

Ethical issues and medical practice in resource-limited settings

Understanding your limits and role

Medical professionals of all levels are often brimming with enthusiasm and excitement when they work abroad. They are eager to put their energy and skills to work to make a meaningful contribution to the medical needs of the host sites. Sometimes medical professionals mistake the lack of resources for a lack of knowledge or capability of the in-country staff, which can cause confusion and unintended insult. It is important to remember that, in many cases, you will be the one learning from those you are working beside. The in-country staff will have deep knowledge of how to practice in their setting with its particular resources, and it will be important to observe and

understand their medical culture in order to be most effective. Many professionals have offended their hosts unintentionally because they have quickly tried to teach methods and approaches from home without consideration of the local practices and the reasons behind them.

Medical trainees working in regions where well-trained healthcare professionals are scarce may find themselves in a position in which they are asked or feel expected to perform duties beyond their level of training and/or without adequate supervision. Although the need may be great, it is inappropriate for trainees to take on responsibilities for which they have not been adequately trained. Remember the maxim: First, do no harm. (Pinto & Upshur, 2009; Elit *et al.*, 2011).

Medical malpractice

Trainees and clinicians should check with their home institution regarding insurance and malpractice coverage abroad. In the event that coverage is not provided, individuals may decide to purchase a separate insurance plan for the trip or travel without insurance.

Table 4.2 Common prophylactic antimalarial medications for travelers.

Medication	Adult dosing	Advantages	Disadvantages
Atovaquone/ proguanil (Malarone)	1 tablet (250 mg/100 mg) p.o. once daily Start 1–2 days before travel Continue for 7 days after returning	Side effects uncommon Pediatric tablets available Need to start only 1–2 days before travel and continue only 1 week after travel	Usually more expensive than other antimalarials Cannot be used while pregnant or breastfeeding a child <5 kg Cannot be taken in severe renal impairment
Chloroquine	300 mg (base) p.o. once weekly Start 1–2 weeks before travel Continue for 4 weeks after travel	Can be used in pregnancy	Cannot be used in areas with chloroquine or mefloquine resistance May exacerbate psoriasis
Doxycycline	100 mg p.o. once daily Start 1–2 days before travel Continue for 4 weeks after travel	Usually least expensive antimalarial Need to start only 1–2 days before travel Can prevent other infections (e.g., rickettsiae and leptospirosis), so may be useful for individuals hiking, camping, or exposed to fresh water	Cannot be used while pregnant or in children <8 years Common potential side effects: sun sensitivity, nausea, pill-induced esophagitis, and increased risk in women of vaginal yeast infections
Mefloquine (Lariam)	250 mg p.o. once weekly Start at least 2 weeks prior to travel Continue for 4 weeks after travel	Can be used in pregnancy	Cannot be used in areas with mefloquine resistance Common potential side effects: vivid dreams, visual disturbances Cannot be used in patients with certain psychiatric conditions, seizure disorders, or cardiac conduction abnormalities

Source: Adapted from Centers for Disease Control (2011).

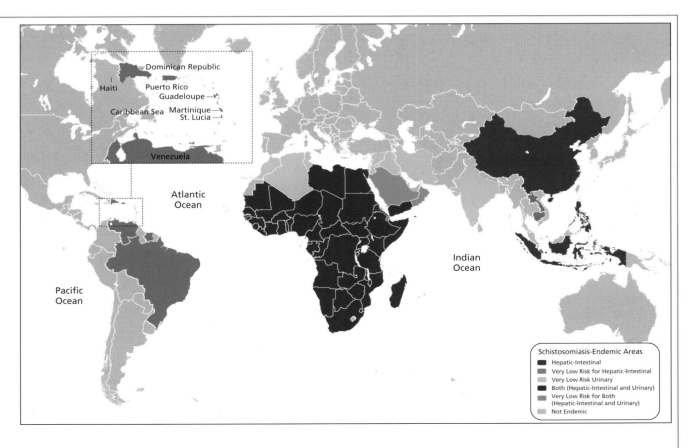

Figure 4.5 Geographic distribution of schistosomiasis. *Source*: CDC Public Health Image Library.

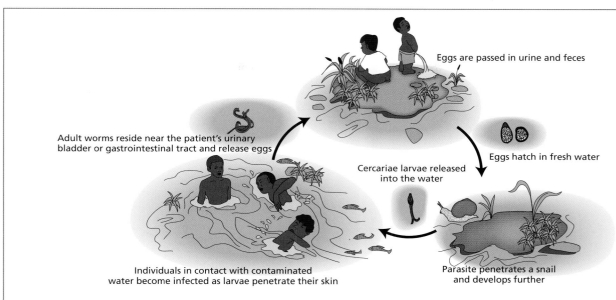

Eggs are passed in urine and feces

Eggs hatch in fresh water

Adult worms reside near the patient's urinary bladder or gastrointestinal tract and release eggs

Cercariae larvae released into the water

Parasite penetrates a snail and develops further

Individuals in contact with contaminated water become infected as larvae penetrate their skin

Figure 4.6 Schistosomiasis transmission cycle.

Table 4.3 Risk of transmission of blood-borne pathogens by exposure type.

	HIV	Hepatitis B	Hepatitis C
Percutaneous	0.2–0.5%	6–30%	0–7%
Mucosal	0.006–0.5%	Risk unknown, transmission documented	Risk unknown, transmission documented
Non-intact skin	<0.1%	Transmission has not been documented	Transmission has not been documented

Source: Data from Beltrami *et al*. (2000) and Weber *et al*. (2013).

Box 4.4 HIV post-exposure management

1. Cleanse exposed area with soap and water (or water only for mucous membranes or eyes)
2. Assess HIV status of source
3. Seek urgent medical evaluation
4. Consider initiation of post-exposure prophylaxis
5. HIV testing at baseline and repeat at 6 weeks, 3 months, and 6 months

Source: Centers for Disease Control (2014).

Writing and photography

Writing can be an excellent way to reflect on your experiences and to share them with family and friends. However, this is also an area where even the most thoughtful, well-intentioned providers frequently run into trouble. For those planning to share their writing, it is first and foremost essential to uphold the same principles of professionalism and patient confidentiality that are expected at your home institution. This means that no patient information should ever be shared in public settings, such as blogs or internet posts, or privately, such as in letters or emails. It is also important to keep in mind the risks to sharing information about colleagues or organizations (e.g., a local hospital, non-governmental organization, or government program) with whom you work as a poorly stated comment could jeopardize important relationships or your reputation.

With respect to photographs, adherence to the same high standards of patient privacy is essential. Taking photos of patients in the hospital is typically unacceptable. If there is a patient or family with whom you have become close, you should obtain permission for a photograph just as you would if you were on the wards back at home. In addition, some cultures may be sensitive about photographs in general (especially government buildings, police, military, airports, etc.). In general, it is a good idea to inquire about the acceptability of taking photographs from local colleagues. If unsure, always ask permission first.

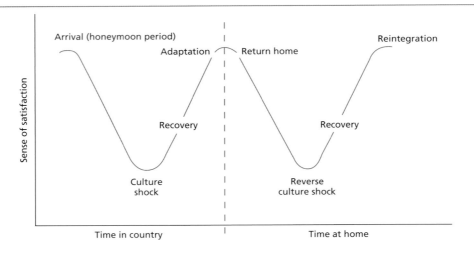

Figure 4.7 The "W" model of culture shock.

Clinical experience

"Early in my fourth year of medical school, I was involved with a research project about neonatal resuscitation in Haiti. My role was to observe nurses providing newborn care in the delivery room to understand what resuscitation techniques were being implemented. Although I was familiar with the resuscitation algorithm, I had personally never resuscitated a newborn before. One evening, a woman in her 26th week of pregnancy arrived to the hospital in labor. As soon as the baby was delivered, the nurse asked me to determine whether the baby was alive while she tended to the mother. I was unable to detect a heartbeat, nor had the nurse been able to shortly before the baby was delivered. As I stood there holding the baby, I realized that the nurse was focused on the mother and not planning to try to resuscitate the child. I wasn't sure what to do. While it seemed that the child was stillborn, I was not confident in making such a call myself and believed that resuscitation should be attempted in case

the child's life could be saved. However, I was supposed to be an observer, not a provider of clinical care, and I also did not feel confident that I could perform the steps in the algorithm well. With only a split second to decide, I ended up trying to resuscitate the child myself. I did the best that I could, but I was never able to detect a heartbeat. Reflecting on the experience, many questions linger. How had my presence affected how the nurse responded to the situation? Would she have done more for the child if I hadn't been there? Or did she think I was naive to even attempt to resuscitate a very premature newborn in this setting? If my resuscitation technique had been less clumsy, would the baby have had a chance of living? Although I may always have some questions, it has been incredibly helpful to debrief with mentors and colleagues about this experience."

Ariel, medical student working in Haiti

Conclusion

When approached thoughtfully and safely, an international experience can be incredibly transformative. It can change the life of the visiting clinician as well as the lives of those served. To make the most of your experience, plan ahead for your trip, ask for guidance and support along the way, be cautious while traveling and working abroad, and approach your experience with a sense of humility and gratitude.

Additional resources

- US State Department information on international travel. Available at http://travel.state.gov/travel/travel_1744.html
- Centers for Disease Control and Prevention (CDC). Country-specific travel information. Available at http://wwwn.cdc.gov/travel/destinationList.aspx
- Centers for Disease Control and Prevention (2014) *The Yellow Book: CDC Health Information for International Travel*

2014. New York: Oxford University Press. Available at http://wwwnc.cdc.gov/travel/page/yellowbook-home-2014
• Centers for Disease Control and Prevention (2005) Updated US Public Health Service guidelines for the management of occupational exposures to HIV and recommendations for postexposure prophylaxis. *MMWR Recomm Rep* 54, No. RR-9. Available at http://www.cdc.gov/mmwr/pdf/rr/rr5409.pdf

• World Health Organization section on international health and travel. Available at http://www.who.int/ith/en/
• Demographic and Health Surveys. Available at http://www.measuredhs.com
• Crump JA, Sugarman J (2010) Ethics and best practice guidelines for training experiences in global health. *Am J Trop Med Hyg* 83:1178–82.

REFERENCES

Beltrami EM, Williams IT, Shapiro CN, Chamberland ME (2000) Risk and management of blood-borne infections in health care workers. *Clin Microbiol Rev* 13:385–407.

Centers for Disease Control (2011) Choosing a drug to prevent malaria. Available at http://www.cdc.gov/malaria/travelers/drugs.html

Centers for Disease Control (2013) Latent tuberculosis infection: a guide for primary health care providers. Available at http://www.cdc.gov/TB/publications/LTBI/pdf/TargetedLTBI.pdf

Centers for Disease Control (2014) *The Yellow Book: CDC Health Information for International Travel 2014.* New York: Oxford University Press. Available at http://wwwnc.cdc.gov/travel/page/yellowbook-home-2014

Elit L, Hunt M, Redwood-Campbell L, Ranford J, Adelson N, Schwartz L (2011) Ethical issues encountered by medical students during international health electives. *Med Educ* 45:704–11.

Pinto AD, Upshur RE (2009) Global health ethics for students. *Dev World Bioeth* 9:1–10.

Pruss-Ustun A, Rapiti E, Hutin Y (2005) Estimation of the global burden of disease attributable to contaminated sharps injuries among health-care workers. *Am J Ind Med* 48:482–90.

Weber DJ, Rutala WA, Eron J (2013) Management of healthcare workers exposed to hepatitis B virus or hepatitis C virus. Available at http://www.uptodate.com/contents/management-of-healthcare-workers-exposed-to-hepatitis-b-virus-or-hepatitis-c-virus

World Health Organization (2005) WHO/Roll Back Malaria and UNICEF. World Malaria Report 2005. Available at http://rbm.who.int/wmr2005

World Health Organization (2010) Working to overcome the global impact of neglected tropical diseases: first WHO report on neglected tropical diseases, 2010. Map available via Global Health Observatory Map Gallery at http://gamapserver.who.int/mapLibrary/Files/Maps/Global_dengue_2008.png

Part 2
Newborn and
Child Health

CHAPTER 5
Overview of Child Health

Suzinne Pak-Gorstein[1] and Melanie Anspacher[2]
[1]University of Washington, Harborview Medical Center, and Seattle Children's Hospital, Seattle, Washington, USA
[2]Children's National Medical Center and George Washington University, Washington, DC, USA

Key learning objectives

- Describe the epidemiology of under-five mortality and compare developed to least-developed countries.
- Outline the underlying socioeconomic and geopolitical determinants of child health.
- Identify evidence-based, cost-effective interventions to decrease under-five mortality at different levels of care within a healthcare system.
- Describe the WHO Integrated Management of Childhood Illnesses (IMCI) guidelines and how they are implemented in developing countries.

Abstract

Each year, nearly 7 million children under 5 years old die worldwide, and most of these deaths are considered preventable. Beyond the neonatal period, during which approximately 40% of under-five deaths occur, diarrhea and pneumonia are the most commonly implicated diseases, and malnutrition contributes to a significant proportion of deaths. Disparities in child health persist both between and within countries and are associated with socioeconomic factors such as poverty, food insecurity, and lack of maternal education. Improvements in child health can be accomplished through implementation of essential evidence-based interventions such as immunizations, micronutrient supplementation, breastfeeding, and use of antibiotics. However, many children in low- and middle-income countries still do not receive these life-saving interventions. Strategies that integrate preventive and curative solutions have been developed to improve child health, starting at the community level up through the healthcare facility.

Key words: child health, child mortality, under-five mortality, newborn mortality, immunizations, vaccine-preventable diseases, health inequities, essential interventions, infections, social determinants of health

Essential Clinical Global Health, First Edition. Edited by Brett D. Nelson.
© 2015 John Wiley & Sons, Ltd. Published 2015 by John Wiley & Sons, Ltd.
Companion website: www.essentialseries.com/globalhealth

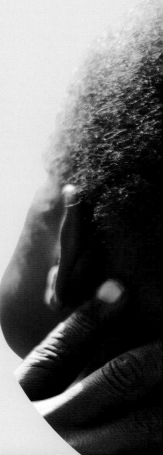

Introduction and epidemiology

In 2011, an estimated 7 million children under 5 years old died worldwide – far too many, but a dramatic improvement from an estimated 12 million in 1990 (UNICEF, 2012a). However, progress in reducing child mortality has not occurred evenly around the world (Figure 5.1). Most of the countries with high under-five mortality are in sub-Saharan Africa, where a child is 20 times more likely to die before his or her fifth birthday than in a developed country. Also concerning is that much of the progress in child health has been limited to improving survival outside the newborn period and, as a result, deaths within the first month of life account for a growing proportion of under-five mortality.

The vast majority of childhood deaths are caused by infections that are preventable, the most common of which are diarrhea and pneumonia (Figure 5.2). In contrast, in developed countries child deaths from infections are less common, and injuries and congenital malformations account for higher proportions of under-five deaths. In Africa, malaria and AIDS account for almost 20% of all under-five deaths (Liu et al., 2012). Undernutrition has been implicated in up to half of under-five deaths, due to the impact of inadequate caloric intake and micronutrient deficiencies on the immune system, and the toll recurrent illnesses take on the child's ability to take in and absorb adequate calories and nutrients.

Child health should not be assessed based on mortality rates alone. Children surviving illness are often left with disability, burdening their families and decreasing future economic productivity. Neonatal disorders, recurrent infections, nutritional deficiencies, and neglected tropical diseases are leading causes of disability in children younger than 5 years old, while injuries, musculoskeletal disorders, chronic respiratory disease, and mental health problems contribute more in older children (Vos et al., 2012).

Socioeconomic determinants of child health in developing countries: roots of health inequities

> This unequal distribution of health-damaging experiences is not in any sense a "natural" phenomenon but is the result of a toxic combination of poor social policies and programmes, unfair economic arrangements, and bad politics.
> *Closing the Gap Report* (WHO, 2008)

While life expectancy and overall health are gradually improving for many people around the world, there remain populations for whom this progress is not occurring equitably. Such disparities in health are reflected not only by differences in child mortality rates between countries, but also by differences between different populations within the same country. In Bolivia, for example, the infant mortality rate is greater than 100 per 1000 live births among children born to mothers with no education, while it is 40 per 1000 among children born to mothers with at least secondary education (WHO, 2008). Similarly, the child mortality rate in Nigeria is 87 per 1000 births for children in the highest wealth quintile, while it is 219 per 1000 for children living in the lowest quintile (UN Inter-Agency Group for Child Mortality Estimation, 2011). The socioeconomic factors that underlie health disparities are significant and reflect a family's risk for disease and malnutrition as well as access to a safe living environment and quality health services.

In response to increasing concern about these persisting and widening inequities, the World Health Organization (WHO) established the Commission on Social Determinants of Health (CSDH). The Commission's final report, launched in 2008, called for increasing the investment in training of health practitioners, policy-makers, and the public about the social determinants of health. The report made the appeal for countries to strengthen governmental social protection policies with emphasis on early child development, education, and empowerment of girls and women.

> Education and training on the social determinants of health for relevant professionals is vital (*Closing the Gap Report*, WHO, 2008).

Greater recognition that the underlying causes of childhood diseases have socioeconomic roots has led to an emphasis on training clinicians about the "upstream" determinants of health and community-based interventions, rather than focusing solely on hospital-based treatments. Physicians working in resource-constrained settings may look at approaches to address the underlying causes of poor health when faced with questions: Why does a 5-year-old girl return to the hospital with pneumonia just months after being discharged for dehydration from diarrhea? What are the factors in her home and community that place her at increased risk of dying from these common childhood infections?

The immediate, underlying, and basic structural causes of disease, malnutrition, and disability are outlined in Figure 5.3. Despite advances in preventive and curative interventions aimed at the more immediate causes of poor health, unless the

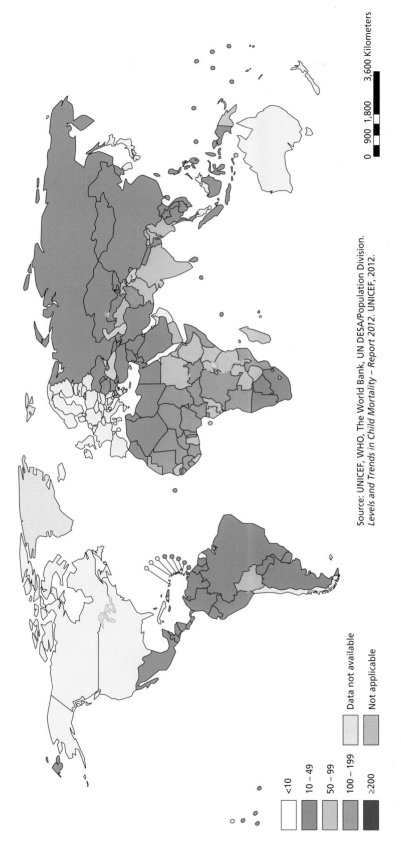

Figure 5.1 Under-five mortality rate (deaths per 1000 live births), 2011. *Source:* WHO (2012). Reproduced with permission of the World Health Organization.

Source: UNICEF, WHO, The World Bank, UN DESA/Population Division. *Levels and Trends in Child Mortality – Report 2012.* UNICEF, 2012.

<10
10 – 49
50 – 99
100 – 199
≥200

Data not available

Not applicable

0   900 1,800   3,600 Kilometers

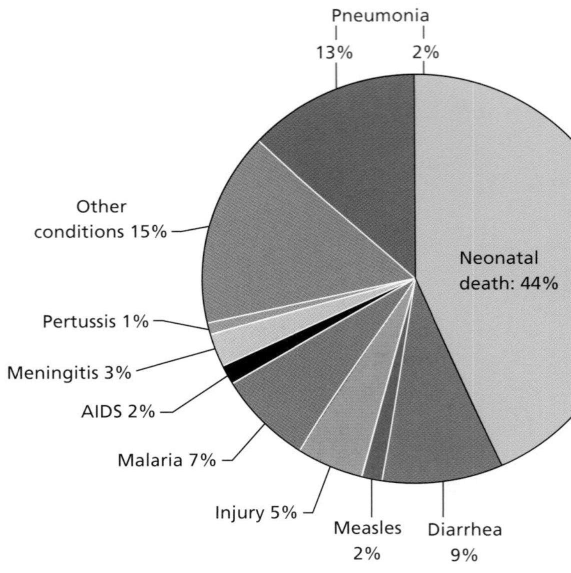

Figure 5.2 Causes of under-five and neonatal mortality worldwide in 2012. *Sources*: CHERG and WHO, Global Health Observatory http://www.who.int/gho/child_health/mortality/causes/en/ and Lawn *et al*. 2012. Reproduced with permission.

basic and underlying determinants of health are addressed, inequities in mortality and morbidity rates will persist.

Essential interventions

Estimates suggest that most of the 7 million annual deaths in children younger than five could be averted by increasing coverage of proven low-cost interventions (Table 5.1) (UN Inter-agency Group for Child Mortality Estimation, 2011). Childhood deaths from diarrheal illness and pneumonia can be prevented by simple measures such as vaccinations and exclusive breastfeeding until 6 months of age. Deaths related to undernutrition, which predisposes children to infectious diseases, may be prevented by proper infant and young child feeding practices, micronutrient supplementation, and community-based screening and management of malnutrition.

Vaccine-preventable diseases

An estimated 1.5 million under-five deaths each year are due to vaccine-preventable diseases (WHO, 2014). Top contributors are pneumococcus and rotavirus, followed by *Haemophilus influenzae* type B (Hib), measles, pertussis, and tetanus. The WHO Expanded Program on Immunization (EPI) has resulted in a dramatic reduction in deaths, illness, and disability from

many of these diseases, as well as the near elimination of poliomyelitis. Recommendations for routine immunizations have continued to grow with the development of new vaccines that have demonstrated significant life-saving potential in industrialized countries (Table 5.2 and Box 5.1).

Vaccines are highly effective in improving child survival. However, rates of coverage are very low in many developing countries, and some life-saving vaccines are not available in many countries. In some cases, it takes years for immunizations introduced in developed countries to be made affordable and available to developing countries and to be incorporated into the national vaccine policy and infrastructure. In other cases, the vaccine is available but does not reach the child. In 2013, it was estimated that 21.8 million children did not receive all three recommended doses of DTP, and 16% of children did not receive a measles vaccine by their second birthday (WHO, 2014).

Reaching every child

Immunizations are not the only interventions that have failed to attain universal coverage. Oral rehydration therapy has been the evidence-based intervention of choice for dehydration from diarrheal illness since the 1970s (see Chapter 9). However, four decades later, fewer than half of children under five with diarrheal illness receive this treatment (UNICEF, 2012b). What impacts whether one child will receive a life-saving intervention while another will not? Characteristics of the healthcare system, social context, and political climate impact whether universal coverage can be reached for evidence-based essential interventions such as those in Table 5.1. Figure 5.5 shows the relationship and interplay of factors impacting coverage of an intervention that should be considered when it is discovered that children are not receiving the most basic, cost-efficient, and well-studied life-saving interventions.

Effective delivery strategies: integrated management of childhood illness

Weak health systems impede the ability of countries to deliver cost-effective interventions and life-saving health messages for children. Such systems are characterized by insufficient numbers of health workers, low-quality training and supervision, and poorly functioning supply chains. While efforts to support child health often focus on improving health service delivery at a single level such as the health facility, effective and lasting improvements can only be achieved with the integration of delivery at all levels, such as adequate referrals and follow-up between community, clinic, and health facility. Other important life-saving strategies include outreach services (e.g., mass immunization and Vitamin A campaigns) and community-based health promotion activities (Figure 5.6).

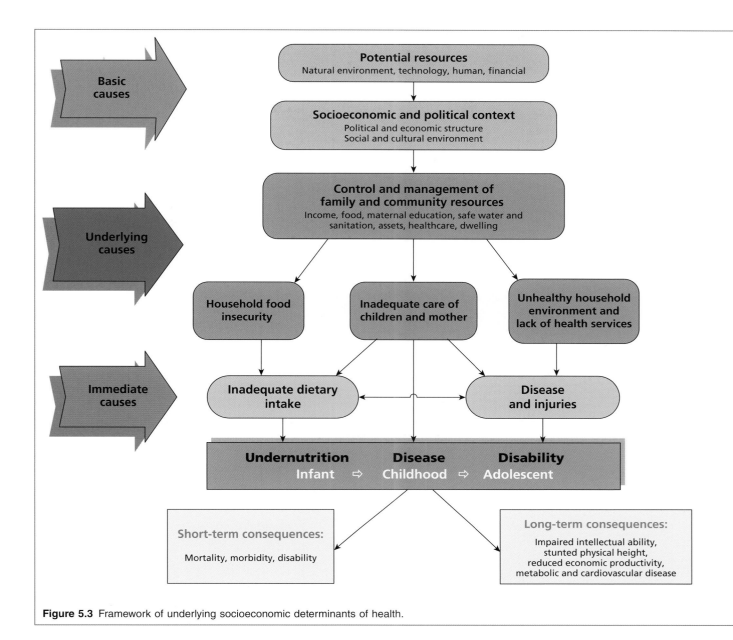

Figure 5.3 Framework of underlying socioeconomic determinants of health.

Community-based interventions are effective in extending healthcare delivery, are low cost, improve healthcare-seeking behavior, and can reduce infant and child mortality and morbidity (Lehmann & Sanders, 2007; Lewin *et al.*, 2010; McCord *et al.*, 2012). Community health workers (CHWs) are members of a community without formal medical training chosen to provide basic health and medical care to their community. CHWs may screen and manage mild to moderate cases of undernutrition, diarrheal disease and pneumonia, and refer serious cases in a timely manner to healthcare facilities. They may promote proper infant and young child feeding, as well as hand-hygiene practices to prevent disease.

The lack of integration of vertical programs that deliver individual interventions results in missed opportunities. Children may receive immunizations from one health worker at one encounter, but go somewhere else to obtain oral rehydration solution for diarrheal illness and yet elsewhere for treatment of malnutrition. Past programs focused on a single disease and set of interventions, while most children present with overlapping signs and symptoms to first-level health facilities with limited diagnostic tools such as laboratories or radiography.

Table 5.1 Essential interventions to improve child survival.

General preventive interventions

- Early and exclusive breastfeeding through 6 months of age
- Continued breastfeeding and complementary feeding from 6 months of age
- Vitamin A supplementation from 6 to 59 months
- Water, sanitation, and hygiene

Disease-specific interventions

Disease or condition	Prevention	Treatment
Birth asphyxia	Maternal intrapartum care and monitoring Skilled delivery	Newborn resuscitation
Newborn infections	Maternal tetanus vaccination Antibiotics for premature rupture of membranes Clean delivery Clean cord care	Antibiotics Case management of sepsis, meningitis, and pneumonia
Complications related to prematurity	Antenatal steroids Intermittent preventive treatment for malaria	Thermal care (kangaroo mother care) Feeding support for small and preterm newborns Surfactant administration Continuous positive airway pressure (CPAP) Treatment of jaundice
Diarrhea/dehydration	Rotavirus vaccination	Oral rehydration solution Zinc supplementation Continued feeding
HIV	Prevention of mother-to-child transmission	Highly active antiretroviral therapy (HAART)
Malaria	Insecticide-treated bednets	Antimalarials
Measles	Measles vaccination	Vitamin A supplementation
Meningitis	Meningococcal/Hib/pneumococcal vaccination	Antibiotics Case management
Pneumonia	Hib/pneumococcal vaccination	Antibiotics Case management
Tetanus	Tetanus vaccination Clean delivery	

Hib, *Haemophilus influenzae* B.
Source: Jones *et al.* (2003) and Partnership for Maternal, Newborn and Child Health (2011).

Box 5.1 Child health cards

Children in most countries will have an immunization or child health card (Figure 5.4), such as the WHO's "Road to Health" card that their guardian carries with them. This is the best way to check a child's immunization history.

These cards may also serve as a portable medical record, charting growth, medical visits, and treatment of HIV in some locations.

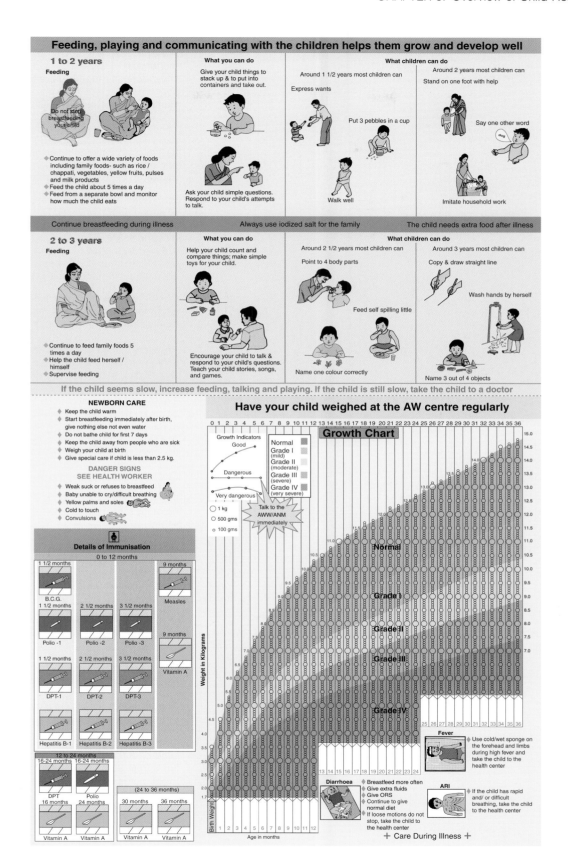

Figure 5.4 An example of a child health card. Adapted from a card produced by the Ministry of Health and Child Welfare (Zimbabwe).

Table 5.2 Routine immunizations recommended by the World Health Organization as of 2014.

Vaccine	Birth	6 weeks	10 weeks	14 weeks	9–12 months	Booster	Considerations
BCG (Bacillus Calmette–Guérin)	✓						Prevents severe tuberculosis (TB) and TB meningitis Only recommended in TB-endemic countries Contraindicated in HIV-positive children
DTP (diphtheria, tetanus, and pertussis)		✓	✓	✓		Yes	Whole cell pertussis vaccine still used in many countries "DTP3" (receiving all three doses in the primary series) is a commonly used marker of vaccination coverage
Hepatitis B	✓	✓	✓	✓			Birth dose recommended for prevention of perinatal transmission Premature newborns <2 kg may not respond well Three doses needed for immunity, but can receive four if necessary when combined with other routine vaccinations
OPV (oral polio vaccine)		✓	✓	✓			OPV is used in many developing countries due to low cost, ease of administration, and resulting herd immunity An additional birth dose is recommended only in highest-risk countries As of 2014, the WHO recommends that *all* children get at least one dose of inactivated polio vaccine (IPV), which can be given at earliest 14 weeks when maternal antibodies wane. A different schedule exists for IPV (inactivated polio vaccine), which creates less herd immunity and is only recommended in low-risk countries
Hib (*Haemophilus influenzae* B)		✓	✓	✓			Important cause of pneumonia and meningitis especially among children <2 years
Measles					*Option 1* 9 months *Option 2* 12 months	*Option 1* 15–18 months *Option 2* 15 months to 4 years	All children should get two doses of measles vaccine High-transmission/high-mortality countries should start at 9 months to decrease mortality
Pneumococcus (PCV10 or 13)		✓	✓*	✓		* Yes, if not given at 10 weeks	Important cause of pneumonia, sepsis, and meningitis
Rotavirus		✓	✓	✓			Need for third dose depends on vaccine brand Rotavirus kills >400,000 children annually In 2011, only implemented in 31 countries
Rubella					9–12 months with measles vaccine		Goal is to prevent congenital rubella syndrome (CRS) More than 80% coverage is needed to avoid increasing risk for CRS by continued presence of unimmunized pregnant women who were not exposed as children

6-, 10-, and 14-week schedule based on WHO recommendation to start at 6 weeks for many routine immunizations, with minimum 4 weeks between subsequent doses.

Source: adapted from WHO recommendations for routine immunization: summary tables. Available at http://www.who.int/immunization/policy/immunization_tables/en/

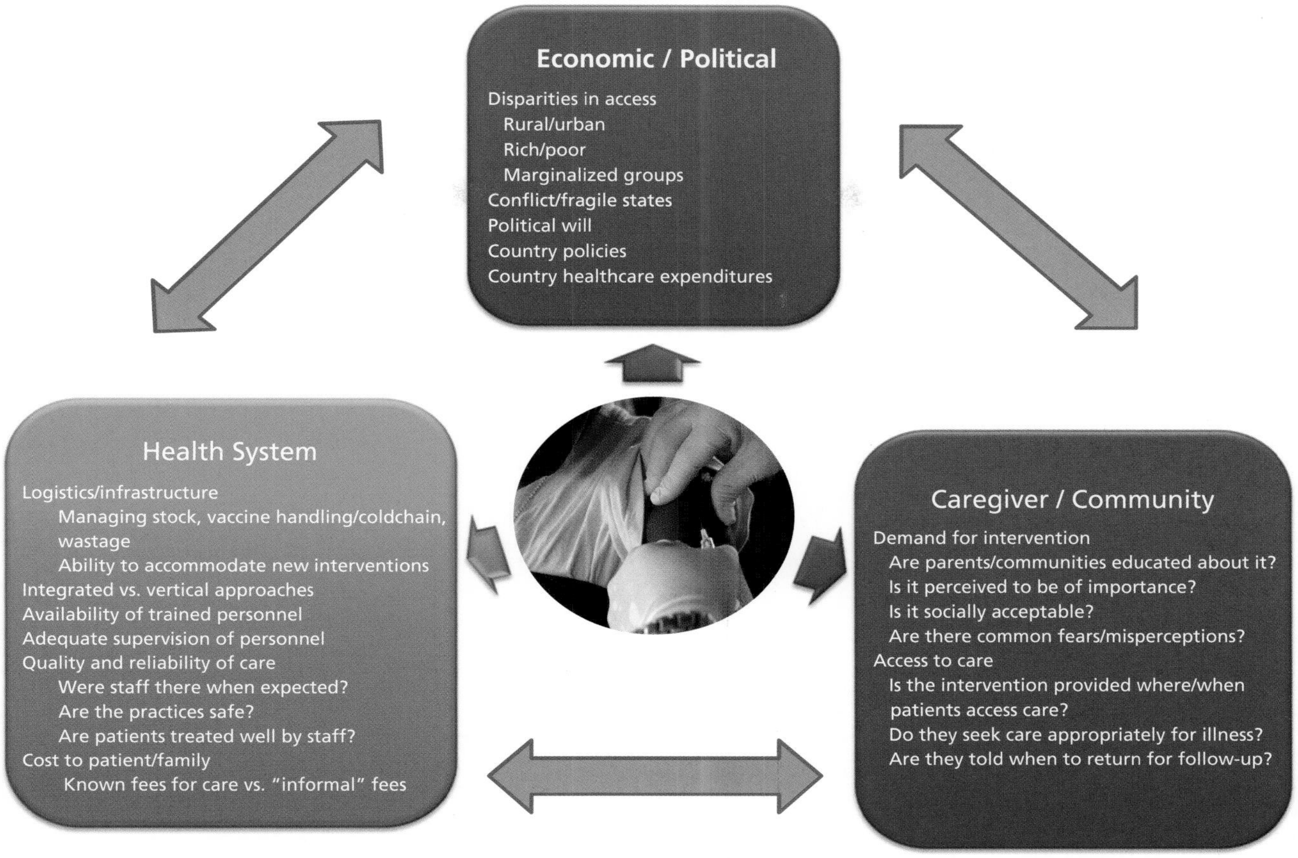

Economic / Political

Disparities in access
  Rural/urban
  Rich/poor
  Marginalized groups
Conflict/fragile states
Political will
Country policies
Country healthcare expenditures

Health System

Logistics/infrastructure
  Managing stock, vaccine handling/coldchain,
  wastage
  Ability to accommodate new interventions
Integrated vs. vertical approaches
Availability of trained personnel
Adequate supervision of personnel
Quality and reliability of care
  Were staff there when expected?
  Are the practices safe?
  Are patients treated well by staff?
Cost to patient/family
  Known fees for care vs. "informal" fees

Caregiver / Community

Demand for intervention
  Are parents/communities educated about it?
  Is it perceived to be of importance?
  Is it socially acceptable?
  Are there common fears/misperceptions?
Access to care
  Is the intervention provided where/when
  patients access care?
  Do they seek care appropriately for illness?
  Are they told when to return for follow-up?

Figure 5.5 Factors influencing coverage of interventions.

The Integrated Management of Childhood Illnesses (IMCI) is an approach to reduce child death, illness, and disability and to promote improved growth and development. IMCI includes both preventive and curative elements with guidelines that are implemented by families and communities as well as by providers at health facilities. One key component of IMCI is to train CHWs to identify signs of common childhood illness and to decide when a child needs referral to a health facility. IMCI trains CHWs to instruct parents on home management of ill children including oral rehydration solution and zinc for diarrhea, antimalarial medicine for febrile children who test positive for malaria, and antibiotics for children with signs of pneumonia. CHWs can schedule follow-up visits for ill children. They also promote use of bednets, hand-washing, and proper infant and young child feeding.

While IMCI guidelines are useful tools proven to reduce under-five mortality (Figure 5.7), the resources for CHW training and supervision, supply of medications, and referral are often limited or completely absent (Goga & Muhe, 2011). More efforts are needed to integrate delivery of services between all levels of care while empowering communities to identify and manage childhood illnesses properly (Box 5.2).

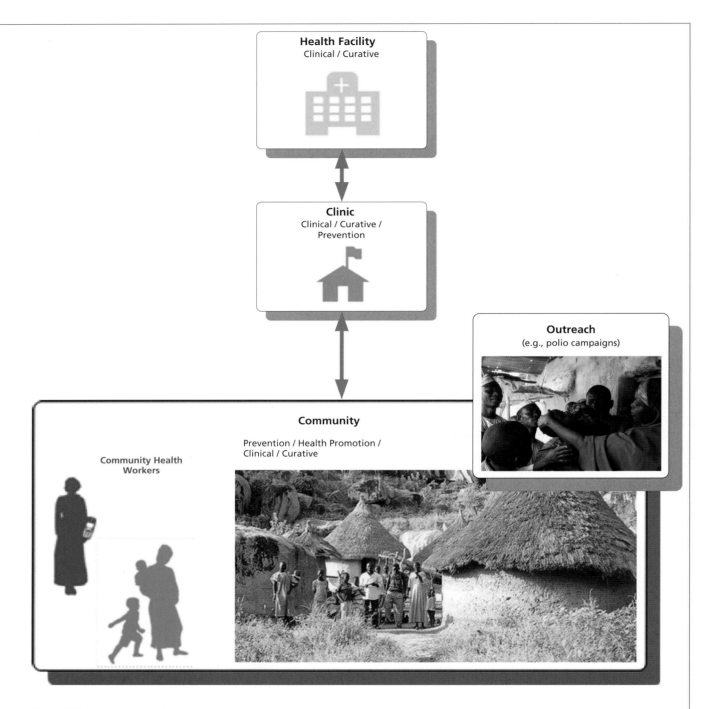

Figure 5.6 Health services delivery systems.

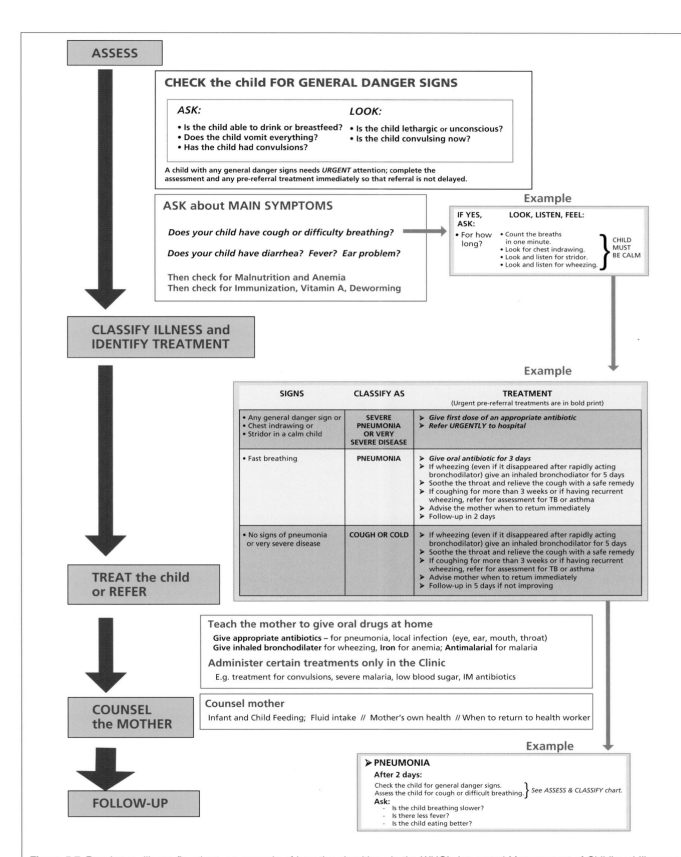

Figure 5.7 Respiratory illness flowchart: an example of how the algorithms in the WHO's Integrated Management of Childhood Illnesses can be applied.

Box 5.2 Case study: the interrelationship between disease, nutrition, and socioeconomic context

You are working with local healthcare staff at a hospital serving an impoverished district. You admit a 3-year-old girl for pneumonia and severe acute malnutrition. Despite a high case fatality rate for such children in the hospital, this child improves and is able to be discharged home. You note statistics that show a high mortality rate for children after being discharged, and you reflect on your training that emphasizes the importance of proper discharge instructions. You also want to ensure that you have comprehensively addressed all medical issues before discharge since you know that she will not receive any primary care follow-up. You consider the following questions.

Identification of other infections and disease prevention
- Has this child been screened for HIV? What is HIV prevalence in the area where you are working?
- Has this child's immunization status been checked and updated?

Prevention of malnutrition and other illnesses
- Has the mother received any nutritional counseling?
- Has the child received routine Vitamin A supplementation?
- Is she anemic? Has she received antihelminthic treatment?
- How will this child's undernourished state impact her risk of infection when she returns to the community?

Follow-up plan
- What is the follow-up plan for this child, who is responsible for implementing this plan, what are the challenges, and how will follow-up be monitored?

Socioeconomic determinants of health and disease
- What is the socioeconomic context to which this child will return, and how does that place her at risk for mortality upon her return as she continues her convalescence at home?
- What have been the direct and indirect costs of this hospitalization on the family? What are the mechanisms and resources for the family to recover from the financial impact of this hospital admission?

Home visit
You accompany a CHW to visit the child in her community after discharge. It is a 20-minute drive and 30-minute walk into the rural community. On arrival at the home, you observe that the side of the house serves as an open latrine. You observe that the mother is working much of the day harvesting a corn crop, with little supervision of the girl and her two siblings at home.

- What are the factors in her community and in her social situation that might influence how the mother accesses care when one of her children is sick?
- How could this child's condition have been initially addressed in the community to prevent her from becoming so severely ill that it warranted her being admitted?
- What are the risk factors for this girl's other young siblings to also fall ill?
- What role might a traditional healer play in providing ongoing care for infants and children in the community? What are the potential benefits and risks of this role?
- What is the role that CHWs can play in providing appropriate nutrition and disease counseling to parents, as well as in identifying and treating illnesses within the community? How might CHWs be supported in the community to carry out this role?
- What other social services and community resources are available to strengthen the families' ability to keep their children healthy? Are there micro-loan programs, kitchen gardening activities, etc.?

Additional resources

- UNICEF. Monitoring the situation of children and women. Available at www.childinfo.org
- UNICEF. State of the World's Children annual report. Available at http://www.unicef.org/sowc/
- Countdown to 2015. Maternal, newborn, and child survival. Available at http://www.countdown2015mnch.org/
- World Health Organization. Child health. Available at http://www.who.int/topics/child_health/en/
- World Health Organization. Integrated Management of Childhood Illness. Available at http://www.who.int/maternal_child_adolescent/documents/imci_community_care/en/index.html
- World Health Organization. *Pocket Book of Hospital Care for Children*, 2nd edn, 2013. Available at http://www.who.int/maternal_child_adolescent/documents/9241546700/en/index.html
- World Health Organization. Recommendations for routine immunizations. Available at http://www.who.int/immunization/policy/immunization_tables/en/

- World Health Organization. National immunization schedules. Available at http://www.who.int/immunization_monitoring/data/data_subject/en/
- World Health Organization. Essential interventions, commodities, and guidelines for reproductive, maternal, newborn and child health. Available at http://www.who.int/pmnch/topics/part_publications/essential_interventions_18_01_2012.pdf?ua=1

REFERENCES

Goga A, Muhe LM (2011) Global challenges with scale-up of the integrated management of childhood illness strategy: results of a multi-country survey. *BMC Public Health* 1:503.

Jones G, Steketee RW, Black RE, Bhutta ZA, Morris SS (2003) How many child deaths can we prevent this year? *Lancet* 362:65–71.

Lawn JE, Kinney MV, Black RE et al. (2012) Newborn survival: a multi-country analysis of a decade of change. *Health Policy Plan* 27(Suppl. 3):iii6–28.

Lehmann U, Sanders D (2007) Community health workers: what do we know about them? The state of the evidence on programmes, activities, costs and impacts on health outcomes of using community health workers. Evidence and information for policy. Available at http://www.who.int/hrh/documents/community_health_workers.pdf

Lewin S, Munabi-Babigumira S, Glenton C et al. (2010) Lay health workers in primary and community health care for maternal and child health and the management of infectious diseases. *Cochrane Database Syst Rev* (3):CD004015.

Liu L, Johnson HL, Cousens S et al. (2012) Global, regional, and national causes of child mortality: an updated systematic analysis for 2010 with time trends since 2000. *Lancet* 379:2151–61.

McCord G, Liu A, Singh P (2012) Deployment of community health workers across rural sub-Saharan Africa: financial considerations and operational assumptions. *Bull WHO* 91:244–53.

Partnership for Maternal, Newborn and Child Health (2011) Essential interventions, commodities, and guidelines for reproductive, maternal, newborn, and child health. Geneva: PMNCH. Available at http://www.who.int/pmnch/topics/part_publications/essential_interventions_18_01_2012.pdf?ua=1

UN Inter-agency Group for Child Mortality Estimation (2011) Levels and trends in child mortality, 2011. Available at http://www.unicef.org/media/files/Child_Mortality_Report_2011_Final.pdf

UNICEF (2012a) Committing to child survival: a promise renewed. Available at http://www.apromiserenewed.org/

UNICEF (2012b) UNICEF global databases 2012, based on multiple indicator cluster surveys, demographic and health surveys and other national surveys. Available at http://www.childinfo.org/diarrhoea_progress.html

Vos T, Flaxman AD, Naghavi M et al. (2012) Years lived with disability (YLDs) for 1160 sequelae of 289 diseases and injuries 1990–2010: a systematic analysis for the Global Burden of Disease Study 2010. *Lancet* 380:2163–96.

WHO (2008) Closing the Gap in a Generation: Health Equity Through Action on the Social Determinants of Health. Final Report of the Commission on Social Determinants of Health. Geneva: World Health Organization. Available at http://whqlibdoc.who.int/publications/2008/9789241563703_eng.pdf

WHO (2014) Global immunization data, July 2014. Available at http://www.who.int/immunization_monitoring/Global_Immunization_Data.pdf

CHAPTER 6
Newborn Care

Joy E. Lawn[1,2], Helen Brotherton[3], and Anne C.C. Lee[4]

[1]MARCH, London School of Hygiene Tropical Medicine, London, UK
[2]Saving Newborn Lives/Save the Children, Cape Town, South Africa
[3]Royal Hospital for Sick Children, Edinburgh, UK
[4]Brigham and Women's Hospital and Harvard Medical School, Boston, MA, USA

Key learning objectives

- Understand the major causes of neonatal mortality globally and efforts for improving newborn survival.
- Describe the basic principles of essential newborn care.
- Understand special care for preterm and sick newborns when neonatal intensive care is not available.
- Consider some of the ways that newborn health could become a higher priority and how to help accelerate progress.

Abstract

Forty-four percent of under-five deaths occur during the neonatal period, with mortality predominantly due to prematurity, infections, and intrapartum hypoxia ("birth asphyxia"). There are simple solutions that can immediately reduce deaths, even among preterm newborns in the lowest-income settings, such as early and exclusive breastfeeding, chlorhexidine application to the umbilical cord, kangaroo mother care, and treatment of infections. However, higher-impact facility-based care is also needed and is dependent on nurses and others with skills in caring for small and sick newborns. Starting with intensive care will fail if simple hygiene, careful attention to feeding, and other basic building blocks are not first in place. Although few resource-limited countries can rapidly scale up neonatal intensive care in a short time, no country can afford to neglect the provision of simple care measures for every newborn, especially those who are preterm, while developing increased health systems capacity. Importantly, 71% of neonatal deaths can be prevented without full neonatal intensive care.

Key words: newborn, neonatal, preterm birth, neonatal sepsis, neonatal jaundice, kangaroo mother care, essential newborn care, breastfeeding, low-resource settings

Essential Clinical Global Health, First Edition. Edited by Brett D. Nelson.
© 2015 John Wiley & Sons, Ltd. Published 2015 by John Wiley & Sons, Ltd.
Companion website: www.essentialseries.com/globalhealth

Introduction and epidemiology

Each year, 2.9 million newborns die in the neonatal period (first 28 days of life). Newborn health is increasingly important for child survival since 44% of global under-five deaths occur in the critical first month of life. The average annual rate of change of neonatal mortality rate (NMR) has accelerated since 2000 compared with the 1990s, associated with the increased focus on Millennium Development Goal 4 to reduce child mortality by two-thirds between 1990 and 2015. However, annual progress in neonatal mortality reduction (2.0%) is still slower than for 1–59 month child deaths (3.4%) and maternal deaths (2.6%) (Lawn *et al.*, 2014). In addition, since 2000 the poorest regions of the world are being left further behind, with high-income countries reducing NMR at an annual rate of 3.0%, while in Africa the reduction is only 1.5% per year (Box 6.1).

The main causes of newborn deaths are complications of preterm birth, intrapartum- or childbirth-related complications (including birth asphyxia, discussed in Chapter 7), and neonatal infections (Figure 6.1). Worldwide, more than 1 million newborns die each year directly because they were born preterm (<37 weeks), and around three-quarters of all newborn deaths are among those who are preterm, small for gestational age, or both (Blencowe *et al.*, 2012; Lee *et al.*, 2013).

All the approximately 135 million newborns born worldwide each year are vulnerable given that birth and the following few days hold the highest concentrated risk of death of any time in the human lifespan (Figure 6.2). Birth and the early neonatal period are also a time of high risk for neurodevelopmental injury that can result in long-term impairment. Hence, this period is one of the most critical and cost-effective for intervention. It represents an opportunity for major reductions in child mortality in many low-income countries. With recent increased coverage in facility-based births, there are even greater opportunities to reach women and their newborns with better care. However, it is also critical to remember the 50 million home births each year, which often occur among the poorest families. Community-based care and approaches, such as women's groups, have been shown to save lives and also to increase facility-based births and access to care.

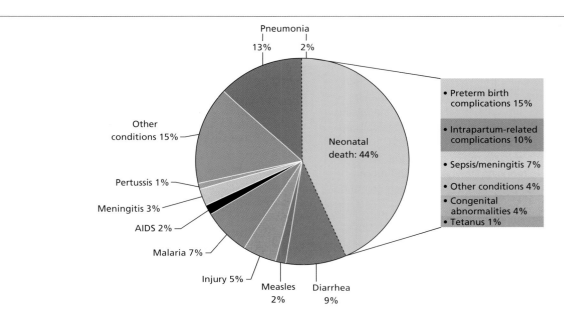

Figure 6.1 Causes of under-five and neonatal mortality worldwide in 2012. *Source*: CHERG and WHO, Global Health Observatory http://www.who.int/gho/child_health/mortality/causes/en/ and Lawn *et al*. 2012. Reproduced with permission.

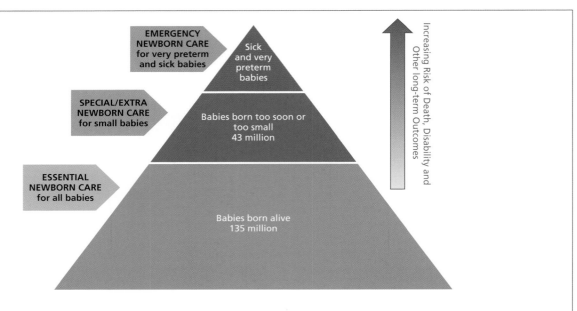

Figure 6.2 Pyramid of 135 million births with need for various levels of care.

Box 6.1 Clinical relevance of improving neonatal care in low-income countries

At the current rate of change, it will be 110 years before a newborn in Africa has the same survival chance as one born in the US or UK. Yet the US and UK reduced NMR by this magnitude 50 years ago and three times faster, despite more knowledge now of essential newborn care (breastfeeding, hygiene) and more innovation (antenatal corticosteroids, simplified resuscitation, kangaroo mother care). Therefore, progress should be faster in low-resource contexts, not slower. Indeed, many neonatal intensive care units in high-income settings are de-intensifying care, increasing use of CPAP, and this makes even comprehensive care more transferable. Some countries have made remarkable progress despite major challenges, for example Rwanda is reducing newborn deaths more than four times faster than neighboring African countries (Lawn *et al.*, 2014).

All newborns need essential newborn care

Every baby needs essential newborn care (Table 6.1 and Box 6.2), ideally with their mothers providing warmth, breastfeeding, and cleanliness. Essential newborn care begins immediately at birth and must extend with safe care at home.

Thermal care

Simple methods to maintain a newborn's temperature after birth include immediate drying and wrapping, increasing the ambient temperature (if able), covering the newborn's head (e.g., with a knitted cap), skin-to-skin contact with the mother, and covering both the mother and newborn with a blanket (McCall *et al.*, 2005). Delaying the newborn's first bath is encouraged, but there is a lack of evidence as to how long to delay or how significant the impact is of this practice, especially if the bath can be warm and in a warm room (Penny-MacGillivray, 1996).

Early and exclusive breastfeeding

Early initiation of breastfeeding within 1 hour after birth is associated with reduced neonatal mortality (Edmond *et al.*, 2006; Bhutta *et al.*, 2008). Unless the newborn or the mother has serious illnesses, or the mother is HIV-positive and has decided on replacement feeding, all newborns should be put to the breast within 1 hour of birth. "Exclusive" breastfeeding means that the child receives only breast milk and no additional food, water, or other fluids (with the exception of medicines and vitamins, if needed). Exclusive breastfeeding is recommended for the first 6 months of life. Newborns should be breastfed as often as they want, day and night. This will be at least eight times in 24 hours (typically every 2–3 hours). Breastfeeding is natural, but mothers need help and support, especially first-time mothers and those with preterm newborns or multiple births. Details on positioning and attachment during breastfeeding are shown in Panel 6.1.

Table 6.1 Packages of newborn care (Lawn *et al.*, 2013).

Risk for all newborns, especially preterm	Essential care for all newborns	Extra care for preterm/small newborns	Emergency care for newborns with complications
Hypothermia (low body temperature): increased risk of infections, mortality and, for preterm newborns, increased risk of respiratory distress syndrome (RDS)	Thermal care: drying, warming, skin-to-skin, and delayed bathing	Extra thermal care: continuous skin-to-skin care, Kangaroo Mother Care, newborn hats, blankets, overhead heaters, incubators	Maintain normothermia: head/body cooling not recommended for neonatal encephalopathy
Hypoglycemia (low blood sugar): increased risk of impairment or death	Early and exclusive breastfeeding	Extra support for breastfeeding (e.g., expressing and cup or tube feeding, supplemented breast milk if indicated) Lack of breast milk is a risk factor for necrotizing enterocolitis in preterm newborns	Continue breastfeeding where possible Nasogastric/intravenous fluids when appropriate
Hypoxia (low oxygen levels): increased risk of impairment or death and, for preterm newborns, higher risk of RDS and intracranial bleeding	Neonatal resuscitation if not breathing at birth: bag-and-mask resuscitation with room air is sufficient for >99% of newborns not breathing at birth	Safe oxygen use: monitored oxygen use (e.g., in head box or with nasal cannula) using pulse oximeters	Safe oxygen management: supportive care for RDS including CPAP and/or surfactant if available
Infection: cord and skin infections, neonatal sepsis	Hygienic cord and skin care at birth and home care practices Hand washing and other hygiene Delayed cord clamping Consider chlorhexidine	Extra attention to infection prevention and skin care Consider chlorhexidine and emollients	Case management of newborns with signs of infection Case management of significant jaundice

Source: Lawn et al. (2013)

Box 6.2 The Every Newborn Action Plan

The Every Newborn Action Plan marks a historic global commitment to ending preventable newborn mortality. It sets a target to end all preventable newborn deaths by 2035 and achieve universal coverage of key services. Specifically, the Every Newborn Action Plan calls for:

- Fewer than ten newborn deaths per 1,000 live births and ten stillbirths per 1,000 total births in and within each country by 2035, resulting in a global average of seven newborn deaths per 1,000 live births and eight stillbirths per 1,000 total births by 2035
- 95% of women to give birth with skilled attendance by 2025
- 75% of babies who do not breathe at birth to be resuscitated by 2025
- 75% of preterm babies to receive kangaroo mother care by 2025

- 75% of newborn babies with bacterial infection to receive antibiotics by 2025
- 90% of women and newborns to receive good-quality postnatal care within two days of birth by 2025, with tracking of content and outcomes such as 50% exclusive breastfeeding.

At the 67th World Health Assembly in May 2014 health ministers of 194 countries endorsed the Every Newborn Action Plan and made commitments to put in practice recommended actions. The Director General of the United Nations has been requested to monitor progress and report to the World Health Assembly periodically until 2030.

Source: WHO and UNICEF (2014) Every Newborn: an action plan to end preventable deaths.
Available at http://www.everynewborn.org

👁 Panel 6.1 Feeding and fluid management

Status of newborn	Feeding plan / type of fluid	Feeding details (volume, frequency, and clinical pearls)
Stable term newborn able to suck and swallow	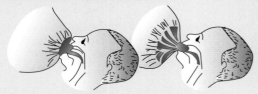 Good attachment Poor attachment Good and poor attachment. *Source*: Breastfeeding counselling: a training course. WHO/UNICEF. Reproduced with permission.	***Breastfeeding*** Ensure good position and attachment (latch) Newborn should be able to sustain active feeding with observed sucking/swallowing for at least 5 min every 2–3 hours Signs of good latch: • Mouth open • Lower lip turned outwards like fish • Chin touching breast • Large part of areola in the mouth
Preterm or sick newborn and cannot suck well	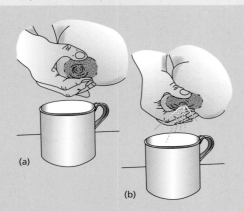 (a) (b)	***Hand expression of breast milk*** • Choose a cup, glass, or jar with a wide opening • Clean the container with soap and water and allow it to air dry in the sun • When preparing to use the container, pour boiling water into the container and leave it for a few minutes • When ready to express the breast milk, pour the water out of the cup • Place the thumb at 12 o'clock and index finger at 6 o'clock on the outside border of the dark areola • Press inwards toward the chest wall • Then press the areola behind the nipple between the thumb and index finger together ***Feeding the newborn by cup*** • Place the newborn in an upright position on the mother's lap • Support the newborn's back and neck with one hand • Place the cup close to the newborn's mouth so the cup almost touches the newborn's upper lip • Observe to see if the newborn extrudes his/her tongue to lick the milk or suckle at the cup • The cup may be gently tipped so that the newborn may lap the milk with his/her tongue or drink the milk. Observe whether the newborn sputters the milk out and whether the newborn can swallow the milk without coughing, choking, or sputtering • If the newborn is unable to swallow milk without coughing or choking, a nasogastric or orogastric tube needs to be inserted.

◉ Panel 6.1 Feeding and fluid management (*Continued*)

Status of newborn	Feeding plan / type of fluid	Feeding details (volume, frequency, and clinical pearls)
Preterm or sick newborn unable to swallow (coughs or sputters when attempts to cup feed)	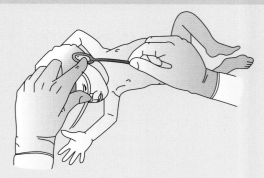	***Inserting a nasogastric or orogastric tube*** • For <2 kg, 5-French; >2 kg, 8-French • Estimate the required length of insertion by holding the tube from the nostril/mouth to lower edge of earlobe to the stomach just below the lowest rib • Mark the distance on the tube with a pen • When inserting a nasogastric tube, flex the newborn's neck slightly and pass the tube through the nostril until the marked spot • Secure the tube with tincture of benzoin and tape • If you have resistance, try the other nostril ***Confirm placement of NG tube*** • Fill syringe with 1–2 mL of air and connect to end of tube. Use stethoscope to listen over stomach as air is injected. If whistling sound not heard over stomach, tube is incorrectly positioned, *or* • Use litmus paper to test pH of aspirate. If it turns pink, then tube is correctly positioned. If it remains blue, tube needs to be repositioned • Target feeding volumes for a term newborn are shown by day of life in Table 6.3
Unstable newborn or cannot be fed (e.g., respiratory distress, poor tone, immature swallow, necrotizing enterocolitis)	Intravenous fluids 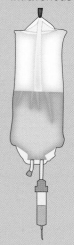 **1 mL = 60 microdrops = 20 drops**	***Intravenous fluids*** • Intravenous fluid management is complex in a newborn and changes daily depending on the newborn's oral intake, age in days, and urine output. It is described in detail in the WHO Managing Newborn Problems Manual. Here we only describe fluid management in the term >2500 g infant. For more details refer to the WHO manual (WHO, 2003a) • The initial fluid type should be D10W (10% glucose) for the first 3 days of life. On day 4, if the newborn is urinating, the fluids should be changed to D10W in quarter normal saline • The newborn's daily weight should be monitored closely, and the newborn should be observed for swelling and overhydration • Use a microdropper and calculate microdrops/minute • Target intravenous fluid volumes are shown by day of life in Table 6.2

Exclusive breastfeeding for the first 6 months of life is recommended for newborns of HIV-positive women in low-resource settings, and recent guidelines advise extending breastfeeding to 12 months if the mother is on antiretroviral therapy. To avoid increased risk of diarrheal disease, formula milk should not be used unless it is acceptable, feasible, affordable, sustainable, and safe (WHO, 2010).

Hygienic care at birth

Clean birth practices in both health facilities and the community will reduce maternal and neonatal mortality and morbidity from infection-related causes, including tetanus (Blencowe et al., 2011). The WHO recommends the six "cleans" for safe birth (WHO, 2006).

- Clean hands of the attendant (clean gloves).
- Clean surface upon which to deliver.
- Clean blade for cutting cord.
- Clean cord tie.
- Clean towels to dry the baby and then wrap the baby.
- Clean cloth to wrap the mother.

To prevent infection, all equipment used for childbirth must be sterile, including suction catheters, forceps, scissors, hemostats, and cord ties. Additionally, hand cleansing, using soap and water or a hand sanitizer, among hospital staff and family members is especially critical in nurseries and neonatal care units.

Cord care at birth

Tie or clamp the umbilical cord using hemostats, sterile string, rubber bands, or plastic cord clamps.

1. Tie or clamp the cord 3 cm (the width of two fingers) from the newborn's abdomen.
2. Tie or clamp another 3 cm further along the cord.
3. Cut the cord between the two ties or clamps with sterile scissors or a sterile blade. If using hemostats, tie or clamp the cord and remove the hemostats. If using a plastic clamp on the umbilical cord, check that the clamp is securely in place. If using sterile string or rubber bands, use two on the newborn's umbilical cord stump to prevent bleeding in the case that one tie comes loose. Even a small amount of bleeding is dangerous.

Delayed cord clamping

A simple and effective intervention, especially for preterm newborns, is delaying cord clamping by 2–3 minutes or until the cord stops pulsating, while keeping the newborn below the level of the placenta. This reduces the risk of intracranial bleeding, anemia, and need for blood transfusions. The Cochrane review of recent-evidence statements by obstetric societies supports delayed cord clamping for several minutes in all uncomplicated births (McDonald et al., 2013).

Chlorhexidine to cord if appropriate

Recent cluster-randomized trials have shown some benefit from topical application of chlorhexidine to the newborn's cord with no identified adverse effects. To date, about half of the trials have shown a significant neonatal mortality effect especially for preterm newborns and with early application, which may be challenging for home births (Arifeen et al., 2012; Soofi et al., 2012; Mullany et al., 2006). There are currently no trials evaluating chlorhexidine cord care in facility settings.

Neonatal resuscitation

See Chapter 7 on neonatal resuscitation for details on immediate care of the newborn after birth. It is estimated that immediate newborn assessment and resuscitation can reduce intrapartum-related and preterm deaths by 15–30% (Lee et al., 2011).

Pre-discharge teaching and examination

Implementation of a systematic pre-discharge teaching and physical examination of mothers and their newborns is an opportunity to identify risk factors, prevent complications, and increase care-seeking behavior. Teaching should include advising mothers on healthy newborn home care, common newborn problems, important danger signs, and when families should bring their newborn to a healthcare provider.

Preterm newborns need extra care

Preterm newborns are especially vulnerable to temperature instability, feeding difficulties, low blood sugar, infections, and breathing difficulties (see Table 6.1) (Lawn et al., 2013). Recognition of small newborns and distinguishing which ones are preterm is an essential first step in identifying the highest risk newborns: those who are both preterm and growth restricted. The gold standard for determining gestational age is a first-trimester ultrasound assessment, but this is not available for most of the world's pregnant women. Other options include last menstrual period, using birthweight as a surrogate, or clinical estimation of gestational age using the Eregie (2000) method or New Ballard examination (http://www.ballardscore.com/). In settings where weight and clinical estimations are not possible, foot length may serve as a surrogate for low birth weight. Foot length less than 8 cm may identify newborns less than 2500 g with high sensitivity in the African settings (Marchant et al., 2010).

Thermoregulation

Kangaroo mother care (KMC) is defined in Panel 6.2 and has been shown to halve neonatal mortality in newborns under 2000 g. The positive trials so far are all in hospital facilities, where feeding support, antibiotic case management of infections, and other care were also available. Despite the evidence of its cost-effectiveness, KMC is underutilized. Nevertheless, it is a rare example of a medical innovation moving from the southern

Panel 6.2 Kangaroo mother care (KMC)

What is it?

KMC was developed in the 1970s by a Colombian pediatrician, Edgar Rey, who sought a solution to incubator shortages, high infection rates, and abandonment among preterm births in his hospital (Rey & Martinez, 1983; Charpak et al., 2005).

With KMC, the premature newborn is put in early and continuous direct skin-to-skin contact with her mother or another family member to provide stable warmth and to encourage frequent and exclusive breastfeeding. Additional attention is paid to support breastfeeding and for early identification of any complications.

There is an increased probability of earlier discharge, but a very premature newborn and her mother may stay as an inpatient until feeding well and stable and then continue KMC at home. The median length of stay in Malawi is 5 days but is up to 5 weeks for newborns who are very preterm.

What is the evidence?

A systematic review and meta-analysis of several randomized controlled trials found that KMC is associated with a 51% reduction in neonatal mortality for stable newborns weighing <2000 g if started in the first week, compared with incubator care (Lawn et al., 2010).

An updated Cochrane review also reported a 40% reduction in risk of post-discharge mortality, about a 60% reduction in neonatal infections, and an almost 80% reduction in hypothermia. Other benefits included increased breastfeeding, weight gain, mother–newborn bonding, and developmental outcomes (Conde-Agudelo et al., 2011).

In addition to being more parent and newborn friendly, KMC is more health system friendly by reducing hospital stay and nursing load and therefore results in cost savings (Lima et al., 2000).

KMC was endorsed by the World Health Organization in 2003 when it developed a program implementation guide (WHO, 2003b). Some studies and program protocols have a lower weight limit for KMC (e.g., not below 800 g), but in contexts where no intensive care is available, some newborns under 800 g do survive with KMC and more research is required before setting a lower cut-off.

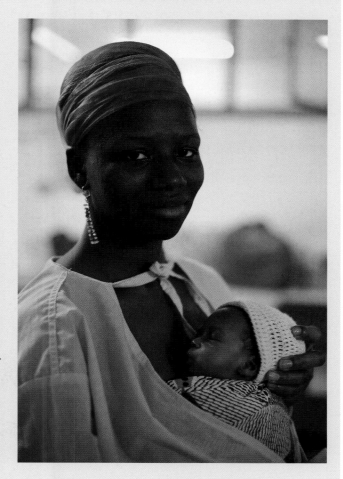

Bamako, Mali: Aminata Sangaré (18) and baby Maimouna Bagayogo (girl) 50 days old, in the Kangaroo Care center at the Gabrielle Traoré Hospital in Bamako, Mali, January 8, 2010. The baby girl was born 5 weeks premature and weighed 1 kg (2.2 pounds). *Source*: Joshua Roberts for Save the Children. Reproduced with permission of Save the Children.

(Continued)

◉ Panel 6.2 Kangaroo mother care (KMC) *(Continued)*

What are the principles for practice?

Countries that are making more rapid progress have a national policy for KMC (in which newborns receive KMC, feeding support, discharge criteria, etc.), a plan for national implementation, a learning site, national champions, and have integrated essential newborn care and resuscitation training into pre-service medical and nursing education.

KMC can be safely delivered by trained patient attendants under the supervision of nurses, allowing nurses to look after the sickest neonates, a successful example of task-shifting.

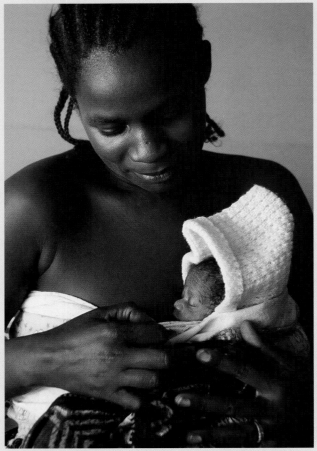

Grace, a mother in Malawi, holds Tuntufye, her baby girl who was born 2 months early, weighing only 1 kg (2.2 pounds). Through a Save the Children program, Grace learned to provide KMC, keeping the baby close to her skin to stay warm and breastfeeding every hour. After 1 week, Tuntufye gained 100 g (3.5 ounces). *Source*: Mark Amann/NCI Communications. Reproduced with permission of Save the Children.

hemisphere to Europe and North America, where KMC is now being included in intensive care (Lawn *et al.*, 2010). Other warming techniques include warming pads or warming cots, radiant heaters, or incubators. However, these require additional nursing skills and equipment maintenance (WHO, 1997). There are several trials suggesting benefit for plastic wrappings, but these have only been tested in very preterm newborns in neonatal intensive care units (Duman *et al.*, 2006).

Supplemental feeding and fluid management

Preterm newborns benefit from breast milk nutritionally, immunologically, and developmentally (Callen & Pinelli,

2005). The short-term and long-term benefits compared with formula feeding are well established, with lower incidence of infection and necrotizing enterocolitis and improved neurodevelopmental outcome (Edmond *et al.*, 2007; Hurst, 2007). Most preterm newborns require extra support for feeding by using a cup, spoon, or an oral or nasal gastric tube (Lawn *et al.*, 2001; WHO, 2011). The mother also requires support for expressing her breast milk. Where expressed breast milk is insufficient or not possible, donor milk is recommended (WHO, 2011), although in populations with high HIV prevalence, feasible solutions for pasteurization are critical. Table 6.2 shows recommended volumes, frequency, and fluids for supplemental feeding.

Table 6.2 Recommended total daily fluid volumes* for term or >2500 g newborns according to age in days.

Day of life	1	2	3	4	5	6	7+
Milliliters of feeds and/or intravenous fluid per kg body weight	60	80	100	120	140	150	160+

*Total feeds are the recommended total *combined* oral and intravenous volume per kilogram per 24 hours.
* Recommended feeding volumes for preterm and/or low-birthweight newborns are different and generally higher. For feeding volumes in these newborns, please refer to WHO (2003a).

Table 6.3 Diagnosis and management of neonatal infection.

Diagnosis

Symptomatic diagnosis based on assessment for signs of possible severe bacterial infection (based on WHO IMCI young infant algorithm):
- History of difficulty feeding
- Movement only when stimulated
- Temperature <35.5 or >37.5°C
- Respiratory rate >60
- Severe chest indrawing
- History of convulsions

Investigations

Complete blood count with white blood cell differential
If available, blood culture and cerebrospinal fluid culture (if bulging fontanelle)

Antibiotic management

If meningitis, treat for 2 weeks
Possible severe bacterial infection should be treated for 7–10 days
Ampicillin (or penicillin) and gentamicin (see Table 6.5 for doses)

Supportive care

Oxygen/respiratory support
Nasogastric feeds or intravenous fluids if unable to feed
Phenobarbital if seizures

Extremely preterm newborns under 1000 g and newborns who are ill may require intravenous fluids or even total parenteral nutrition, but this requires meticulous attention to volume and flow rates (Tables 6.2 and 6.3). For detailed instructions on recommended feeding for preterm infants see WHO (2003a). Routine supplementation of human milk given to preterm newborns is not currently recommended by the WHO. A recent WHO review also does not recommend any vitamin or mineral supplements (WHO, 2011), although other WHO guidelines have recommended Vitamin K at birth for low-birthweight newborns and iron supplementation for preterm newborns (WHO, 2003a, 2012a).

Sick and very small newborns need emergency care

Respiratory support, especially for preterm newborns

Optimal respiratory support of preterm newborns may include surfactant, nasal continuous positive airway pressure (CPAP), and mechanical ventilation, although there has been a recent shift in high-income countries towards less invasive ventilation with CPAP to deliver pressurized, humidified, warmed air and/or oxygen (Sankar *et al.*, 2008). Some health centers may also utilize elective intubation and surfactant at birth of moderately preterm newborns followed by non-invasive respiratory support. These less invasive approaches may be feasible for wider use in middle-income countries and for some low-income countries that have stronger support systems. However, the mainstay of respiratory support of both term and preterm newborns in many low-income countries is prone positioning, oxygen, bag-mask ventilation, aminophylline for apnea, and careful fluid management.

Simplified CPAP technologies such as "bubble CPAP" (see Chapter 26, Figure 26.2) are being developed specifically for low-income countries but need to be tested for durability, reliability, and safety (Brown *et al.*, 2013). To be effective and safe, CPAP-assisted ventilation requires skill, training, and supportive equipment such as an oxygen source, oxygen-monitoring device, and a suctioning device.

Oxygen is provided by oxygen concentrators, cylinders and, rarely, piped oxygen and can be delivered via nasal prongs, nasal catheters, head box, or directly into an incubator. Safe oxygen management is crucial, and any newborn receiving continuous oxygen therapy should be monitored with a pulse oximeter (Duke *et al.*, 2009). Particular care should be taken in preterm newborns to avoid oxygen toxicity, which can cause lung and retinal damage. Current literature suggests titrating oxygen delivery to achieve newborn oxygen saturation of 91–95% (BOOST II United Kingdom, Australia, and New Zealand Collaborative Groups, 2013).

Care of newborns with signs of infection

Serious newborn infections present at any age, can rapidly deteriorate, and have clinical features such as poor feeding, no spontaneous movement, fever, lethargy, respiratory distress, convulsions, and a bulging fontanelle (The Young Infants

Table 6.4 Diagnosis and management of superficial infections of the skin, umbilicus, and eyes.

	Skin pustules	Cellulitis/abscess	Umbilical infection	Conjunctivitis
Diagnosis	Solitary pustules or blisters in clusters around neck, axillae, umbilicus, groin with or without signs of sepsis	Red swollen skin Tender fluctuant swelling	Red and swollen umbilicus Foul-smelling or draining pus Abdominal distension	Red swollen eye draining pus
Investigations	Open pustule with sterile lancet Swab for culture and sensitivity Blood culture if available	If abscess drained, send material for culture and sensitivity	Swab of discharge material for culture and sensitivity	Swab for culture and sensitivity
Antibiotic management (refer to Table 6.5 for doses)	If <10 pustules: observe with or without oral cloxacillin (5 days) If >10 pustules: cloxacillin i.m. (5 days) If signs of sepsis: cloxacillin i.v. plus gentamicin i.v. (5–10 days)	Cloxacillin i.v. If improving after 5 days, change to oral cloxacillin for 5 days If no improvement after 5 days, add gentamicin for 10 days	Cloxacillin i.v. Gentamicin i.v. (5 days)	*S. aureus:* 1% tetracycline ointment (5 days) Gonorrhea: ceftriaxone i.m. single dose *Chlamydia:* erythromycin oral (14 days), 1% tetracycline ointment If no organism identified Age <7 days: ceftriaxone i.m. Age >7 days: erythromycin oral
Supportive care	Wash skin with antiseptic solution Swab pustules with 0.5% gentian violet solution	Drain abscess if fluctuant swelling	Clean umbilicus with antiseptic solution Swab area with 0.5% gentian violet solution	Clean eyelids with normal saline Wash face daily with cooled boiled water

Clinical Signs Study Group, 2008). In many low-income settings, laboratory testing (e.g., blood counts, blood cultures, or cerebrospinal fluid studies) may not be possible. Therefore, possible severe newborn infections are instead defined by clinical signs and symptoms, most commonly using the WHO approach to possible severe bacterial infection, with a low threshold for treating with antibiotics. These protocols have been incorporated into WHO's Integrated Management of Childhood Illness (Table 6.3) (WHO, 2003a; The Young Infants Clinical Signs Study Group, 2008). Improved survival is dependent on early detection of the danger signs and rapid treatment with antibiotics (WHO, 2005). Identification is complicated by atypical signs in ill newborns, such as a low temperature rather than fever. The WHO recommends that all newborns with danger signs be referred to a hospital. Where referral is not possible, then treatment at the primary care center can be life-saving.

Nosocomial infections are a significant cause of mortality and morbidity, especially in preterm and low-birthweight newborns. Cleaning of cots and incubators, hand-washing, and disinfecting reusable items such as nasal cannulas are all essential. Keeping potentially infected newborns away from stable preterm or low-birthweight newborns is also important, and many units have a separate "feeding and growing" section to avoid cross-infection.

Although major progress has been made in reducing neonatal tetanus deaths, with many countries reaching elimination status, this high case-fatality condition remains a reality, especially among the poorest families. Tetanus can present with poor feeding, fever, and spasms, and management consists of human antitetanus toxoid, benzylpenicillin, nasogastric feeds, pain management, diazepam for spasms, and minimal handling in a quiet low-stimulus environment. It is also critical to ensure the mother is immunized to prevent her next child being affected as well.

Superficial infections

Superficial infections (e.g., skin/umbilical infections, conjunctivitis) in newborns may be very contagious (Table 6.4). Observe strict infection prevention practices to avoid spread to other newborns in the nursery.

Care of newborns with jaundice

Jaundice is very common in newborns and may be physiological or due to hemolysis (e.g., ABO incompatibility, rhesus disease, or glucose 6-phosphate dehydrogenase deficiency), sepsis, and other causes. It is important to assess and treat jaundice promptly due to the risk of bilirubin encephalopathy (kernicterus) and long-term disability (Table 6.6). Preterm

Table 6.5 Common drugs used in newborns.

Drug	Dose	Indications
Aminophylline	Loading dose 6 mg/kg i.v./oral Maintenance 2.5–4 mg/kg every 12 hours	Apnea in preterm newborns
Ampicillin	50 mg/kg i.v. every 12 hours during first 7 days, every 8 hours in weeks 2–4	Possible severe bacterial infection Pneumonia, meningitis
Benzylpenicillin	50,000 U/kg per dose (30 mg/kg per dose) every 12 hours during first 7 days, every 6 hours in weeks 2–4 100,000 U/kg per dose (60 mg/kg per dose) every 12 hours	Possible severe bacterial infection Pneumonia, meningitis Tetanus
Ceftriaxone	50 mg/kg i.m. one-time dose (max. 150 mg)	Conjunctivitis (gonococcus)
Cloxacillin	25–50 mg/kg i.v. every 12 hours during first 7 days, every 8 hours in weeks 2–4	Skin, umbilical infections
Diazepam	0.1–0.3 mg/kg every 1–4 hours	Convulsions and management of neonatal tetanus
Erythromycin	12.5 mg/kg every 12 hours	Conjunctivitis (*Chlamydia*)
Gentamicin	First 7 days • Weight <2.5 kg: 3 mg/kg once daily i.m./i.v. • Weight >2.5 kg: 5 mg/kg once daily i.m./i.v. 2–4 weeks • 7.5 mg/kg once daily i.m./i.v.	Possible severe bacterial infection Pneumonia, meningitis Severe skin, umbilical infections
Phenobarbital	Loading dose 20 mg/kg i.v./i.m./oral Repeated at 10 mg/kg to max. 40 mg/kg Maintenance dose 5 mg/kg i.v./i.m./oral	Seizures

Table 6.6 Diagnosis and management of neonatal jaundice.

Diagnosis

Signs of abnormal/pathologic/non-physiologic jaundice
• Jaundice noticed on the first day of life
• Severe, deep jaundice: palms and soles of newborn deep yellow
• Jaundice with fever
• Jaundice lasting >14 days in term newborn or >21 days in preterm newborn
Bilirubin encephalopathy due to severe jaundice
• Convulsions, opisthotonus, and/or floppiness in a severely jaundiced newborn

Investigations (if available)

Serum bilirubin level or consider icterometer
Hemoglobin or hematocrit
Blood type of newborn and mother and Coombs test
If concern for infection, white blood cell count, neutrophil-band count, and/or blood culture
If available, consider syphilis serology, G6PD*, thyroid function tests

Specific care

Treat with phototherapy if jaundice is severe, occurs with fever, is present on first day of life or if serum bilirubin level is available (see Table 6.7 for level requiring treatment)
Exchange transfusion if very severe jaundice or bilirubin encephalopathy

Supportive care

Ensure good hydration, frequent and adequate breastfeeding
Treat suspected infection

*G6PD, glucose 6-phosphate dehydrogenase.

newborns are at increased risk of jaundice and infection and have more permeable blood–brain barriers, compounding risks for death and disability (Mwaniki *et al.*, 2012). If LED phototherapy units are not available, simple phototherapy units can be made using ultraviolet or fluorescent lights on a wooden frame (Figure 6.3). Exchange transfusion should be done if the serum bilirubin passes a given threshold (Table 6.7), using donated O-negative blood or blood that is compatible with the newborn's blood type. Estimate the total blood volume as 80 mL/kg for term and 100 mL/kg for preterm newborns. Remove and replace blood in 5–15 mL aliquots, depending on the weight of the newborn, using a three-way tap connected to an umbilical venous catheter.

Care of newborns with neonatal encephalopathy

Neonatal encephalopathy resulting from birth complications and intrapartum hypoxia is one of the leading causes of neonatal mortality and morbidity and has multiple contributing factors, including maternal infections such as chorioamnionitis. Further details on the diagnosis and management of neonatal encephalopathy are shown in Table 6.8, although it can be challenging to manage in a low-resource setting. Long-term prognosis for severe brain injury and poor long-term neurodevelopmental outcomes can be predicted by 1 week of age with newborns who are floppy, spastic, unresponsive, or unable to suckle.

Newborn care: where to start?

Community

It is critical to ensure that women and communities are enabled and informed about being prepared for birth, obtaining essential newborn care, and seeking care for themselves and their newborns if sick. It is important that caregivers can recognize signs of illness, especially in preterm newborns, and are ready and able to seek medical care.

Home-visit packages by community health workers during pregnancy and after birth provide an opportunity to empower women to have better outcomes themselves and for their newborns (WHO, 2009). An early postnatal visit by a community health worker (within 2 days of birth) is one of only seven coverage indicators along the continuum of care selected by the United Nations Commission on Information and Accountability and tracked by the Countdown to 2015 (Commission on Information and Accountability for Women's and Children's Health, 2011; Requejo *et al.*, 2012). This early postnatal visit by a community health worker is critical for survival and health and an important opportunity to identify preterm and sick newborns. Novel methods for identification of preterm newborns include community health workers using foot size to identify those newborns likely to be preterm and then providing extra visits, breastfeeding support, and referral to a facility if needed (Marchant *et al.*, 2010). Womens' groups offering peer counseling and community mobilization have

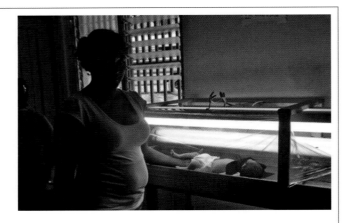

Figure 6.3 A hand-made phototherapy box in Nicaragua for the treatment of neonatal jaundice. This box was developed by pediatric and internal medicine residents during their global health electives. *Source*: Drs A. Bjorklund, J. Nordell, and T. Slusher. Reproduced with permission of A. Bjorklund.

Table 6.7 Treatment of jaundice based on serum bilirubin level.

	Phototherapy				Exchange transfusion			
	Healthy term newborn		**With risk factors***		**Healthy term newborn**		**With risk factors***	
Age	**mg/dL**	**μmol/L**	**mg/dL**	**μmol/L**	**mg/dL**	**μmol/L**	**mg/dL**	**μmol/L**
Day 1	Any visible jaundice				15	260	13	220
Day 2	15	260	13	220	25	425	15	260
Day 3	18	310	16	270	30	510	20	340
Day 4 +	20	340	17	290	30	510	20	340

*Risk factors are preterm, birthweight <2.5 kg, hemolysis, or sepsis. If jaundice present on day 1, start phototherapy immediately while awaiting bilirubin result (WHO, 2003a).

Table 6.8 Diagnosis and management of neonatal encephalopathy.

Diagnosis

History of possible intrapartum hypoxic events:
- Fetal distress
- Obstructed or prolonged labor
- Other risk factors (non-vertex presentation, preeclampsia, placental abruption, meconium, abruption, intrauterine growth restriction, multiple gestation)
- Neonatal depression at birth (low Apgar score)

Newborn with signs of (starting within first week of life):
- Convulsions/seizures
- Apnea or irregular respiratory pattern
- Inability to suck and poor feeding
- Abnormal neurologic tone, either hypotonia or hypertonia/spasticity

Investigations

Blood sugar to rule out hypoglycemia as cause of seizure
If available and suspicion of infection, consider blood culture and/or cerebrospinal fluid culture

Specific care

Neonatal resuscitation at the time of birth
With onset of neonatal encephalopathy/seizures, phenobarbital for seizure (see Table 6.5 for dosing)
Body and head cooling is currently not yet recommended in low- and middle-income settings and studies are forthcoming

Supportive care

Respiratory support: bag-mask ventilation in cases of apnea, aminophylline if available, and oxygen as needed
Feeding support and nasogastric tube feedings or intravenous fluids if unable to feed
Avoid fluid overload given risk of SIADH*
Avoid hyperthermia (unmonitored under radiant warmer)

*SIADH, syndrome of inappropriate antidiuretic hormone.

Box 6.3 Practical tips for where to start saving newborns in a facility

Who?
Training of nurses with skills for essential newborn care, neonatal resuscitation, KMC, and infection case management. A mixed skills team with patient attendants and other less trained cadres can be very successful, especially if these staff do not have to rotate and can build skills over time.

Where?
In the labor ward, there needs to be a surface for newborn resuscitation and basic equipment ready at all times. In the postnatal or pediatric ward, have at a minimum a "newborn corner" with a table and overhead heater, basic equipment, oxygen, and clinical charts and guidelines posted on the wall. This can be near a set of beds used for mothers practicing KMC. If a room is used for a special newborn care unit, this room should be kept at a warmer ambient temperature and be more carefully equipped with pulse oximeters and other essentials for safe newborn care.

What?
Basic equipment includes bag-and-mask resuscitation devices, different-sized face masks, suction devices, resuscitation training mannequins, nasogastric tubes, neonatal intravenous catheters, and feeding cups. Essential drugs, especially antibiotics, and intravenous dextrose. Phototherapy devices. Basic diagnostics to test for anemia and hyperbilirubinemia.

Source: adapted from UNICEF (2009) and WHO (2012b).

---

been shown to have a significant effect on reducing neonatal mortality in at least half of the trials in Asia and Africa to date (Lassi *et al.*, 2010; Prost *et al.*, 2013).

Health facilities

Addressing newborn care in public district hospitals is a key priority for improving newborn survival and health. In most countries, district hospitals are understaffed and poorly resourced compared with teaching hospitals. Examples of improved newborn care in district hospitals include targeted quality improvement initiatives with mentors, accreditation programs, standard guidelines, training courses, and alternative cadres of clinical aides specially trained in newborn care and

restricted from rotations to other wards (Sen *et al.*, 2007; Opondo *et al.*, 2009). Design and implementation of context-specific hospital newborn care packages is critical, especially as more births occur in facilities (Box 6.3).

Shortages of qualified health workers and inadequate training and skills for the care of newborns are a major reason for poor progress in reducing neonatal deaths (Knippenberg *et al.*, 2005; Victora & Rubens, 2010). Nurses or midwives with skills in critical areas such as resuscitation, KMC, safe oxygen management, and breastfeeding support are the frontline workers who provide the vast majority of newborn care, yet in the whole of sub-Saharan Africa there are no known neonatal nurse training courses. Urgent systematic attention is required for pre-service and in-service training, non-rotation of nurses with skills in neonatal care, rewards for those who work against the odds in hard-to-serve areas, and, where appropriate, the development of a neonatal nurse cadre.

Table 6.9 Tools, technologies, and innovations required for the care of newborns.

Priority packages and interventions	Current technology/tools	Technological innovations required
All babies		
Essential newborn care and extra care for preterm babies Thermal care (drying, warming, skin-to-skin, and delayed bathing) Early initiation of exclusive breastfeeding Hygienic cord and skin care	Protocols for care, training materials and job aids Materials for counseling, health education, and health promotion Weighing scales Cord clamp and scissors, clean birth kit if appropriate Vitamin K for low-birthweight newborns	Generic communications and counseling toolkit for local adaptation Generic modular training kit for adaptation, novel methods (e.g., cell phone prompts) Birth kits for frontline workers Chlorhexidine preparations for application to the umbilical cord Simplified approaches to identifying preterm newborns such as footsize
Neonatal resuscitation for newborns who do not breathe at birth	Materials for training and job aids Training mannequins Newborn resuscitation devices (bag-and-mask) Suction devices Resuscitation stations with overhead heater Clock with large face and second hand	Wide-scale novel logistics systems to increase availability of devices for basic resuscitation and training mannequins Additional innovation for resuscitation devices (e.g., upright bag-and-mask, adaptable, lower-cost resuscitation stations)
Preterm babies		
Kangaroo mother care (KMC) for small newborns (birthweight <2000 g)	Cloth or wrap for KMC Newborn hats	Generic communications and counseling toolkit for local adaptation Innovation to address cultural, professional barriers Generic modular training kit and job aids for local adaptation
Care of preterm babies with complications, including: • extra support for feeding preterm and small babies • case management of babies with signs of infection • safe oxygen management and supportive care for RDS • case management of babies with significant jaundice • management of seizures	Nasogastric tubes, feeding cups, breast milk pumps Blood sugar testing sticks Intravenous fluids including glucose and more accurate giving sets Syringe drivers Injection antibiotics, 1-mL syringes/27G needles, preloaded syringes Oxygen supply/concentrators Nasal prongs, head boxes, other oxygen-delivery systems Pulse oximeters to assess blood oxygen levels with reusable cleanable neonatal probes Bilirubinometers (table-top and transcutaneous) Phototherapy lamps and eye shades, exchange transfusion kits Hot cots, overhead heaters	Lower cost and more robust versions of: • Blood sugar testing for newborns on low-volume samples, heel pricks • Oxygen condensers, including portable options • Pulse oximeters and robust probes, including with alternative power options • Syringe drivers able to take a range of syringes • Bilirubin testing devices including lower-cost transcutaneous devices • Hemoglobin, blood grouping, and rhesus point-of-care tests • CRP/procalcitonin point-of-care test • Apnea alarm • Phototherapy devices such as portable "bilibed" to provide both phototherapy treatment and heat
Neonatal intensive care	Continuous positive airway pressure (CPAP) devices with standardized safety features	Lower-cost robust CPAP equipment with standardized settings Neonatal intensive care context-specific "kits" (e.g., for district hospital with ongoing support for quality use and for equipment maintenance) Surfactant as more stable lower-cost preparations

CRP, C-reactive protein; RDS, respiratory distress syndrome.

Comprehensive neonatal care moving toward intensive care

Seven low- and middle-income countries have halved their neonatal deaths within a decade. These countries are Sri Lanka, Turkey, Belarus, Croatia, Ecuador, El Salvador, Oman, and China. Some of these countries also had fertility rate reductions, which may have contributed, but the likely explanation is national focus on improved obstetric and neonatal care and systematic establishment of referral systems with higher capacity of neonatal care units, staff, and equipment, helped in some cases by larger national budgets. Over time, as neonatal care increases in scope, provider skills, commodities, and equipment become more critical and, at an NMR below 15 per 1000 live births, intensive care plays an increasing role. Hence, low- and middle-income countries should be able to halve the risk of their newborns dying by ensuring they have the right people and the right basic commodities. Investing in frontline workers and their training is crucial to building their life-saving skills and overcoming nervousness of many workers when looking after tiny newborns. A phased approach, for example using KMC as an entry point to show that newborns weighing under 1000 g at birth can and do survive and thrive, can be a turning point for clinical staff as well as hospital management.

Starting from existing program platforms at the community level (e.g., home visit packages, womens' groups) and at the facility level to ensure effective care for all births at health facilities is cost-effective and more likely to show early results. However, as long as families remain unreached, for example because of financial barriers to facility birth care, these service gaps often mean those most at risk are excluded.

While most newborns can be saved with the right people and simple care, for more extremely preterm newborns additional skills, equipment, and commodities are critical, ranging from bag-and-mask devices and controlled intravenous fluid giving sets to CPAP and surfactant (Table 6.9). The UN Commission on Life-saving Commodities for Women and Children has prioritized high-impact neglected commodities, and these include several for the care of newborns: chlorhexidine, injectable antibiotics, antenatal corticosteroids, and resuscitation equipment.

Future steps

Globally, progress is being made in reducing maternal and child deaths after the first month of life. Progress for neonatal deaths is slower but even deaths among preterm newborns born outside facilities in the lowest-income settings can be reduced. However, higher-impact facility-based care is needed and is dependent on nurses and others with skills in caring for small and sick newborns and can be phased in over time to add increased level of care. Starting with intensive care will fail if simple hygiene, careful attention to feeding, and other basic building blocks are not first in place. Although few resource-limited countries can afford to rapidly scale up neonatal intensive care in a short time, 71% of neonatal deaths can be prevented without full neonatal intensive care. (Bhutta *et al.*, Lancet 2014). No country can afford to miss doing the simple things well for every newborn and investing extra attention in survival and health of newborns, especially those who are preterm, while developing increased health systems capacity.

Additional resources

- Every Newborn Action Plan. Available at http://www.everynewborn.org/
- Healthy Newborn Network for latest numbers, guidelines, and many resources. Available at http://www.healthynewborn network.org
- Helping Babies Breathe. Newborn resuscitation training program. Available at http://www.helpingbabiesbreathe.org
- World Health Organization. Born too soon: the global action report on preterm birth. Available at http://www.who.int/maternal_child_adolescent/documents/born_too_soon/en/index.html
- World Health Organization. Essential Newborn Care Course. Available at http://www.who.int/maternal_child_adolescent/documents/newborncare_course/en/
- World Health Organization. *Pocket Book of Hospital Care for Children*, 2nd edn, 2013. Available at http://www.who.int/maternal_child_adolescent/documents/9241546700/en/index.html
- World Health Organization. Managing newborn problems: a guide for doctors, nurses, and midwives. http://www.who.int/maternal_child_adolescent/documents/9241546220/en/index.html

REFERENCES

Arifeen SE, Mullany LC, Shah R *et al.* (2012) The effect of cord cleansing with chlorhexidine on neonatal mortality in rural Bangladesh: a community-based, cluster-randomised trial. *Lancet* 379:1022–8.

Bhutta ZA, Ahmed T, Black RE *et al.* (2008) What works? Interventions for maternal and child undernutrition and survival. *Lancet* 371:417–40.

Bhutta ZA, Das JK, Bahl R, *et al.* (2014) Can available interventions end preventable deaths in mothers, newborn babies, and stillbirths, and at what cost? *Lancet* 384(9940):347–70.

Blencowe H, Cousens S, Mullany LC *et al.* (2011) Clean birth and postnatal care practices to reduce neonatal deaths from sepsis and tetanus: a systematic review and Delphi estimation of mortality effect. *BMC Public Health* 11(Suppl. 3):S11.

Blencowe H, Cousens S, Oestergaard MZ, Chou D, Moller AB (2012) National, regional, and worldwide estimates of preterm birth rates in the year 2010 with time trends since 1990 for selected countries: a systematic analysis and implications. *Lancet* 379:2162–72.

BOOST II United Kingdom, Australia, and New Zealand Collaborative Groups (2013) Oxygen saturation and outcomes in preterm infants. *N Engl J Med* 368:2094–104.

Brown J, Machen H, Kawaza K *et al.* (2013) A high-value, low-cost bubble continuous positive airway pressure system for low-resource settings: technical assessment and initial case report. *PLoS ONE* 8(1):e53622.

Callen J, Pinelli J (2005) A review of the literature examining the benefits and challenges, incidence and duration, and barriers to breastfeeding in preterm infants. *Adv Neonatal Care* 5:72–88.

Charpak N, Ruiz JG, Zupan J *et al.* (2005) Kangaroo Mother Care: 25 years after. *Acta Paediatr* 94:514–22.

Commission on Information and Accountability for Women's and Children's Health (2011) Keeping promises, measuring results. Available at http://www.everywomaneverychild.org/images/content/files/accountability_commission/final_report/Final_EN_Web.pdf

Conde-Agudelo A, Belizan JM, Diaz-Rossello J (2011) Kangaroo mother care to reduce morbidity and mortality in low birthweight infants. *Cochrane Database Syst Rev* (3):CD002771.

Duke T, Subhi R, Peel D, Frey B (2009) Pulse oximetry: technology to reduce child mortality in developing countries. *Ann Trop Paediatr* 29:165–75.

Duman N, Utkutan S, Kumral A, Koroglu TF, Ozkan H (2006) Polyethylene skin wrapping accelerates recovery from hypothermia in very low-birthweight infants. *Pediatr Int* 48:29–32.

Edmond KM, Zandoh C, Quigley MA, Amenga-Etego S, Owusu-Agyei S, Kirkwood BR (2006) Delayed breastfeeding initiation increases risk of neonatal mortality. *Pediatrics* 117:e380–6.

Edmond KM, Kirkwood BR, Amenga-Etego S, Owusu-Agyei S, Hurt LS (2007) Effect of early infant feeding practices on infection-specific neonatal mortality: an investigation of the causal links with observational data from rural Ghana. *Am J Clin Nutr* 86:1126–31.

Eregie CO (2000) A new method for maturity determination in newborn infants. *J Trop Pediatr* 46:140–4.

Hurst NM (2007) The 3 M's of breast-feeding the preterm infant. *J Perinat Neonatal Nurs* 21:234–9.

Knippenberg R, Lawn JE, Darmstadt GL *et al.* (2005) Systematic scaling up of neonatal care in countries. *Lancet* 365:1087–98.

Lassi ZS, Haider BA, Bhutta ZA (2010) Community-based intervention packages for reducing maternal and neonatal morbidity and mortality and improving neonatal outcomes. *Cochrane Database Syst Rev* (11):CD007754.

Lawn JE, McCarthy BJ, Ross SR (2001) *The Healthy Newborn: A Reference Guide for Program Managers.* Atlanta, GA: CDC and CARE.

Lawn JE, Mwansa-Kambafwile J, Horta BL, Barros FC, Cousens S (2010) "Kangaroo mother care" to prevent neonatal deaths due to preterm birth complications. *Int J Epidemiol* 39(Suppl. 1):i144–54.

Lawn JE, Davidge R, Paul VK, *et al.* (2013) Born too soon: care for the preterm baby. *Reprod Health* 10(Suppl. 1):S5.

Lawn JE, Blencowe H, Oza S, *et al.* (2014) Every Newborn: progress, priorities, and potential beyond survival. *Lancet* 384(9938):189–205.

Lee AC, Cousens S, Wall SN, Niermeyer S, Darmstadt GL (2011) Neonatal resuscitation and immediate newborn assessment and stimulation for the prevention of neonatal deaths: a systematic review, meta-analysis and Delphi estimation of mortality effect. *BMC Public Health* 11(Suppl. 3):S12.

Lee AC, Katz J, Blencowe H *et al.* (2013) National and regional estimates of term and preterm babies born small for gestational age in 138 low-income and middle-income countries in 2010. *Lancet Global Health* 1:e26–36.

Lima G, Quintero-Romero S, Cattaneo A (2000) Feasibility, acceptability and cost of kangaroo mother care in Recife, Brazil. *Ann Trop Paediatr* 20:2–26.

Marchant T, Jaribu J, Penfold S, Tanner M, Armstrong Schellenberg J (2010) Measuring newborn foot length to identify small babies in need of extra care: a cross sectional hospital based study with community follow-up in Tanzania. *BMC Public Health* 10:624.

McCall EM, Alderdice FA, Halliday HL, Jenkins JG, Vohra S (2005) Interventions to prevent hypothermia at birth in preterm and/or low birthweight babies. *Cochrane Database Syst Rev* (1):CD004210.

McDonald SJ, Middleton P, Dowswell T, Morris PS (2013) Effect of timing of umbilical cord clamping of term infants on maternal and neonatal outcomes. *Cochrane Database Syst Rev* (7):CD004074.

Mullany LC, Darmstadt GL, Khatry SK, *et al.* (2006) Topical applications of chlorhexidine to the umbilical cord for prevention of omphalitis and neonatal mortality in southern Nepal: a community-based, cluster-randomised trial. *Lancet* 367(9514):910–8.

Mwaniki MK, Atieno M, Lawn JE, Newton CR (2012) Long-term neurodevelopmental outcomes after intrauterine and neonatal insults: a systematic review. *Lancet* 379:445–52.

Opondo C, Ntoburi S, Wagai J *et al.* (2009) Are hospitals prepared to support newborn survival? An evaluation of eight first-referral level hospitals in Kenya. *Trop Med Int Health* 14:1165–72.

Penny-MacGillivray T (1996) A newborn's first bath: when? *J Obstet Gynecol Neonatal Nurs* 25:481–7.

Prost A, Colbourn T, Tripathy P, Osrin D, Costello A (2013) Analyses confirm effect of women's groups on maternal and newborn deaths. *Lancet* 381:e15.

Requejo J, Bryce J, Deixel A, Victora C (2012) Accountabiliy for maternal, newborn and child survival: an update on progress in priority countries. Available at http://www.who.int/pmnch/knowledge/publications/201203_accountability_for_mnc_survival/en/

Rey E, Martinez H (1983) *Manejio racional del Nino Prematuro*. Medicina Fetal, Bogota, Colombia: Universidad Nacional, Cursode.

Sankar MJ, Sankar J, Agarwal R, Paul VK, Deorari AK (2008) Protocol for administering continuous positive airway pressure in neonates. *Indian J Pediatr* 75:471–8.

Sen A, Mahalanabis D, Singh AK, Som TK, Bandyopadhyay S, Roy S (2007) Newborn aides: an innovative approach in sick newborn care at a district-level special care unit. *J Health Popul Nutr* 25:495–501.

Soofi S, Cousens S, Imdad A, Bhutto N, Ali N, Bhutta ZA (2012) Topical application of chlorhexidine to neonatal umbilical cords for prevention of omphalitis and neonatal mortality in a rural district of Pakistan: a community-based, cluster-randomised trial. *Lancet* 379:1029–36.

The Young Infants Clinical Signs Study Group (2008) Clinical signs that predict severe illness in children under age 2 months: a multicentre study. *Lancet* 371:135–42.

UNICEF (2009) Toolkit for setting up special care newborn units, stabilisation units and newborn care corners. Available at http://www.unicef.org/india/SCNU_book1_April_6.pdf

Victora CG, Rubens CE (2010) Global report on preterm birth and stillbirth (4 of 7): delivery of interventions. *BMC Pregnancy Childbirth* 10(Suppl. 1):S4.

WHO (1997) Thermal protection of the newborn: a practical guide. Available at http://www.who.int/maternal_child_adolescent/documents/ws42097th/en/

WHO (2003a) Managing newborn problems: a guide for doctors, nurses and midwives. Available at http://apps.who.int/iris/bitstream/10665/42753/1/9241546220.pdf?ua=1

WHO (2003b) Kangaroo mother care: a practical guide. Available at http://www.who.int/maternal_child_adolescent/documents/9241590351/en/

WHO (2005) Handbook IMCI: Integrated management of childhood illness. Available at http://www.who.int/maternal_child_adolescent/documents/9241546441/en/

WHO (2006) Opportunities for Africa's newborns: Practical data, policy and programmatic support for newborn care in Africa. Available at http://www.who.int/pmnch/media/publications/oanfullreport.pdf

WHO (2009) WHO-UNICEF Joint Statement. Home visits for the newborn child: a strategy to improve survival. Available at http://www.unicef.org/spanish/health/files/WHO_FCH_CAH_09.02_eng.pdf

WHO (2010) Guidelines on HIV and infant feeding: Principles and recommendations for infant feeding in the context of HIV and a summary of evidence. Available at http://www.who.int/maternal_child_adolescent/documents/9789241599535/en/

WHO (2011) Guidelines on optimal feeding of low birth weight infants in low and middle income countries. Available at http://www.who.int/maternal_child_adolescent/documents/infant_feeding_low_bw/en/

WHO (2012a) Recommendations for management of common childhood conditions: Evidence for technical update of pocket book recommendations. Available at http://www.who.int/maternal_child_adolescent/documents/management_childhood_conditions/en/

WHO (2012b) Born too soon: the global action report on preterm birth. Available at http://www.who.int/pmnch/media/news/2012/201204_borntoosoon-report.pdf

WHO and UNICEF (2014) Every Newborn: an action plan to end preventable deaths. Available at www.everynewborn.org

CHAPTER 7
Birth Asphyxia

Brett D. Nelson[1] and Elizabeth Nowak[2]
[1]Harvard Medical School and Massachusetts General Hospital, Boston, MA, USA
[2]Ben-Gurion University and Columbia University, Israel

Key learning objectives

- Understand the large burden of birth asphyxia in resource-limited settings.
- Learn what needs to be prepared prior to every delivery.
- Learn what to do for newborns immediately after delivery.
- Learn how to help a newborn if it is not breathing after birth.

Abstract

Intrapartum-related complications, or commonly called "birth asphyxia," is one of the leading causes of neonatal mortality worldwide. However, most of these asphyxia-related deaths are preventable using existing, simple, cost-effective interventions. Approximately 10% of newborns will require some form of assistance in breathing during the first seconds and minutes of life. There have been several new advancements in resuscitation for resource-limited settings that have been proven to increase access to care and prevent death. Some of these advances include low-cost equipment and a simple algorithm for training skilled birth attendants in the steps of newborn resuscitation. This chapter explores the global burden of birth asphyxia and the practical measures that can be used to prevent asphyxia-related deaths. It includes a summary of the Helping Babies Breathe program that is used to train skilled birth attendants around the world.

Key words: birth asphyxia, perinatal asphyxia, intrapartum-related complications, newborn resuscitation, newborn health, newborn mortality, Helping Babies Breathe program

Introduction and epidemiology

A leading cause of newborn mortality worldwide involves intrapartum-related complications, commonly called "birth asphyxia," which involves the inability of the newborn to effectively take the first breaths of life. Asphyxia is often the result of fetal hypoxia prior to or during the delivery process. Every year, it is estimated that intrapartum-related complications are responsible for approximately 1 million neonatal deaths and 1 million stillbirths worldwide. In addition to this significant mortality, surviving newborns may face considerable lifelong morbidity, including cerebral palsy, mental impairment, and blindness (Lee et al., 2011a).

The vast majority of asphyxia-related perinatal and neonatal deaths occur in low- and middle-income countries. Many of these deaths can be easily prevented using existing cost-effective interventions (Lawn et al., 2011). For example, studies suggest a reduction of 30–40% or more in early neonatal mortality with the introduction of newborn resuscitation (Lee et al., 2011b; Msemo et al., 2013). However, one challenge faced in addressing asphyxia-related mortality is providing mothers and newborns with access to proven interventions and skilled birthing care.

In many low- and middle-income countries, mothers are more likely to receive intrapartum care outside of established health facilities and from traditional or unskilled birth attendants (Herbert et al., 2012). On the other hand, mothers who are assisted in their delivery by skilled birth attendants are more likely to be referred for complications and have lower incidences of stillbirth and newborn death (Sibley et al., 2007; Bhutta et al., 2011). To some extent, these results are dependent on the birth attendant's level of training. Interventions that target providers' understanding of birth asphyxia can greatly reduce the risk of perinatal death. This is true for both community- and health facility-based practitioners (Lee et al., 2011b). Yet in a National Service Assessment of six African countries, for example, only 2–12% of birth-related practitioners were trained in newborn resuscitation practices (Wall et al., 2009).

In the following sections we will discuss simple and effective approaches to reduce perinatal deaths due to birth asphyxia.

Preparing for delivery

Newborns regularly need help to take the first breaths of life, with approximately 1 in 10 newborns requiring more than the basic warming and drying. For some newborns, the need for resuscitation may be anticipated; for instance, in the setting of maternal illness, preterm delivery, prolonged labor, non-reassuring fetal heart tones, or meconium-stained amniotic fluid, newborns are more likely to require resuscitation. However, in many cases it is not always possible to predict prior to delivery which newborns will need immediate help breathing. Therefore it is necessary to have trained personnel and essential equipment present at every delivery. Panel 7.1 lists the newborn personnel and equipment essential at every birth.

Newborn resuscitation in developing countries

Life-saving approaches have long existed for preventing deaths from birth asphyxia. In developed countries, birth attendants use well-established evidence-based algorithms such as newborn resuscitation guidelines from the American Academy of Pediatrics, American Heart Association, European Resuscitation Council, and the International Liaison Committee on Resuscitation. However, the approaches that are effective in high-income countries have not always been easily implemented in settings with significantly less resources and fewer trained staff

(Lawn et al., 2005, 2006; Darmstadt et al., 2009). Furthermore, some clinical guidelines may not be appropriate in resource-limited settings, particularly for care outside tertiary referral centers. For example, newborn resuscitation recommendations for low- and middle-income countries frequently stop short of chest compressions, intubation, and other advanced resuscitative efforts due to inadequate resources and poor access to supportive critical care.

In recent years, there has been a renewed commitment to improving newborn health worldwide, and significant progress is being made in the management of perinatal asphyxia in resource-limited settings. This progress includes advances in setting-appropriate algorithms, devices, and training equipment.

A new initiative known as Helping Babies Breathe (HBB) was introduced in 2010 by the American Academy of Pediatrics, in collaboration with the US Agency for International Development, Save the Children, the US National Institute of Child Health and Development, World Health Organization (WHO), and other partners. HBB was designed as an evidence-based educational approach that uses a concise algorithm (Figure 7.1) to teach newborn resuscitation to birth attendants in resource-limited settings (International Liaison Committee on Resuscitation, 2006; American Academy of Pediatrics, 2014). The program stresses the critical importance of skilled birth attendance, newborn assessment, temperature control, stimulation to breathe, and assisted ventilation when needed

👁 Panel 7.1 Newborn personnel and equipment needed at each delivery

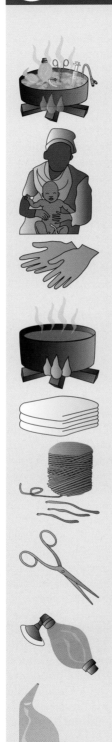

Sterilization: all reusable newborn equipment (e.g., newborn bag–mask device, bulb suction, scissors) should be sterilized or boiled for 10 minutes between each patient

Birth attendant trained in newborn resuscitation: at the delivery of every newborn, there should be present a birth attendant who is properly trained in newborn resuscitation

Gloves: birth attendants should wear gloves to protect the mother, the newborn, and the provider from infection

Clean water: prepare clean water for every delivery. Water can be cleaned ahead of time through boiling, chlorination, or solar distillation. Clean water is used for washing the provider's hands, washing the mother's perineum, and for emergency interventions such as uterine balloon tamponade for postpartum hemorrhage (see Chapter 17)

Several clean cloths: it is important to dry the newborn with multiple clean cloths and to wrap the newborn in another dry cloth. Clean cloths may also be needed in the control of maternal bleeding

Cord clamps or ties: prepare umbilical cord clamps or two to three pieces of string to tie the umbilical cord before the cord is cut

Scissors or blade: use sterile scissors or blade to cut the umbilical cord after it is properly tied

Bag–mask device: also called an Ambu bag, this device is used to provide assisted ventilation if the newborn does not breathe effectively on her own

Bulb suction: this item removes fluid from the newborn's mouth and nose as needed after birth

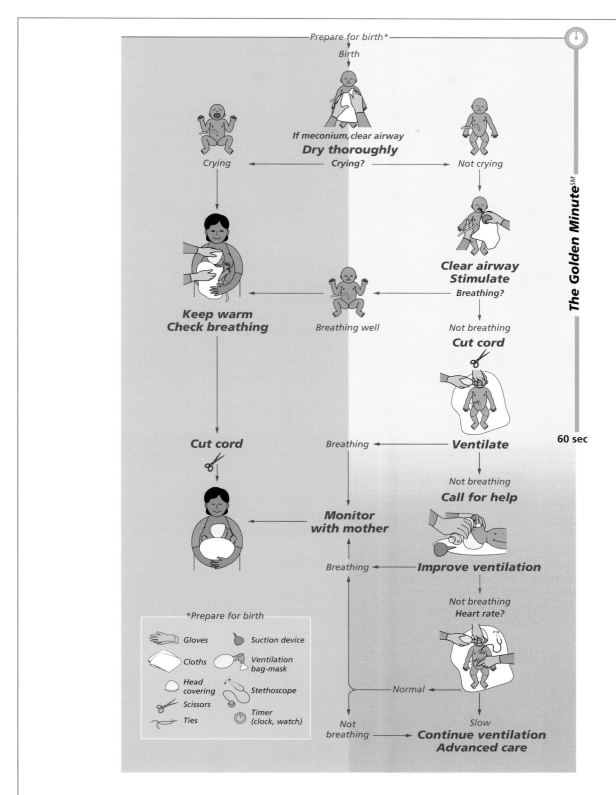

Figure 7.1 Helping Babies Breathe algorithm. Used with permission of the American Academy of Pediatrics, Guide for implementation of Helping Babies Breathe (2011).

for every newborn within the so-called "golden minute" of life. Since its introduction, HBB has received wide endorsement and has quickly become a central global strategy for reducing newborn mortality and achieving Millennium Development Goal 4 (UNICEF, 2007).

Clinical experience

"We were at a rural health facility in South Sudan, where I was helping a US pediatrician train local midwives in basic newborn resuscitation. In the middle of our training, local hospital staff came running in and eagerly beckoned us to the OB/GYN operating theater. A baby had just been delivered by C-section but was not breathing. We arrived and found the baby blue, limp, and with no signs of life. Using the simple steps we had just been teaching, we helped the hospital staff resuscitate the baby. After just a minute or two, a shout of excitement went up from the staff as the baby began breathing and crying on her own! It was so rewarding to me and our trainees to witness firsthand the incredible effectiveness of these steps. A baby who would otherwise have probably passed away, instead quickly received simple life-saving resuscitation and was now a healthy newborn."

Ellie, medical student working in South Sudan

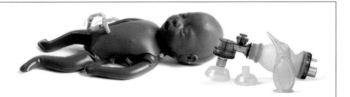

Figure 7.2 Innovative newborn resuscitation training mannequin (NeoNatalie) and equipment. *Source*: Laerdal Global Health. Reproduced with permission of Laerdal Global Health.

Facilitating the HBB program are several important innovations in affordable resuscitative devices and training equipment. Historically, implementation and dissemination of newborn resuscitation management were significantly limited by inaccessible and prohibitively expensive equipment. Bag–mask resuscitation devices and bulb suction devices that are used in developed countries are frequently single-use items and relatively costly. Similarly, conventional newborn training mannequins are exorbitantly expensive, costing hundreds or thousands of US dollars, and are therefore also impractical for large-scale implementation in resource-limited settings (PATH & USAID, 2010).

To address these barriers, Laerdal Global Health recently developed cost-effective resuscitative equipment designed specifically for resource-limited settings and that include a reusable bag–mask device, bulb suction, and newborn training resuscitator (Figure 7.2). The bag–mask device and bulb suction are boilable after each use and cost a fraction of previous equipment. Laerdal's training resuscitator, named NeoNatalie, can be inflated with air or filled with water and includes functional lungs and umbilical cord pulse, depending on the model. Together these make resuscitation training and equipment provision much more accessible to healthcare facilities and providers in low- and middle-income countries.

Overview of newborn resuscitation

Arguably one of the most impactful and effective interventions in medicine is newborn resuscitation for the management of perinatal asphyxia. Simple resuscitative procedures, such as warming, drying, stimulating, and ventilating, are sufficient for managing the overwhelming majority of asphyxiated newborns (Kattwinkel, 2006; Kattwinkel *et al.*, 2010). The following are the basic steps in newborn resuscitation (Figure 7.3).

Warming and drying

When first delivered, a newborn should always be immediately warmed and dried (Figure 7.3a). Wet newborns are at very high risk of losing critical body heat. Warming and drying of the

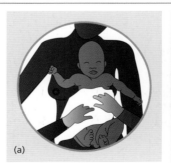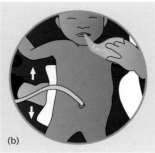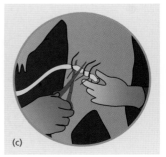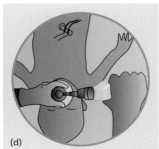

(a)   (b)   (c)   (d)

Figure 7.3 The basic steps in newborn resuscitation: (a) warming and drying; (b) bulb suction and stimulation; (c) cutting the umbilical cord; and (d) bag–mask ventilation.

newborn is accomplished by using multiple dry cloths (removing wet cloths) and can be performed while the newborn is placed on the mother's abdomen and before cutting of the umbilical cord.

Bulb suction and stimulation

If the newborn is not breathing well after warming and drying, the provider should clear secretions from the newborn's mouth and then nose using a bulb suction (or the corner of a clean cloth if bulb suction is not available). Secretions in the newborn's upper airway can impede breathing and possibly lead to aspiration of secretions into the lungs. However, if the newborn is crying and breathing well, the newborn does not typically need bulb suctioning.

A newborn that is not breathing well after quickly warming, drying, and bulb suctioning needs additional stimulation to breathe (Figure 7.3b). This stimulation is achieved by further rubbing the newborn's back with a dry cloth. By now, the overwhelming majority of newborns will be breathing well with good tone, color, and heart rate (>100 beats per minute). If the newborn does not improve with stimulation, it is important to move quickly to the next step in resuscitation.

The issue of meconium

Before delivery, while *in utero*, some newborns expel fetal stool, or meconium, which may be an indicator that the newborn was under stress. If inhaled into the lungs upon the newborn's first breath, meconium can be dangerous and possibly lead to meconium aspiration syndrome. Therefore, if meconium is present at delivery and the newborn has not yet cried or taken a breath, the likelihood of meconium aspiration may be decreased by clearing the newborn's mouth and nose with a bulb suction before drying or stimulating the newborn. (See section Advanced resuscitation for the approach to meconium in resource-rich settings.) Once the newborn has taken that first breath, however, prevention of meconium aspiration is no longer the aim and providers should follow typical newborn resuscitation steps.

Cutting the umbilical cord

After the initial resuscitative steps, which should all occur within the first 30 seconds of life, the newborn will either be breathing well on her own or will require immediate additional resuscitative steps. If additional resuscitation is needed, the umbilical cord should be quickly tied and cut (Figure 7.3c) so that the newborn can be taken to the mother's side or another clean surface for further resuscitation. However, if the newborn is breathing well, there is no urgency in tying and cutting the umbilical cord; it can be cut between 1 and 3 minutes of life.

In either case, cutting the umbilical cord needs to be done in a clean manner since the newborn can become extremely ill if the scissors, razor blade, umbilical ties, or hands of the birth attendant are unclean. Before cutting the cord, two to three ties should be firmly placed a couple of centimeters above the abdominal skin such that, when the cord is cut between them, there remains one to two firm ties on the newborn's umbilical stump and one tie on the cord segment attached to the placenta (see Chapter 6).

Bag–mask ventilation

If the newborn is not breathing well or crying after initial warming, drying, and stimulating, the newborn needs immediate ventilation with a bag–mask device, or Ambu bag (Figure 7.3d). In fact, all newborns should either be breathing well or receiving assisted ventilation within 30–60 seconds of birth.

The newborn bag–mask device is placed over the newborn's nose and mouth and should be properly sized to reach from the bridge of the nose to the tip of the chin. The mask is held tightly to the face using a C-shaped grip, with thumb and index finger on the mask and the remaining fingers on the newborn's mandible. The newborn's chin should be tilted slightly upward into the "sniffing position" to maximize airway patency. The provider then uses the other hand to squeeze the bag at a rate of 40–60 breaths per minute while observing the newborn's chest for adequate chest rise. If air is heard escaping from around the mask or if there is inadequate chest rise, the provider should reposition and try again.

Bag–mask ventilation is continued until the newborn is breathing well without assistance (or after 10–20 minutes of proper resuscitation without response). Advanced providers may use the newborn's heart rate, along with spontaneous breaths, as an indicator for continued bag–mask ventilation. A newborn that is breathing well should have a heart rate greater than 100 beats per minute. A heart rate less than 100 means that the newborn still needs assisted ventilation. One of the easiest ways to assess the newborn heart rate is to feel for a pulse by gently pinching the base of the umbilical stump.

When to discontinue resuscitation

There is increasing evidence that basic resuscitation can prevent around 30% of the neonatal deaths caused by intrapartum complications (Wall *et al.*, 2009). Unfortunately in some cases, newborns will have absent heartbeats and lack spontaneous breaths despite adequate resuscitation efforts. The decision to end resuscitation efforts can pose difficult emotional challenges for care providers and families.

Guidelines from HBB and the WHO suggest that resuscitation should end after 10 minutes of correct resuscitation. if there is no detectable heart rate and no spontaneous breathing. In newborns with heart rates remaining below 60 beats per minute after 20 minutes of correct resuscitation, resuscitative efforts should then stop. There is very little evidence to suggest that efforts extending beyond these time frames are effective, and most newborns will suffer significant morbidity and mortality as a result (Kapoor & Kapoor, 2007).

There are circumstances in which resuscitation may be withheld altogether. This is the case when a newborn suffers from a condition that will almost certainly result in early mortality. Typically, these are newborns with extreme prematurity, low birthweight, or fatal congenital anomalies. Individual cases should be discussed with the health team and family members to determine the best course of action. Definitions of what constitutes extreme prematurity and birthweight can vary, so it is best to follow local standards in the decision-making process (Wall *et al.*, 2009).

Clinical pearl: discussing traditional birth practices

During your work abroad, you may come across a variety of traditional clinical practices. Traditional practitioners are frequently central, respected members of a community who can be strong partners in your efforts. They often have not had the opportunity of formal health training but will often welcome learning new approaches.

In many rural areas of developing countries, a large majority of deliveries still occur outside of health facilities among community-based traditional birth attendants (TBAs). TBAs may still use traditional practices that run counter to evidence-based medical practice. Practices for managing birth asphyxia that do not help the newborn and can actually be dangerous include holding the newborn upside down, slapping the newborn on its back, splashing water on the newborn, and making loud noises above the newborn to stimulate breathing.

Ask local practitioners what traditional practices are in use in your area. Whenever possible, build relationships with key stakeholders and TBAs. In a non-judgmental way, explain that some practices may have been widely used but have been shown to be less effective or even dangerous. Express confidence and excitement in the evidence-based newborn resuscitation interventions in this chapter. Traditional practitioners are equally committed to helping the newborn and will become excited about these approaches as they witness their effectiveness.

Advanced resuscitation

In resource-rich settings, such as in North America and Europe, trained providers utilize advanced resuscitative procedures that are not frequently used in resource-limited settings. These advanced procedures include intubating the newborn airway to improve assisted ventilation. Chest compressions are initiated when the heart rate remains particularly low (<60 beasts per minute) despite proper assisted ventilation. Medications such as epinephrine (adrenaline) can also be administered as needed.

In the specific case of meconium, trained providers in resource-rich settings will momentarily intubate and suction the airway of meconium-stained newborns if they have not yet cried or taken their first breath. Using a laryngoscope, a newborn endotracheal tube is inserted past the epiglottis, suction is applied to remove any meconium present, and the tube is then immediately removed. Newborn resuscitation is subsequently continued as usual.

However, in the overwhelming majority of developing settings, where resources and training are frequently limited, these advanced resuscitative procedures and elective intubation for meconium are usually not recommended. An exception may be at tertiary referral centers that have trained staff and critical care units for resuscitated newborns.

Additional resources

- American Academy of Pediatrics. Helping Babies Breathe. Available at http://www.helpingbabiesbreathe.org
- World Health Organization. Guidelines on basic newborn resuscitation. Available at http://www.who.int/maternal_child_adolescent/documents/basic_newborn_resuscitation/en/index.html
- American Academy of Pediatrics and American Heart Association (2010) *Textbook of Neonatal Resuscitation*, 6th edn. Elk Grove Village, IL: American Academy of Pediatrics and American Heart Association.
- Wall SN, Lee AC, Niermeyer S *et al.* (2009) Neonatal resuscitation in low-resource settings: what, who, and how to overcome challenges to scale up? *Int J Gynaecol Obstet* 107(Suppl. 1):S47–62, S63–4.

REFERENCES

American Academy of Pediatrics (2014) Helping Babies Breathe. Available at http://www.helpingbabiesbreathe.org/

Bhutta ZA, Soofi S, Cousens S et al. (2011) Improvement of perinatal and newborn care in rural Pakistan through community-based strategies: a cluster-randomised effectiveness trial. *Lancet* 377:403–12.

Darmstadt GL, Yakoob MY, Haws RA, Menezes EV, Soomro T, Bhutta ZA (2009) Reducing stillbirths: interventions during labour. *BMC Pregnancy Childbirth* 9(Suppl. 1):S6.

Herbert HK, Lee AC, Chandran A, Rudan I, Baqui AH (2012) Care seeking for neonatal illness in low- and middle-income countries: a systematic review. *PLoS Med* 9(3):e1001183.

International Liaison Committee on Resuscitation (2006) The International Liaison Committee on Resuscitation (ILCOR) consensus on science with treatment recommendations for pediatric and neonatal patients: pediatric basic and advanced life support. *Pediatrics* 117:e955–77.

Kapoor SH, Kapoor D (2007) Review article: Neonatal resuscitation. *Indian J Crit Care Med* 11:81–9.

Kattwinkel J (ed.) (2006) *Textbook of Neonatal Resuscitation*, 5th edn. Elk Grove Village, IL: American Academy of Pediatrics and American Heart Association.

Kattwinkel J, Perlman JM, Aziz K *et al.* (2010) Neonatal resuscitation: 2010 American Heart Association Guidelines for Cardiopulmonary Resuscitation and Emergency Cardiovascular Care. *Pediatrics* 126:e1400–13.

Lawn JE, Cousens S, Zupan J (2005) Lancet neonatal survival steering team. 4 million neonatal deaths: when? where? why? *Lancet* 365:891–900.

Lawn JE, Cousens SN, Darmstadt GL *et al.* (2006) Lancet Neonatal Survival Series steering team. 1 year after Lancet Neonatal Survival Series: was the call for action heard? *Lancet* 367:1541–7.

Lawn JE, Bahl R, Bergstrom S *et al.* (2011) Setting research priorities to reduce almost one million deaths from birth asphyxia by 2015. *PLoS Med* 8(1):e1000389.

Lee AC, Cousens S, Darmstadt GL *et al.* (2011a) Care during labor and birth for the prevention of intrapartum-related neonatal deaths: a systematic review and Delphi estimation of mortality effect. *BMC Public Health* 11(Suppl. 3):S10.

Lee AC, Cousens S, Wall SN *et al.* (2011b) Neonatal resuscitation and immediate newborn assessment and stimulation for the prevention of neonatal deaths: a systematic review, meta-analysis and Delphi estimation of mortality effect. *BMC Public Health* 11(Suppl. 3): S12.

Msemo G, Massawe A, Mmbando D *et al.* (2013) Newborn mortality and fresh stillbirth rates in Tanzania after Helping Babies Breathe training. *Pediatrics* 131:e353–60.

PATH & USAID (2010) Practical selection of neonatal resuscitators, version 3: a field guide. Available at http://www.path.org/publications/detail.php?i=1565

Sibley LM, Sipe TA, Brown CM, Diallo MM, McNatt K, Habarta N (2007) Traditional birth attendant training for improving health behaviours and pregnancy outcomes. *Cochrane Database Syst Rev* (3): CD005460.

UNICEF (2007) MDG 4: Reduce child mortality: newborn care. Available at http://www.unicef.org/progressforchildren/2007n6/index_41806.htm

Wall SN, Lee AC, Niermeyer S, *et al.* (2009) Neonatal resuscitation in low-resource settings: what, who, and how to overcome challenges to scale up? *Int J Gynaecol Obstet* 107(Suppl. 1):S47–62, S63–4.

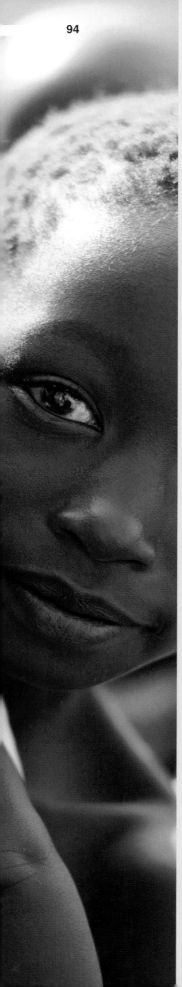

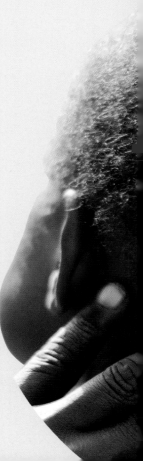

CHAPTER 8
Acute Respiratory Infections

Nancy E. Ringel[1], Tabish Hazir[2], Sylvia V. Romm[3], and Shamim A. Qazi[4]
[1]Harvard Medical School, Boston, MA, USA
[2]Pakistan Institute of Medical Sciences, Islamabad, Pakistan
[3]Boston University School of Medicine and Massachusetts General Hospital, Boston, MA, USA
[4]World Health Organization, Geneva, Switzerland

Key learning objectives

■ Understand the global burden and epidemiology of acute respiratory infections.

■ Understand that childhood pneumonia must be diagnosed and treated in a timely manner to prevent death.

■ Understand how to diagnose pneumonia in children.

■ Learn other important causes of acute respiratory infections in children, including croup, epiglottitis, bronchiolitis, and acute otitis media.

■ Realize the importance of preventing acute respiratory infection in resource-limited settings.

Abstract

Acute respiratory infections (ARIs) are illnesses caused by an acute infection of the respiratory tract, usually with a virus or bacterium. ARIs are extremely common in children and contribute significantly to childhood morbidity and mortality around the world. Pneumonia is a leading cause of mortality in children aged 1–5 and requires prompt diagnosis and treatment to prevent death. Management of pneumonia varies depending on the severity of illness; many cases may be appropriately treated with community-based interventions, although care at higher-level health facilities may be necessary with more severe infections. Other ARIs that contribute significantly to global child morbidity and mortality include croup, epiglottitis, bronchiolitis, and acute otitis media. Risk factors for children developing ARIs include lack of vaccination, poor nutritional status, and environmental exposures such as indoor cooking smoke. Since controlling these risk factors can significantly reduce the burden of ARIs in children, medical personnel must consider integrating respiratory protection strategies into the healthcare maintenance of their patients.

Key words: acute respiratory infections, pneumonia, croup, epiglottitis, bronchiolitis, acute otitis media, bronchitis, child mortality

Introduction and epidemiology

Acute respiratory infections (ARIs) are illnesses caused by an acute infection of the respiratory tract, which includes the nose, sinuses, pharynx, larynx, trachea, bronchi, bronchioles, and the alveoli. ARIs are classified by which part of the respiratory tract is infected, and different types of infections are more common in certain locations (Figure 8.1).

The number of pneumonia deaths is estimated to be 1 million each year (WHO *et al.*, 2013b; WHO, 2014a). ARIs are the leading cause of morbidity and mortality in young children outside the neonatal period, comprising nearly half of all illnesses in children less than 5 years old and one-third of illnesses in children aged 5–12 years. Children under 5 have an average of three to six ARIs each year, and these infections comprise 30–40% of childhood hospital admissions (Nair *et al.*, 2013). Most significantly, ARIs are responsible for over 1.2 million deaths among children under the age of 5 each year, more than the combination of AIDS, malaria, and tuberculosis (WHO/UNICEF, 2013a).

Risk factors for children developing ARIs include being unvaccinated against common pathogens, poor nutritional status, and environmental exposures such as indoor cooking smoke. Controlling these risk factors can significantly reduce the burden of ARIs in children.

A number of different pathogens are known to commonly cause ARIs in children. These are largely airborne microbes, mostly viruses and bacteria, and are easily spread in communities from one person to another. *Streptococcus pneumoniae* and *Haemophilus influenzae* type B are the two most common bacterial causes of childhood pneumonia and yet are also vaccine-preventable (Rudan *et al.*, 2013). Respiratory syncytial virus (RSV) and influenza are the two most common viral organisms responsible for ARIs in children (Nair *et al.*, 2010).

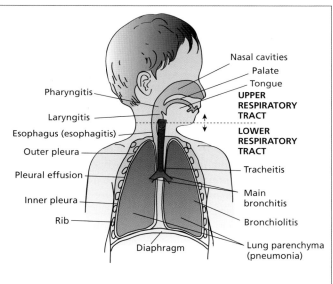

Figure 8.1 Infections of the respiratory tract.

Pneumonia presentation

Children with pneumonia often present with tachypnea, fever, and cough. As young children are often unable to communicate their symptoms, mothers and caregivers often notice signs of a child seeming "unwell," which manifests differently depending on the age of the child.

In neonates, an unwell child is often identified first by the parent, who may provide a history of the child acting "sick," having a tactile fever, breathing unusually quickly, or acting lethargic. In older children, similar signs are often recognized, but the child may also be able to communicate that he or she is feeling unwell. The child may also have more typical respiratory symptoms, such as having a cough and/or wheezing; however, a presentation with wheezing should be considered carefully as wheeze is often indicative of other respiratory conditions such as bronchiolitis or asthma. Features suggestive of pneumonia include fever, sick contacts, and malaise.

Severe pneumonia is defined as pneumonia with at least one of the following additional features:

- central cyanosis;
- oxygen saturation <90% on pulse oximetry;
- severe respiratory distress;
- inability to breastfeed/feed;
- lethargy/unconsciousness;
- convulsions;
- severe malnutrition.

Early recognition of severe pneumonia is essential in order to provide appropriate treatment for what can be a life-threatening illness.

Diagnosis of pneumonia

The diagnosis of pneumonia in children typically depends on the setting (e.g., community or facility level), available resources, as well as the age of the child. A brief discussion follows of how pneumonia is initially assessed and diagnosed in both the community and healthcare facility settings.

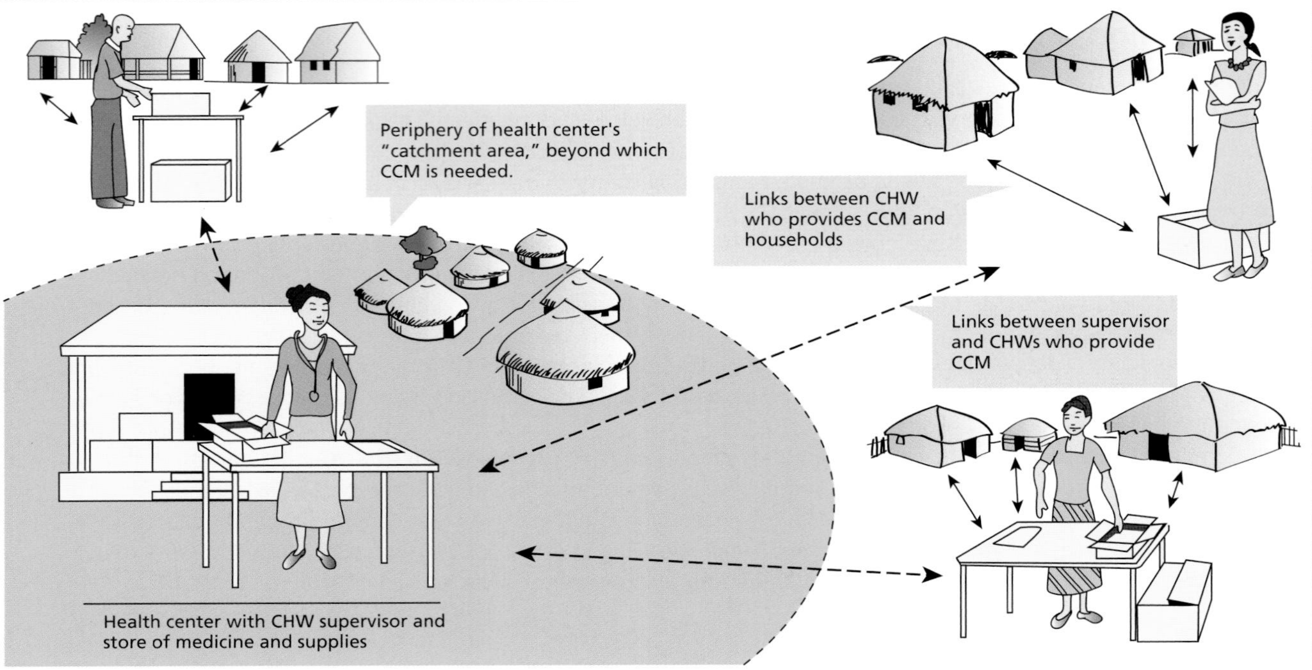

Figure 8.2 Community health workers (CHWs) play a critical role in the identification and community case management (CCM) of ARIs and other health conditions. *Source*: World Health Organization/United Nations Children's Fund (2012). Reproduced with permission of the World Health Organization.

Community-based assessment and case management

Most ARIs are first detected in the community setting. Community health workers should be able to correctly assess infection severity and subsequently choose the appropriate treatment for that severity. The World Health Organization (WHO) and UNICEF report that only 60% of caregivers actively seek care for suspected pneumonia in children (WHO & UNICEF, 2013a), thereby making properly trained community-based health workers a critical element for an effective pneumonia management strategy (Figure 8.2). As treatment of severe pneumonia requires care in a health facility, community-based providers must be able to differentiate severe pneumonia from less severe ARIs. Integrated community case management (iCCM) algorithms were designed to assist community-based workers in appropriately triaging care and beginning treatment of ARI at the community level.

Facility-based assessment and case management

Most cases of pneumonia can be correctly diagnosed and treated effectively by community health workers. However, some children will require referral to a nearby health facility for further evaluation.

While iCCM algorithms were developed for community-based management, the Integrated Management of Childhood Illness (IMCI) guidelines are designed for the facility-based

management of common childhood illnesses by healthcare providers, including managing ARIs at outpatient clinics and first-level facilities. IMCI treatment approaches for pneumonia differ in newborns up to 2 months of age compared with older children. Figure 8.3 displays two examples of IMCI algorithms that illustrate the recommended management of newborns and older children who present with acute respiratory symptoms.

Some children may also require further evaluation (chest X-ray, laboratory tests, etc.) or treatment that cannot be provided at home, such as injectable antibiotics, oxygen, and inhaled bronchodilators through a nebulizer. Treatment of severe pneumonia in a hospital should be considered if IMCI algorithms indicate that higher-level care may be needed, or if "general danger signs" are present, as discussed in the following section.

Physical examination

On physical examination, many findings can be helpful in diagnosing and determining the severity of pneumonia. Signs suggestive of pneumonia (Figure 8.4) include:

- increased respiratory rate ($\geq$60 breaths/min in children <2 months, $\geq$50 breaths/min in children 2–11 months, and $\geq$40 breaths/min in children 1–5 years);
- lower chest wall indrawing;
- grunting, nasal flaring, audible wheeze;

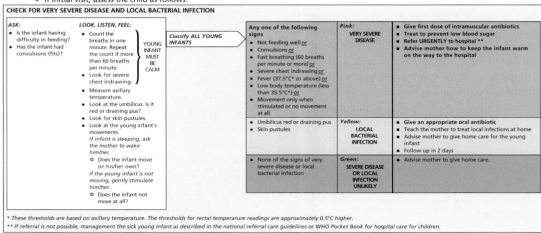

ASSESS AND CLASSIFY THE SICK YOUNG INFANT

ASSESS	CLASSIFY	IDENTIFY TREATMENT

ASK THE MOTHER WHAT THE CHILD'S PROBLEMS ARE

- Determine if this is an initial or follow-up visit for this problem.
    - if follow-up visit, use the follow-up instructions on TREAT THE CHILD chart.
    - if initial visit, assess the child as follows:

USE ALL BOXES THAT MATCH THE CHILD'S SYMPTOMS AND PROBLEMS TO CLASSIFY THE ILLNESS

CHECK FOR GENERAL DANGER SIGNS

Ask:
- Is the child able to drink or breastfeed?
- Does the child vomit everything?
- Has the child had convulsions?

Look:
- See if the child is lethargic or unconscious.
- Is the child convulsing now?

URGENT attention

• Any general danger sign	**Pink:** VERY SEVERE DISEASE	■ Give diazepam if convulsing now ■ Quickly complete the assessment ■ Give any pre-referal treatment immediately ■ Treat to prevent low blood sugar ■ Keep the child warm ■ Refer URGENTLY.

A child with any general danger sign needs *URGENT* attention; complete the assessment and any pre-referral treatment immediately so referral is not delayed.

THEN ASK ABOUT MAIN SYMPTOMS:
Does the child have cough or difficult breathing?

If yes, ask:
- For how long?

Look, listen, feel*:
- Count the breaths in one minute.
- Look for chest indrawing.
- Look and listen for stridor.
- Look and listen for wheezing.

CHILD MUST BE CALM

If wheezing with either fast breathing or chest indrawing:
Give a trial of rapid acting inhaled bronchodilator for up to three times 15-20 minutes apart. Count the breaths and look for chest indrawing again, and then classify.

If the child is:
2 months up to 12 months

12 Months up to 5 years

Fast breathing is:
50 breaths per minute or more

40 breaths per minute or more

Classify COUGH or DIFFICULT BREATHING

• Any general danger sign or • Stridor in calm child.	**Pink:** SEVERE PNEUMONIA OR VERY SEVERE DISEASE	■ Give first dose of an appropriate antibiotic ■ Refer URGENTLY to hospital**
• Chest indrawing or • Fast breathing.	**Yellow:** PNEUMONIA	■ Give oral Amoxicillin for 5 days*** ■ If wheezing (or disappeared after rapidly acting bronchodilator) give an inhaled bronchodilator for 5 days**** ■ If chest indrawing in HIV exposed/infected child, give first dose of amoxicillin and refer. ■ Soothe the throat and relieve the cough with a safe remedy ■ If coughing for more than 14 days or recurrent wheeze, refer for possible TB or asthma assessment ■ Advise mother when to return immediately ■ Follow-up in 3 days
• No signs of pneumonia or very severe disease.	**Green:** COUGH OR COLD	■ If wheezing (or disappeared after rapidly acting bronchodilator) give an inhaled bronchodilator for 5 days**** ■ Soothe the throat and relieve the cough with a safe remedy ■ If coughing for more than 14 days or recurrent wheeze, refer for possible TB or asthma assessment ■ Advise mother when to return immediately ■ Follow-up in 5 days if not improving

*If pulse oximeter is available, determine oxygen saturation and refer if < 90%.

** If referral is not possible, manage the child as described in the pneumonia section of the national referral guidelines or as in WHO Pocket Book for hospital care for children.

***Oral Amoxicillin for 3 days could be used in patients with fast breathing but no chest indrawing in low HIV settings.

**** In settings where inhaled bronchodilator is not available, oral salbutamol may be tried but not recommended for treatment of severe acute wheeze.

(a)

ASSESS AND CLASSIFY THE SICK CHILD

ASSESS	CLASSIFY	IDENTIFY TREATMENT

DO A RAPID APRAISAL OF ALL WAITING INFANTS
ASK THE MOTHER WHAT THE YOUNG INFANT'S PROBLEMS ARE

- Determine if this is an initial or follow-up visit for this problem.
    - if follow-up visit, use the follow-up instructions.
    - if initial visit, assess the child as follows:

USE ALL BOXES THAT MATCH THE INFANT'S SYMPTOMS AND PROBLEMS TO CLASSIFY THE ILLNESS

CHECK FOR VERY SEVERE DISEASE AND LOCAL BACTERIAL INFECTION

ASK:
- Is the infant having difficulty in feeding?
- Has the infant had convulsions (fits)?

LOOK, LISTEN, FEEL:
- Count the breaths in one minute. Repeat the count if more than 60 breaths per minute.
- Look for severe chest indrawing.
- Measure axillary temperature.
- Look at the umbilicus. Is it red or draining pus?
- Look for skin pustules.
- Look at the young infant's movements. *If infant is sleeping, ask the mother to wake him/her.*
    - Does the infant move on his/her own? *If the young infant is not moving, gently stimulate him/her.*
    - Does the infant not move at all?

YOUNG INFANT MUST BE CALM

Classify ALL YOUNG INFANTS

Any one of the following signs • Not feeding well or • Convulsions or • Fast breathing (60 breaths per minute or more) or • Severe chest indrawing or • Fever (37.5°C* or above) or • Low body temperature (less than 35.5°C*) or • Movement only when stimulated or no movement at all.	**Pink:** VERY SEVERE DISEASE	■ Give first dose of intramuscular antibiotics ■ Treat to prevent low blood sugar ■ Refer URGENTLY to hospital ** ■ Advise mother how to keep the infant warm on the way to the hospital
• Umbilicus red or draining pus • Skin pustules	**Yellow:** LOCAL BACTERIAL INFECTION	■ Give an appropriate oral antibiotic ■ Teach the mother to treat local infections at home ■ Advise mother to give home care for the young infant ■ Follow up in 2 days
• None of the signs of very severe disease or local bacterial infection	**Green:** SEVERE DISEASE OR LOCAL INFECTION UNLIKELY	■ Advise mother to give home care.

* These thresholds are based on axillary temperature. The thresholds for rectal temperature readings are approximately 0.5°C higher.

** If referral is not possible, management the sick young infant as described in the national referral care guidelines or WHO Pocket Book for hospital care for children.

(b)

Figure 8.3 IMCI algorithm for the facility-based management of ARIs in (a) young infants up to 2 months of age and (b) children 2 months to 5 years.

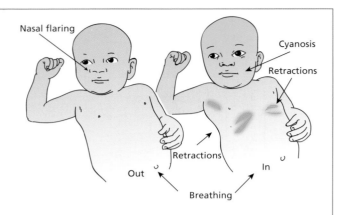

Figure 8.4 Signs suggestive of pneumonia in children.

- stridor;
- cyanosis;
- tachycardia;
- crackles, decreased air entry, or bronchial breath sounds heard in lung fields on auscultation.

The presence of any general danger signs is cause for referral to a higher-level health facility. These signs are used by IMCI practitioners to identify very ill children and include:

- a child who is unable to drink or breastfeed;
- a child who is vomiting all intake;
- a child with convulsions/seizures with the current illness;
- a child who is lethargic or unconscious.

Imaging

In most cases in resource-limited settings, a diagnosis of pneumonia is made clinically. However, when available, a chest X-ray may be helpful in establishing a diagnosis. Chest X-ray can also be useful in the management of a patient who has not had improvement of symptoms or has had worsening of symptoms after initial antibiotic management. While chest X-rays often confirm the diagnosis of pneumonia, some serious infections may have normal imaging, such as in HIV-positive patients or those infected with *Pneumocystis jiroveci* pneumonia (commonly known as PCP). Figure 8.5 shows illustrations of chest X-ray findings consistent with pneumonia.

Laboratory studies

Several laboratory studies and clinical data points can be used to support a diagnosis of pneumonia.

- Pulse oximetry helps to detect hypoxia and can guide when to start and stop oxygen therapy.

- Complete blood count can demonstrate evidence of infection and confirm or exclude other causes of shortness of breath such as anemia.
- Bacterial studies, including sputum Gram stains, cultures, and various antigen tests, although these are often unavailable in low-resource settings.

Differential diagnosis

As with any clinical presentation, it is important to consider not just the signs and symptoms that are consistent with pneumonia but also what other conditions those signs and symptoms may represent (Table 8.1). If the cough has been persistent for more than 2 weeks, the WHO recommends evaluating for chronic illnesses, including tuberculosis. Tuberculosis may be endemic in many areas and therefore it is important to keep this diagnosis on the differential (WHO, 2013).

Pneumonia treatment

The ideal treatment for pneumonia involves appropriate antibiotic therapy, supportive care, and clinical follow-up after initiation of therapy. However, adherence to this treatment course is often limited by long distances between patients and clinics, lack of transportation, drug stock-outs at health facilities, shortage of diagnostic equipment, insufficient access to clean water for rehydration, and numerous other hurdles that vary from community to community. The WHO has established guidelines for the treatment of pneumonia that all health systems should strive to achieve, but the persistent prevalence of morbidity and mortality from pneumonia in children is evidence that there is still progress to be made in the efforts to make access to this care universal.

WHO guidelines for pneumonia and severe pneumonia

Outpatient management is recommended for pneumonia that does not fall under the category of "severe" (Figure 8.6). Outpatient management includes at-home administration of oral amoxicillin 40 mg/kg twice daily for 3–5 days (3 days is sufficient for uncomplicated pneumonia, but a 5-day course should be used in HIV settings). Supportive care in the home with rest and hydration with clean water is also recommended in non-exclusively breast fed children. The caregiver of a sick child should also be instructed to immediately report to a health facility with the child if the child displays any signs of severe pneumonia and to also follow up within 3 days of diagnosis regardless of the child's clinical status (WHO, 2013).

For severe pneumonia, children need to be treated in the inpatient setting. Patients should be admitted to a hospital where their airways can be monitored and where intubation is available should the child show signs of respiratory compromise.

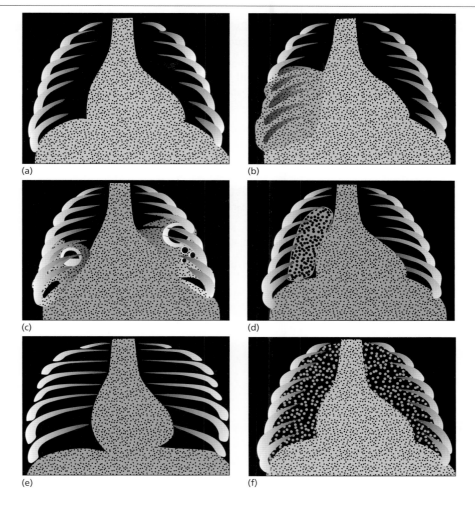

Figure 8.5 Chest X-rays with findings consistent with pneumonia. (a) Normal chest X-ray: the lungs are clear and there are no consolidations. (b) Lobar pneumonia: note the consolidation in the right lower lobe (consolidations can occur in any of the lobes of the lung). (c) Staphylococcal pneumonia: a serious bacterial pneumonia shown here with fluid-filled abscesses and pneumatoceles. (d) Pneumothorax: while not a type of pneumonia, collapse of a lung can cause shortness of breath. An X-ray of a pneumothorax may show a more transparent margin without lung markings around the periphery of the collapsed lung, and the collapsed lung may also appear more dense, as illustrated here. Whereas, a non-collapsed lung will have lung markings all the way to the periphery. (e) Hyperinflated chest X-ray: features are an increased transverse diameter, ribs running more horizontally, a small contour of the heart, and flattened diaphragm. (f) Miliary tuberculosis: tuberculosis can cause symptoms similar to pneumonia but typically looks different on chest X-ray. Note the small patchy consolidations diffusely throughout the lung.

Use of oxygen

Oxygen therapy is also often required in cases of severe pneumonia when a patient's pulse oximetry measures less than 90% and the patient has signs of respiratory distress. In resource-limited settings, affordable delivery systems for oxygen therapy may be unavailable.

Two options for oxygen therapy include oxygen tanks and concentrators, each having their own benefits and drawbacks. Tanks have a finite supply of oxygen; they therefore need to be refilled regularly and are not always a sustainable choice for all health facilities. Concentrators, on the other hand, produce concentrated oxygen from room air, so they are more practical in areas that lack refilling capabilities; however, they are dependent on electricity or a generator, and many health facilities do not have consistent access to these resources. These limitations illustrate that new advances in oxygen delivery systems are needed in resource-limited settings.

Antibiotics

Increasing access to treatment is necessary to decrease the current levels of morbidity and mortality associated with pneumonia. According to the WHO, only 31% of children with suspected pneumonia receive antibiotics (WHO & UNICEF, 2013a). While the antibiotics used to treat the most common bacterial causes of pneumonia in children are affordable and a part of the WHO Essential Medicines List, stock-outs within

Table 8.1 Differential diagnosis of pneumonia.

Condition	Characteristic signs and symptoms that distinguish from pneumonia
Asthma	History of asthma in patient and/or family member Wheezing heard on auscultation Respiratory distress improves with trial dose of bronchodilators
Bronchiolitis	Age less than 2 years Wheeze not responding to inhaled bronchodilators is a predominant symptom Usually, child does not have fever It is a self-limiting infection, usually not needing antibiotics
Pertussis	Bouts of severe cough leading to cyanosis, vomiting, and a characteristic whooping sound Child usually not vaccinated with DTP Relatively unremarkable chest X-ray
Croup	Presence of inspiratory stridor is the diagnostic hallmark Must be differentiated from epiglottitis, which is a pediatric emergency
Diphtheria	Mostly an unvaccinated child for DTP Child sick and toxic On examination of the throat, there is a characteristic membrane, the extent of which varies
Malaria	Cyclic fevers with shaking chills in a child living in an endemic area History of mosquito bite(s) Fast breathing is also present, so malaria is important to consider in a child presenting with this symptom, especially in areas where falciparum is endemic
Severe anemia	Pallor Slow onset of fast breathing Weakness, malaise
Foreign body aspiration	Sudden onset of respiratory distress usually preceded by a violent bout of cough in an otherwise well child A high level of suspicion must mandate an emergency bronchoscopy
Cardiac conditions (e.g., heart failure, congenital heart disease)	Fast breathing accompanied by tachycardia Careful auscultation of the heart and examination of the pulses is essential In congenital heart disease there is a prolonged history

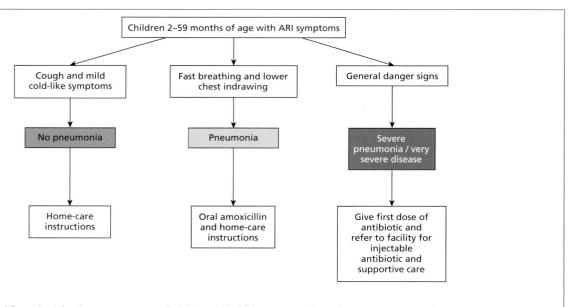

Figure 8.6 A general flow chart for the management of children with ARI symptoms, based on symptom severity.

Table 8.2 Recommended antibiotic therapy for pneumonia and severe pneumonia.

Disease classification	First-line therapy	Second-line therapy
Pneumonia (fast breathing only and/or lower chest indrawing)	Oral amoxicillin 80 mg/kg/day twice daily for 5 days For settings with low HIV prevalence, 3-day treatment is sufficient and therefore recommended	If patient deteriorates, refer to health facility for injectable therapy
Severe pneumonia (presence of general danger signs)	Referral to a health facility Injectable antibiotics: injectable ampicillin 50 mg/kg for 5+ days or benzylpenicillin 50,000 U/kg i.m./i.v. every 6 hours and injectable gentamicin 7.5 mg/kg i.m./i.v. once a day for 5+ days	Injectable ceftriaxone 80 mg/kg i.m./i.v. once daily for 10 days or injectable gentamicin 7.5 mg/kg i.m./i.v. once daily and cloxacillin 50 mg/kg i.m./i.v. every 6 hours for 10 days
Pneumonia in child with HIV or with suspected HIV infection	First-line and second-line treatments are the same as for severe pneumonia, but for 10 days In a child <12 months, or if there are clinical or radiographic signs of PCP in a child 12–59 months of age, also add high-dose co-trimoxazole (8 mg/kg trimethoprim/40 mg/kg sulfamethoxazole i.v. every 8 hours or orally three times daily for 3 weeks)	

facilities are common. Age-appropriate formulations of medicines for children are also not always available, and dosing can be difficult without the ability to accurately measure a child's weight or calculate proper doses of medications.

Practitioners should therefore have a broad spectrum of knowledge regarding appropriate antibiotics and alternatives for treating the most common pathogens, as well as the ability to determine appropriate dosing with existing resources. Inappropriate treatment can lead to clinical worsening and increased complications, so the ultimate goal is for improved supply chain management and delivery of appropriate therapy.

Table 8.2 lists the antibiotics that are considered priority for treatment of pneumonia and other ARIs in children. While these specific antibiotics are recommended in the general WHO guidelines, individual countries and communities may have slightly different antibiotics and treatment algorithms. It is important to adapt treatment choices in a way that considers local needs and available resources.

As indicated, amoxicillin is the primary antibiotic choice for uncomplicated pneumonia in the outpatient setting. Paracetamol (acetaminophen) should also be provided to address mild discomfort and fever. However, if a child does not respond to this treatment or if a child initially presents with general danger signs, then injectable antibiotics and care in a health facility are necessary. First-line injectable antibiotics for pneumonia are ampicillin or benzylpenicillin (Table 8.2). Additionally, adding gentamicin is recommended for children with general danger signs. If the child has a poor response to therapy after 48 hours, treatment should be changed to injectable ceftriaxone as a second-line drug (alternatively, gentamicin plus cloxacillin). In the case of penicillin hypersensitivity, erythromycin is recommended (WHO, 2013).

For pneumonia in children who are, or suspected to be, HIV-positive, first-line treatment is similar to treatment for severe pneumonia, specifically ampicillin plus gentamicin,

but in this case for 10 days. If the patient does not improve within 48 hours, treatment should be changed to ceftriaxone (or gentamicin plus oxacillin if ceftriaxone is not available). If the child is less than 12 months of age, or if there are clinical or radiographic signs of PCP in a child aged 12–59 months, also give high-dose co-trimoxazole (trimethoprim/sulfamethoxazole). See Chapter 18 for details on PCP prophylaxis with co-trimoxazole for HIV-exposed and HIV-infected children.

Pneumonia with complications

Complications of pneumonia include pleural effusion, empyema, lung abscess, pneumothorax, septicemia, and seeding of other organs with infection. All of these complications are extremely serious and require management in a health facility.

Other acute respiratory infections

While pneumonia is of great importance in the world of pediatric ARIs, other respiratory infections also contribute significant morbidity to children around the globe. Table 8.3 summarizes the key features of several important respiratory conditions commonly seen in children. It is critical to also consider these respiratory infections when caring for a child with respiratory symptoms, in order to provide appropriate treatment.

Prevention

Although case management continues to be a major component of our global approach to ARIs, there has been a significant shift in the last decade from a case management-centric approach to a more coordinated pneumonia control strategy

Table 8.3 Features of other common respiratory infections in children.

Condition	Description	Presentation	Diagnosis	Treatment	Vaccine
Acute bronchitis	Viral or bacterial infection causing inflammation of the large bronchi or medium-sized airways, usually lasting days to weeks	Cough, shortness of breath, wheeze, sputum production	Clinical, sputum culture, Gram stain	Supportive care, appropriate antibiotics for sputum with positive Gram stain or culture	No
Common cold	Acute viral infection of the upper respiratory tract, including the nose, sinuses, pharynx, or larynx	Cough, nasal discharge, sore throat, sneezing, low grade fever	Clinical	Supportive care	No
Influenza	Viral infection with aerosol transmission, usually occurring in seasonal epidemics	Chills, fever, nasal discharge, sore throat, headache, cough, fatigue, nausea, vomiting	Clinical, cell culture, molecular assays, rapid tests	Supportive care, oseltamivir for severe cases	Yes
Respiratory syncytial virus (RSV) and bronchiolitis	Viral infection causing inflammation of bronchioles, usually occurring in children <2 years old	Cough, wheezing, shortness of breath	Clinical, rapid RSV testing	Supportive care, oxygen therapy, hypertonic saline	No
Croup	Acute viral infection of the upper airway	"Barking" cough, stridor, hoarseness	Clinical	Single dose of oral steroids	No
Epiglottitis	Bacterial infection and inflammation of the epiglottis, interferes with breathing	Fever, drooling, difficulty swallowing, stridor, hoarseness; later cyanosis and asphyxiation	Clinical via visualization of a red swollen epiglottis; laryngoscopy	Antibiotics (second- or third-generation cephalosporins with penicillin or ampicillin)	Yes (*Haemophilus influenzae* type B vaccine)
Acute otitis media	Infection of the upper airways that leads to blockage of the eustachian tube, which then leads to bacterial infection of the middle ear	Ear pain, irritability, fever, cough, nasal discharge	Clinical; middle ear effusion and inflammation of tympanic membrane	Symptom management with analgesics, conservative therapy, antibiotics, tympanostomy tube in chronic cases	Yes (*Streptococcus pneumoniae, Haemophilus influenzae* type B vaccine)

(WHO & UNICEF, 2014b). The framework to approach pneumonia from a "Protect, Prevent, and Treat" strategy was developed by the WHO and UNICEF, and articulated in the Integrated Global Action Plan for Pneumonia and Diarrhoea (GAPPD). GAPPD aims to reduce morbidity and mortality from both pneumonia and diarrheal illness by utilizing a three-part focus: protecting children by establishing good health practices from birth such as exclusive breastfeeding and adequate complementary feeding; by preventing children from becoming ill by elimination of risk factors and vaccination; and treating children with standard case management.

Vaccinations against ARI-causing pathogens

Vaccinations are a key component of the strategy to prevent pneumonia-associated morbidity and mortality. Vaccine-preventable pneumonias (e.g., those caused by pathogens such as *Streptococcus pneumoniae, Haemophilus influenzae*, and the influenza virus) account for at least one-third of severe pneumonia episodes, and two-thirds of deaths from pneumonia (Walker *et al.*, 2013). Additionally, *Haemophilus influenzae* and *Streptococcus pneumoniae* are responsible for up to 85% of all types of bacterial childhood pneumonia in developing countries. Vaccinations for pertussis and measles are also available, which can prevent other common causes of ARIs in children. *Streptococcus pneumoniae* and *Haemophilus influenzae* type B (Hib) are the two most common bacterial causes of childhood pneumonia, and use of vaccines against these pathogens substantially reduces the disease burden and deaths associated with these infections (WHO & UNICEF, 2013a).

Elimination of risk factors by improved nutrition

Improving childhood nutrition is classified as a "protective" strategy for combating acute respiratory infections, and it is an important preventive strategy for numerous childhood illnesses. Exclusive breastfeeding for 6 months and continued breastfeeding with appropriate complementary feeding has been shown to reduce the onset and severity of pneumonia in infants (Boccolini *et al.*, 2011). There are many other health benefits to exclusive breastfeeding, although effectively implementing behavior change strategies of any form can be very difficult to accomplish and takes time. Only 39% of infants less than 6 months of age are exclusively breastfed according to UNICEF; therefore, continuing to promote this important behavior will be pivotal to pneumonia prevention until there is widespread adoption.

Lessening exposure to environmental risk factors

Addressing indoor air pollution, for example by avoiding unclean-burning fuels and using newer clean-burning stoves, is a high-priority prevention strategy for combating childhood pneumonia. Reduction of household air pollution with improved stoves has been shown to reduce cases of severe pneumonia, which is the major contributor of mortality in pediatric ARIs (Smith *et al.*, 2011). Additionally, safer and more energy-efficient stoves prevent burns, save time, save costs on fuel, and contribute to better development opportunities for households and communities. As the benefits of reducing household air pollution are broad, prevention efforts are strongly emphasizing this tactic.

HIV prevention

HIV infection in children greatly increases their susceptibility to ARI. Thus, prevention of HIV is considered an integral part of the pneumonia prevention strategy and is discussed in detail in Chapter 18. For individuals who are HIV-positive, tuberculosis and PCP are two additional respiratory infections that commonly cause morbidity and mortality.

REFERENCES

Boccolini C, Carvalho M, Oliveira M, Boccolini M (2011) Breastfeeding can prevent hospitalization for pneumonia among children under 1 year old. *J Pediatr (Rio J)* 87:399–404.

Nair H, Nolkes DJ, Gessner BD *et al.* (2010) Global burden of acute lower respiratory infections due to respiratory syncytial virus in young children: a systematic review and meta-analysis. *Lancet* 375:1545–55.

Nair H, Simoes EAF, Rudan I *et al.* (2013) Global and regional burden of hospital admissions for severe acute lower respiratory infections in young children in 2010: a systematic analysis. *Lancet* 381: 1380–90.

Rudan I, O'Brien KL, Nair H *et al.* (2013) Epidemiology and etiology of childhood pneumonia in 2010: estimates of incidence, severe morbidity, mortality, underlying risk factors and causative pathogens for 192 countries. *J Glob Health* 3(1):010401.

Smith K, McCracken J, Weber M *et al.* (2011) Effect of reduction in household air pollution on childhood pneumonia in Guatemala (RESPIRE): a randomized controlled trial. *Lancet* 378:1717–26.

Walker C, Rudan I, Liu L *et al.* (2013) Global burden of pneumonia and diarrhoea. *Lancet* 381:1405–16.

WHO (2013) *Pocket Book of Hospital Care for Children: Guidelines for the Management of Common Illnesses With Limited Resources*, 2nd edn. Geneva: World Health Organization.

WHO/UNICEF (2012) Integrated Community Case Management (iCCM). Geneva: World Health Organization/United Nations Children's Fund.

WHO & UNICEF (2013a) Ending preventable child deaths from pneumonia and diarrhoea by 2025: Global Action Plan for Pneumonia and Diarrhoea (GAPPD). Geneva: World Health Organization/United Nations Children's Fund.

WHO, UNICEF, The World Bank, United Nations Population Division (2013b) Maternal, newborn, child and adolescent health. Levels and Trends in Child Mortality: Report 2013. Available at http://www.who .int/maternal_child_adolescent/documents/levels _trends_child_mortality_2013/en/

WHO & UNICEF (2014a) Integrated Management of Childhood Illnesses. Geneva: World Health Organization/United Nations Children's Fund.

WHO (2014b) Global Health Observatory. Child health. Available at http://www.who.int/gho/child_health/en/ index.html

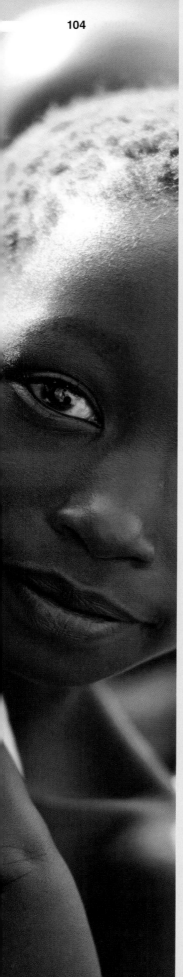

CHAPTER 9
Diarrheal Illness and Rehydration

Ana A. Weil[1], Mohammod Jobayer Chisti[2], and Jason B. Harris[1]

[1]Massachusetts General Hospital, and Harvard Medical School, Boston, MA, USA
[2]International Centre for Diarrhoeal Disease and Research, Dhaka, Bangladesh

Key learning objectives

- Recognize the morbidity and mortality of diarrheal disease in resource-limited settings.
- Understand differences between acute watery, invasive, and persistent diarrhea.
- Understand the clinical assessment and treatment of dehydration.
- Understand the importance of preventing and treating malnutrition in children with diarrhea.
- Understand how to modify treatment of diarrhea among children with severe malnutrition.
- Recognize major complications and comorbidities associated with childhood diarrhea.

Abstract

After newborn causes and acute respiratory infections, diarrheal disease is the third most common cause of death in children under 5 years old. Prompt assessment and treatment of dehydration greatly reduces the mortality of diarrhea in children, and most patients can be effectively treated with oral rehydration solution. Antibiotics are not needed for most causes of acute watery diarrhea but should be given and directed against shigellosis in children with invasive diarrhea. Adjunctive treatment with zinc reduces the severity of diarrheal illness and prevents subsequent episodes of diarrhea. Nutritional support in children with dehydrating diarrhea speeds recovery and prevents malnutrition. Children with preexisting severe malnutrition presenting with diarrhea have a high mortality rate, which may be greatly reduced through a standardized approach involving treatment of comorbid infections (including pneumonia and sepsis) and prevention of complications.

Key words: diarrheal illness, cholera, dysentery, rehydration, oral rehydration solution, malnutrition

Essential Clinical Global Health, First Edition. Edited by Brett D. Nelson.
© 2015 John Wiley & Sons, Ltd. Published 2015 by John Wiley & Sons, Ltd.
Companion website: www.essentialseries.com/globalhealth

Introduction

After newborn causes and acute respiratory infections, diarrheal disease is the third most common cause of death in resource-limited settings in children under 5 years old (Figure 9.1). Diarrheal disease is common and can range from mild disease to severe episodes that cause life-threatening dehydration. The World Health Organization (WHO) defines diarrhea as three or more loose stools in 24 hours. Malnourished children have a higher risk of death in acute diarrheal illness (Pelletier *et al.*, 1995). Prompt treatment of diarrheal disease, including rehydration and nutritional management, reduces the morbidity and mortality of childhood diarrheal illness (World Health Organization, 2005a).

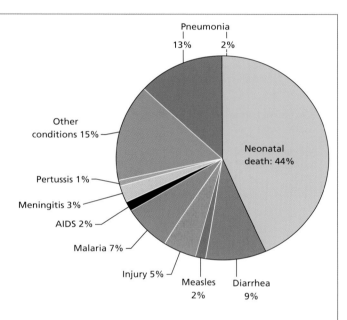

Figure 9.1 Causes of under-five and neonatal mortality worldwide in 2012. *Source*: CHERG and WHO, Global Health Observatory http://www.who.int/gho/child_health/mortality/causes/en/ and Lawn *et al*. 2012. Reproduced with permission.

Epidemiology

Approximately 1 million diarrhea-related deaths occur each year in children under 5 years old, and nearly all take place in developing countries (Liu *et al.*, 2012). Infants in developing countries experience approximately six episodes of diarrhea per year, and children have a median of three episodes per year (Kosek *et al.*, 2003). Risk factors for death from diarrhea include malnutrition, younger age, unsafe food and water, and absence of breastfeeding. Recurrent episodes of diarrhea can lead to a cycle of malnutrition and chronic diarrhea that results in childhood growth deficits (Guerrant *et al.*, 1992).

Most acute diarrheal disease in the developing world is caused by infectious gastroenteritis. While determination of the cause is not always needed to treat diarrheal illness, it is helpful to understand the major causes of childhood diarrhea (Table 9.1).

In a recent study of diarrhea in young children, rotavirus, *Cryptosporidium*, *Shigella*, and enterotoxigenic *Escherichia coli* (ETEC) were among the most important causes in all seven study locations in Asia and Africa (Kotloff *et al.*, 2013). Other causes of diarrhea were only significant in some locations. For example, *Campylobacter jejuni* and *Aeromonas* were major causes of diarrhea in Asia, and *Vibrio cholerae* was a major cause of diarrhea in Asia and in Africa. Age is also an important factor in diarrheal illness. Rotavirus is the most common cause of diarrhea in children aged under 2 years, while *Shigella* is the most common cause of diarrhea in children aged 2–5 years (Kotloff *et al.*, 2013).

Approach to the patient with diarrhea

The approach to the patient with diarrheal illness involves the following five steps:

1. classification of diarrheal illness (acute watery, invasive, or persistent);
2. assessment and management of dehydration;
3. management and prevention of malnutrition;
4. antibiotic treatment of underlying cause of illness, in select cases;
5. identification and management of complications and comorbid conditions.

Classification

Diarrhea can be classified as acute watery diarrhea, invasive diarrhea, or persistent diarrhea (lasting for ≥14 days). This classification is based on important differences in etiologies, and optimal management differs in each category of diarrheal illness.

Table 9.1 Common causes of infectious diarrhea in resource-limited settings.

	Cause of diarrhea	Comments
Pathogens associated with acute watery diarrhea	Rotavirus	Vaccine-preventable illness, yet responsible for the largest burden of disease in infants
	Enterotoxigenic *Escherichia coli* (ETEC)	Common cause of disease in older children, associated with increased risk of death
	Cryptosporidium	Increasingly recognized cause of diarrhea in infants, associated with increased risk of death
	Norovirus	Acute onset, associated with outbreaks
	Vibrio cholerae	Associated with rapid dehydration. Often occurs in large epidemics
	Other viruses	Adenovirus, astrovirus, sapovirus
Pathogens associated with bloody diarrhea[a]	*Shigella* species	Leading cause of invasive diarrhea. Associated with serious systemic and abdominal complications
	Salmonella	Can cause disseminated infection in infants
	Amebiasis	Parasitic infection that can mimic bacterial invasive diarrhea
	Campylobacter species	Can mimic appendicitis and be complicated by Guillain–Barré syndrome
	Enterohemorrhagic *Escherichia coli* (EHEC)	Acute onset, often occurs in small outbreaks, and complicated by hemolytic–uremic syndrome

[a] Most pathogens associated with bloody diarrhea may also cause mild cases of watery diarrhea.

Acute watery diarrhea

Acute watery diarrhea leads to rapid losses of fluids and electrolytes in the stool (Figure 9.2a) and vomitus. In most cases of acute watery diarrhea, it is not necessary to identify a specific cause, and antibiotics are not routinely given. An exception to this is *Vibrio cholerae* infection, which often occurs in epidemics (Box 9.1).

Invasive diarrhea

Invasive diarrhea, also known as dysentery, is diagnosed by the presence of visible blood in the stool. Invasive diarrhea is most often the result of invasive bacterial infection. In invasive diarrhea, the stool may also contains mucus (Figure 9.2b). Fever is common and results from the inflammatory response. The major cause of invasive diarrhea is shigellosis, and empiric antibiotic therapy is aimed at *Shigella* species. However, it is important to recognize that shigellosis cannot be distinguished from other causes of invasive diarrhea solely on clinical grounds.

Persistent diarrhea

Diarrhea lasting 2 weeks or more is classified as persistent diarrhea. In some cases, persistent diarrhea is associated with specific causes of infection such as enteroaggregative *E. coli* or *Cryptosporidium*. However, many cases of persistent diarrhea are thought to be triggered by acute infectious gastroenteritis. In persistent diarrhea, the intestinal injury is long-standing and leads to chronic enteropathy, resulting in failure to absorb nutrients, including the sugar lactose. Persistent diarrhea is also associated with malnutrition and should raise suspicion for HIV infection. In HIV-infected children, unexplained persistent diarrhea is an AIDS-defining illness.

Assessment and management of dehydration

Assessment

The assessment of hydration status must occur immediately in patients presenting with diarrhea. The recognition and treatment of dehydration is critical in reducing deaths due to childhood diarrheal illness. The mainstay of rehydration is oral rehydration solution (ORS), which is comprised of water and equimolar concentrations of sugar and salt to allow the most optimized absorption of fluid via glucose and sodium cotransport in the intestine.

By examining the child's general appearance, skin, eyes, and behavior, the level of dehydration is rapidly estimated

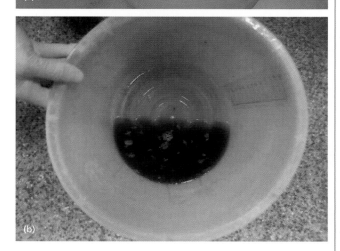

Figure 9.2 (a) Rice-water stool, consistent with cholera. (b) Blood/mucus stool, consistent with dysentery. *Source:* Photo (a) courtesy of Jason Harris and (b) courtesy of Mohammod Jobayer Chisti.

Box 9.1 Recognizing a cholera outbreak

An outbreak of cholera can emerge quickly and spread rapidly. Areas of crowding where sewage may contaminate the water supply, such as refugee camps or unplanned urban areas, are at risk for cholera outbreaks. Severe cholera is characterized by massive fluid losses and the rapid onset of dehydration. If a healthy child older than 5 years or a healthy adult becomes severely dehydrated or dies of a rapidly dehydrating diarrheal illness within 24 hours of the onset of symptoms, cholera should be considered. A presumptive diagnosis of cholera can also be made using a rapid test (Crystal VC®, Span Diagnostics) or by the presence of motile vibrios, which appear as "shooting stars" on dark-field microscopy.

Cholera outbreaks may cause panic in the population and even among healthcare providers. Rapid mobilization of resources to ensure safe water sources for surrounding areas and local access to oral rehydration therapy is essential. Aggressive management of rehydration is also needed to save lives in a cholera outbreak. The Cholera Outbreak and Shigellosis Training Program (COTS, www.cotsprogram .com) is a useful web resource in such a scenario.

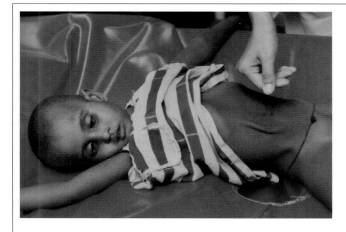

Figure 9.3 Child with delayed skin pinch recovery and sunken eyes.

using a combination of signs and symptoms (Figure 9.3 and Table 9.2). Using a combination of signs and symptoms is essential, because the absence of any single sign or symptom does not exclude the possibility of dehydration.

Patients usually do not show physical signs of dehydration until they have lost 5% of their total body weight in fluids. Laboratory measures have not been shown to provide substantial predictive benefit beyond the clinical examination and are not necessary to estimate the degree of dehydration.

Management

The approach to rehydration depends on initial estimated degree of dehydration. There are two components of hydra-

tion therapy: replacement and maintenance. Replacement involves replacing fluids lost before the patient came to medical attention, and maintenance involves replacement of ongoing losses. In patients with signs of dehydration, both replacement and maintenance hydration need to occur simultaneously.

Table 9.2 Assessment and treatment of dehydration.

Degree of dehydration	None	Some (if two or more criteria below are present)	Severe (if two or more criteria below are present)
General appearance	Alert, well	Restless, irritable	Lethargic or unconscious
Eyes	Normal	Sunken	Very sunken
Thirst	Drinks normally or no thirst	Thirsty, drinks eagerly	Drinks poorly or unable to drink
Skin pinch	Retracts quickly	Retracts slowly ($\geq$2 seconds)	Retracts very slowly ($\geq$3 seconds)
Percent body fluid loss	<5%	5–10%	>10%
Estimated fluid deficit	<50 mL/kg	50–100 mL/kg	>100 mL/kg
General treatment plan	Maintenance: ORS to match stool volume	Hydration with ORS and observation	Rapid intravenous hydration and ORS if possible. Close monitoring

Source: World Health Organization (2005a).

Clinical experience

"During a cholera outbreak, I worked with nurses to register patients as they arrived in a treatment center. A child was carried in who could not open her eyes, and she was vomiting more than five times per hour. She had only been sick with diarrhea for one day, but her skin looked dull and stiff. She would not even cry. Healthcare workers felt no pulse and placed two intravenous catheters in her arm veins before she was even out of her father's arms. After receiving intravenous fluids for an hour, she was awake. A few hours later, after more treatment, she was smiling brightly and eating a banana. I was amazed that this small child arrived completely lifeless and, in a few hours with one simple treatment, seemed like a healthy child."

Kayla, working in Haiti

No signs of dehydration

Patients who do not have obvious signs or symptoms of dehydration have lost less than 5% of their total body water. These patients may be sent home after a period of observation to ensure that they are matching ongoing fluid losses by drinking fluids. Ideally, ORS is given as a maintenance fluid to replace ongoing fluid and electrolyte losses.

For most patients, thirst should be sufficient to guide the volume of ORS administered. However, a simple approximation is that children under 2 years should receive approximately 50–100 mL of ORS, and children over 2 years should receive 100–200 mL of ORS for each episode of diarrhea or vomiting.

Table 9.3 Estimated replacement fluid volume in children with some dehydration.

Age	Weight (kg)	Fluid (mL)
<4 months	<5	200–400
4–12 months	5–8	400–600
1–2 years	8–11	600–800
2–4 years	11–16	800–1200
5–14 years	16–30	1200–2200

Source: World Health Organization (2005a).

Some dehydration

Patients with some signs of dehydration are approximately 5–10% dehydrated. The ideal treatment for most patients with some signs of dehydration is replacement therapy with ORS in a closely monitored setting. The goal is to replace an estimated 75 mL/kg of fluid within 3–4 hours of presentation. The amount of replacement fluids can also be rapidly estimated based on the age of the patient (Table 9.3).

If ongoing stool losses are profound, the volume of these losses should be added to the fluids given over the first 4 hours. While it is best to measure stool output, for example by using a cholera cot (Figure 9.4), ongoing fluid losses can also be estimated as 10–20 mL/kg body weight for each stool.

Frequent reassessment of hydration status is essential to care for patients with any signs of dehydration. Replacement fluids should be continued until all signs of dehydration are absent. This may often require more fluids than initially estimated. Once all signs and symptoms of dehydration have

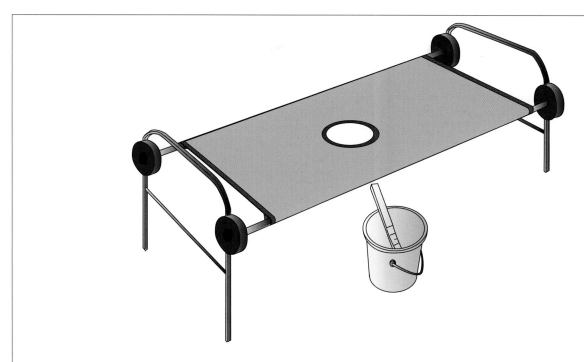

Figure 9.4 Cholera cot used for measuring ongoing stool output.

resolved and the patient has urinated, maintenance fluids are continued to match ongoing losses.

Patients with profound ongoing stool losses or frequent vomiting may fail to improve after oral rehydration or may even progress to severe dehydration. This occurs in approximately 5% of patients. Such patients require immediate intravenous fluids for management of severe dehydration.

Severe dehydration

Patients with signs of severe dehydration are over 10% dehydrated. Patients with severe dehydration are in hypovolemic shock and must be given intravenous fluids urgently in order to restore circulation and prevent imminent death. These fluids should be given as quickly as possible, often through multiple sites of intravenous access or through a nasogastric tube (Figure 9.5 and Box 9.2). Important exceptions to aggressive intravenous fluid resuscitation is children with septic shock in resource limited settings with a high prevalence of malnutrition and anemia (Box 9.3 and see Chapter 26 for further discussion).

Only isotonic intravenous fluids should be used to restore fluid volume. Of the commonly available isotonic fluids, lactated Ringer's or Ringers' lactate with 5% dextrose is preferred, although normal saline is an acceptable alternative. Colloids, blood products, or hypotonic fluids can be harmful and should never be administered since these may cause irreversible cellular injury in patients with severe dehydration.

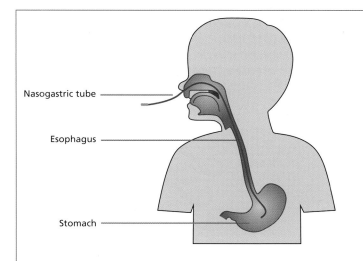

Figure 9.5 Nasogastric tube placement.

ORS should be initiated in addition to intravenous fluids as soon as the patient can drink because commonly available intravenous fluids (lactated Ringer's or normal saline) replace water and sodium but do not replace glucose, potassium, or other electrolyte losses as effectively as ORS (Figure 9.6). Children without severe malnutrition who can take fluids by mouth and have less than three stools in 24 hours can be safely

Box 9.2 Fluids via nasogastric tube

When intravenous fluids are not available or intravenous access cannot be established, patients with severe dehydration can be given fluids via nasogastric tube. Patients should be monitored for abdominal distension. If neither of these approaches is possible, fluids may be administered by mouth directly at a rate of 20 mL/kg per hour for up to 6 hours. This is suboptimal due to the risk of aspiration but preferable to no fluid therapy. Comatose patients receiving oral fluids should be monitored for vomiting and aspiration, in which case the rate of administration should be slowed until fluids are tolerated.

Other rehydration methods have also been applied to resource-limited settings. These include intraosseous, subcutaneous (hypodermoclysis), and intraperitoneal hydration (Rouhani *et al.*, 2011). Intraosseous administration is often utilized during acute emergencies when intravenous access is needed but not quickly obtained. Subcutaneous infusion has been effectively used for non-emergent rehydration when intravascular access is difficult to obtain.

Box 9.3 Case study: dehydration in severely malnourished children

Severely malnourished children with diarrhea are more prone to develop complications including electrolyte imbalance, heart failure, and bacterial infections. A mid-upper arm circumference measurement is a quick tool used to screen for malnutrition (see Chapter 12). Treatment requires an individualized approach including gradual rehydration over a period of 10–12 hours and avoidance of intravenous fluids unless frank shock is observed.

The ability to accurately predict the degree of dehydration in malnourished patients based on the standard WHO clinical criteria is limited. For example, the lack of subcutaneous fat, the presence of edema, and the presence of baseline apathy interfere with assessment of

skin turgor and mental status as indicators of dehydration and intravascular volume. Cool or clammy extremities, diminished pulses, and diminished urine output are all signs that suggest poor perfusion and indicate that additional fluids are needed to replace intravascular volume losses secondary to dehydration and/or sepsis.

Intravenous fluids should only be used in severely malnourished patients in the setting of overt shock. ReSoMal (ORS for severely malnourished children) is preferred for malnourished children, when available. Oral rehydration, broad-spectrum antibiotics, and conservative nutritional support (fluid volume 120 mL/kg per 24 hours with an average energy of 80 kcal/kg per 24 hours) should be immediately instituted to avoid complications.

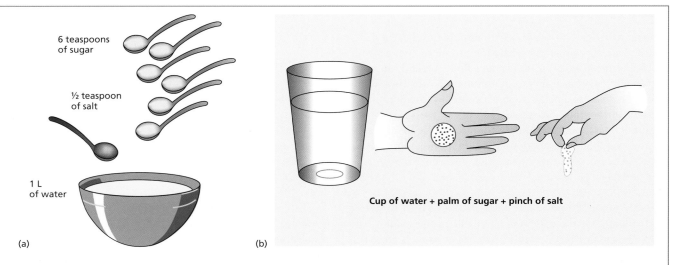

6 teaspoons of sugar

½ teaspoon of salt

1 L of water

(a)

Cup of water + palm of sugar + pinch of salt

(b)

Figure 9.6 Oral rehydration solution recipes. When pre-packaged sachets are not readily available, home-made oral rehydration solution can be mixed (a) in a 1-liter bowl or (b) in a drinking glass.

Table 9.4 Fluids used for rehydration (values in mmol/L).

		Na+	K+	Cl−	HCO₃−	Carbohydrate	Comments
Intravenous therapy	Lactated Ringer's solution	130	4	109	28	— (278 if D5LR available)	Lactated Ringer's solution is preferred over normal saline because it contains potassium and bicarbonate
	Normal saline	154	0	154	0	—	
Oral rehydration therapy[a]	ORS (WHO 2002)	75	20	65	10	75 glucose	A home-made preparation of ORS is inferior because it lacks potassium and bicarbonate, but it is effective in correcting dehydration
	Rice-based ORS (e.g., CeraORS 75®)	75	20	65	10	27 g of rice syrup solids	
	Home-made ORS[b]	~75	0	~75	0	~75	

[a] For patients without signs of dehydration, ORS is always preferred, but acceptable alternatives include fluids with salt such as salted yogurt drinks, broth, coconut or rice water, unsweetened weak tea, and unsweetened fruit juice. Unacceptable alternatives include coffee and medicinal teas, which can have diuretic effects, and carbonated beverages and sweetened juice, which may worsen diarrhea.
[b] Use a half teaspoon of salt with six teaspoons sugar dissolved in 1 L of clean water.

Box 9.4 Response to an outbreak of severe acute watery diarrhea

Rapid assessment of dehydration and initiation of treatment are crucial for an outbreak treatment center. Other important roles include:

- provision of large amounts of clean water for ORS;
- recording of information including what treatments are given and monitoring of ongoing fluid losses;
- providing soap and water purification materials to patients and families;
- ensuring high-calorie safe foods are available to well-nourished patients, and moderate-calorie foods to malnourished patients;
- communication of educational messages to the affected community, including water purification, proper sanitation, and teaching recognition of dehydration.

discharged. Distance of family's home from healthcare facilities should be taken into consideration when deciding when discharge is appropriate.

A summary of the fluids used for dehydration is given in Table 9.4. Important points to consider during an outbreak of severe acute watery diarrhea are listed in Box 9.4.

🔍 Clinical pearl

For patients who present with acute diarrhea with no or mild to moderate signs of dehydration, ORS is better than intravenous hydration because it lowers the risk of complications such as hypoglycemia and serious electrolyte imbalances (such as hypokalemia).

Management and prevention of malnutrition during diarrheal illness

Prompt nutritional support in children with dehydrating diarrhea speeds recovery and prevents malnutrition. Infants who are breastfeeding should continue to breastfeed while taking in ORS throughout both the rehydration and recovery stages (World Health Organization, 2011). Infants under 6 months of age or non-breastfed infants under 6 months of age using formula should continue to take undiluted formula in addition to ORS during rehydration and maintenance treatment for dehydration. Even in cases of severe dehydration and vomiting, patients should be encouraged to eat when the initial fluid deficit is corrected, especially after the correction of metabolic acidosis (rapid and deep breathing due to massive loss of bicarbonate in severe diarrhea), ideally within 4 hours of presentation. In well-nourished patients, the resumption of a high-calorie diet, even while diarrhea continues, may prevent several complications including electrolyte abnormalities, low blood sugar, and malnutrition (Chowdhury et al., 2010). Foods with high energy content should be offered frequently as long as diarrhea continues.

Zinc reduces the severity of diarrheal episodes and prevents subsequent episodes of diarrhea (Lukacik et al., 2008). For children under 5 years of age with diarrhea, the WHO recommends supplementation (10 mg/day for 10 days for children aged 2–6 months and 20 mg/day for 10 days for children aged 6 months to 5 years). Children with diarrhea who are at risk of Vitamin A deficiency, severe malnutrition, or recent measles should receive high-dose Vitamin A supplementation (50,000 IU for children 1–6 months, 100,000 IU for children 6–12 months, and 200,000 IU for children over 12 months).

🔍 Clinical pearl

For patients with acute diarrhea who are able to feed (e.g., breast milk, formula, or foods), never withhold feeding and give zinc supplementation.

Box 9.5 Empiric antibiotics for childhood diarrhea

- Suspected shigellelosis (invasive diarrhea): oral ciprofloxacin 30 mg/kg daily (divided twice daily) for 3 days or oral azithromycin 15 mg/kg on day 1 and 10 mg/kg daily during days 2–5 (World Health Organization, 2005b).
- For severe and refractory infections: ceftriaxone 50–100 mg/kg i.v./i.m. daily (once daily) for 2–5 days (World Health Organization, 2005c).
- Suspected cholera: azithromycin 20 mg/kg daily in one dose. Do not exceed 1 g (Saha *et al.*, 2006).

Note that pathogen resistance to antibiotics can occur and changes over time. Microbiologic confirmation of sensitivity testing is needed for appropriate treatment in a specific area.

Red flag

Patients with severe malnutrition require an alternate approach to rehydration because of the serious risk of fluid overload and electrolyte imbalances.

Antibiotic treatment and other therapies

Antibiotic therapy should only be used in certain cases of diarrheal illness (Box 9.5); it is not recommended for mild watery diarrhea when cholera is not suspected. However, in confirmed and suspected cases of cholera, antibiotics reduce the duration of illness, total volume losses, and in-hospital care needs. Invasive diarrhea should also be treated with antibiotic therapy directed at shigellosis, and resistant organisms or alternative diagnoses should be considered if improvement does not occur within 48 hours.

Antimotility agents and antiemetics can have effects that can interfere with rehydration. These agents may be harmful in young children with acute diarrhea and should not be given.

Clinical pearl

In areas where stool cultures are not possible, antibiotics should be aimed toward shigellosis for children with invasive (bloody) diarrhea. Reassess response after 48 hours.

Management and prevention of complications

Electrolyte abnormalities can complicate the treatment of dehydration in infants and children. Diarrhea can cause an imbalance in sodium levels, and this is more common when using intravenous fluid to correct dehydration. Hypokalemia or low potassium is secondary to stool potassium losses and may present as ileus, profound weakness, or muscle cramping. Severe hypoglycemia can occur and is more common in malnourished children. If seizures occur, hypoglycemia should be rapidly treated with a dextrose infusion, and hyponatremia or hypernatremia should be suspected. Oral rehydration results in a more gradual correction of fluid and electrolyte losses compared with intravenous rehydration and is therefore less likely to cause complications of electrolyte disarray.

Identification and management of common comorbid conditions

The presence of acute watery diarrhea does not exclude other potentially life-threatening infections that may be part of a greater systemic disease. If the child has a fever, difficulty breathing, or severe abdominal pain, diarrhea could be part of an infection such as pneumonia, sepsis, or malaria. Surgical emergencies, such as intussusception or appendicitis, may also present with diarrhea. Concomitant pneumonia is an important cause of mortality in patients presenting with diarrheal illness. Tachypnea occurs frequently in children with dehydration, but typically resolves after rehydration therapy. Cough, fever, or an abnormal pulmonary examination should further raise suspicion for pneumonia. Infants and children with dehydration should be reevaluated for the presence of pneumonia after rehydration, especially in cases of comorbid malnutrition.

Prevention

The provision of safe food and water will prevent most acute diarrheal illness in developing countries. Unfortunately, safe water and sanitation remain out of reach for 1 billion of the world's people. To prevent spread of diarrheal disease, handwashing should be conducted after defecation, after disposing of stool, and before and after eating or preparing meals. Latrines should be located more than 10 m and downhill from drinking water sources. The WHO also recommends the rotavirus vaccine be included in all national immunization programs.

Additional resources

- World Health Organization. First steps for managing an outbreak of acute diarrhea. Available at https://extranet.who.int/iris/restricted/handle/10665/69073
- Cholera outbreak Training and Shigellosis. Free materials available in several languages for diarrheal outbreak treatment and prevention. Available at http://www.cotsprogram.com
- World Health Organization (2005) *The Treatment of Diarrhea: A Manual for Physicians and Other Senior Health Workers*, 4th revision. Geneva: WHO. Available at http://whqlibdoc.who.int/publications/2005/9241593180.pdf

REFERENCES

Chowdhury F, Khan AI, Faruque ASG, Ryan ET (2010) Severe, acute watery diarrhea in an adult. *PLoS Negl Trop Dis* 4(11):e898.

Guerrant RL, Schorling JB, McAuliffe JF, de Souza MA (1992) Diarrhea as a cause and an effect of malnutrition: diarrhea prevents catch-up growth and malnutrition increases diarrhea frequency and duration. *Am J Trop Med Hyg* 47(1 Pt 2):28–35.

Kosek M, Bern C, Guerrant RL (2003) The global burden of diarrhoeal disease, as estimated from studies published between 1992 and 2000. *Bull WHO* 81:197–204.

Kotloff KL, Nataro JP, Blackwelder WC *et al.* (2013) Burden and aetiology of diarrhoeal disease in infants and young children in developing countries (the Global Enteric Multicenter Study, GEMS): a prospective, case-control study. *Lancet* 382:209–22.

Lawn JE, Kinney MV, Black RE *et al.* (2012) Newborn survival: a multi-country analysis of a decade of change. *Health Policy Plan* 27(Suppl. 3):iii6–28.

Liu L, Johnson HL, Cousens S *et al.* (2012) Global, regional, and national causes of child mortality: an updated systematic analysis for 2010 with time trends since 2000. *Lancet* 379:2151–61.

Lukacik M, Thomas RL, Aranda JV (2008) A meta-analysis of the effects of oral zinc in the treatment of acute and persistent diarrhea. *Pediatrics* 121:326–36.

Pelletier DL, Frongillo EA Jr, Schroeder DG, Habicht JP (1995) The effects of malnutrition on child mortality in developing countries. *Bull WHO* 73:443–8.

Rouhani S, Meloney L, Ahn R, Nelson BD, Burke TF (2011) Systematic literature review of alternative rehydration methods: lessons for resource-limited care. *Pediatrics* 127:e748–57.

Saha D, Karim MM, Khan WA, Ahmed S, Salam MA, Bennish ML (2006) Single-dose azithromycin for the treatment of cholera in adults. *N Engl J Med* 354:2452–62.

World Health Organization (2005a) The treatment of diarrhea: a manual for physicians and other senior health workers, 4th revision. Available at http://whqlibdoc.who.int/publications/2005/9241593180.pdf

World Health Organization (2005b) Guidelines for the control of shigellosis, including epidemics due to *Shigella dysenteriae* type1. Available at http://whqlibdoc.who.int/publications/2005/9241592330.pdf

World Health Organization (2005c) Guidelines for the control of shigellosis, including epidemics due to *Shigella dysenteriae* 1. Available at http://www.who.int/cholera/publications/shigellosis/en/

World Health Organization (2011) Treatment of the patient with cholera. Emerging and other Communicable Diseases, Surveillance and Control. Available at http://www.who.int/csr/resources/publications/cholera/whocddser9115rev1.pdf

CHAPTER 10
Malaria

Ryan W. Carroll[1,2,3], Danny A. Milner Jr[3,4], and Hans C. Ackerman[5]

[1]Global Health Collaborative, MUST, Uganda
[2]Massachusetts General Hospital, Boston, MA, USA
[3]Harvard Medical School, Boston, MA, USA
[4]Brigham and Women's Hospital, Boston, MA, USA
[5]National Institute of Allergy and Infectious Diseases, Rockville, MD, USA

Key learning objectives

- Understand the diversity of malaria species that cause human infection and the spectrum of disease encountered.

- Understand the life cycle of malaria parasites and how it relates to infection, disease, treatment, and prevention strategies.

- Understand the tools available to diagnose malaria.

- Understand the principles of malaria treatment, including geographic considerations and species-specific approaches.

- Be able to formulate a prevention plan for a given population based on geography, availability of drugs and vaccines, and species encountered.

Abstract

Malaria is one of the oldest diseases of humans and is shared by almost all vertebrate animals. Five species of *Plasmodium* cause disease in humans, and symptoms range from asymptomatic carriage to severe illness and death. Malaria claims up to 500,000 to 1 million deaths per year, a result of up to 250 million infections per year, and poses a tremendous socioeconomic burden to individuals and families in endemic areas. Clinical diagnosis of malaria should be suspected in any person with a fever in an endemic area, and confirmatory diagnosis, which can be made by light microscopy or rapid test, is advised before treatment. Malaria has been targeted for elimination. Efforts include patient and community education, preventive measures at the individual and population levels, rapid access to diagnosis and increasingly effective treatment, and the development of vaccines.

Key words: malaria, cerebral, anemia, mosquito, *Plasmodium*

Essential Clinical Global Health, First Edition. Edited by Brett D. Nelson.
© 2015 John Wiley & Sons, Ltd. Published 2015 by John Wiley & Sons, Ltd.
Companion website: www.essentialseries.com/globalhealth

Introduction

Malaria is caused by infection with *Plasmodium* parasites that are acquired through the bite of a female *Anopheles* mosquito. Currently, more than 2 billion people live in malaria-endemic areas, and malaria is responsible for up to 500,000 to 1 million deaths per year, as a result of up to 250 million infections per year (data for 2012; WHO Malaria Fact Sheet, 2013). Malaria is not only a leading health issue worldwide, it also creates a tremendous socioeconomic burden to individuals, families, and communities in endemic areas.

Malaria is part of our evolutionary past, infecting our primate ancestors and early humans, and expanding with human populations as agriculture was developed about 10,000 years ago. Early descriptions of the disease appear in 4500-year-old texts, and DNA from *Plasmodium* has been detected in Egyptian mummies and remains of ancient Romans (Cox, 2002). Our historical coexistence with the *Plasmodium* parasite and the *Anopheles* mosquito vector has shaped the human genome, and has given rise to genetic diseases such as sickle cell anemia and thalassemia. The interplay between parasite, mosquito, and human populations has helped shape history, politics, and economics, and today leaves many of the world's most vulnerable people at risk for this deadly disease.

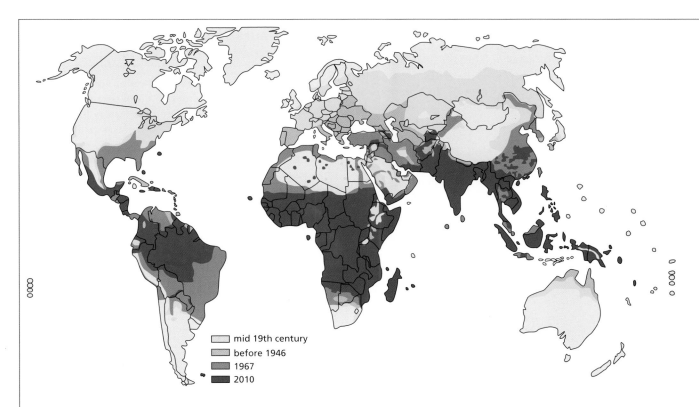

Figure 10.1 Distribution of malaria over time. *Source*: Roll Back Malaria Partnership (2011), figure E.1, p. 9. Reproduced with permission of Roll Back Malaria.

Geographic distribution and economic impact of malaria

Malaria infections most commonly occur in tropical areas of the world, including sub-Saharan Africa, Southeast Asia, Oceania, and South America. *Plasmodium falciparum* is responsible for most virulent infections worldwide, although *P. vivax* also causes substantial disease burden outside of Africa. *Plasmodium malariae* and *P. ovale* also cause malaria symptoms in humans. *P. knowlesi* is a fifth species that causes malaria in humans, comes from its primary host the macaque, and is prevalent in parts of Southeast Asia.

Malaria eradication efforts from the 1930s to 1970s succeeded in Europe and the United States but not in Central and South America, India, and Indonesia. Sub-Saharan Africa was not included in these major eradication efforts and today still bears the greatest disease burden (Figure 10.1). The economic and sociopolitical implications of malaria are pervasive: for

Africa, gross domestic product loss is in the tens of billions of US dollars, and person-days lost due to malaria infection is in the billions. Likely not coincidentally, the global maps of malaria burden and poverty are overlapping (Figure 10.2), reflecting the cycle wherein illness decreases productivity and leads to poverty, while poverty makes treatment and elimination programs difficult to access and sustain.

Human genetic resistance or susceptibility to malaria

Genetic variants that affect the red blood cell (RBC), adhesion to vascular endothelium, and the regulation of immune responses have been associated with protection from or susceptibility to malaria (Kwiatkowski, 2005). One example of conferred protection is found within Africa, wherein the distribution of malaria overlaps with the distribution of sickle cell trait (Figure 10.3). Other genetic polymorphisms in RBCs that confer various levels of protection against malaria have arisen and remain fixed in populations where malaria remains endemic. It is not entirely clear how these RBC and hemoglobin variants confer protection, however. In brief, genetic variants that confer protection or susceptibility involve the following (Driss *et al.*, 2011):

- hemoglobinopathies (e.g., HbC, HbE, HbS, α-thalassemia, β-thalassemia);
- RBC enzyme deficiencies (e.g., glucose 6-phosphate dehydrogenase and pyruvate kinase deficiencies);
- RBC membrane and morphology abnormalities (e.g., ovalocytosis, elliptocytosis, glycophorins);
- RBC surface proteins (e.g., ABO blood group);
- haptoglobin variants;
- nitric oxide synthase 2 variants;
- heme oxygenase 1 variants.

Life cycle

Malaria transmission occurs when a female *Anopheles* mosquito takes a blood meal from an infected person (Figure 10.4). Male and female gametocytes, which emerge from human RBCs, cross-fertilize and develop into ookinetes in the midgut of the mosquito. The ookinetes must evade mosquito immune mechanisms, and typically only one to ten survive to become oocysts. The population expands when each oocyst gives rise to about 1000 sporozoites. These motile sporozoites travel through the hemolymph (mosquito blood) to the mosquito salivary glands, where they prepare to enter the next host. The mosquito stage of the *Plasmodium* life cycle takes about 1–2 weeks.

When a malaria-infected mosquito probes the skin looking for a blood meal, sporozoites are released into the skin of the host. Using molecular motors and specialized proteins, sporozoites invade blood or lymphatic vessels and reach the liver within 2 hours. The parasite uses a cholesterol receptor to gain entry into a liver hepatocyte, where each sporozoite grows and multiplies into about 10,000–100,000 merozoites. These merozoites emerge in the bloodstream 1–2 weeks later. The merozoites invade RBCs, digesting the protein contents of the cell as they develop and multiply 24- to 32-fold before reemerging 48 hours later to invade the next RBCs. As the parasite number climbs, the symptoms of malaria begin with paroxysms of fever as merozoites burst out of infected RBCs. During the peak of the blood-stage infection, the number of parasites may climb into the trillions. A fraction of these blood-stage parasites develop into gametocytes, which are taken up by another mosquito and the cycle begins again. The majority of the released parasites, schizonts, invade RBCs, and the erythrocytic cycle begins again.

Pathophysiology, presentation, and clinical course of infection with *P. falciparum*

By the time fever and chills have begun, an infection with *P. falciparum* is advanced, with billions of parasites circulating in the bloodstream. There are multiple factors that influence the severity and outcome of a malaria parasite infection (Figure 10.5).

An individual's symptoms stem from an immune response to exposed parasites. Most people experience waves of fever, chills, muscle aches, nausea, and vomiting associated with parasites rupturing out of cells and triggering an inflammatory response. However, individuals who have disease-controlling immunity can harbor circulating parasites without feeling ill.

The human spleen is an excellent filter for RBCs and can detect infected cells that are too rigid, irregularly shaped, or clumped. Immune cells in the spleen remove and digest irreversibly damaged RBCs. To complete its blood-stage life cycle, the parasite must evade destruction in the spleen by adhering to the wall of a blood vessel.

As the maturing parasite reaches the late trophozoite or schizont stage, the RBC becomes more noticeably altered and susceptible to splenic clearance. The parasite exports adhesion molecules to the surface of the RBC to anchor it to the vessel wall. The most important of these molecules is PfEMP1 (*Plasmodium falciparum* erythrocyte membrane protein 1) that is encoded by the *var* genes, which are highly variable not only across a population of parasites but also within a single parasite. The size and diversity of the repertoire of PfEMP1 proteins is a testament to the importance of endothelial adhesion for parasite survival. The adhesion of parasite-infected RBCs to vascular endothelium makes it difficult to determine the density of parasites infecting a particular patient because the density of parasites counted in a blood sample does not reflect the parasites that are adherent to vessel walls.

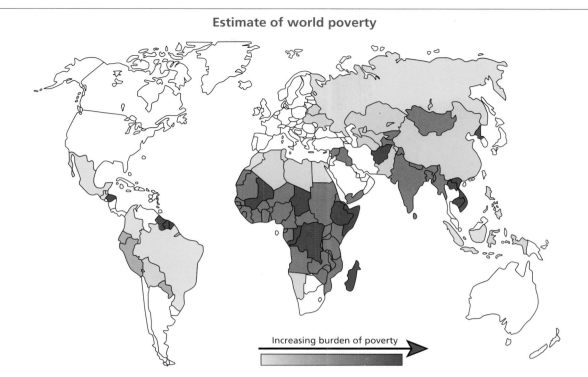

Estimate of world poverty

Increasing burden of poverty

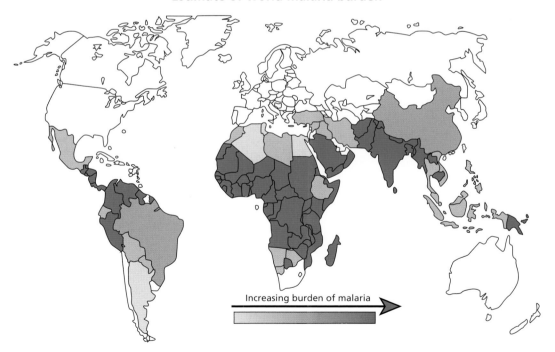

Estimate of world malaria burden

Increasing burden of malaria

Figure 10.2 Estimation of world malaria burden compared with estimations of world poverty showing strongly overlapping distributions. Similar maps appear for HIV and tuberculosis; world poverty is influenced by multiple factors in addition to malaria. *Source*: RBM data. Jeffrey Sachs 1990, Reproduced with permission of Jeffrey Sachs.

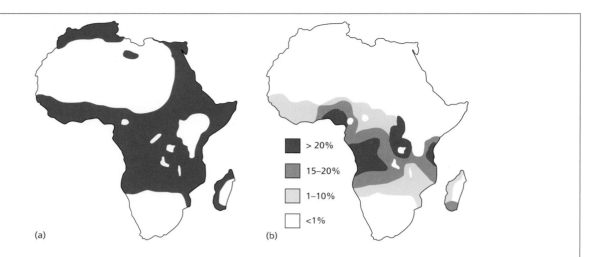

Figure 10.3 Distribution of malaria in Africa (a) compared with distribution of percent of the population heterozygous for hemoglobin S (b). *Source*: Wikimedia © Anthony Allison. Reproduced under the Creative Commons license.

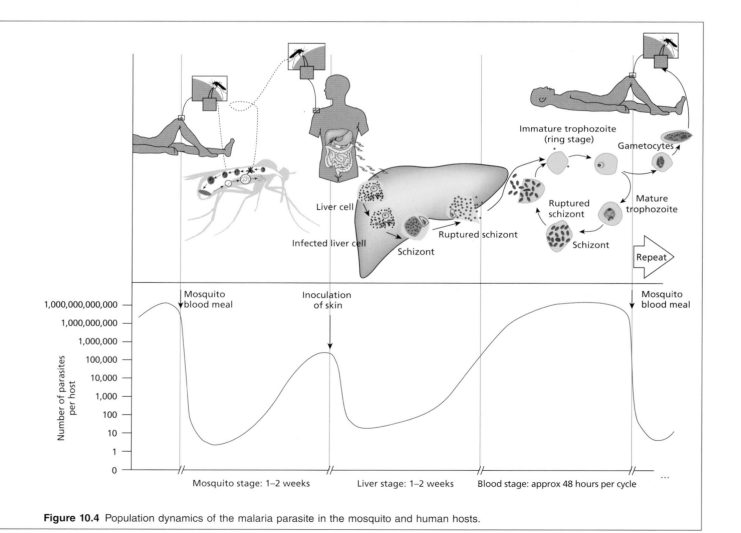

Figure 10.4 Population dynamics of the malaria parasite in the mosquito and human hosts.

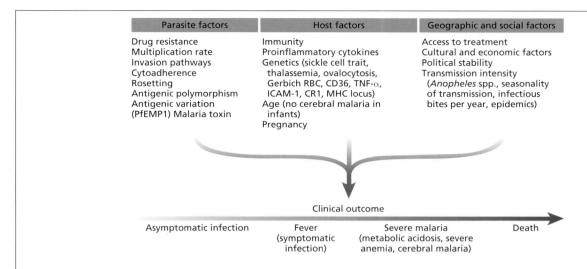

Parasite factors	Host factors	Geographic and social factors

Drug resistance
Multiplication rate
Invasion pathways
Cytoadherence
Rosetting
Antigenic polymorphism
Antigenic variation
(PfEMP1) Malaria toxin
	Immunity
	Proinflammatory cytokines
	Genetics (sickle cell trait,
	  thalassemia, ovalocytosis,
	  Gerbich RBC, CD36, TNF-α,
	  ICAM-1, CR1, MHC locus)
	Age (no cerebral malaria in
	  infants)
	Pregnancy
		Access to treatment
		Cultural and economic factors
		Political stability
		Transmission intensity
		  (*Anopheles* spp., seasonality
		  of transmission, infectious
		  bites per year, epidemics)

Clinical outcome

Asymptomatic infection — Fever (symptomatic infection) — Severe malaria (metabolic acidosis, severe anemia, cerebral malaria) — Death

Figure 10.5 Parasite, host, geographic, and social factors determine the severity and outcome of a malaria infection. *Source*: Miller *et al*. (2002), figure 1, p. 673. Reproduced with permission from *Nature*.

Clinical studies of patients who are hospitalized for malaria have identified three major overlapping syndromes that together account for most of the life-threatening manifestations of malaria: severe malaria-related anemia, respiratory distress, and cerebral malaria. The World Health Organization (WHO) groups signs and symptoms together to define uncomplicated and severe malaria (Table 10.1). Patients who meet the clinical definition of severe malaria should be hospitalized and receive parenteral antiparasite medication and supportive care. Although it is estimated that only 1% of malaria infections progress to severe malaria, this still results in more than 5 million severe malaria cases and more than 500,000 deaths in sub-Saharan Africa each year.

Severe anemia is common in young children (1–3 years of age) with malaria. Children often present with fever and lethargy and have profound anemia, with hemoglobin levels often as low as 2–5 g/dL. The causes of the anemia are multifactorial and involve a combination of accelerated destruction of RBCs and inadequate production of new RBCs. Excess inflammation and oxidative stress is thought to prevent the production or release of new RBCs from the bone marrow. Anemia leads to inadequate oxygen delivery and demands very high cardiac output that is unsustainable and eventually leads to death. However, with careful blood transfusion and timely antiparasitic drugs, more than 95% of children with severe malarial anemia will recover.

Respiratory distress describes the elevated respiratory rate and increased respiratory effort of children with severe malaria-induced metabolic acidosis. Although the precise source of the acidosis is unknown, it may come from the increased anaerobic glycolysis in the host tissues, impaired clearance of lactate, and possibly from lactate generated by the parasite. No specific therapies have improved the outcome of patients with respiratory distress from lactic acidosis and the mortality is 10–30%. Judicious use of intravenous fluid is recommended, as a recent trial demonstrated worse outcomes in patients receiving boluses up to 40 mL/kg (Maitland *et al*., 2012). Transfusing patients who have concomitant severe anemia as well as treatment with antiparasitic drugs are the mainstays of therapy.

Cerebral malaria (CM) is defined clinically as coma attributed to malaria infection. Parents often bring their child to medical attention after seeing an abrupt loss of consciousness or witnessing a seizure. Clinicians determine the depth of malarial coma using the Blantyre Coma Scale (BCS) (Table 10.2), which is a modification of the Glasgow Coma Scale (see Chapter 25). The BCS is a summation of motor, verbal, and eye responses to a painful stimulus and ranges from 0 (unresponsive) to 5 (normal). Any score less than 5 is associated with an increased risk of death and therefore these children should be monitored closely. A BCS of 2 or less is part of the criteria for CM. Examination of the retina demonstrates hemorrhages, vessel color changes (orange or white), and areas of ischemia (white patches) that are further diagnostic of CM. The pathophysiology of CM is multifactorial and appears to involve sequestration of parasites in the brain, disruption of the endothelial lining of blood vessels with microscopic blood clots and small hemorrhages, and swelling of the brain due to edema or engorgement of blocked vessels. Mortality from CM ranges from 15 to 35% in most studies. Patients with CM should receive prompt antimalarial medications, as well as supportive care measures, including treatment of hypoglycemia and seizure control.

Neurological sequelae are common in survivors of CM. The incidence is 10–40% and can include gross and/or fine motor dysfunctions, persistent seizure disorders, and/or cognitive and behavioral abnormalities (Birbeck *et al*., 2010).

Table 10.1 Classification of malaria by severity of symptoms.

	Definition	Mortality
Asymptomatic parasitemia	Detection of parasite in blood in the absence of symptoms. Quoted incidence: 17%, 37%, 47%, depending on population and type of tool used (Nsobya et al., 2004; Males et al., 2008)	0% (incidental finding)
Uncomplicated malaria	Fever and parasitemia with any of the following: • Headache without abnormal neurologic signs • Chills • Joint or muscle pain • Abdominal pain and loss of appetite • Nausea, vomiting, or diarrhea • Splenomegaly	<1%
Severe malaria	Any of following symptoms increase the risk of death in children: • Coma (BCS ≤2) • Severe malaria anemia (hemoglobin <5 g/dL) • Respiratory distress/lactic acidosis • Impaired consciousness (BCS <5) • Renal failure • Hypoglycemia • Shock • Coagulation dysfunction • Jaundice • Hyperparasitemia These symptoms demand parenteral treatment: • Vomiting and cannot take oral medications • Dehydration • Prostration (inability to sit up in a child who previously achieved this milestone) • Parasitemia >2%	P. falciparum: in children, mortality is 15–35% with CM, 10–30% with respiratory distress, <5% with SMA. Mortality can be 20–40% in adults with CM, ARDS, and/or renal failure P. vivax: <1%, all ages
Placental malaria	Adhesion and sequestration of parasitized RBCs involving the syncytiotrophoblast (the epithelial lining of the placental intervillous space); especially problematic for primigravidae women; results in maternal anemia, low birthweight, and preterm infants (Mockenhaupt et al., 2006)	50% of low birthweights attributable to placental malaria; 100,000 infant deaths annually (Umbers et al., 2011)

ARDS, acute respiratory distress syndrome; CM, cerebral malaria; SMA, severe malaria-related anemia.

Table 10.2 The Blantyre Coma Scale (BCS) is used to assess for malarial coma in children who are too young to follow verbal commands or speak a language, which is the typical age group affected by cerebral malaria. Coma is defined by a BCS ≤ 2.

Motor	2	Localizes painful stimuli
	1	Withdraws from painful stimuli
	0	No response
Verbal	2	Appropriate verbal response (normal cry or speech) to painful stimuli or verbal prompt
	1	Inappropriate verbal response (abnormal cry or grunt) to painful stimuli or verbal prompt
	0	No response
Eye	1	Opens eyes *and* focuses on evaluator
	0	No response, or eyes open but not focusing or following

Source: Molyneux et al. (1989).

Rehabilitating patients with neurological sequelae poses a tremendous burden to families and communities within resource-limited settings.

Other complications of malaria include renal dysfunction, bleeding diathesis, heart failure, respiratory failure, and bacterial co-infections. Patients with malaria are predisposed to bacterial infection with non-typhoidal salmonellae, *Escherichia coli*, and other Gram-negative organisms, with anemia being a strong predisposing factor for developing such an infection (Olupot-Olupot *et al.*, 2013).

Diagnosis

Light microscopy is considered the gold-standard technique for diagnosing a *Plasmodium* species infection and is used to determine the specific *Plasmodium* species and stage of infection. However, this requires a skilled microscopist and the appropriate equipment and stains. In addition, low levels of parasitemia (50–100 parasites/μL) and mixed infections can be missed. This technique involves taking a drop of blood from the patient and performing a thick and/or thin smear. A thick smear is processed in such a way that multiple layers of RBCs and parasitized RBCs (pRBCs) can be seen, providing a general metric of parasitemia (often denoted as 0, +, ++, +++, or ++++). A thin smear is a monolayer of RBCs and pRBCs, stained with Giemsa, Wright-Giemsa, or Field stain. It is used for a more accurate quantification of parasite load and allows the operator to determine the species and stage of *Plasmodium* (Panel 10.1). However, smears created from blood obtained from peripheral blood will not accurately reflect the sequestered parasite load. A more detailed description of malaria blood smear procedures can be found in Chapter 31.

Rapid diagnostic testing is often used as a screening tool or may be the only way to diagnose *Plasmodium* infection in a resource-poor area in which a microscopist and appropriate staining tools are not available. Rapid diagnostic tests are based on a simple antibody reaction and include a built-in positive control. Some utilize *Plasmodium* lactate dehydrogenase (PLDH), which is used to diagnose an infection with any *Plasmodium* species, or *Plasmodium falciparum*-specific histidine-rich protein 2 (PfHRP2), used to diagnose an infection with *P. falciparum*, the most concerning infection clinically. The sensitivity and specificity of rapid diagnostic tests are 88–94% and 71–88%, respectively, depending on the manufacturer and which antigen is being targeted (Hendriksen *et al.*, 2011).

Polymerase chain reaction (PCR) is also used to diagnose malaria and can accurately identify a species as well as quantify parasite density, including parasite density levels well below those detected by light microscopy (Lucchi *et al.*, 2013). However, there are some pitfalls with PCR: it is expensive, not readily available in endemic areas, and may detect DNA fragments that remain after an infection has cleared, generating a false-positive result.

Not all patients with fever have malaria. Asymptomatic incidental parasitemia has been reported to occur in 17–47%, of patients. Therefore, it is important to consider all potential non-malaria causes of a febrile illness, even in patients with smears positive for parasites. Another issue to consider, malaria is often diagnosed without a confirmatory rapid diagnostic test or smear and patients are treated with antimalarials, reducing local supplies and cultivating resistance, while potentially leading to a missed diagnosis.

Treatment

The treatment of symptomatic malaria is paramount in any patient in order to decrease the risk for progression to severe disease, prevent transmission to mosquitoes, and to improve a patient's condition. Antimalarial medications are the mainstay of treatment, with the goal of clearing parasites as quickly as possible. The chemotherapeutic treatment for a given *Plasmodium* species depends primarily on geography. Quinine, a natural product found in cinchona trees, was the primary drug for malaria for hundreds of years and remains effective in intravenous form. Chloroquine, a derivative, has been the mainstay of therapy for the last 90 years and remains useful in areas where chloroquine resistance is uncommon (e.g., Caribbean, Central America). Within 20 years of use, chloroquine resistance emerged and spread quickly across the globe. Several additional drugs were subsequently developed for malaria treatment (sulfadoxine/pyrimethamine, atovaquone, mefloquine) but populations of parasites have since developed resistance.

Currently, for uncomplicated malaria, oral combination therapy (the use of two drugs simultaneously) is the recommended frontline treatment. More specifically, artemisinin combination therapy is recommended, which involves using artemisinin with an additional antimalarial such as lumefantrine, amodiaquine, mefloquine, or sulfadoxine/pyrimethamine (Laufer *et al.*, 2012). Optimal drug regimens vary depending on antimalarial availability, local resistance patterns, and government-supported programs. For severe malaria, intravenous antimalarial treatment is recommended and, in this case, artesunate is used. Artesunate is a water-soluble injectable artemisinin derivative and has been found to be more effective than traditional treatment with intravenous quinine (Sinclair *et al.*, 2012). Reports now show that artemisinin resistance has occurred, so the quest to find new drugs continues (Dondorp *et al.*, 2009; Miller *et al.*, 2013).

Non-chemotherapeutic treatments are required for certain clinical manifestations. Specifically, severe anemia (hemoglobin <5 g/dL) requires immediate blood transfusion, if available. Other supportive care includes airway management, seizure management, judicious fluid resuscitation for patients with evidence of intravascular depletion or frank dehydration, correction of low glucose, and diagnosis and treatment of suspected co-infections (see Box 10.1 regarding advanced interventions and diagnostics for malaria).

To date, there are no known effective adjuvant therapies, but several are being explored for use in severe and cerebral malaria populations, including inhaled nitric oxide, L-arginine

👁 Panel 10.1 Illustrations of *Plasmodium* species and stages

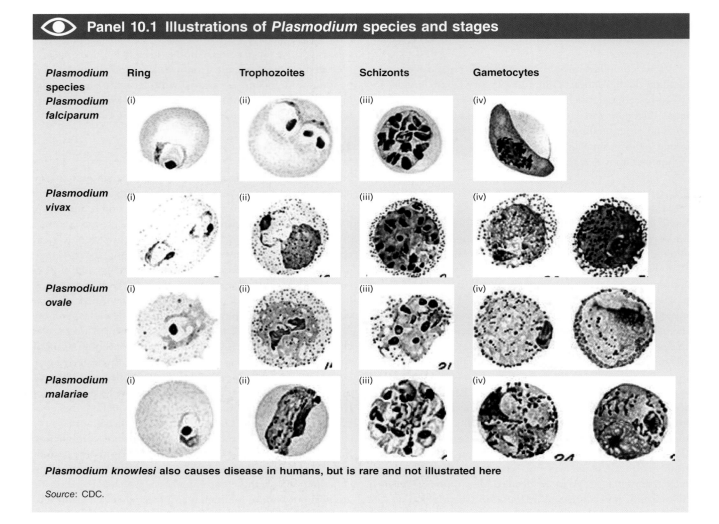

Plasmodium species	Ring	Trophozoites	Schizonts	Gametocytes
Plasmodium falciparum	(i)	(ii)	(iii)	(iv)
Plasmodium vivax	(i)	(ii)	(iii)	(iv)
Plasmodium ovale	(i)	(ii)	(iii)	(iv)
Plasmodium malariae	(i)	(ii)	(iii)	(iv)

Plasmodium knowlesi also causes disease in humans, but is rare and not illustrated here

Source: CDC.

Box 10.1 Advanced interventions and diagnostics for malaria

Tertiary care interventions and diagnostics that may be available in more developed settings

- Exchange transfusion is uncommon in resource-limited settings. However, it is used for rapid removal of parasitized RBCs and may improve RBC flow and reduce inflammatory molecules and cytokines. This is often used when parasitemia levels reach 10% and/or there are worsening clinical signs, such as CM or respiratory distress. There have been no randomized controlled trials to assess the benefits of exchange transfusion, although there has been a recent retrospective cohort study demonstrating safety in adults (Auer-Hackenberg *et al.*, 2012).
- Mechanical ventilation could be used when a patient no longer protects his or her airway in the face of severe neurological dysfunction, as seen in CM or unremitting seizures. This mode of assistance is not often available in resource-poor settings and requires a high level of surveillance, personnel, and infrastructure.
- Renal replacement therapy could be utilized in the face of oliguric or anuric renal failure, utilizing known thresholds for initiating such treatment.

Advanced imaging

Based on availability, advanced imaging (MRI and/or CT) has been used in severe malaria. Early data have demonstrated a mixture of white-matter and gray-matter disease, including cerebral edema and impending herniation. However, a pattern of parenchymal involvement specific to malaria has yet to be identified. Other modes of imaging and monitoring that have been used include ultrasound of the optic nerve sheath, transcranial Doppler for cerebral vascular tone and flow, and near-infrared spectroscopy monitoring.

supplementation, and levetiracetam. Others have been tested but proven to be ineffective or even dangerous. For an in-depth review of treatment of severe malaria, see Pasvol (2006).

Prevention

Transmission of parasites from one person to another requires the *Anopheles* mosquito, the vector, to be in close proximity to infected humans. Malaria researchers developed the concept of "vectorial capacity" to describe the ability of a mosquito to transmit malaria (Box 10.2).

Box 10.2 Understanding parasite transmission using vectorial capacity

"Vectorial capacity," V, is the number of infective mosquito bites generated from a single infected person in one day. It depends on several factors: the number of mosquitoes, m, available to bite a single person; the fraction of mosquitoes that actually bite a human, a; the fraction of mosquitoes that can support the parasite, i.e., "vector competence," b; the probability, p, that the mosquito will live through 1 day; and the number of days, n, the parasite must develop inside the mosquito.

$$v = \frac{m \cdot a^2 \cdot b \cdot p^n}{-\ln p}$$

It becomes apparent that two terms – the fraction of mosquitoes that bite a human, a, and the probability that a mosquito survives 1 day, p, – are especially important in determining vectorial capacity since they are raised to the second and nth powers. Therefore, strategies that decrease the number of mosquito bites or decrease mosquito survival will be particularly effective at reducing transmission.

The rate at which disease prevalence changes in a population can be described by another equation: the basic reproductive rate (R). When R is greater than 1, the disease is increasing; when it is less than 1, the disease prevalence is decreasing. R can be estimated by multiplying the number of infective bites, v, generated from one infected person times the chance that a bitten person will become infected, c, and divided by the chance that an ill person will recover, r.

$$R = \frac{v \cdot c}{r}$$

In this way, we can consider different malaria control measures in terms of how they affect these variables. (For a more detailed discussion, see Ribeiro & Valenzuela, 2011.)

Strategies to reduce mosquito bites and mosquito survival

By reducing the number of mosquitoes that can bite a person, transmission is reduced by decreasing the chance of biting an infected person and by reducing the chance of that infected mosquito biting an uninfected person. Likewise, decreasing the survival of biting mosquitoes decreases vectorial capacity exponentially because mosquitoes must live long enough to support the development of the parasite over 1–2 weeks. In contrast, reducing the number of mosquitoes in a population will only produce a linear reduction in vector capacity. The following interventions affect vector capacity in different ways.

Insecticide-treated bednets

Insecticide-treated bednets (ITNs) are used to cover sleeping areas, and are impregnated with insecticides (predominantly pyrethroids) by either the manufacturer or the consumer. These can be provided to specific vulnerable populations such as pregnant women and children. ITNs are inexpensive, have been shown to reduce a family's burden of disease by 20%, and prevent transmission on two fronts: first, by preventing mosquitoes from feeding on infected individuals and, second, by protecting healthy individuals from infective bites. However, ITNs require strict compliance; they must be used at all times, cannot have holes, cannot touch the user during sleep (mosquitoes can bite through the mesh), and will only be effective if the mosquito population bites primarily at night. The user also needs to reapply insecticide periodically to maintain effectiveness.

Indoor residual spraying

Indoor residual spraying involves the coating of human dwelling walls with DDT (or other insecticide) that kills mosquitoes. Indoor spraying is relatively simple, inexpensive, and may provide durable killing of susceptible mosquito populations. It targets mosquitoes that are most likely to bite humans and limits DDT exposure to other animals. Reducing the average survival of the mosquito decreases vectorial capacity exponentially, so even partial killing may be effective at reducing transmission. However, many mosquito populations have developed resistance to DDT, and local testing for susceptibility may need to be performed with kits available from the WHO. Effectiveness is dependent on a high level of household participation. Some individuals or groups may consider the hazard of DDT in the environment to be greater than the threat of malaria.

Mosquito larvae control

Mosquito larvae control involves removing, draining, or securely covering standing water sources around a home or compound. Included in this strategy is coating water sources with a thin layer of oil, treating water with larvae-specific toxins, or introducing animals that feed on mosquito larvae. Larvae control is simple, involves durable interventions that can be implemented by each household in response to public health regulations, and can be enforced by inspections with a fee or reward incentive program (Gorgas, 1909). However, it may be difficult to eliminate all uncovered outdoor sources of water (e.g., hoofprints), and water sources away from the home may continue to support mosquito populations. A larvae control approach also requires a high rate of killing to decrease vectorial capacity. Some feel that DDT treatment of larvae should be discouraged since it is less effective than indoor spraying, causes more environmental contamination, and still increases mosquito resistance to the insecticide.

Malaria-resistant mosquitoes

Malaria-resistant mosquitoes have been developed by conventional breeding techniques or by molecular genetic modification in the laboratory. Because malaria infection decreases the fitness of mosquitoes, a malaria-resistant mosquito population might outcompete a malaria-susceptible population. Another approach is to release a population of sterile male mosquitoes that mate with female mosquitoes but produce no viable offspring. This approach could reduce or eliminate mosquito transmission of malaria by reducing the ability of a mosquito to support the development of the malaria parasite. However, there are challenges related to breeding and releasing modified mosquitoes. The parasite may adapt to the modified vector or to other existing vectors. There could be unintended consequences of introducing genetically modified organisms into the environment, such as transfer of drug-resistance genes or reversion to being competent vectors.

Drug treatments that kill the parasite

Chemoprophylaxis and intermittent presumptive treatment are ways to kill parasites in vulnerable populations.

Pharmacological prophylaxis or chemoprophylaxis

Pharmacological prophylaxis or chemoprophylaxis is recommended for individuals visiting endemic regions (see Chapter 4). By maintaining therapeutic levels of an efficacious antiparasite drug, chemoprophylaxis kills parasites when they enter the blood. This prevents the visitor from becoming ill. This strategy can be problematic because most chemoprophylactic regimens are expensive and adherence can be difficult. In addition, chemoprophylaxis is too expensive for persistent indigenous use.

Intermittent presumptive treatment

Intermittent presumptive treatment involves at-risk infants and pregnant women (see Chapter 17). Treatment of all infants in a community without prior diagnostic testing can significantly reduce the burden of disease in high-transmission areas. A typical regimen involves an appropriate antimalarial taken once every 2 months for a total of three doses. A similar approach can be effective at preventing the complications of malaria in pregnant women. This treatment interval does not impede the development of immunity. These approaches can decrease malaria morbidity in mothers, infants, and newborns. Like all drug-based interventions, the local parasite population must be susceptible to the drug employed.

Immunity that kills the parasite or prevents transmission

Human vaccination against malaria is currently being investigated and tested. Humans develop immunity to malaria over time in endemic regions. The immunity decreases the appearance or severity of clinical symptoms, but is generally short-lived (approximately 5 years). Vaccine strategies use common antigens displayed by the parasite to generate immunity capable of eliminating infection, reducing clinical disease, or preventing human transmission. Vaccination lowers the chance of infection and increases the rate of recovery. Transmission-blocking vaccines that elicit antibodies against gametocytes also decrease the capacity of the vector to transmit the disease. Vaccines are relatively inexpensive to administer to a population, and enhanced immunity could have multiple additional benefits, including preventing transmission, illness, and death. However, no vaccine is currently available for malaria. Immunity to one strain might not convey protection against other strains of the parasite. A single parasite can change its antigens to evade the immune system, and a population of parasites can evolve new antigens that a vaccinated individual will not recognize.

Conclusion

Malaria continues to affect millions of individuals per year, stunting socioeconomic growth in endemic regions, and ultimately claiming up to 1 million lives per year, mostly children. Antimalarial medications are at risk of becoming ineffective as parasites rapidly develop resistance. Preventive measures hold promise but require tremendous amounts of effort, time, money, and vigilance to work. Vaccination development also holds promise, and if proven to be beneficial will take years to be put into effect. Eradicating this terrible disease requires the minds, skills, and financial support of the global community.

Additional resources

- World Health Organization. Insecticide-treated mosquito nets: a WHO position statement. Available at http://www.who.int/malaria/publications/atoz/itnspospaperfinal.pdf
- World Health Organization. This annually updated resource provides statistics, up-to-date data, and current accepted guidelines for treatment and diagnosis of malaria. Available at http://www.who.int/topics/malaria/en/

- Centers for Disease Control and Prevention. This constantly updated resource provides information on diagnosis and treatment for all malaria infections in multiple languages. Available at http://www.cdc.gov/malaria/ and http://www.cdc.gov/malaria/resources/pdf/clinicalguidance.pdf
- RDT Info. This website is dedicated to rapid diagnostic tests for malaria with updates, literature, etc. Available at http://www.wpro.who.int/malaria/sites/rdt/
- Making Malaria History. This organization presents updates on policies and global initiatives for eliminating/eradicating malaria. Available at http://www.makingmalariahistory.org

- Miller LH, Ackerman HC, Su X-Z, Wellems TE (2013) Malaria biology and disease pathogenesis: insights for new treatments. *Nat Med* 19:156–67.
- Milner DA (2010) Rethinking cerebral malaria pathology. *Curr Opin Infect Dis* 23:456–63.
- Kappe SHI, Vaughan AM, Boddey JA, Cowman AF (2010) That was then but this is now: malaria research in the time of an eradication agenda. *Science* 328:862–6.
- Crompton PD, Pierce SK, Miller LH (2010) Advances and challenges in malaria vaccine development. *J Clin Invest* 120:4168–78.

REFERENCES

Auer-Hackenberg L, Staudinger T, Bojic A *et al.* (2012) Automated red blood cell exchange as an adjunctive treatment for severe *Plasmodium falciparum* malaria at the Vienna General Hospital in Austria: a retrospective cohort study. *Malar J* 11:158–65.

Birbeck GL, Molyneu ME, Kaplan PW *et al.* (2010) Blantyre Malaria Project Epilepsy Study (BMPES) of neurological outcomes in retinopathy-positive paediatric cerebral malaria survivors: a prospective cohort study. *Lancet Neurol* 9:1173–81.

Cox F (2002) History of human parasitology. *Clin Microbiol Rev* 15:595–612.

Dondorp AM, Nosten F, Yi P *et al.* (2009) Artemisinin resistance in *Plasmodium falciparum* malaria. *N Engl J Med* 361:455–67.

Driss A, Hibbert JM, Wilson NO, Iqbal SA, Adamkiewicz TV, Stiles JK (2011) Genetic polymorphisms linked to susceptibility to malaria. *Malar J* 10:271.

Gorgas WC (1909) Sanitation of the tropics with special reference to malaria and yellow fever. *JAMA* 52:1075–7.

Hendriksen IC, Mtove G, Pedro AJ *et al.* (2011) Evaluation of a PfHRP2 and a pLDH-based rapid diagnostic test for the diagnosis of severe malaria in 2 populations of African children. *Clin Infect Dis* 52:1100–7.

Kwiatkowski DP (2005) How malaria has affected the human genome and what human genetics can teach us about malaria. *Am J Hum Genet* 77:171–92.

Laufer MK, Thesing PC, Dzinjalamala FK *et al.* (2012) A longitudinal trial comparing chloroquine as monotherapy or in combination with artesunate, azithromycin or atovaquone-proguanil to treat malaria. *PLoS ONE* 7(8):e42284.

Lucchi NW, Oberstaller J, Kissinger JC, Udhayakumar V (2013) Malaria diagnostics and surveillance in the post-genomic era. *Public Health Genomics* 16:37–43.

Maitland K, Kiguli S, Opoka RO *et al.* (2012) Mortality after fluid bolus in African children with severe infection. *N Engl J Med* 364:2483–95.

Males S, Gaye O, Garcia A (2008) Long-term asymptomatic carriage of *Plasmodium falciparum* protects from malaria attacks: a prospective study among Senegalese children. *Clin Infect Dis* 46:516–22.

Miller LH, Baruch DI, Marsh K, Doumbo OK (2002) The pathogenic basis of malaria. *Nature* 415:673–9.

Miller LH, Ackerman HC, Su X-Z, Wellems TE (2013) Malaria biology and disease pathogenesis: insights for new treatments. *Nat Med* 19:156–67.

Mockenhaupt FP, Bedu-Addo G, von Gaertner C *et al.* (2006) Detection and clinical manifestation of placental malaria in southern Ghana. *Malar J* 5:119–29.

Molyneux ME, Taylor TE, Wirima JJ, Borgstein A (1989) Clinical features and prognostic indicators in paediatric cerebral malaria. A study of 131 comatose Malawian children. *Q J Med* 265:441–59.

Nsobya SL, Parikh S, Kironde F *et al.* (2004) Molecular evaluation of the natural history of asymptomatic parasitemia in Ugandan children. *J Infect Dis* 189:2220–6.

Olupot-Olupot P, Urban BC, Jemutai J *et al.* (2013) Endotoxemia is common in children with *Plasmodium falciparum* infection. *BMC Infect Dis* 13:117.

Pasvol G (2006) The treatment of complicated and severe malaria. *Br Med Bull* 75–76:29–47.

Ribeiro J, Valenzuela JG (2011) Vector biology. In: Guerrant RL, Walker DH, Weller PF (eds) *Tropical Infectious Diseases: Principles, Pathogens and Practice*, 3rd edn. Philadelphia: Saunders Elsevier.

Sinclair D, Donegan S, Isba R, Lalloo DG (2012) Artesunate versus quinine for treating severe malaria. *Cochrane Database Syst Rev* (6):CD005967.

Umbers AJ, Aitken EH, Rogerson SJ (2011) Malaria in pregnancy: small babies, big problem. *Trends Parasitol* 27:168–75.

WHO (2013) Malaria Fact Sheet 2013. http://www.who.int/malaria/media/world_malaria_report_2013/en/

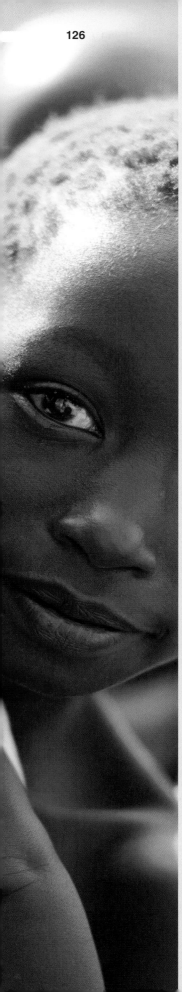

CHAPTER 11
Measles

Alejandro J. Candelario and Elizabeth R. Wolf
Seattle Children's Hospital and the University of Washington, Seattle, WA, USA

Key learning objectives

- Understand the global burden of measles.
- Learn the classic physical findings associated with measles.
- Understand how to manage both uncomplicated and complicated measles.
- Learn the key elements of measles control.

Abstract

Measles is a highly contagious virus that affects hundreds of thousands of children every year and remains a leading cause of vaccine-preventable death. Although widespread control efforts have decreased the incidence of measles dramatically, measles outbreaks continue to occur in places where vaccination coverage is limited and total herd immunity has not yet been achieved. Measles is characterized by fever, cough, conjunctivitis, and an erythematous maculopapular rash. Measles complications occur in many organ systems and can be devastating. The management of uncomplicated measles consists of supportive care and Vitamin A.

Key words: measles, Koplik, fever, rash, conjunctivitis, pneumonia, encephalitis, vaccine, Vitamin A

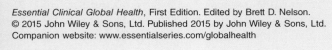

Essential Clinical Global Health, First Edition. Edited by Brett D. Nelson.
© 2015 John Wiley & Sons, Ltd. Published 2015 by John Wiley & Sons, Ltd.
Companion website: www.essentialseries.com/globalhealth

Introduction and epidemiology

Prior to the introduction of the measles vaccine in the 1960s, measles illness was nearly universal. However, since the implementation of global measles immunization, the incidence of measles has plummeted (WHO, 2013a) (Figure 11.1). In fact, a recent study found that global measles mortality decreased approximately 74% from 2000 to 2010 (Simons *et al.*, 2012). Yet measles remains one of the leading causes of vaccine-preventable death (Duke & Mgone, 2003) and affects hundreds of thousands of children every year (WHO, 2013a). The majority of outbreaks now occur in Africa and Southeast Asia, where herd immunity has been difficult to achieve (Figure 11.2). Since measles is extremely contagious, very high levels of vaccination coverage (>90%) are required to interrupt transmission (Fox, 1983). Countries with inadequate healthcare systems or remote populations are often unable to reach these levels of vaccine coverage.

Measles epidemics can also occur in regions with high vaccination rates. For example, migratory populations and non-vaccine-responders represent risk groups that can serve as niduses for outbreaks. Furthermore, the use of a single vaccine dose at 9 months of age, although driven by public health realities, results in lower rates of seroconversion (Gans *et al.*, 2001; Redd *et al.*, 2004; Halsey *et al.*, 1985). Children with HIV also have higher rates of primary vaccine failure (i.e., insufficient antibody response to the vaccine) and secondary vaccine failure (i.e., previously adequate antibody levels that have decreased over time) (Breña *et al.*, 1993; Moss *et al.*, 2007).

Despite these challenges, the characteristics of the measles virus make it well suited for global elimination, and many public health resources are devoted to this very purpose (Moss & Griffin, 2006). Measles has no animal reservoir, there are sensitive and specific laboratory tests to diagnose the virus, and there is an effective vaccine that can prevent the disease.

Measles is one of the most contagious pathogens known to humans. Indeed, the R_0 (the basic reproductive number, or the average number of additional cases one case generates) is higher in a susceptible population than that of smallpox (Ferguson *et al.*, 2003). Transmission of measles occurs through infectious droplets encountering the respiratory tract. These droplets can persist in the environment hours after an infectious patient has left. The infectious period lasts from 4 days before to 4 days after the onset of rash.

Classically, measles has been a disease of infancy. However, in populations with high vaccination coverage, older children and adolescents with primary or secondary vaccine failure are also commonly affected (Moss & Griffin, 2012). In the first six months of life, infants lose their passive protection by maternal antibodies (Leuridan *et al.*, 2010) and enter an extremely vulnerable period in which they have lost maternal antibodies but are still too young for the vaccine. HIV-exposed infants experience decreased transfer of maternal antibodies (Scott *et al.*, 2007) and thus are vulnerable to measles for a longer period of time.

Clinical course, physical examination, and diagnosis

The classic course of the disease includes prodromal, exanthematous, and recovery phases (Table 11.1). Following an asymptomatic incubation period of 8–12 days, the prodromal period of measles begins with fever, conjunctivitis, runny nose (coryza), cough, and fussiness. Measles conjunctivitis usually occurs with non-purulent lacrimation and may be accompanied by photophobia (Cherry, 2009). During this prodromal phase, pathognomonic lesions known as Koplik spots (Figure 11.3) may appear along the hard or soft palate and across from the molar teeth in the buccal mucosa (Bernstein & Schiff, 1998). These lesions appear as 1- to 3-mm elevations, consisting of an erythematous base and a raised central white hue.

On approximately the fourth day of illness, an erythematous maculopapular rash (Figure 11.4) emerges and lasts between 4 and 7 days (Griffin & Bellini, 1996). The rash first appears on the face or behind the ears and then spreads cephalocaudally to the trunk and upper and lower extremities. The palms and soles are typically spared. It is common for the exanthem to become confluent in areas where it first appears, such as the face and neck. In severe cases, the rash may include petechiae or appear hemorrhagic (Abramson *et al.*, 1995). During the exanthematous phase of the illness, the patient may continue to be febrile and suffer from pharyngitis and conjunctivitis. These symptoms usually begin to improve as the exanthem fades to dark, brownish, desquamating patches (Suringa *et al.*, 1970).

The recovery phase of the illness may include a cough persisting 1–2 weeks, with resolution of other clinical stigmata. Immunocompetent individuals begin to produce antiviral IgG,

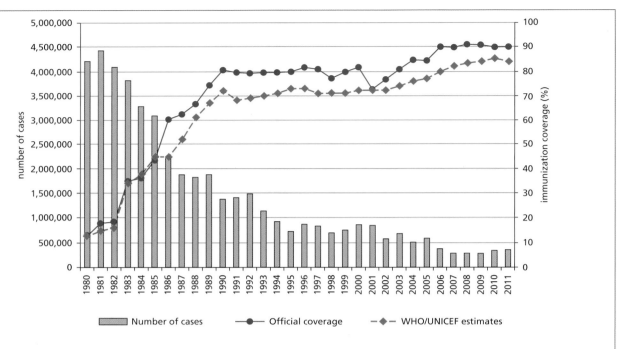

Figure 11.1 Number of annual measles cases and percent coverage by first measles vaccine (MCV1), 1980–2011. *Source:* WHO (2013b). Reproduced with permission of the World Health Organization.

which usually confers lifelong immunity (Griffin & Bellini, 1996).

Of note, a milder form of measles may occur in children with preexisting partial immunity (either from passive maternal antibodies, partial vaccination response, or previous measles disease). It is characterized by mild respiratory symptoms, with or without a rash or fever (Cherry, 2009).

The diagnosis of measles within the context of an outbreak is usually straightforward and based on the clinical criteria mentioned above. Cases that appear early in the epidemic or in patients with atypical presentations (such as the severely immunocompromised) can be more challenging for clinicians to diagnose. In such situations, establishing laboratory diagnosis with measles IgM can be helpful (Helfand *et al.*, 1997). Often, measles IgM is run concurrently with rubella IgM as the rubella rash can be easily confused with measles. The measles IgM assay has a sensitivity of 83–92% and a specificity of 87–100% (Ratnam *et al.*, 2000). Other diseases that should be included in the differential diagnosis of measles include erythema infectiosum (parvovirus B19), Epstein–Barr virus infection, Kawasaki disease, *Mycoplasma pneumoniae*, rubella, roseola, and drug rash (Cherry, 2009).

Management of uncomplicated measles

There is strong evidence that Vitamin A supplementation reduces morbidity and mortality associated with measles, espe-

cially in areas where Vitamin A deficiency is endemic (Hussey & Klein, 1990; Huiming *et al.*, 2005). The World Health Organization (WHO) recommends age-specific "loading doses" of Vitamin A on day 1 and day 2 of illness. If the child exhibits signs of Vitamin A deficiency or if the child lives in an area where Vitamin A deficiency is endemic, a third dose is recommended 2–4 weeks later (Table 11.2). Signs and symptoms of Vitamin A deficiency include night blindness, Bitot spots (gray or white triangular spots of keratinized epithelium on the conjunctivae; Figure 11.5), xerosis (dryness) of conjunctivae and cornea, pruritus, and growth retardation (Hussey & Klein, 1990; Semba & Bloem, 2004).

Besides giving Vitamin A, the management of uncomplicated measles is largely supportive. It includes the use of antipyretics for fever and discomfort as well as nasogastric or intravenous fluids for dehydration. In the developed world, ribavirin can also be given to severely immunocompromised patients (Banks & Fernandez, 1984; Krasinski & Borkowsky, 1989).

Complications

The rate of complications with measles is quite variable and ranges from 10 to 40%, depending on the population studied (Orenstein *et al.*, 2004). Groups at higher risk of complications include the immunocompromised (such as individuals infected with HIV), pregnant women, malnourished children

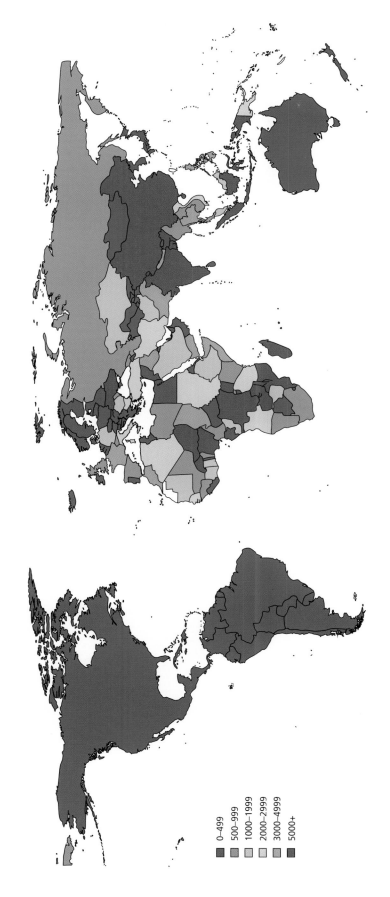

Figure 11.2 Mean annual incidence of measles over the past 10 years. Cases are by country report, as listed by the World Health Organization (WHO, 2013a). *Source:* Emily Carnahan at the Institute for Health Metrics and Evaluation, based on data from WHO (2013a). Reproduced with permission of the World Health Organization.

0–499
500–999
1000–1999
2000–2999
3000–4999
5000+

Table 11.1 Clinical phases of measles.

Phase	Time course	Clinical features
Incubation	8–12 days	Usually asymptomatic
Prodrome	2–3 days	Fever, cough, conjunctivitis, and coryza Pathognomonic Koplik spots may appear on oral mucosa (Figure 11.3)
Exanthem	4–7 days	Maculopapular rash, beginning on face with cephalocaudal (head to toe) spread to trunk and lower extremities Other symptoms may include lymphadenopathy, pharyngitis, and conjunctivitis
Recovery	1–2 weeks	Resolution of fevers, but cough may persist Rash begins to fade to dark brown spots and may desquamate Immunocompetent individuals usually develop lifelong immunity

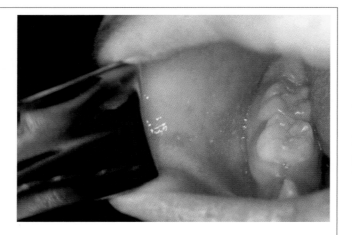

Figure 11.3 Koplik spots. *Source*: CDC Public Health Image Library.

Table 11.2 Vitamin A dosing for treatment of measles.

Vitamin A on days 1 and 2[a]

200,000 IU orally for children ≥12 months of age
100,000 IU orally for infants 6–11 months of age
50,000 IU orally for infants <6 months of age

[a] A third age-specific dose should be given 2–4 weeks later to children with clinical signs and symptoms of Vitamin A deficiency. In areas where Vitamin A deficiency is endemic, this third dose should be given even in the absence of the aforementioned symptoms of deficiency.
Source: WHO (2004) and information is summarized in WHO (2013c), p. 178. Reproduced with permission of the World Health Organization.

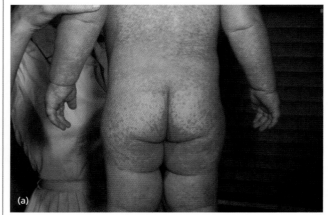

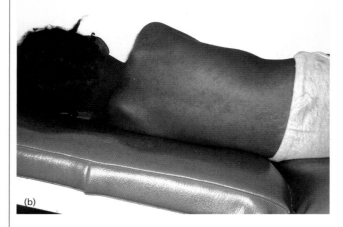

Figure 11.4 (a, b) Classic measles rashes in a lightly pigmented child (a) and a more darkly pigmented child (b). *Source*: (a) CDC Public Health Image Library; (b) Wikimedia © Mike Blyth. Reproduced under the Creative Commons license.

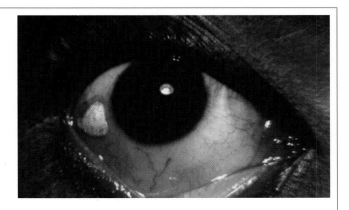

Figure 11.5 Bitot spot. *Source*: The University of Iowa, Iowa, USA and EyeRounds.org. Used with permission of The University of Iowa and EyeRounds.org

(particularly those with Vitamin A deficiency), infants, and the elderly. The most common complications in children are pneumonia, otitis media, gastroenteritis, and croup (Bernstein & Schiff, 1998). The WHO estimates the case fatality rate of measles to be as high as 6% in some developing countries, with the highest fatality rates in unimmunized children under the age of 5 years (Stein *et al.*, 2003; Nandy *et al.*, 2006; Wolfson *et al.*, 2009). Mortality in complex humanitarian emergencies can be even higher.

Children in developing nations commonly suffer from measles-associated respiratory disease, manifesting as pneumonia, bronchiolitis, or croup (Strebel *et al.*, 2008). Pneumonia is the most common fatal complication of measles and accounts for approximately 85% of measles-related deaths in the developing world (Beckford *et al.*, 1985). Although measles-associated pneumonia is usually a sequela of the primary viral infection, some children will develop a secondary bacterial superinfection with *Streptococcus pneumoniae*, *Staphylococcus aureus*, or *Haemophilus influenzae* (Quiambao *et al.* 1998).

Ophthalmologic complications of measles can be devastating. In fact, measles is the leading cause of pediatric blindness in developing countries (Semba & Bloem, 2004). The spectrum of ophthalmologic complications includes xerophthalmia (dry eyes), Bitot spots, keratitis, corneal ulceration, night blindness, and total blindness (M'garrech *et al.*, 2013).

A child with altered mental status or convulsions may be suffering from a neurologic complication of measles. Neurologic complications include acute viral encephalitis, acute disseminated encephalomyelitis (ADEM), and subacute sclerosing panencephalitis (SSPE). Approximately 1 in 1000 children with measles suffer from acute viral encephalitis during the exanthematous phase of the disease (Cherry, 2009). Of these cases, 15% progress rapidly to death and 25% suffer long-term neurodevelopmental sequelae. Measles-associated ADEM

presents later in the course of illness, usually within 2 weeks of the exanthem phase. Much like measles-associated encephalitis, post-measles ADEM has a high mortality rate, estimated to be 10–20% (Johnson *et al.*, 1984). Surviving children often suffer from residual neurologic complications, such as developmental delay, epilepsy, and motor deficits. SSPE occurs in 4–11 of 100,000 cases of measles and typically presents 7–10 years after an acute measles infection (Bellini *et al.*, 2005). It is a uniformly fatal and incurable disease that progresses from personality and behavior changes to myoclonic jerks, dementia, vegetation, and death (Bellini *et al.*, 2005). The gravity of these neurologic complications underscores the importance of measles prevention.

Management of measles complications
(Table 11.3)

Measles-associated pneumonia

Children with measles should be closely monitored for pneumonia (see Chapter 8). There is limited evidence to support prophylactic antibiotics to prevent pneumonia in children with measles and therefore it is not routine practice (Kabra *et al.*, 2008; Shann *et al.*, 2008). Antibiotics are certainly indicated, however, once a secondary bacterial pneumonia is suspected.

Measles-associated conjunctivitis

Measles conjunctivitis usually presents with non-purulent watery discharge. As such, ophthalmologic antibiotic ointments are not necessary unless a bacterial superinfection or ophthalmologic complication is suspected (WHO, 2004). In these cases, the WHO recommends tetracycline eye ointment three times a day for 7 days. Steroid eye ointments and traditional local remedies should be avoided, as these may worsen ophthalmologic disease.

Measles croup

The recommended management of measles croup is similar to other types of viral croup. Supportive care and nebulized epinephrine are appropriate, as indicted. However, the WHO recommends against corticosteroids because of the theoretical concern that they may worsen measles-related immunosuppression.

Measles-associated ADEM

No formal clinical trials of any therapeutic agent have been published to provide definitive recommendations for treating measles-associated ADEM. However, there have been case reports of successful treatment of ADEM with corticosteroids, plasma exchange, and IVIG. Current expert opinion guidelines include treating ADEM with methylprednisolone 30 mg/kg (maximum 1 g) i.v. daily for 3 days, followed by a 4–8 week taper of oral steroids (Tenembaum *et al.*, 2002; Bennetto & Scolding, 2004). If the patient's condition continues to deteriorate, it is recommended to administer IVIG 2 g/kg over 3–5

Table 11.3 Management of measles complications.

Uncomplicated measles	Supportive care including nutrition, fluids, antipyretics for fever/discomfort Vitamin A loading dose on days 1 and 2 of illness and third dose 2–4 weeks later if evidence or suspicion of Vitamin A deficiency Clinical monitoring for complications as detailed below
Measles pneumonia	Oxygen and respiratory support as necessary If bacterial superinfection is suspected, antibiotics that target S. pneumoniae, H. influenzae, and/or S. aureus
Measles conjunctivitis	Usually no treatment is needed If purulent fluid or ophthalmologic complication is present, treat with tetracycline ophthalmologic ointment three times a day for 7 days Ophthalmologic involvement beyond expected viral conjunctivitis is considered an emergency and an ophthalmologist should be consulted Avoid steroid eyedrops or ointments
Measles croup	Supportive care and nebulized epinephrine as indicated Avoid corticosteroids if possible
Measles encephalitis	Supportive care, including antiepileptics if needed
Measles ADEM	Methylprednisolone 30 mg/kg (1 g max) i.v. daily for 3 days, followed by 4–8 weeks of oral steroid taper
Measles SSPE	Supportive care Antispasmodics for symptomatic relief

days. If this is not sufficient, plasma exchange may be performed every other day for 14 days. Unfortunately, these additional therapies are usually not available for the patients at highest risk in developing countries.

Vaccination and measles control

In most countries in the developing world, the measles vaccine is given as a single live-attenuated vaccine. About 84% of the world's children received one dose of measles vaccine by age 1 in 2012 (WHO, 2014). The vaccine is also available in combination with mumps, rubella, and/or varicella. The distribution of these combination vaccines is increasing with the help of GAVI (Global Alliance for Vaccines and Immunisation) (GAVI Alliance, 2013).

The measles vaccine is recommended for all children, with the exception of the severely immunocompromised (e.g., HIV-infected individuals over 5 years of age with absolute CD4

counts <200 lymphocytes/mm^3 or HIV-infected individuals at any age with CD4 count <15%) (McLean et al., 2013). In practice, the vaccine is often given universally in the developing world, as the benefits of the measles vaccine are felt to outweigh any potential risks.

In areas with frequent outbreaks, the first dose of the measles vaccine is typically given at 9 months of age. Although the rates of seroconversion are lower at 9 months than at 12 months, early administration improves protection during the most vulnerable period of infancy. In non-endemic areas, the first dose is given at 12–15 months of age for a higher likelihood of seroconversion (95–98% vs. 87%) (Watson et al., 1998; Redd et al. 2004). As part of the global measles eradication plan, the WHO now recommends a second dose of measles vaccine for all children. In countries with strong healthcare infrastructure, this is typically achieved through a scheduled second dose of the measles vaccine. The schedule for this second dose varies by country and depends on the rates of endemic measles transmission and goals for measles control (WHO, 2009). Countries with weaker healthcare infrastructure tend to rely on supplementary immunization activities for delivery of the second dose. The second dose of the measles vaccine should be given no less than 28 days from the first dose (Red Book, 2012).

To control the extent of measles outbreaks, affected individuals should be kept in isolation, either at home or in measles-specific isolation wards of hospitals. A case of measles provides an opportunity for checking the vaccination status of family members and healthcare personnel. All measles cases should be reported to national ministries of health, which in turn report to the WHO. Supplementary immunization activities should also be undertaken in a prompt fashion to augment standard vaccination regimens. These campaigns can integrate other public health interventions, such as deworming and Vitamin A supplementation to reduce childhood mortality.

Measles vaccination, particularly with the two-dose series, usually confers long-term immunity (several decades) in immunocompetent individuals (Anders et al., 1996). HIV-infected individuals (particularly those who are severely immunosuppressed) have high rates of primary and secondary vaccine failure (Breña et al., 1993; Moss et al., 2007).

Additional resources

- Measles and Rubella Initiative. Global partnership of the American Red Cross, the United Nations Foundation, the US Centers for Disease Control and Prevention, UNICEF and the World Health Organization. Available at http://www.measlesinitiative.org
- World Health Organization (2009) Measles vaccine: WHO position paper. *Weekly Epidemiol Rec* 84:349–60.
- Centers for Disease Control and Prevention. Measles: questions and answers about disease and vaccine. Available at http://www.cdc.gov/vaccines/vpd-vac/measles/faqs-dis-vac-risks.htm

REFERENCES

Abramson O, Dagan R, Tal A, Sofer S (1995) Severe complications of measles requiring intensive care in infants and young children. *Arch Pediatr Adolesc Med* 149:1237–40.

Anders JF, Jacobson RM, Poland GA, Jacobsen SJ, Wollan PC (1996) Secondary failure rates of measles vaccines: a metaanalysis of published studies. *Pediatr Infect Dis J* 15:62–6.

Banks G, Fernandez H (1984) Clinical use of ribavirin in measles: a summarized review. In: Smith R, Knight V, Smith J (eds) *Clinical Applications of Ribavirin*. New York: Academic Press, p. 203.

Beckford A, Kaschula R, Stephen C (1985) Factors associated with fatal cases of measles. A retrospective autopsy study. *S Afr Med J* 68:858–63.

Bellini WJ, Rota JS, Lowe LE et al. (2005) Subacute sclerosing panencephalitis: more cases of this fatal disease are prevented by measles immunization than was previously recognized. *J Infect Dis* 192:1686–93.

Bennetto L, Scolding N (2004) Inflammatory/postinfectious encephalomyelitis. *J Neurol Neurosurg Psychiatry* 75(Suppl. 1):i22–28.

Bernstein D, Schiff G (1998) Measles. In: Gorbach S, Bartlett J, Blacklow N (eds) *Infectious Diseases*. Philadelphia: WB Saunders, p. 1296.

Breña AE, Cooper ER, Cabral HJ, Pelton SI (1993) Antibody response to measles and rubella vaccine by children with HIV infection. *J Acquir Immune Defic Syndr* 6:1125–9.

Cherry J (2009) Measles virus. In: Feigin R, Cherry J, Demmler-Harrison G (eds) *Textbook of Pediatric Infectious Diseases*, 6th edn. Philadelphia: Saunders, p. 2427.

Duke T, Mgone CS (2003) Measles: not just another viral exanthem. *Lancet* 361:763–73.

Ferguson NM, Keeling MJ, Edmunds WJ et al. (2003) Planning for smallpox outbreaks. *Nature* 425:681–5.

Fox JP (1983) Herd immunity and measles. *Rev Infect Dis* 5:463–6.

Gans H, Yasukawa L, Rinki M et al. (2001) Immune responses to measles and mumps vaccination of infants at 6, 9, and 12 months. *J Infect Dis* 184:817–26.

GAVI Alliance (2013) Measles–rubella vaccine support Available at http://www.gavialliance.org/support/nvs/measles-rubella/

Griffin D, Bellini W (1996) Measles virus. In: Fields B, Knipe D, Howley P (eds) *Fields' Virology*. Philadelphia: Lippincott-Raven, p. 1267.

Halsey NA, Boulos R, Mode F et al. (1985) Response to measles vaccine in Haitian infants 6 to 12 months old. Influence of maternal antibodies, malnutrition, and concurrent illnesses. *N Engl J Med* 313:544–9.

Helfand R, Heath J, Anderson L, Maes EF, Guris D, Bellini WJ (1997) Diagnosis of measles with an IgM capture EIA: the optimal timing of specimen collection after rash onset. *J Infect Dis* 175:195–9.

Huiming Y, Chaomin W, Meng M (2005) Vitamin A for treating measles in children. *Cochrane Database Syst Rev* (4):CD001479. doi: 10.1002/14651858.CD001479.pub2.

Hussey GD, Klein M (1990) A randomized, controlled trial of vitamin A in children with severe measles. *N Engl J Med* 323:160–4.

Johnson R, Griffin D, Hirsch R et al. (1984) Measles encephalomyelitis: clinical and immunologic studies. *N Engl J Med* 310:137–41.

Kabra SK, Lodha R, Hilton DJ (2008) Antibiotics for preventing complications in children with measles. *Cochrane Database Syst Rev* (3):CD001477.

Krasinski K, Borkowsky W (1989) Measles and measles immunity in children infected with human immunodeficiency virus. *JAMA* 261:2512–16.

Leuridan E, Hens N, Hutse V, Ieven M, Aerts M, Van Damme P (2010) Early waning of maternal measles antibodies in era of measles elimination: longitudinal study. *BMJ* 340:c1626.

McLean HQ, Fiebelkorn AP, Temte JL, Wallace GS (2013) Prevention of measles, rubella, congenital rubella syndrome, and mumps, 2013: summary recommendations of the Advisory Committee on Immunization Practices (ACIP). *MMWR Recomm Rep* 62(RR-04):1.

M'garrech M, Gendron G, de Monchy I et al. (2013) Corneal manifestations of measles in the unvaccinated adult: two typical cases during an epidemic. *J Fr Ophtalmol* 36:197–201.

Moss WJ, Griffin DE (2006) Global measles elimination. *Nat Rev Microbiol* 4:900–8.

Moss WJ, Griffin DE (2012) Measles. *Lancet* 379:153–64.

Moss WJ, Scott S, Mugala N et al. (2007) Immunogenicity of standard-titer measles vaccine in HIV-1-infected and uninfected Zambian children: an observational study. *J Infect Dis* 196:347–55.

Nandy R, Handzel T, Zaneidou M et al. (2006) Case-fatality rate during a measles outbreak in eastern Niger in 2003. *Clin Infect Dis* 42:322–8.

Orenstein WA, Perry RT, Halsey NA (2004) The Clinical Significance of Measles: A Review. *J Infect Dis* 189 (Supplement 1):S4–16.

Quiambao B, Gatchalian S, Halonen P et al. (1998) Coinfection is common in measles-associated pneumonia. *Pediatr Infect Dis J* 17:89–93.

Ratnam S, Tipples G, Head C, Fauvel M, Fearon M, Ward B (2000) Performance of indirect immunoglobulin M

(IgM) serology tests and IgM capture assays for laboratory diagnosis of measles. *J Clin Microbiol* 38:99–104.

Red Book (2012) Measles. In: Pickering LK, Baker CJ, Kimberlin DW, Long SS (eds) *Red Book. 2012 Report of the Committee on Infectious Diseases*, 29th edn. Elk Grove, IL: American Academy of Pediatrics, pp. 489–99.

Redd SC, King GE, Heath JL, Forghani B, Bellini WJ, Markowitz LE (2004) Comparison of vaccination with measles–mumps–rubella vaccine at 9, 12, and 15 months of age. *J Infect Dis* 189(Suppl. 1):S116–22.

Scott S, Moss WJ, Cousens S *et al.* (2007) The influence of HIV-1 exposure and infection on levels of passively acquired antibodies to measles virus in Zambian infants. *Clin Infect Dis* 45:1417–24.

Semba R, Bloem M (2004) Measles blindness. *Surv Ophthalmol* 49:243–55.

Shann F, D'Souza R, D'Souza R (2008) Antibiotics for preventing pneumonia in children with measles. *Cochrane Database Syst Rev* (3):CD001477. doi: 10.1002/14651858.CD001477.pub3

Simons E, Ferrari M, Fricks J *et al.* (2012) Assessment of the 2010 global measles mortality reduction goal: results from a model of surveillance data. *Lancet* 349:2173–8.

Stein CE, Birmingham M, Kurian M, Duclos P, Strebel P (2003) The global burden of measles in the year 2000: a model that uses country-specific indicators. *J Infect Dis* 187(Suppl. 1):S8–14.

Strebel PM, Papania MJ, Dayan GH, Halsey N (2008) Chapter 18. Measles vaccines. In: Plotkin SA, Orenstein WA, Offit PA, editors. *Vaccines*. Philadelphia, PA: Saunders/Elsevier, pp. 353–98.

Suringa D, Bank L, Ackerman A (1970) Role of measles virus in skin lesions and Koplik's spots. *N Engl J Med* 283:1139–42.

Tenembaum S, Chamoles N, Fejerman N (2002) Acute disseminated encephalomyelitis: a long-term follow-up study of 84 pediatric patients. *Neurology* 59:1224–31.

Watson JC, Hadler SC, Dykewicz CA, Reef S, Phillips L (1998) Measles, mumps, and rubella: vaccine use and strategies for elimination of measles, rubella, and congenital rubella syndrome and control of mumps. Recommendations of the Advisory Committee on Immunization Practices (ACIP). *MMWR Recomm Rep* 47(RR-8):1–57.

WHO (2004) *Treating Measles in Children*. Geneva: World Health Organization.

WHO (2009) Measles vaccine: WHO position paper. *Wkly Epidemiol Rec* 35:349–60.

WHO (2012) Measles and rubella status report: progress, challenges and lessons. Meeting of the WHO Strategic Advisory Group of Experts 7 November 2012. Geneva: World Health Organization Available at http://www.who.int/immunization/sage/meetings/2012/november/2_Measles_Figueroa.pdf

WHO (2013a) Measles surveillance data. Available at http://www.who.int/immunization/monitoring_surveillance/burden/vpd/surveillance_type/active/measles_monthlydata/en/

WHO (2013b) Measles. Statistics on measles. Available at http://www.who.int/immunization/monitoring_surveillance/burden/vpd/surveillance_type/active/measles/en/

WHO (2013c) *Pocketbook of Hospital Care for Children*, 2nd edn. Geneva: World Health Organization.

WHO (2014) Measles immunization coverage. Available at http://www.who.int/gho/immunization/measles/en/

Wolfson LJ, Grais RF, Luquero FJ, Birmingham ME, Strebel PM (2009) Estimates of measles case fatality ratios: a comprehensive review of community-based studies. *Int J Epidemiol* 38:192–205.

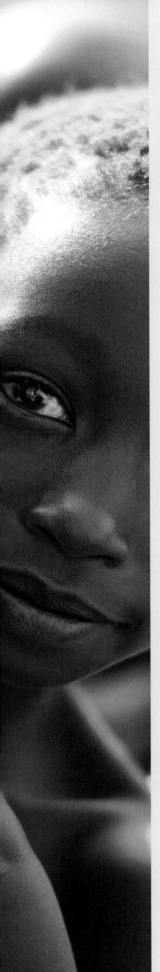

CHAPTER 12

Malnutrition and Micronutrient Deficiencies

Sandra K. Schumacher[1,2] and Sarah E. Messmer[1]
[1]Harvard University Medical School, Boston, MA, USA
[2]Boston Children's Hospital, Boston, MA, USA

Key learning objectives

- Identify the different types of malnutrition and their implications for morbidity and mortality.
- Perform anthropometric measurements and classify a child's growth.
- Understand how to treat acute malnutrition, both inpatient and outpatient.
- Recognize micronutrient deficiencies and their clinical manifestations.
- Understand the broader socioeconomic context of malnutrition and its impact on developing programs to combat child malnutrition.

Abstract

Childhood malnutrition is prevalent worldwide, most notably in resource-limited countries. Up to 50% of child deaths are linked to nutrition-related factors. Malnutrition consists of macronutrient and micronutrient deficiencies and can be acute or chronic. For macronutrient deficiencies, anthropometric measurements are used to determine the type and degree of malnutrition. Mid-upper arm circumference is also used as a rapid screening tool for severe acute malnutrition. Treatment of malnutrition is focused on intensive feeding, with increasing emphasis on community-based treatment models.

Key words: malnutrition, micronutrient, mid-upper arm circumference, severe acute malnutrition, stunting, wasting, kwashiorkor, marasmus

Essential Clinical Global Health, First Edition. Edited by Brett D. Nelson.
© 2015 John Wiley & Sons, Ltd. Published 2015 by John Wiley & Sons, Ltd.
Companion website: www.essentialseries.com/globalhealth

Introduction and epidemiology

Child malnutrition is prevalent worldwide, particularly in resource-limited countries, and carries a great disease burden: an estimated 50% of child deaths have been linked to nutrition-related factors (Caulfield *et al.*, 2004). A lack of adequate nutrition leads to poor growth, a weakened immune system, and impairments in cognitive function (UNICEF-WHO-World Bank, 2012).

A joint report by the World Health Organization (WHO), United Nations Children's Fund (UNICEF), and the World Bank analyzed the growth of children under 5 years old worldwide in 2011. Per this report, approximately 165 million children (26%) in this age group were stunted, with over 90% of stunted children living in Africa and Asia. An estimated 16% were underweight, and 8% met criteria for wasting, with over 70% of wasted children living in Asia. On the other hand, 7% of children under 5 years old were classified as overweight, a 54% increase from 1990 (UNICEF-WHO-World Bank, 2012). The geographic distribution of disease burden due to malnutrition can be seen in the world maps in Figure 12.1.

The underlying causes of child malnutrition are complex. Food insecurity, poverty, inequality, gender roles, local feeding practices, disease, and natural disasters are all factors that contribute to malnutrition (Frongillo *et al.*, 1997; Black *et al.*, 2008). In cases of severe malnutrition, underlying illness such as HIV infection, congenital heart disease, or a metabolic syndrome should be excluded.

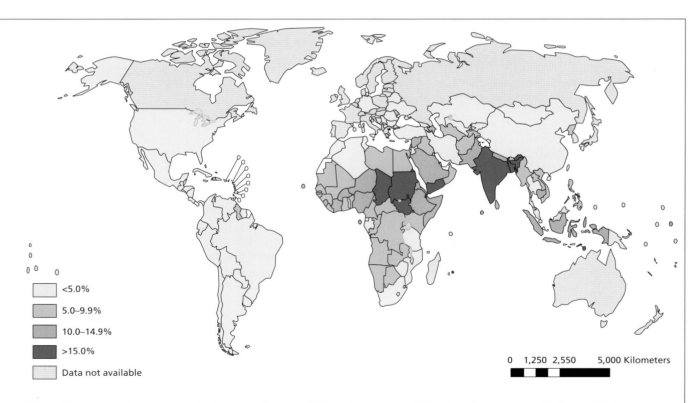

Figure 12.1 By-country estimates of rates of wasting (weight-for-height) among children less than 5 years old. *Source*: World Health Organization (2012), figure 2, p. 10. Reproduced with permission of the World Health Organization.

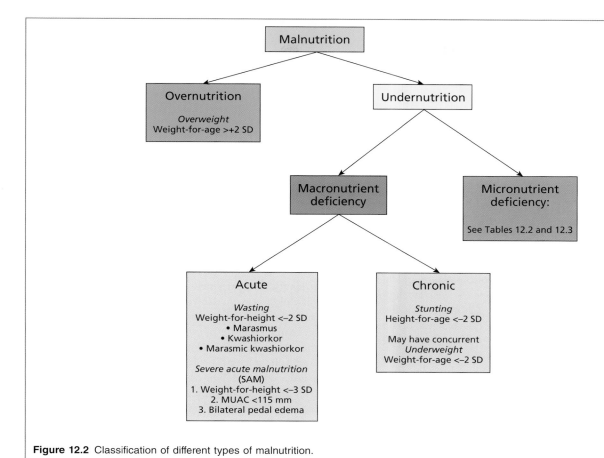

Figure 12.2 Classification of different types of malnutrition.

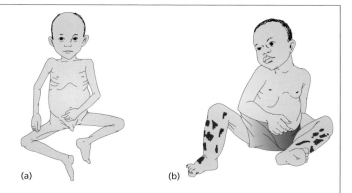

(a)   (b)

Figure 12.3 Phenotypes of acute malnutrition: (a) marasmus and (b) kwashiorkor. Marasmic kwashiorkor may also occur as a mixture of the two phenotypes.

Presentation

Types of malnutrition

Malnutrition can be secondary to macronutrient or micronutrient deficiencies (Figure 12.2). A macronutrient deficiency refers to a lack of total calories, consumed as protein, carbo-

hydrates, and fat, that can occur acutely (as wasting) or chronically (as stunting). At the other end of the spectrum, overnutrition and child obesity are increasing concerns, although they will not be the focus of this chapter. A micronutrient deficiency refers to a lack of a particular vitamin or mineral and will be discussed at the end of the chapter.

Acute malnutrition phenotypes: marasmus, kwashiorkor, and marasmic kwashiorkor

Acute malnutrition (wasting), when severe, may present as one of the following phenotypes: kwashiorkor, marasmus, or marasmic kwashiorkor (Figure 12.3). If a child shows clinical signs of any of these phenotypes, it is an indication for urgent evaluation.

Marasmus is a general nutritional deficiency presenting as a non-edematous form of severe acute wasting. The child often has a "skin and bones" appearance, visible ribs, an "old man" face due to loss of subcutaneous fat, and "baggy pants" due to sagging skin around the buttocks. Although physically these children appear acutely ill, they often remain active, with fewer behavioral changes than other forms of severe malnutrition (World Health Organization, 2008).

Kwashiorkor is predominantly a protein deficiency resulting in an edematous form of severe acute wasting, with the

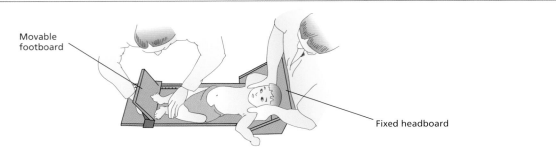

Figure 12.4 For a child under 2 years of age, measure length using a simple length board.

edema often masking the degree of wasting. The low protein may cause reduced intravascular oncotic pressure and hence edema. Skin discoloration and peeling as well as thinning and discolored hair may also occur. Children with kwashiorkor often have significant behavioral changes, becoming irritable, withdrawn, and refusing to eat (World Health Organization, 2008).

In some cases, children have features of both kwashiorkor and marasmus; this is classified as marasmic kwashiorkor. Children with this condition may have a wasted upper body but bilateral pitting edema, although other causes of edema need to be excluded such as heart failure and nephrotic syndrome (World Health Organization, 2008).

 Clinical pearl

Any child with bilateral pitting edema needs further evaluation and treatment. Edema may cause the child's weight to be elevated and artificially reassuring, masking the true degree of malnutrition.

Chronic malnutrition: stunting

Stunting generally presents in a very subtle way: children appear healthy but are short for their age. In areas where stunting is highly prevalent, stunted children appear to be growing well because they are "average" height in their community; however, on plotting their growth on standardized growth curves, the degree of malnutrition becomes evident.

Diagnosis

To diagnose and classify the type of malnutrition, accurate anthropometric measurements are necessary.

Measuring weight

For infants, nude weight should be recorded if possible. For older children, shoes and any heavy clothing should be removed.

Measuring height or length

Height/length is an extremely important data point for monitoring a child's growth. However, it can be difficult to accurately measure the height or length of young children. Children younger than 24 months old should be measured while supine, with the carer helping to calm the child. The child should be measured using a length board, making sure to straighten the child's head while keeping the knees from bending (Figure 12.4). Children 24 months and older should be measured standing, ensuring that the child's heels are pressed against the wall with the feet together.

Screening: mid-upper arm circumference

Another anthropometric measurement used for children in resource-poor settings is the mid-upper arm circumference (MUAC). The MUAC measurement is useful for children aged 6 months to 5 years and is a rapid way to screen for acute malnutrition. The measurement is taken halfway between the elbow and shoulder with the arm relaxed (Figure 12.5). Easy-to-use MUAC tapes are available with four colors corresponding to different triage categories: likely properly nourished (green), at risk (yellow), moderately malnourished (orange), and acutely malnourished (red). Children with an MUAC less than 115 mm have a significantly elevated risk of death and require urgent attention (World Health Organization & United Nations Children's Fund, 2009).

Classifying degree and type of malnutrition based on anthropometric measurements

Once accurate weight and height measurements have been made, they should be plotted on WHO growth curves based on age (WHO Multicentre Growth Reference Study Group, 2006). The definitions of different types of malnutrition are based on WHO child growth standards, using a z-score as a measurement in standard deviations (SD) of a sample from the median value of the reference population. The z-score determines the degree of difference of the child's weight or height from the median at that age.

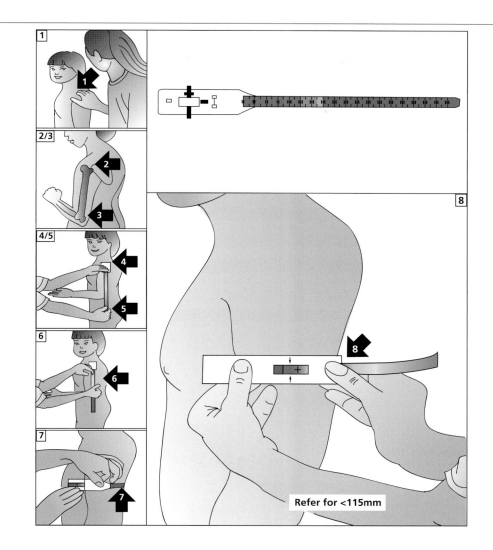

Figure 12.5 Mid-upper arm circumference (MUAC) is a useful screening tool for severe acute malnutrition.

Different classes of malnutrition are defined as follows.

- Stunting (chronic malnutrition): height-for-age z-score 2 SD or more below the median.
- Underweight: weight-for-age z-score 2 SD or more below the median.
- Wasting (acute malnutrition): weight-for-height z-score 2 SD or more below the median. Weight-for-height rather than weight-for-age is used to define wasting because weight-for-age may be artificially low due to concurrent stunting.

Severe acute malnutrition (SAM) is a category of acute malnutrition that requires urgent attention. The diagnostic criteria for SAM include:

- weight-for-height 3 SD or more below the median;
- MUAC <115 mm; or
- bilateral pedal edema (World Health Organization, 2008).

Treatment

Treatment of malnutrition is an evolving field, with increasing focus on community-based treatments and ready-to-use therapeutic foods (RUTF). Acute malnutrition, particularly SAM, and chronic malnutrition are approached very differently.

Acute malnutrition

Children with SAM require immediate attention. Children with weight-for-height z-scores 3 SD below the median have a risk of death ninefold higher than children with weight-for-height z-scores 1 SD below the median, emphasizing the need for urgent treatment (Black *et al.*, 2008; World Health Organization & United Nations Children's Fund, 2009). Treatment of SAM may be community-based or inpatient, depending on the severity. If the child has any medical complications or is not eating, inpatient treatment is required. If no medical

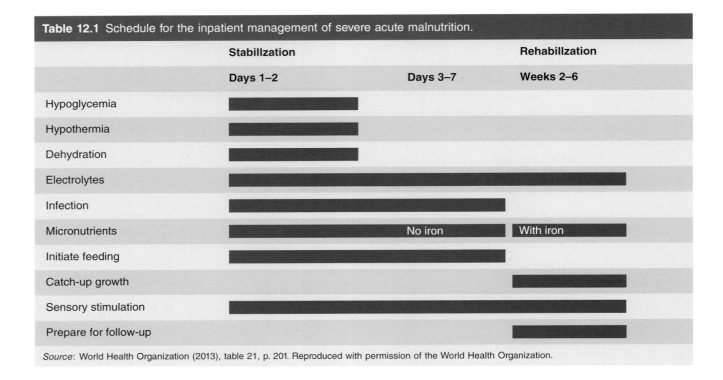

Table 12.1 Schedule for the inpatient management of severe acute malnutrition.

	Stabilization		Rehabilization
	Days 1–2	Days 3–7	Weeks 2–6
Hypoglycemia	████		
Hypothermia	████		
Dehydration	████		
Electrolytes	████████████████████		
Infection	████████████		
Micronutrients	████	No iron	With iron
Initiate feeding	████████████		
Catch-up growth			████
Sensory stimulation	████████████████████		
Prepare for follow-up			████

Source: World Health Organization (2013), table 21, p. 201. Reproduced with permission of the World Health Organization.

complications are present and the child has an appetite, community-based treatment is preferred (World Health Organization & United Nations Children's Fund, 2009).

Inpatient management

Algorithms guide inpatient treatment of SAM (Ashworth *et al.*, 2003). Treatment is divided into three phases: initial treatment (management of life-threatening medical complications such as infections, dehydration, and metabolic abnormalities), rehabilitation (intensive feeding to recover weight loss), and follow-up (post-discharge monitoring to prevent relapse) (Table 12.1).

In the initial phase, a common life-threatening condition is dehydration, often precipitated by diarrheal illness. Oral rehydration solution (ORS) is an effective life-saving solution to dehydration. However, it is important to keep in mind that severely malnourished children are deficient in potassium, while having abnormally elevated sodium levels. Therefore, a special ORS called ReSoMal has been developed specifically for treating dehydration in children with SAM. ReSoMal is available commercially, but its composition is publically available and can be replicated locally. To treat dehydration, give about 70–100 mL/kg of ReSoMal over 12 hours, starting with 5 mL/kg orally or by nasogastric tube every 30 min for the first 2 hours, and then 5–10 mL/kg per hour for the next 10 hours (World Health Organization, 1999).

Feeding also begins in the initial phase. Two formulas have been developed for the treatment of SAM: F-75 and F-100 (Figure 12.6). The F-75 formula includes 75 kcal per 100 mL,

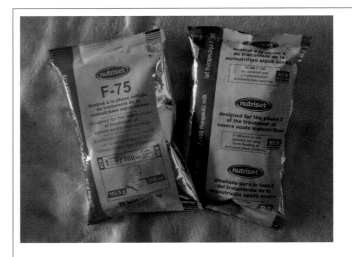

Figure 12.6 Packets of F-75 and F-100 formulas for the treatment of severe acute malnutrition. *Source*: B.D. Nelson, Harvard Medical School, Boston, Massachusetts, USA. Reproduced with permission of B.D. Nelson.

whereas F-100 includes 100 kcal per 100 mL. F-75, as it is less dense, is used for initial treatment, with a goal of 80–100 kcal/kg per day (World Health Organization, 1999).

Once the child has been stabilized medically, the rehabilitation phase begins. During the first 2 days of the rehabilitation phase, the child is transitioned to an equivalent volume of F-100 instead of F-75. The feeding size is then gradually increased with a goal of 150–220 kcal/kg per day. Solid foods may also be reintroduced during the rehabilitation phase for children over 2 years old. Once the child has a good appetite, he or she may be transitioned to community-based management (see below) with continued monitoring at home (World Health Organization, 1999).

As mentioned, a third crucial stage is the follow-up stage. It is important to assess the child's home environment and the factors that led to SAM. Often, children who suffer from SAM are chronically malnourished, and acute illness leads them to become critically ill.

A thorough guide to inpatient management of SAM can be found in World Health Organization (1999), and a toolkit with practical checklists to guide management of patients with SAM is available in World Health Organization (2010).

Community-based management

Whenever possible, community-based management is preferred, as it is generally more acceptable to families and allows the child to remain with the parents. RUTFs have been developed to make home therapy possible. The original RUTFs, such as Plumpy'nut, were developed based on F-100 but with the addition of peanut butter, which resulted in a paste instead of a powder. These types of food supplements have gained popularity because of their long shelf-life and the fact that they do not need to be prepared with water, lowering the risk of a waterborne illness. A variety of RUTFs is available, including some locally produced versions. When choosing an RUTF, it is most important to find one that is both culturally acceptable and readily available locally.

Chronic malnutrition

Chronic malnutrition presents subtly, with stunting contributing to developmental delays and impaired immunity (UNICEF-WHO-World Bank, 2012). Many argue that stunted children can regain height if treated before 24 months of age; however, growth and developmental delays are irreversible outside this critical window (UNICEF, 2013). When developing programs to combat chronic malnutrition, there is a growing focus on the importance of adequate nutrition during the first 1000 days of a child's life, including prenatally to 2 years of age. Successful programs focus on this window by improving mothers' nutrition during pregnancy, supporting exclusive breastfeeding for the first 6 months, educating families about appropriate complementary foods, and providing micronutrient supplementation when needed (UNICEF, 2013). It is important to recognize that chronic malnutrition is usually multifactorial, with its roots in poverty, inequality, and food insecurity. To address this problem adequately, the socioeconomics of the community must be examined, and increased awareness through counseling and education must occur. To assist with treating chronic malnutrition, the WHO has developed a guide to nutrition assessments and education that targets breastfeeding and complementary feeding, and is available in World Health Organization (2008).

Micronutrient deficiencies

Micronutrient deficiencies refer to the lack of a particular vitamin or mineral, often due to an inadequate diet or poor absorption. These deficiencies have certain clinical manifestations, which are shown in Tables 12.2 and 12.3. Of these micronutrient deficiencies, lack of Vitamin A and zinc has been found to contribute most significantly to the global disease burden, leading to approximately 0.6 million and 0.4 million child deaths, respectively, as well as 9% of childhood disability-adjusted-life-years (DALYs) combined (Black et al., 2008). Iron and iodine deficiencies, although resulting in few child deaths, contribute 0.2% of global childhood DALYs (Black et al., 2008).

Vitamin A deficiency can lead to blindness and is therefore an extremely important deficiency to address. It is

Table 12.2 Clinical manifestations of vitamin deficiencies.

Vitamin A (retinol)	Most common worldwide cause of blindness in children
Vitamin B_1 (thiamine)	Beri beri (cardiomegaly, tachycardia, muscle weakness, peripheral paralysis, mental confusion)
Vitamin B_2 (riboflavin)	Anemia, angular stomatitis, seborrheic dermatitis
Vitamin B_3 (niacin)	Pellegra (diarrhea, dermatitis, dementia)
Vitamin B_6 (pyridoxine)	Neuropathy
Vitamin B_9 (folate)	Macrocytic anemia
Vitamin B_{12} (cyanocobalamin)	Pernicious anemia (a form of macrocytic anemia)
Vitamin C (ascorbic acid)	Scurvy (poor wound healing, bleeding gums, leg tenderness)
Vitamin D	Rickets (craniotabes, widened physes of wrists/ankles, femoral/tibial bowing, enlarged costochondral joints)
Vitamin E (tocopherol)	Hemolytic anemia in very young children with prolonged deficiency, neuropathy, muscle weakness
Vitamin K (phylloquinone)	Hemorrhagic disease of newborns

Table 12.3 Clinical manifestations of mineral deficiencies.

Calcium (Ca)	Seizures, arrhythmias, tetany
Copper (Cu)	Anemia, neutropenia, thrombocytopenia, neuropathy
Iodine (I)	Hypothyroidism
Iron (Fe)	Microcytic anemia
Magnesium (Mg)	Muscle weakness, arrhythmias
Potassium (K)	Muscle weakness, arrhythmias
Phosphorus (P)	Muscle weakness
Sodium (Na)	Seizures, cerebral edema, arrhythmias
Zinc (Zn)	Acrodermatitis enteropathica (dry skin, poor wound healing, perioral rashes)

Clinical experience

"While emergency food aid saves lives, it alone cannot solve the long-term challenges that children with malnutrition and their families face. Handouts can sustain patients for a limited time, but health facilities do not have the capacity to meet the long-term nutritional needs of patients, or their families. Many children will fall into a cycle of malnutrition and poor health, and return to health centers with more serious illnesses. We have developed a program that works in close partnership with local health centers, so that children diagnosed with malnutrition not only get the short-term food aid they need, but their families also receive seeds, livestock and education to help their children stay healthy and to produce more nutritious food over the long term. We believe that agriculture can be used as a key driver for community health in rural areas, rather than a practice that contributes to chronic hunger."

Eve, public health professional working in Rwanda

recommended to give a large oral dose of Vitamin A to all severely malnourished children (World Health Organization, 1999). Children younger than 6 months should receive 50,000 IU per dose, children aged 6–12 months should receive 100,000 IU per dose, and children older than 12 months should receive 200,000 IU per dose on the first day of malnutrition treatment, unless there is definitive evidence that a dose of Vitamin A was already given in the month preceding treatment. If there are clinical signs of Vitamin A deficiency such as night blindness, these age-specific doses should be repeated again on the second day of treatment, and again 2 weeks later (World Health Organization, 1999).

Treatment of anemia is also very important to ensure adequate growth and cognitive development. Iron and folic acid supplementation should be provided. In many countries, a powder-based formula including both iron and folic acid has been developed that parents can mix into food, making the supplements more palatable for children. Note that children undergoing treatment for SAM should not be given iron supplementation during the initial phase of treatment as it can make some infections worse, serving as a metabolic source for bacteria. Prescribing iron during this initial phase has been shown to result in increased deaths (World Health Organization, 1999).

Additional resources

- World Health Organization (2008) Training course on child growth assessment. Available at http://www.who.int/childgrowth/training/en/
- World Health Organization (2010) Improving the inpatient management of severe acute malnutrition. Toolkit to monitor current management of severe acute malnutrition. Available at http://www.who.int/nutrition/publications/severemalnutrition/Toolkit_to_monitor_current_SAM.pdf.
- World Health Organization. The WHO child growth standards. Available at http://www.who.int/childgrowth/standards/en/
- Centers for Disease Control and Prevention (2010) Growth charts, based on the WHO child growth standards. Available at http://www.cdc.gov/growthcharts/who_charts.htm
- World Health Organization, the World Food Programme, the United Nations System Standing Committee on Nutrition, the United Nations Children's Fund (2007) Community-based management of severe acute malnutrition. Available at http://www.who.int/nutrition/publications/severemalnutrition/978-92-806-4147-9_eng.pdf

REFERENCES

Ashworth A, Khanum S, Jackson A, Schofield C (2003) Guidelines for the inpatient treatment of severely malnourished children. Available at http://www.who.int/nutrition/publications/guide_inpatient_text.pdf

Black RE, Allen LH, Bhutta ZA *et al.* (2008) Maternal and child undernutrition: global and regional exposures and health consequences. *Lancet* 371:243–60.
Caulfield LE, de Onis M, Blossner M, Black RE (2004) Undernutrition as an underlying cause of child deaths

associated with diarrhea, pneumonia, malaria, and measles. *Am J Clin Nutr* 80:193–8.

Frongillo EA, de Onis M, Hanson KMP (1997) Socioeconomic and demographic factors are associated with worldwide patterns of stunting and wasting of children. *J Nutr* 127:2302–9.

UNICEF (2013) Improving child nutrition: the achievable imperative for global progress. Available at http://www.unicef.org/publications/files/Nutrition_Report_final_lo_res_8_April.pdf

UNICEF-WHO-World Bank (2012) UNICEF-WHO-World Bank joint child malnutrition estimates: levels and trends in child malnutrition. Available at http://www.who.int/nutgrowthdb/jme_unicef_who_wb.pdf?ua=1

WHO Multicentre Growth Reference Study Group (2006) WHO child growth standards: length/height-for-age, weight-for-age, weight-for-length, weight-for-height and body mass index-for-age: methods and development. Available at http://www.who.int/childgrowth/publications/technical_report_pub/en/index.html

World Health Organization (1999) Management of severe malnutrition: a manual for physicians and other senior health workers. Available at http://whqlibdoc.who.int/hq/1999/a57361.pdf

World Health Organization (2008) Training course on child growth assessment. Available at http://www.who.int/childgrowth/training/en/

World Health Organization (2010) Improving the inpatient management of severe acute malnutrition. Toolkit to monitor current management of severe acute malnutrition. Available at http://www.who.int/nutrition/publications/severemalnutrition/Toolkit_to_monitor_current_SAM.pdf.

World Health Organization (2012) Levels and trends in child malnutrition. Available at http://www.who.int/nutgrowthdb/jme_unicef_who_wb.pdf

World Health Organization (2013) *Pocket Book of Hospital Care for Children: Guidelines for the Management of Common Childhood Illnesses*, 2nd edn. Geneva: WHO. Available at http://www.who.int/maternal_child_adolescent/documents/child_hospital_care/en/

World Health Organization & United Nations Children's Fund (2009) WHO child growth standards and the identification of severe acute malnutrition in infants and children. Available at http://whqlibdoc.who.int/publications/2009/9789241598163_eng.pdf

CHAPTER 13
Child Development

Elizabeth Peacock-Chambers[1] and Judith Palfrey[2]
[1]Boston University School of Medicine, Boston, MA, USA
[2]Harvard Medical School, Boston, MA, USA

Key learning objectives

- Understand why child development is important.
- Learn the basics of normal child development.
- Build a toolkit of age-appropriate games and activities.
- Identify potential community resources for children with developmental disability.

Abstract

Hundreds of millions of children fail to reach their developmental potential around the world each year. Both genetic and environmental factors contribute to this problem, although children living in poverty are at increased risk. Ultimately, poor development can lead to lower educational attainment, poor health outcomes, and limited economic success. Healthcare workers have the opportunity to identify children failing to meet developmental milestones and determine whether there are treatable causes or appropriate developmental therapies. By teaching caregivers about child development, simple interventions can prevent developmental delay during critical periods of brain development. Model programs around the world demonstrate how to integrate such interventions into the existing healthcare infrastructure. Further work is needed to increase awareness of child development among healthcare providers and caregivers around the world in order to reach larger populations of children.

Key words: child development, developmental delay, brain development, play, activities, developmental screening

Introduction

More than 200 million children under 5 years of age in low- and middle-income countries (LMICs) do not reach their full developmental potential (Grantham-McGregor *et al.*, 2007). The first 5 years of life is a critical time for development of brain structure and function because of the rapid rate of neuronal growth and networks (First & Palfrey, 1994; Grantham-McGregor *et al.*, 2007). During this period of early child development (ECD), the brain is particularly receptive to positive stimulation and equally vulnerable to toxic stress and neglect (Garner *et al.*, 2012; Shonkoff *et al.*, 2012). Brain development is, therefore, mediated by complex interactions between genetics, biology, and environment (Figure 13.1) (Grantham-McGregor *et al.*, 2007). For example, environmental context can create modifications of DNA that are passed down through generations (Shonkoff *et al.*, 2012). Disruptions to the developing brain may go on to have profound effects on a child's adaptive capacity, resulting in poor educational and health outcomes decades later.

Whether one is working in a medical, surgical, educational, or public health capacity, every encounter with a pediatric patient and their family offers the opportunity to provide positive developmental interactions. Idle children in hospital beds or in the long lines of outpatient clinics are a perfect audience. For those wishing to have possibly an even more lasting impact, working with parents and caregivers is an ideal place to start. Ultimately, sustainable change for the advancement of ECD will require motivation and commitment from local communities and governments.

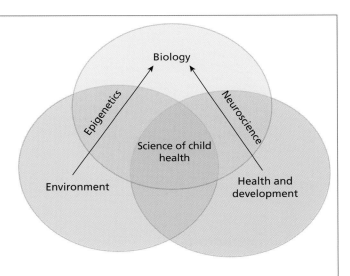

Figure 13.1 The integrated eco-bio-developmental framework: understanding the promotion of health and prevention of disease.

Table 13.1 Risk factors associated with poor growth and development.
Medical
Malnutrition
Toxins
Infections
Prematurity or low birthweight
Perinatal complications (asphyxia)
Congenital syndromes
Social
Poverty
Parental loss
Exposure to violence
Lack of stimulation

Causes of developmental disability

Exact rates of developmental and behavioral problems globally are unknown. Genetic and medical problems, such as birth asphyxia and trauma, continue to be leading causes of severe developmental disability around the world. In LMICs, however, children in general are at an increased risk of poor growth and development since living in poverty-stricken environments exposes children to multiple risk factors (Table 13.1).

Normal child development

Child development can be categorized into three basic domains: fine and gross motor, language, and psychosocial development. Rather than memorizing specific milestones, it can be useful to think about where the child is investing the bulk of his or her developmental energy, as demonstrated in Figure 13.2.

- *0–6 months.* Newborns explore their environment through sensation and visual stimulation. They begin to gain gross motor skills, moving arms and legs, and by 4 months are rolling over and at 6 months are sitting up alone.

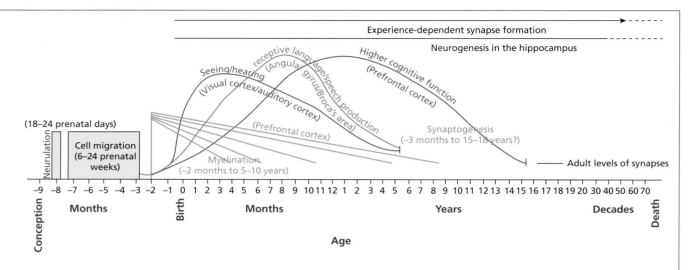

Figure 13.2 Human brain development. Copyright © 2001 by the American Psychological Association. Reproduced with permission from Thompson RA, Nelson CA (2001) Developmental science and the media: early brain development. *Am Psychol* 56:5–15. The use of APA information does not imply endorsement by APA.

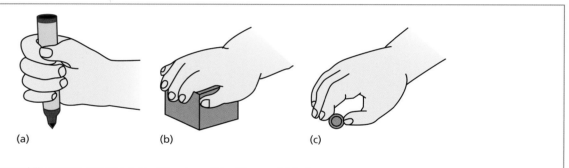

Figure 13.3 Fine motor skills include, progressively, (a) palmar, (b) raking, and (c) pincer grasps.

- *6–12 months.* Gross motor skills continue to advance quickly, first crawling at 8–10 months, then walking by 12–15 months of age. Language becomes increasingly important in this period. By 6 months, an infant displays more babbling with consonant and vowel syllables, such as "bababa," and by 12 months a child may speak his or her first word. Fine motor skills become apparent by children using their fingers in a "pincer grasp" (Figure 13.3) at 11–12 months of age. New understanding of "object permanence" – the fact that an object continues to exist even when it cannot be seen, felt, or heard – allows for new games like "peekaboo" and hiding objects. This may also lead to "stranger anxiety" between 6 and 18 months, a sign of positive attachment with primary caregivers.
- *1–2 years.* The rate of growth in a child's cognitive functioning is at an all-time high during this period. Children are acquiring new skills daily and will want to learn and copy what you do. Drawing, stacking objects, and running/

jumping are new challenges. By 2 years of age, they are starting to put together two-word phrases.
- *3–5 years.* At 3 years, much of a child's speech can be understood, and they ask questions about their surroundings. They enjoy counting and comparing things, for example different shapes or colors. They enjoy learning new songs and stories. This is also the time when children learn to play together instead of in parallel.

🔍 Clinical pearl: play is hard work

For infants and even older children, play can be considered hard work. Newborns and infants can become exhausted after simply making eye contact or copying your expressions. For older children, play is an important part of exploring the world and interacting with others. Allow infants and children to take the lead and look for signs that they may be overstimulated or tired.

Diagnosis and treatment

Development delay is considered failure to reach normal developmental milestones at the expected age, caused by organic, psychological, or environmental factors.

First & Palfrey (1994); American Heritage
Medical Dictionary (2007)

With some basic training, healthcare providers and community members can be empowered to recognize a child with developmental delay. Developmental milestone charts as well as more formal screening questionnaires have been established to assist clinicians in this process. Useful examples of pictorial milestone charts for evaluating and tracking a child's developmental achievements are illustrated in Figure 13.4. These evaluation charts allow longitudinal monitoring of motor, language/cognitive, and psychosocial milestones of a child.

When needed, more rigorous screening tools are also available to assess a child's current level of development. However, finding a culturally appropriate screening tool in resource-limited settings may be a challenge. If a national tool is already in use, it would be the ideal option for the purpose of comparing the development of a specific patient to their local age group. However, the following tools have also been validated in the international settings (see Additional resources for details):

- Ages and Stages Questionnaire (ASQ);
- UNICEF Multiple Indicator Cluster Surveys (MISC);
- UNICEF's Early Child Development Index.

Additionally, Ertem *et al.* (2008) provide an interview-based tool for international use.

Other screening tools, which are more typically used in high-income countries but which could potentially be adapted for other regions, include the Parent Evaluation of Developmental Status (PEDS), Denver II (revised from the Denver Developmental Screening Test, DDST), and the Modified Checklist for Autism in Toddlers (M-CHAT) (see Additional resources section). These tools could be translated and adapted to the local context, while keeping in mind the types of activities and experiences local children typically encounter.

As with all screening tools, no tool is perfect. The sensitivity and specificity of a good child developmental screening tool are often between 70 and 80%.

A toolkit for assessing and fostering child development

Age-appropriate activities with a child can stimulate and foster healthy child development. The World Health Organization (WHO) and the United Nations Children's Fund (UNICEF) have created activity cards called "Care for Child Development" (Figure 13.5). The purpose of these materials is to provide a structure for discussing and teaching age-appropriate activities for children from birth to 5 years. The cards focus on language and play activities. Healthcare providers can use the activities to

interact with children in the clinical setting and to counsel parents on how to encourage child development at home. When talking with parents about child development, a "strengths-based" approach (Box 13.1) has been shown to work best by building on the strengths of both the child and the family.

Having appropriate toys and supplies available is also essential when assessing child development and when modeling developmental activities. Box 13.2 lists useful supplies for a child development toolkit at a healthcare or childcare facility. However, before bringing out the supplies, make sure to create a safe space to play. For infants, a soft clean space without choking or falling hazards is important. For older children, create a space away from traffic, without dangerous chemicals or equipment. Always be aware of any water and the risk of drowning.

When communicating with families and teaching new child development activities or games, remember to incorporate local culture. To understand the local context, consider the following.

- Observe how most parents spend time with their children. How do they view their relationships (e.g., as protector, teacher, disciplinarian)?
- Learn traditional games and songs, if you speak the language.

Clinical experience: child development screening in Guatemala

"While helping with a child nutrition and development project in Guatemala, we quickly realized that the milestones we typically measured did not take into account the local environment or reflect the cultural expectations. For example, on discussing motor milestones with caregivers, it initially seemed that mothers underestimated their child's motor achievements. Almost universally, mothers told us that their walking 12-month-olds had never crawled, but one day the babies could simply walk. I began to connect that mothers continuously carried their young babies wrapped in cloths on their backs. After the babies were about a year old, they were then allowed to walk next to caregivers. Many of the houses had concrete rooms opening onto dirt courtyards and scattered with livestock, fathers' tools, and weaving boards. Mothers did not feel it was safe in this setting to place their young children down to explore their motor abilities. Clearly, the mothers did not underestimate their children's abilities; they simply helped their children grow and learn in safe ways. This realization allowed us to adjust our child development screening tools and then work in partnership with mothers to find new and safe ways for their young babies to explore their world."

Elyse, medical student working in Guatemala

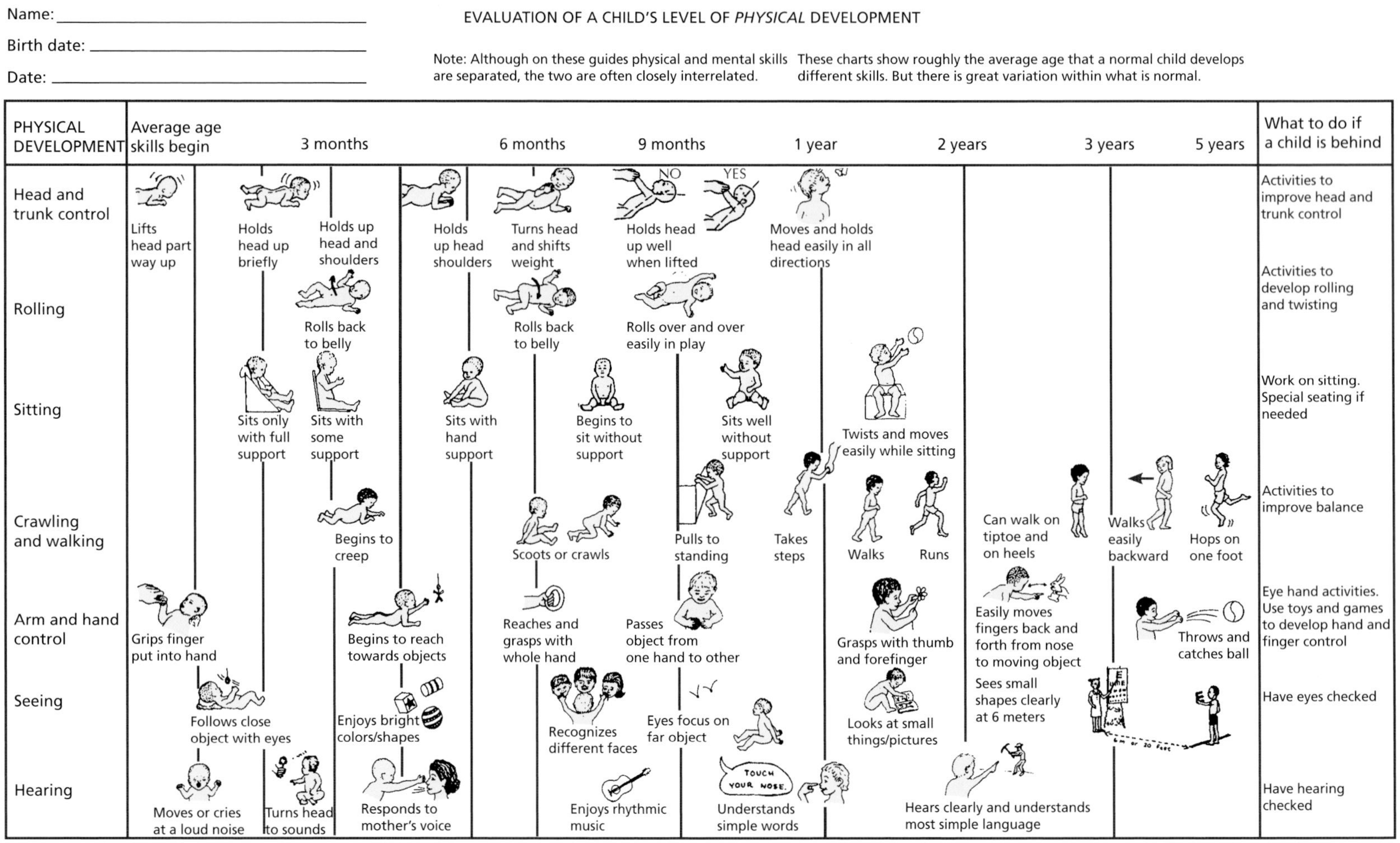

EVALUATION OF A CHILD'S LEVEL OF *PHYSICAL* DEVELOPMENT

Name: _____

Birth date: _____

Date: _____

Note: Although on these guides physical and mental skills are separated, the two are often closely interrelated. These charts show roughly the average age that a normal child develops different skills. But there is great variation within what is normal.

Figure 13.4 Evaluation of normal motor development (a) and language and psychosocial development (b), ages 0–5 years. *Source: Werner (2009). Reproduced with permission of The Hesperian Foundation.

Name: ______________________

Birth date: ______________________

Date: ______________________

EVALUATION OF A CHILD'S LEVEL OF *MFNTAL AND SOCIAL* DEVELOPMENT

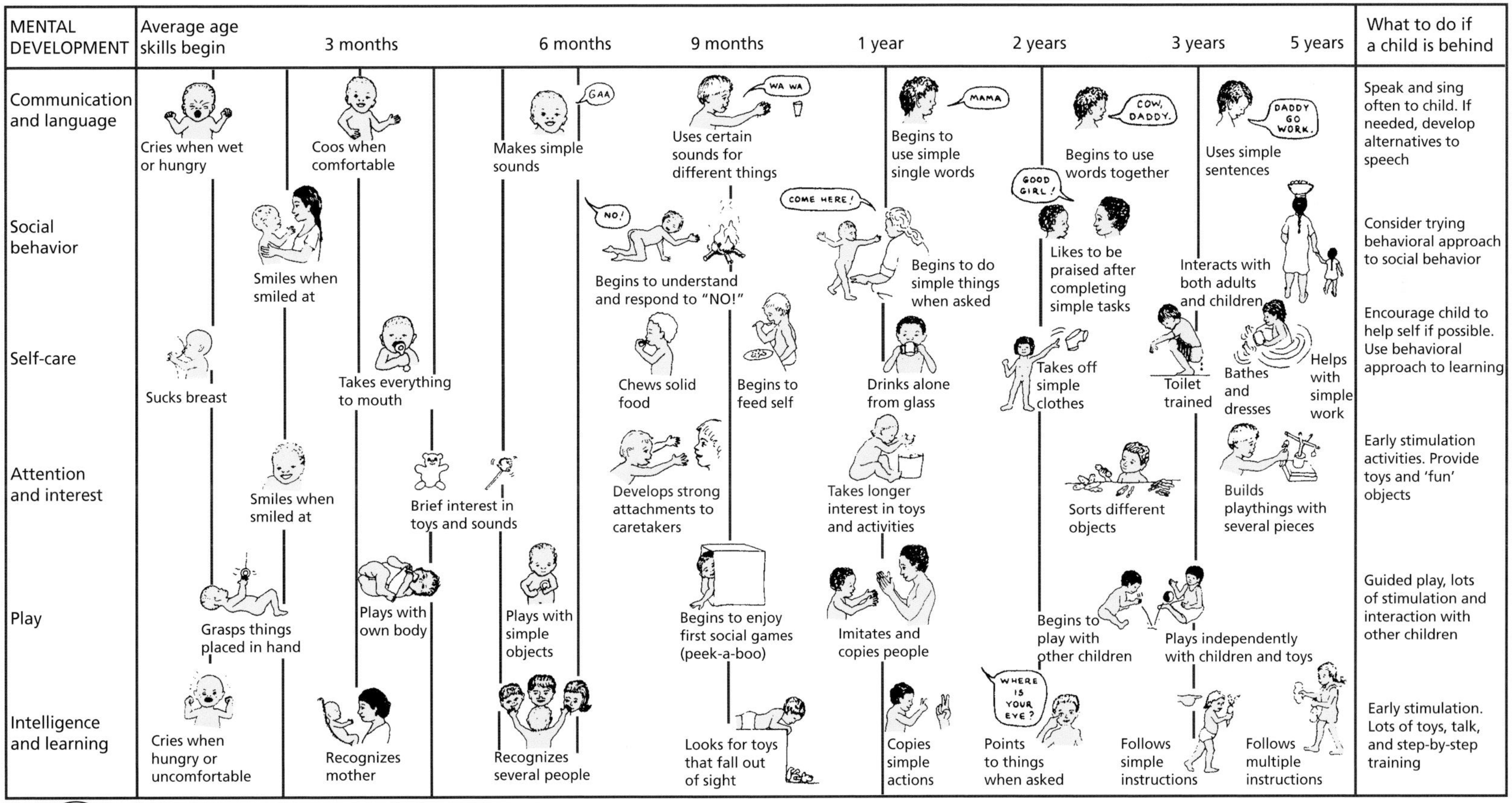
MENTAL DEVELOPMENT
Average age skills begin
3 months
6 months
9 months
1 year
2 years
3 years
5 years
What to do if a child is behind
Communication and language
Cries when wet or hungry
Coos when comfortable
Makes simple sounds
GAA
Uses certain sounds for different things
WA WA
Begins to use simple single words
MAMA
Begins to use words together
COW, DADDY.
Uses simple sentences
DADDY GO WORK.
Speak and sing often to child. If needed, develop alternatives to speech
Social behavior
Smiles when smiled at
Begins to understand and respond to "NO!"
NO!
COME HERE!
Begins to do simple things when asked
GOOD GIRL!
Likes to be praised after completing simple tasks
Interacts with both adults and children
Consider trying behavioral approach to social behavior
Self-care
Sucks breast
Takes everything to mouth
Chews solid food
Begins to feed self
Drinks alone from glass
Takes off simple clothes
Toilet trained
Bathes and dresses
Helps with simple work
Encourage child to help self if possible. Use behavioral approach to learning
Attention and interest
Smiles when smiled at
Brief interest in toys and sounds
Develops strong attachments to caretakers
Takes longer interest in toys and activities
Sorts different objects
Builds playthings with several pieces
Early stimulation activities. Provide toys and 'fun' objects
Play
Grasps things placed in hand
Plays with own body
Plays with simple objects
Begins to enjoy first social games (peek-a-boo)
Imitates and copies people
Begins to play with other children
Plays independently with children and toys
Guided play, lots of stimulation and interaction with other children
Intelligence and learning
Cries when hungry or uncomfortable
Recognizes mother
Recognizes several people
Looks for toys that fall out of sight
Copies simple actions
WHERE IS YOUR EYE?
Points to things when asked
Follows simple instructions
Follows multiple instructions
Early stimulation. Lots of toys, talk, and step-by-step training

Put a (circle) around the level of development that the child is now at in each area.

Put [square] around the skill to the right of the one you circled, and focus training on that skill.

If the child has reached an age and has noi mastered the corresponding level of skill, special training may be needed.

Figure 13.4 *(Continued)*

Recommendations for
Care for Child Development

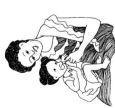

NEWBORN, BIRTH UP TO 1 WEEK	1 WEEK UP TO 6 MONTHS	6 MONTHS UP TO 9 MONTHS	9 MONTHS UP TO 12 MONTHS	12 MONTHS UP TO 2 YEARS	2 YEARS AND OLDER

Your baby learns from birth

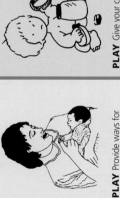

PLAY Provide ways for your baby to see, hear, move arms and legs freely, and touch you. Gently soothe, stroke and hold your child. Skin to skin is good.

PLAY Provide ways for your child to see, hear, feel, move freely, and touch you. Slowly move colorful things for your child to see and reach for. *Sample toys: shaker rattle, big ring on a string.*

PLAY Give your child clean, safe household things to handle, bang, and drop. *Sample toys: containers with lids, metal pot and spoon.*

PLAY Hide a child's favorite toy under a cloth or box. See if the child can find it. Play peek-a-boo.

PLAY Give your child things to stack up, and to put into containers and take out. *Sample toys: Nesting and stacking objects, container and clothes clips.*

PLAY Help your child count, name and compare things. Make simple toys for your child. *Sample toys: Objects of different colors and shapes to sort, stick or chalk board, puzzle.*

COMMUNICATE Look into baby's eyes and talk to your baby. When you are breastfeeding is a good time. Even a newborn baby sees your face and hears your voice.

COMMUNICATE Smile and laugh with your child. Talk to your child. Get a conversation going by copying your child's sounds or gestures.

COMMUNICATE Respond to your child's sounds and interests. Call the child's name, and see your child respond.

COMMUNICATE Tell your child the names of things and people. Show your child how to say things with hands, like "bye bye". *Sample toy: doll with face.*

COMMUNICATE Ask your child simple questions. Respond to your child's attempts to talk. Show and talk about nature, pictures and things.

COMMUNICATE Encourage your child to talk and answer your child's questions. Teach your child stories, songs and games. Talk about pictures or books. *Sample toy: book with pictures*

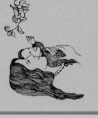
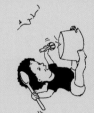
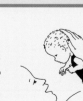

- Give your child affection and show your love
- Be aware of your child's interests and respond to them
- Praise your child for trying to learn new skills

Figure 13.5 Cards for counseling families on child development. *Source:* World Health Organization (2012). Reproduced with permission of the World Health Organization.

Counsel the Family about Problems in **Care for Child Development**

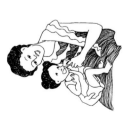

If the mother does not breastfeed, counsel the mother to:

Hold the child close when feeding, look at the child, and talk or sing to the child.

If caregivers do not know what the child does to play or communicate:

- Remind caregivers that children play and communicate from birth.
- Demonstrate how the child responds to activities.

If caregivers feel too burdened or stressed to play and communicate with the child:

- Listen to the caregivers feelings, and help them identify a key person who can share their feelings and help them with their child.
- Build their confidence by demonstrating their ability to carry out a simple activity.
- Refer caregivers to a local service, if needed and available.

If caregivers feel that they do not have time to play and communicate with the child:

- Encourage them to combine play and communication activities with other care for the child.
- Ask other family members to help care for the child or help with chores.

If caregivers have no toys for the child to play with, counsel them to:

- Use any household objects that are clean and safe.
- Make simple toys.
- Play with the child. The child will learn by playing with the caregivers and other people.

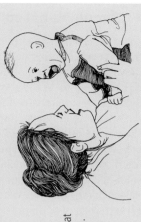

If the child is not responding, or seems slow:

- Encourage the family to do extra play and communication activities with the child.
- Check to see whether the child is able to see and to hear.
- Refer the child with difficulties to special services.
- Encourage the family to play and communicate with the child through touch and movement, as well as through language.

If the mother or father has to leave the child with someone else for a period of time:

- Identify at least one person who can care for the child regularly, and give the child love and attention.
- Get the child used to being with the new person gradually.
- Encourage the mother and father to spend time with the child when possible.

If it seems that the child is being treated harshly:

Recommend better ways of dealing with the child.

- Encourage the family to look for opportunities to praise the child for good behavior.
- Respect the child's feelings. Try to understand why the child is sad or angry.
- Give the child choices about what to do, instead of saying "don't".

Figure 13.4 (*Continued*)

Box 13.1 "Strengths-based" approach to early child development

All families and all children have particular areas of strength as well as challenges they face. Children will frequently advance in one area of development, such as gross motor skills (Figure 13.6), ahead of another area, such as language. A strengths-based approach to child development encourages healthcare providers and parents to first focus on the family's and child's strengths, providing praise and building confidence. The provider–caregiver team can then turn attention to areas of developmental delay while continuing to nurture a child's natural abilities. Caregivers may be naturally interested in nurturing certain skills over others. Helping families become aware of their own strengths and challenges helps frame a plan for developmental interventions.

Developmentally appropriate activities can reflect the culture and community from which children come and can involve simple local materials. For instance, in a seaside community, children can learn naming, counting, shapes, and special relationships by handling objects found on the beach (e.g., shells, starfish, algae).

Simple books that tell stories from the local area can build on community strengths. Reach Out and Read, for example, has developed books in Haitian Creole and Philippine Tagalog. Children identify with the characters and local places as they hear the story being told or read.

Music and art build on community strengths. Coloring mandalas from Southeast Asia and Central America are great activities to teach fine motor skills, shapes, color, and design. Simple local songs teach language, stories, rhythm, and rhyme.

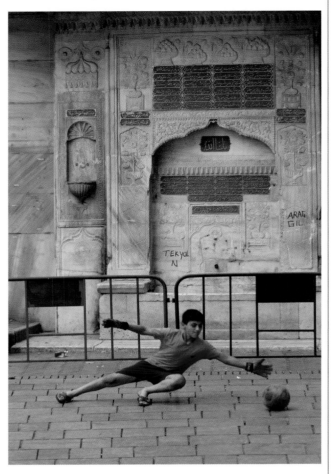

Figure 13.6 Child in Istanbul playing football. *Source*: B.D. Nelson, Harvard Medical School, Boston, Massachusetts, USA. Reproduced with permission of B.D. Nelson.

Box 13.2 Supplies for an early child development tool kit

Books
- Collect donations in your home country or abroad.
- Reading is one of the best language, motor, and social activities for children.

Paper and crayons/pens
- These are a simple intervention but can be incredibly effective.

Balls
- Football/soccer, tennis, rubber balls, anything that fits in your suitcase.

Theater
- Collecting dress-up clothes and props from the community lets older children escape into their imaginations.
- Theater can also be a powerful tool for self-expression, education, and addressing difficult topics.

For infants
- No need for fancy toys.
- Clean stackable objects, cups, cans, or boxes do quite well.
- To prevent choking, ensure that objects are large enough that they do not fit through, for example, a toilet paper roll.

- Incorporate traditional clothing, artwork, or the local environment into your activities. Coastal, farming, or mountain towns each serve as great classrooms for children.
- Be creative! See what toys are commonly used in the community. How can you make a new game out of common toys or materials? Children are much better at making up new games out of common objects, so follow their lead.

Treatment

Treatment options for children with identified developmental delay vary widely within LMICs. Whenever available, accessing and utilizing the local infrastructure is the most sustainable option. Government agencies, public health departments, non-governmental organizations, and private practitioners are all potential resources, depending on the location.

Stakeholders who may be involved in providing care for developmental delay include:

- parents and motivated community members;
- teachers;
- psychologists;
- speech pathologists;
- physical and occupational therapists.

However, in many parts of the world, especially in rural areas, no organized system or programs exist for the promotion of optimal child development or treatment of developmental delay. Developing an ECD program at a local hospital or clinic could therefore provide a long-lasting impact for a larger population.

> ### Clinical pearl
> The key to the most successful and sustainable child development programs involves integration into existing health and education systems.

Each encounter with a family or child can address the "whole child" with a comprehensive approach to child and family health. This may involve, for example, turning an acute medical visit for mild diarrhea into an opportunity to also address signs of malnutrition, review two or three developmental milestones, and assess the caregiver's ability to read infant cues or the bond they have established with their infant. Box 13.3 includes additional strategies for incorporating child development into established child healthcare services.

An effective model for integrating ECD into existing healthcare services includes UNICEF's and WHO's program for integrating ECD into child nutrition services (UNICEF & WHO, 2012).

> ### Box 13.3 Strategies to promote integrated child healthcare
> - Envision the multipurpose use of your healthcare infrastructure
> - Capitalize on waiting time in hospitals and clinics as opportunities for screening and education
> - Train non-medical personnel or community health workers in essential child development
> - Create natural partnerships, for example with nutrition and childcare programs
> - Keep it simple! Example: Give a picture book to a 6-month-old infant and talk to the family about the benefits of reading

Review of successful programs

Various child development interventions have been reviewed for their success in preventing developmental delay and promoting optimal ECD. Some of these programs have been integrated into regional and national health systems. Common themes of successful child development programs include (Engle *et al.*, 2011):

- involvement of both the caregiver and the child in your intervention;
- using participatory or active education strategies to show and promote caregiving behaviors through practice, role play, or coaching to improve parent–child interactions;
- training childcare workers with standardized curricula (see Additional resources section);
- establishing high-quality "center-based learning" (e.g., childcare facilities) for children under 5, which improve cognitive development and school readiness;
- targeting vulnerable populations (e.g., orphans, children with comorbid conditions);
- considering partnering with groups conducting creative interventions outside the healthcare system, such as cash-transfer or micro-loan programs for single mothers, since extreme poverty has been shown to be a significant risk factor for poor development;
- promoting child development media through local radio or internet networks.

For those working at the health systems level, examples of evidence-based interventions have already been developed. Please see the Additional resources section for reviews of successful systems-level interventions as well as strategies for conducting monitoring and evaluation of programs or ECD research internationally (Fernald *et al.*, 2009).

The future of global child development

As countries progress along the spectrum of economic development and improve their rates of under-five child survival, new populations with developmental disability may arise, such as preterm infants or children with perinatal complications who previously may not have survived infancy. Governments will hopefully increasingly recognize the positive economic implications of investing in child development; for example, the economic gain by increasing pre-school enrollment by 50% in LMICs is estimated to be US$33 billion (Engle *et al.*, 2011). Meanwhile, healthcare and educational professionals will need to play a central role in ensuring that children thrive physically as well as emotionally, socially, and developmentally.

Additional resources

Child development groups

- Center on the Developing Child. Global Children's Initiative. Available at http://developingchild.harvard.edu/topics/global_child_development/
- Consultative Group on Early Childhood Care and Development. Available at http://www.ecdgroup.com
- The World Bank. Early Child Development. Available at http://web.worldbank.org/WBSITE/EXTERNAL/TOPICS/EXTCY/EXTECD/0,,menuPK:344945~pagePK:149018~piPK:149093~theSitePK:344939,00.html
- International Society on Early Intervention. Available at http://depts.washington.edu/isei/index.html
- Universal Baby. Available at http://universalbaby.org/

Toolkits

- Care for child development: improving the care for young children. Available at http://www.who.int/maternal_child_adolescent/documents/care_child_development/en/index.html
- ECD Group. "The Essential Package" Toolkit and guides. Available at http://www.ecdgroup.com

Screening tools

- UNICEF. MICS. Available at http://www.childinfo.org/mics.html
- UNICEF. Early child development index (36–59 months). Available at http://www.childinfo.org/ecd_indicators_mics.html
- ASQ. Available at http://agesandstages.com/
- PEDS. Available at http://www.pedstest.com/default.aspx
- Denver II. Available at http://www.denveriionline.com/
- M-CHAT. Available at https://www.m-chat.org/
- Ertem IO, Dogan DG, Gok CG *et al.* (2008) A guide for monitoring child development in low- and middle-income countries. *Pediatrics* 121:e581–9.

Interventions

- UNICEF (2006) Programming experiences in early child development. Available at http://www.unicef.org/earlychildhood/files/programming%20experiences%20in%20early%20childhood.pdf
- UNICEF & WHO (2012) Integrating Early Childhood Development (ECD) activities into nutrition programmes in emergencies: why, what, and how. Available at http://www.who.int/mental_health/emergencies/ecd_note.pdf
- Engle PL, Fernald LCH, Alderman H *et al.* (2011) Strategies for reducing inequalities and improving developmental outcomes for young children in low-income and middle-income countries. *Lancet* 378:1339–53.

Monitoring and evaluation of programs

- Care for child development. A framework for monitoring and evaluating the WHO/UNICEF intervention. Available at http://apps.who.int/iris/bitstream/10665/75149/17/9789241548403_eng_Framework.pdf
- Fernald LCH, Kariger P, Engle P, Raikes A (2009) Examining early child development in low-income countries: a toolkit for the assessment of children in the first five years of life. Washington, DC: The World Bank. Available at http://www.unicef.org/ceecis/Examining_ECD_Toolkit_FULL.pdf

REFERENCES

American Heritage Medical Dictionary (2007) Boston: Houghton Mifflin Company.

Engle PL, Fernald LCH, Alderman H *et al.* (2011) Strategies for reducing inequalities and improving developmental outcomes for young children in low-income and middle-income countries. *Lancet* 378:1339–53.

Ertem IO, Dogan DG, Gok CG *et al.* (2008) A guide for monitoring child development in low- and middle-income countries. *Pediatrics* 121:e581–9.

Fernald LCH, Kariger P, Engle P, Raikes A (2009) *Examining early child development in low-income countries: a toolkit for the assessment of children in the first five years of life.* Washington, DC: The World Bank.

First LR, Palfrey JS (1994) The infant or young child with developmental delay. *N Engl J Med* 330:478–83.

Garner AS, Shonkoff JP, Siegel BS *et al.* (2012) Early childhood adversity, toxic stress, and the role of the pediatrician: translating developmental science into lifelong health. *Pediatrics* 129:e224–31.

Grantham-McGregor S, Cheung YB, Cueto S, Glewwe P, Richter L, Strupp B (2007) Developmental potential in the first 5 years for children in developing countries. *Lancet* 369:60–70.

Shonkoff JP, Garner AA, Siegel BS *et al.* (2012) Toxic stress, brain development, and the early childhood foundations of lifelong health. *Pediatrics* 129:e232–46.

Thompson RA, Nelson CA (2001) Developmental science and the media: early brain development. *Am Psychol* 56:5–15.

UNICEF & WHO (2012) Integrating Early Childhood Development (ECD) activities into nutrition programmes in emergencies: why, what, and how. http://www.who.int/mental_health/emergencies/ecd _note.pdf

Werner D (2009) *Disabled Village Children: A Guide for Community Health Workers, Rehabilitation Workers, and Families*, 2nd edn. Berkley, CA: The Hesperian Foundation.

World Health Organizatin (2012) *Care for Child Development: Improving the Care for Young Children*. Geneva: WHO. Available at http://www.who.int/ maternal_child_adolescent/documents/care_child _development/en/

Part 3
Adolescent,
Reproductive, and
Maternal Health

CHAPTER 14
Adolescent Health

Peter S. Azzopardi[1,2,3], Mick B. Creati[1], and Susan M. Sawyer[1,2,3]
[1]Royal Children's Hospital, Victoria, Australia
[2]Murdoch Childrens Research Institute, Victoria, Australia
[3]University of Melbourne, Melbourne, Victoria, Australia

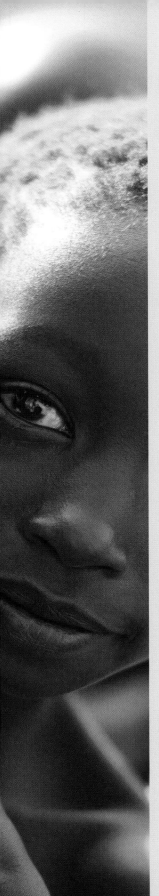

Key learning objectives

- Understand adolescence as an important stage of human development.
- Appreciate how adolescence is relevant to global health.
- Understand the major health issues for adolescents and learn the key skills required to provide quality healthcare for adolescents.
- Learn how to make a health service more adolescent-friendly.

Abstract

Adolescence is increasingly recognized by the global health community as a developmental stage of great opportunity for lasting health gains across the lifecourse. This chapter aims to provide clinicians working in resource-limited settings with the key knowledge and skills to realize these opportunities. The chapter outlines the critical reasons for investing in adolescent health, summarizes adolescent development as it relates to health and well-being, and describes the major health issues that affect young people globally. The chapter then focuses on the core clinical skills that underpin consultations with young people: assuring confidentiality, moving beyond the presenting complaint, and conducting a psychosocial assessment. Beyond individual clinical skills, a wider framework is presented that informs how health services can be made more adolescent-friendly.

Key words: adolescent health, adolescent medicine, youth health, development, well-being, confidentiality, psychosocial assessment, prevention, health promotion, adolescent-friendly health care

Essential Clinical Global Health, First Edition. Edited by Brett D. Nelson.
© 2015 John Wiley & Sons, Ltd. Published 2015 by John Wiley & Sons, Ltd.
Companion website: www.essentialseries.com/globalhealth

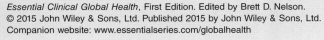

Introduction

Adolescence is increasingly recognized as an age of immense opportunity for global health. Old notions of adolescence as a brief and healthy stage of life are being replaced by new views that highlight both the extent of the burden of disease experienced by adolescents and the opportunities for health across the lifecourse that can be achieved during this developmental stage.

The WHO defines "adolescents" as people aged 10–19 years and "youth" as those aged 15–24 years. The terms "young people" and "adolescents and young adults" are increasingly used to refer to 10–24 year olds, commonly differentiated into three 5-year age bands of early adolescence (10–14 years), late adolescence (15–19 years), and young adults (20–24 years) (Sawyer *et al.*, 2012). In this chapter, we use the terms "adolescents," "adolescents and young adults," and "young people" interchangeably to refer to the 10–24 year old age group.

Today's generation of young people is the largest in human history, with over one-quarter of the world's population aged 10–24 years. In low- to middle-income countries, however, high fertility rates and improvements in child survival result in adolescents representing an even larger proportion of the population. For example, young people comprise well over one-third of the population in many sub-Saharan African and Middle Eastern countries (Figure 14.1) (Sawyer *et al.*, 2012).

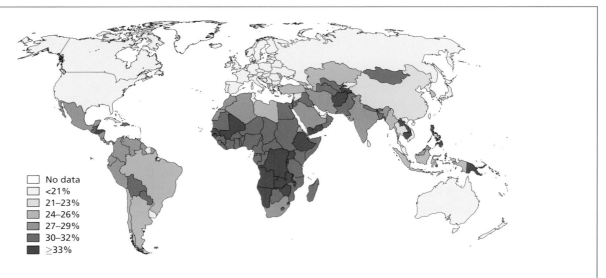

No data
<21%
21–23%
24–26%
27–29%
30–32%
≥33%

Figure 14.1 World map: adolescents and young adults as a proportion of national populations. Reprinted from *The Lancet*, 379, Sawyer SM, Afifi RA, Bearinger LH *et al.* Adolescence: a foundation for future health, 1630–1640 (2012), with permission from Elsevier.

The imperatives to invest in adolescent health

The world is now home to 1.8 billion adolescents aged 10–24 years. While their right to health is a basic human right (Sawyer *et al.*, 2012), there are at least five additional imperatives to invest in the health and well-being of adolescents (UNICEF, 2011).

Firstly, adolescents and their health are critical to the socio-economic development of a community (World Bank, 2007).

Supporting adolescents' access to education and employment is critical to breaking the intergenerational cycle of disadvantage and essential to driving the socioeconomic development of communities (Viner *et al.*, 2012). This will be most effectively realized through empowerment of women and girls and through efforts to reduce current inequities in access to education and employment.

Secondly, adolescence is a period where the health gains from earlier childhood can be consolidated. Significant improvements in the health and well-being of children, characterized by reduced under-five mortality and increasing rates of primary education, can only be fully realized if they are met with appropriate investment in the second decade of life and beyond. Additionally, adolescence is increasingly being recognized as critical to further reducing early childhood mortality and improving child health. Children born to adolescent mothers are at excess risk of mortality, a risk that is compounded by poor maternal nutrition (Black *et al.*, 2013).

Thirdly, adolescence is a period where future patterns of adult health are established; many health-related behaviors (e.g., tobacco and alcohol use) and health-related states (e.g., mental health disorders, overweight, and obesity) have their onset in adolescence and substantially contribute to the burden of non-communicable disease (NCD) in adults. NCDs are now among the leading contributors to the burden of disease globally, not just in the high-income world (Murray *et al.*, 2013).

Fourthly, adolescence provides significant opportunities (and risks) for sexual and reproductive health. Sexual activity usually commences during adolescence. However, early sexual debut (<15 years of age) has broad health implications as young adolescents do not have the knowledge and skills to negotiate safe sex (Patton *et al.*, 2012). Adolescents disproportionately contribute to sexually transmitted infections, including HIV, and are an important population for preventive interventions. Additionally, around 16 million adolescents aged 15–19 years give birth each year, of which 95% are in developing countries (Mangiaterra *et al.*, 2008). Complications related to pregnancy and childbirth are among the leading causes of death of 15- to 19-year-old females, who are twice as likely to die from maternal causes as women in their twenties

and for whom complications such as obstetric fistulae can have lifelong effects on morbidity (Glasier *et al.*, 2006). Early pregnancy can also have profound long-term and intergenerational impacts, contributing to poorer child health outcomes and perpetuating a cycle of gender inequality and poverty (WHO, 2007).

Finally, the developmental aspects of adolescence have many implications for health services providing clinical care and for community agencies focused on prevention and early intervention. While the particular health needs of adolescents are not necessarily met by health services targeting children or adults, neither are health promotional or preventive interventions that are developed for children or adults typically influential for young people.

Adolescent development

Puberty heralds the onset of adolescence, while the social role transitions (such as completion of education, employment, marriage/union, and parenting) usually signify its completion and transition to adulthood (Figure 14.2). Variations in the timing of puberty, the nature of social role changes for males and females, and the hopes and aspirations of adolescents across the globe are widely influenced by the social determinants of health, including distal economic and sociocultural factors and more proximal risk and protective factors derived from family, peers and community (Sawyer *et al.*, 2012).

Understanding adolescent development includes knowledge of the various effects of puberty and neurocognitive maturation (Table 14.1). Puberty is initiated in childhood with a cascade of endocrine changes that, among other changes, leads

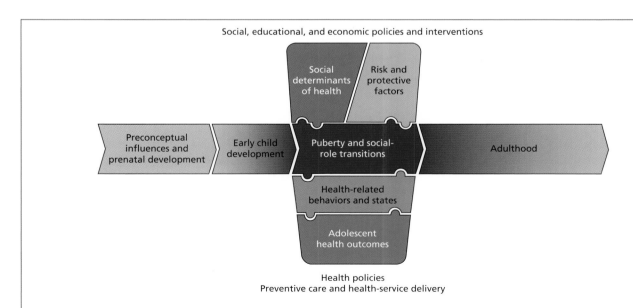

Figure 14.2 Conceptual framework for adolescence. Reprinted from *The Lancet*, 379, Sawyer SM, Afifi RA, Bearinger LH *et al*. Adolescence: a foundation for future health, 1630–1640 (2012), with permission from Elsevier.

Table 14.1 Developmental characteristics of adolescence.

	Physical development	Cognitive development	Social and emotional development
Early adolescence (age 10–14 years)	Puberty: growth of body hair, increased perspiration and oil production in hair and skin; great physical growth (both height and weight); breast and hip development and onset of menstruation (girls); growth of testicles and penis, wet dreams and deepening of voice (boys)	Growth in capacity for abstract thought; mostly interested in present with little thought about the future; expansion of and increased importance placed on intellectual interests; deepening of moral thinking.	Struggle with sense of identity; feel awkward about themselves and their body; worry about being normal; realize that parents are not perfect; have heightened conflict with parents; become increasingly influenced by peer group; have raised desire for independence; return to childish behavior when stressed; are prone to mood swings; test rules and limits; become more private; have a growing interest in sex.
Late adolescence (age 15–19 years)	Physical growth slows for girls but continues for boys	Continued growth in capacity for abstract thought; increased capacity for setting goals; interest in moral reasoning; think about the meaning of life.	Have intense self-involvement, alternating between high expectations and poor self-identity; continue to adjust to changing body worry about being normal; tend to distance themselves from their parents; have a continued drive for independence; are driven to make friends and have a greater reliance on them (popularity can be an important issue); have a heightened capacity for emotional regulation; experience feelings of love and passion; have increasing interest in sex.
Young adulthood	Young women are typically fully developed physically; young men continue to gain height, weight, muscle mass and body hair	Ability to think ideas through from beginning to end; ability to delay gratification; examination of inner experiences; increased concern for the future; continued interest in moral reasoning.	Have a firmer sense of identity, including sexual identity; have increased emotional stability, concern for others and independence and self-reliance; still place importance on peer relationships; regain some interest in social and cultural traditions.

Source: reprinted from *The Lancet*, 379, Sawyer SM, Afifi RA, Bearinger LH *et al*. Adolescence: a foundation for future health, 1630–1640 (2012), with permission from Elsevier.

to sexual maturation and reproductive capacity. Its consequences for health and well-being are profound and paradoxical: while puberty results in physical maturation with peaks in strength and reproductive capacity, it is also accompanied by a rise in emotional and behavioral problems that can have long-lasting effects, such as major affective and anxiety disorders, tobacco and substance use, and functional somatic disorders (e.g., headache, abdominal pain). This has given rise to a view of adolescence as a period of vulnerability due to heightened sensitivity to social and environmental influences that can become manifest as mental and behavioral disorders. Patterns of response can become biologically embedded or "hard-wired" and more resistant to later interventions. There is therefore great interest in how interventions at this critical time, including health interventions, may alter this trajectory (Viner *et al.*, 2012).

Neurocognitive development is a key feature of adolescent development, with brain maturation continuing into the mid-twentiess. Brain connections and signaling mechanisms selectively change during adolescence. Some of the most important changes occur in the prefrontal cortex, the region responsible for planning, decision-making, impulse control, and self-awareness. The prefrontal cortex starts to develop very early in life and continues across adolescence until at least the third decade. In contrast, the limbic system, which governs reward processing, appetite, and pleasure-seeking, matures earlier. The greatest disparity in the maturation of these two systems (limbic and prefrontal cortex) is during early to mid adolescence, which might reflect a developmental imbalance favoring behaviors driven by pleasurable emotional rewards over more rational decision-making. Activities that involve peers are prone to involve greater risk-taking. In situations involving peers, adolescents may engage in risky behaviors despite knowledge of risks that, in the absence of peers, they might otherwise decide not to engage in. Their heightened sensitivity to peers extends to media environments including social networking, which can powerfully shape expectations about adolescent behaviors.

Pubertal and neurocognitive maturation are accompanied by greater emotional regulation and a shifting significance of social relationships that are played out within family, peers, school, and community. The developmental tasks of adolescence are around more mature understandings of autonomy and independence; body self-integrity, sexuality, and personal identity; and educational and vocational goals. These tasks can also be framed in relation to standing out, fitting in, measuring up, and taking hold. "Standing out" refers to young people developing their identity and pursuing activities more autonomously. This includes differentiating themselves from their parents (such as by wearing different clothes). "Fitting in" is about finding comfortable affiliations and gaining acceptance from one's peers (such as by doing similar things, like supporting the same football team, wearing similar jewellery, or getting a tattoo). Adolescence is also the time in which young people wish to "measure up" by developing competence and finding ways to achieve, which can include academic, recreational, and creative pursuits. "Taking hold" refers to the commitments that young people typically make in adolescence to particular goals, activities, beliefs, and values.

Parents remain highly influential in most young people's lives across adolescence (even if young people say otherwise!). However, in most societies, young people no longer simply do what their parents (or healthcare providers) tell them to do but must come to their own understandings of why they do particular things – or not (Box 14.1). While adolescents do not require the same physical protection as younger children, they continue to benefit from "social scaffolding," that is, ensuring that families, schools, and communities provide safe social and emotional (as well as physical) environments for young people. Young people who are given too much autonomy too early, or too little too late, have poorer life and health outcomes.

What makes these developmental changes even more challenging is that they are now played out within communities and countries that are experiencing rapidly changing sociocultural environments due to increased urbanization, globalization, and economic development together with changing gender roles, prolonged periods of education for both girls and boys, and greater access to social media, many of the consequences of which are still unknown.

Major health issues for adolescents

The major health issues for young people are shown in Table 14.2. Many of these health issues reflect the complex interactions between the biology of adolescence and the social determinants of health. Injury and mental health disorders account

---

Box 14.1 Case study 1 (Azzopardi, 2012)

One evening on-call, you answer a knock at your door. As the pediatric doctor on duty, you expected a pediatric emergency. Instead, you find a teenage boy standing in the shadows. "Doc, my girlfriend has just come back, and we are going to have sex, and I need your help." You may seem a little confused, so he continues to explain his situation. "Doc, I know all about ABC. A is for abstinence, but I don't want to abstain. I want to have sex. B is for being faithful. … So I need C, a condom. Can you give me one?" Despite the ABC message being advertised on prominent billboards across town, he tells you that condoms are difficult to find. He hasn't been to the clinic because the nurse there is his *wantok* (from the same village or family), and he doesn't have any money to buy them from the pharmacist.

---

for the majority of the burden of disease experienced by young people. Sexual debut usually occurs during adolescence, and sexually transmitted infection, unplanned pregnancy, and termination of pregnancy are significant contributors to the burden of disease experienced by adolescent females.

Adolescence and young adulthood is the age of onset of health-related behaviors (such as diet, physical activity, smoking, use of alcohol and other substances) that, once stably established, typically persist to impact on NCDs in adulthood (Beaglehole *et al.*, 2011).

In addition, significant improvements in child survival and medical technologies have resulted in more children surviving into adolescence with congenital or early-onset chronic conditions, while adolescence itself is also characterized by development of new chronic conditions and disabilities, such as obesity, type 2 diabetes, HIV/AIDS, and acquired brain injuries following trauma.

Particular groups of young people are at greater risk for poor health and life outcomes (Sawyer *et al.*, 2012). Examples include adolescents and young adults who are socially marginalized and excluded because of ethnic minority or refugee status; homelessness; sexual orientation or sexual behaviors such as gay, lesbian, bisexual and transgender youth, and men who have sex with men; young people who engage in transactional sex; substance users; and youth offenders.

Making health services adolescent-friendly

Many young people experience significant barriers to accessing health services. While such barriers are important in any age group, that many of the health issues experienced by

Table 14.2 Major health issues for adolescent and young people globally.

Health priority	Rationale
Injury (intentional or unintentional)	Road traffic accidents are the leading cause of mortality in 10–24 year olds; 40% of all deaths in this age group are due to either road traffic accidents, homicide, suicide, violence, war, drowning, or fire
Mental health disorders	Mental health disorders are the leading cause of disability and death in 10–24 year olds Self-inflicted injuries are the second leading cause of mortality in 10–24 year olds 75% of adult mental disorders have their onset before 24 years of age, 50% before 14 years
Sexual and reproductive health	Sexual debut usually occurs during adolescence 1 in 8 births in low- and middle-income countries are to 15–19 year olds Over 40% of married 15–19 year olds wish to avoid pregnancy, but two-thirds are not using effective contraception Abortion accounts for 3.7% of the burden of disease experienced by females aged 10–24 years; maternal sepsis accounts for 2.7% HIV/AIDS is the second leading cause of death in 20–24 year olds
Health-risk behaviors relating to adult non-communicable disease (NCD)	NCDs such as cardiovascular disease, diabetes, chronic respiratory disease, and malignancy are leading contributors to the global burden of disease 90% of adult smokers start smoking before 20 years 17% of 13–15 year olds use tobacco; 11% use tobacco other than cigarettes 70% of obese adolescents have more than one risk factor for cardiovascular disease; 23% have more than three
Chronic diseases	1 million 15–24 year olds are infected with HIV annually, accounting for 41% of all new infections Asthma is the most common chronic disease in adolescents There is an emerging epidemic of adolescent-onset type 2 diabetes globally (International Diabetes Federation, 2011)

Source: modified from Sawyer *et al.* (2012), Gore *et al.* (2011) and Patton *et al.* (2009).

young people can be improved with early intervention makes addressing barriers to access especially important (Tylee *et al.*, 2007). Strengthening health systems is complex and largely beyond the scope of healthcare providers. However, much can be done to make health services more adolescent-friendly.

Table 14.3 highlights some relatively simple interventions targeting the community, health services, and healthcare providers that can improve the "adolescent friendliness" of healthcare. These interventions aim to improve accessibility, confidentiality of services, age-appropriateness of services, attitude of staff toward young people, quality of communication, and quality of medical care provided (World Health Organization, 2002; Ambresin *et al.*, 2013).

In almost all settings, adolescents access healthcare though the same services that provide healthcare to the general population. The notion of adolescent-friendly healthcare does not refer to stand-alone services but rather denotes that services provide quality healthcare for adolescents. The principles of adolescent-friendly healthcare echo those of quality health systems for all; healthcare that is effective, efficient, accessible, acceptable, equitable, and safe will also provide quality healthcare to adolescents (WHO, 2002, 2006). How these aspects are implemented is what differentiates healthcare delivery to young people from that of other age groups.

Health services, such as clinics and hospitals, play a key role in improving health outcomes for young people. However, health services represent only part of the broader health system that includes all the organizations, policies, resources, and people whose primary purpose is to improve health (WHO, 2010a). For example, community attitudes, laws, and regulations around access to contraception for unmarried adolescents and the requirement for spousal or parental consent to access contraception have a profound impact on the health of young people. Clinicians need to be familiar with relevant laws and regulations. They are also encouraged to take on wider advocacy roles within their communities to support the attitudinal changes within civil society that are required for protective laws to be appropriately implemented (e.g., access to contraception for unmarried women).

A policy framework should underpin the provision of healthcare. In developing policies for health services for young people, together with attending to laws, it is also important to engage with the community to ensure that health services are culturally acceptable. This is especially important when considering sensitive policies such as young people accessing healthcare without parental or spousal consent and mandatory reporting of abuse. It is also essential to engage and consult with young people to ensure that their rights are not being infringed.

Table 14.3 Improving a health service to make it more adolescent-friendly.

Target	Examples of how to improve a health service to make it more adolescent-friendly
Community	Engage with broader community leaders around how to help young people grow up to be healthy and well Advertise the health service in schools and in any local media accessed by young people Provide targeted outreach to young people, especially those most at risk (homeless youth, transactional sex workers) Support transport to clinic if possible
Health facility	Involve young people in the health service (e.g., advisory committee) Develop access policies respecting sociocultural context (e.g., minimum age, marital status) Provide flexible appointment times, such as after-hours clinic for adolescents in school or work Clearly indicate fees up-front. If possible, reduce or waive fees for young people who come alone Provide adolescent-appropriate health promotion material (e.g., posters) Consider an adolescent-specific waiting area Assure clinic spaces are quiet, private, and clean Identify the capacities of the clinic and develop and streamline appropriate referral linkages Implement policies and practices to ensure commodity supply (e.g., contraceptives) Simplify access to healthcare and commodities (e.g., make condoms available in patient's bathroom) Integrate adolescent health services with existing (or proposed) programs. For example, HPV vaccination as an opportunity for broader health promotion and intervention (Broutet *et al.*, 2013)
Healthcare providers	Provide training to all staff (clerical, clinical, transport) around adolescent health and development Develop policies for all staff that support confidentiality for clients accessing the clinic Encourage staff to take an interest in young people and their lives (i.e., go beyond the presenting health issue) Allow adequate time to explore health issues and to listen to the young person's concerns Communicate health issues clearly and in a non-judgmental way. Avoid jargon Assure confidentiality (and exceptions) at each consultation Provide timely pain management Ensure evidence-based clinical practice using the best available local resources

Source: modified from Ambresin *et al.* (2013), Sawyer *et al.* (2014), Department of Health (2011) and WHO (2010b).

The clinical consultation with a young person: putting it into practice

Key features of a quality consultation with a young person include appropriate engagement, assuring confidentiality, and moving beyond the presenting complaint to explore broader aspects of health and well-being. These are detailed below and summarized in the care plan (Figure 14.3).

Engagement

Engaging adolescents involves building rapport and trust and involving them in decisions about their health. While young people value healthcare providers who treat them with respect and take a broader interest in their lives beyond their health complaint (Ambresin *et al.*, 2013), an equally important reason to engage with them and explore broader aspects of their health is that many of the issues that young people

experience are not perceived by them as issues for which to visit the doctor and are therefore rarely the presenting complaint. Yet many of these issues have great relevance for health and can indeed be assisted by sensitive health consultations (Boxes 14.2 and 14.3).

Young people may come to the health facility accompanied by a parent, friend or spouse. If local laws and customs permit, offer to see the young person alone for part of the consultation, explaining to their parent or spouse that this is an important part of developing a good relationship with the young person. Even if a young person cannot be seen alone (because they are perceived as too young or because local customs do not allow it), it is still important to involve them as much as possible in the consultation. Make a point of speaking with them rather than to their parents or spouse about them. Mid-adolescence (>14 years) usually coincides with young people developing the cognitive maturity to start making health-related decisions autonomously (Weithorn & Campbell, 1982).

Clinical approach to consulting with adolescents

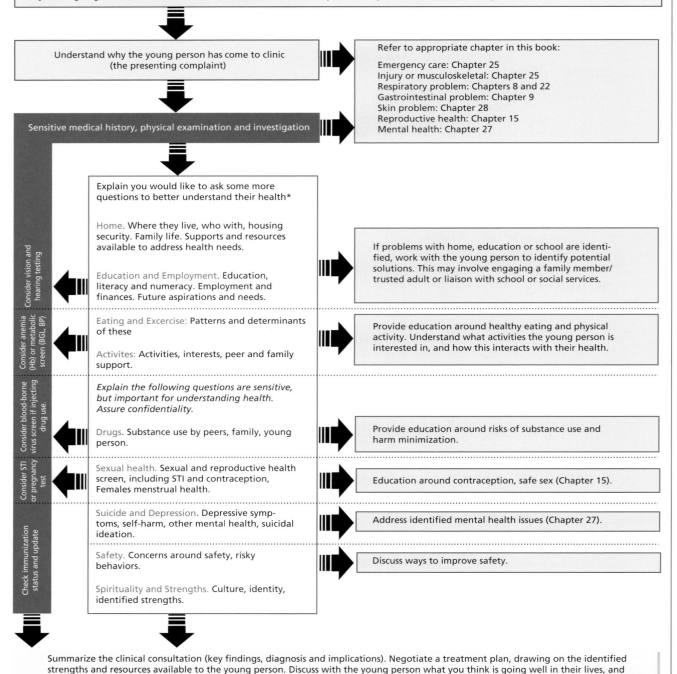

Welcome the young person. Find a private place in the clinic to see them. If the young person is accompanied, offer to see them alone for part or all of the consultation. Consider a staff chaperone. Assure confidentiality: '*Everything we talk about stays between you and me. There however be times when we will need to break this confidentiality, such as if you told me someone is hurting you, you are hurting yourself, or you are going to hurt someone. If we need to break confidentiality, I will tell you and we will do this together.*'

Understand why the young person has come to clinic (the presenting complaint)

Refer to appropriate chapter in this book:

Emergency care: Chapter 25
Injury or musculoskeletal: Chapter 25
Respiratory problem: Chapters 8 and 22
Gastrointestinal problem: Chapter 9
Skin problem: Chapter 28
Reproductive health: Chapter 15
Mental health: Chapter 27

Sensitive medical history, physical examination and investigation

Consider vision and hearing testing

Consider anemia (Hb) or metabolic screen (BGL, BP)

Consider blood-borne virus screen if injecting drug use.

Consider STI or pregnancy test

Check immunization status and update

Explain you would like to ask some more questions to better understand their health*

Home. Where they live, who with, housing security. Family life. Supports and resources available to address health needs.

Education and Employment. Education, literacy and numeracy. Employment and finances. Future aspirations and needs.

If problems with home, education or school are identified, work with the young person to identify potential solutions. This may involve engaging a family member/trusted adult or liaison with school or social services.

Eating and Exercise: Patterns and determinants of these

Activites: Activities, interests, peer and family support.

Provide education around healthy eating and physical activity. Understand what activities the young person is interested in, and how this interacts with their health.

Explain the following questions are sensitive, but important for understanding health. Assure confidentiality.

Drugs. Substance use by peers, family, young person.

Provide education around risks of substance use and harm minimization.

Sexual health. Sexual and reproductive health screen, including STI and contraception, Females menstrual health.

Education around contraception, safe sex (Chapter 15).

Suicide and Depression. Depressive symptoms, self-harm, other mental health, suicidal ideation.

Address identified mental health issues (Chapter 27).

Safety. Concerns around safety, risky behaviors.

Discuss ways to improve safety.

Spirituality and Strengths. Culture, identity, identified strengths.

Summarize the clinical consultation (key findings, diagnosis and implications). Negotiate a treatment plan, drawing on the identified strengths and resources available to the young person. Discuss with the young person what you think is going well in their lives, and where you think the challenges lie. Negotiate with the young person a good time to come back for review.

* Addressing these domains is dependent on the competence of the young person and local protocols for clincal service delivery.
For a detailed description of psychosocial assessment, refer to Table 14.4

Figure 14.3 Care plan.

Box 14.2 Case study 2

Anjali is a 17-year-old girl who has come to see you with her mother. The receptionist tells you she knows Anjali well. "We're from the same village. She has some tummy pain I think." You greet Anjali and her mother in the waiting room and walk with them into the clinic room. As you all sit, Anjali's mother begins to explain, "Doc, we are all so worried about this tummy pain Anjali has – it just won't go away." You listen to Anjali's mother's concern and explain, "It is really good you all came to clinic, and we will do our best to help Anjali." Then, turning to Anjali, you explain further, "Anjali, because you are becoming an adult, I would like to spend some time talking with you alone to better understand your health needs." Anjali and her mother agree, and once you are alone with Anjali you assure her that the consultation is confidential and that you won't tell her mother, the receptionist, or anyone else anything you discuss, unless she is being hurt, hurting herself, or hurting someone else. Anjali seems relieved – she explains she has a slight tummy pain, but that there are other things on her mind too. Using the HEADSS tool (Table 14.4), you begin exploring broader aspects of her life. You start by talking about her home and family, and her friends. Asking permission to ask about some more personal questions, you soon find out Anjali has just recently started having a sexual relationship with a boy and is worried she might be pregnant. She is very distressed about this as she says that if she is pregnant her boyfriend will leave her, her parents will disown her, and she will have to leave school.

Box 14.3 Case study 3

Mo is a 16-year-old adolescent who comes to see you with a sore ankle. He tells you he just twisted it playing football with his friends. It is obviously swollen and looks painful. You help him up on the examination couch and immediately arrange for some pain relief. Mo soon feels more comfortable, and examining his ankle you are confident it is not broken. Talking to Mo, you realize this is his first visit to the clinic. He assures you he is "healthy" but welcomes the opportunity to talk about broader aspects of his health. You reassure him about confidentiality and move beyond the presenting complaint by undertaking a psychosocial assessment. You soon find he smokes "several" cigarettes a day. He is obese, and as part of a physical examination you notice a velvety hyperpigmented rash on his neck. On direct questioning, he agrees that he has been going to the toilet more frequently at night.

Confidentiality

Confidentiality is a particular barrier to young people accessing healthcare (as in the case study described in Box 14.1). Without its guarantee, many adolescents will forgo healthcare around sensitive issues (Ford *et al.*, 2004). Additionally, with increasing maturity, young people have the right to make independent decisions and receive confidential healthcare (Lansdown, 2011). At the beginning of each consultation, assure young people of confidentiality and explain when it may need to be breached. An example of a confidentiality statement is:

> Everything that we discuss will be confidential – that means it stays between you and me. However, we will have to tell someone else if: someone is hurting you; you are hurting yourself; or you are hurting someone else. If we have to tell someone else, we will do it together.

Linked to confidentiality is privacy, which becomes increasingly important during adolescence. If examination of a private area of the body is required, it is important to explain to the young person why this is so. Ask the young person to undress himself or herself and provide them with a sheet or cover so they are in control. Consider a staff chaperone, especially if the young person is of the opposite gender.

Moving beyond the presenting complaint

Young people usually present to health services with a physical health complaint or concern, and it is essential to understand and address this health issue. However, a quality consultation for a young person also involves exploring beyond this primary concern; young people may be reluctant themselves to raise "sensitive" issues relating to mental health or sexual and reproductive health, even if this is their concern (Box 14.2). A commonly used tool to identify comorbidity is the HEADSS psychosocial assessment (Table 14.4). This simple approach promotes assessment of proximal social determinants of health (**h**ome, **e**ducation/**e**mployment, **a**ctivities, and peer connectedness), health-risk behaviors (**a**ctivities, **d**rugs and **s**exual behaviors), and important adolescent health outcomes (anxiety, depression, self-harm, and **s**uicidality). In exploring health-risk behaviors and health outcomes, it provides opportunities around anticipatory guidance (e.g., tobacco and other drugs) and health promotion (e.g., safer sexual activity) (see case study in Box 14.3). The information summarized in Table 14.4 provides some broad guidance to asking young people about psychosocial health. These domains are best assessed by using open-ended questions. It is important to be respectful of sociocultural norms, especially in addressing sensitive health issues. A psychosocial assessment is ideally completed with the young person alone, even if some of these domains have previously been addressed with a parent. Start a HEADSS assessment with a confidentiality statement, similar to the one in the preceding section. The HEADSS approach is structured to begin with less threatening aspects of a young person's life (home) and moves toward more sensitive issues (sexual health, mental

Table 14.4 HEADSS psychosocial assessment.

Domains	Potential topics to discuss	Tips on contextualizing and addressing these domains
Home	Where they live, with whom Housing security (tenure), recent moves Physical environment and resources (e.g., electricity, transport, phone) Social environment, key supports	Physical living arrangements and social and psychological supports available to young persons are all key to understanding and addressing health conditions, especially chronic conditions (such as mental health). Living arrangements of young people can be quite complex, so it is important not to make any assumptions.
Education and employment	Current education/employment Educational performance, literacy, and numeracy Relationships with peers and superiors Employment, finances, and financial security/supports Future aspirations and needs	Education and employment are important determinants of health and well-being. Health status is also a significant determinant of young people's capacity to engage in education and employment. In addressing this domain, it is important to be sensitive. "Telling off" or "scolding" are rarely effective interventions for young people. Rather, explore possible problems, identify goals, and work with them to achieve these.
Eating/exercise	Number and nature of meals Body image; satisfaction, are others concerned? Exercise patterns	Capitalize on the opportunity to address nutrition and exercise: both under- and over-nutrition are important determinants of individual and intergenerational health. Avoid using language like "fat," "chubby," or "bony" – young people are sensitive about their weight and body image, irrespective of their body habitus.
Activities	Activities and interests, including weekends/holidays Family contact, shared activities, supports Friend and peer networks, including social media	Personal, peer, and family activities are all important determinants of health. Interests and hobbies may also provide a lever for change (e.g., ability to play sport may be an incentive to take asthma medication). Marginalized youth may have limited supports and friends, so it is important to ask questions sensitively.
Drugs	Peer and family substance use Individual substance use, recent changes Effects of substance use and regrets Injected substances (blood-borne virus risk) Knowledge gaps	Family, peer, and personal drug use all impact on health outcomes and behaviors. Adolescence is a period of experimentation, and drug use is often modifiable. Before asking these questions, reaffirm confidentiality. Asking first about family and peer substance use helps normalize and contextualize this. Use this opportunity to provide education and advice around harm reduction.
Sexuality	Sexual activity, orientation, and identity Concerns around sex (coercion, unplanned pregnancy, STI) Contraception and safe sex Females: menstrual periods Knowledge gaps	Sexual debut is common during adolescence. STIs and unplanned pregnancy disproportionally affect adolescents. Explain why you are asking these questions, and use the opportunity to educate and promote sexual reproductive health and rights. Do not assume that sexual intercourse only occurs within marriage. Be sensitive; sexual coercion is common in many countries, and not all sexual experiences may be desired or pleasurable.
Suicide and depression	Sleep, appetite, energy, emotions (depression symptom screen) Common mental health problems (anxiety) Self-harm/suicidal thoughts, attempts, plans	Poor mental health is a significant health issue for youth globally but an uncommon reason for accessing healthcare. Additionally, mental health is an important determinant of many other health outcomes. In addressing this domain, be cognizant of the stigma of mental illness; a sensitive approach and reassurance of confidentiality (and its exceptions) are important. There is no evidence that asking about suicide or self-harm increases risk of these behaviors.
Safety	Safety at community, home, school, work Reasons for not feeling safe Personal weapons Seatbelt, bicycle helmet, etc.	Injury is a leading contributor to the burden of disease experienced by young people globally. Health consultations provide an opportunity to identify key risk behaviors and can help the young person identify ways to improve their safety.
Strengths and spirituality	Culture and identity Strengths, both as identified by the individual, and strengths that others identify	Culture and identity are essential to holistic healthcare and can be very powerful protective factors. This domain also promotes a strengths-based approach and may help reassure young people of the skills and strengths they have and the active role they can play in improving their health. Importantly, culture and identity of young people can be different to that of their family or community.

Source: adapted from Azzopardi *et al.* (2012), RACP (2008) and WHO (2010b).

health) as rapport is built. A useful strategy is to ask young people about their friend's behaviors before asking about their own; this helps normalize the question and can place the young person's behaviors in context. HEADSS should be considered as a framework and useful guide to a thorough and sensitive consultation, rather than enacted as a strict checklist when it may feel overly confronting.

Summarizing the key findings and formulating a management plan

At the conclusion of the consultation, summarize the identified health issues using plain language that avoids jargon. Communicate the key findings, diagnosis, and implications and negotiate treatment options in a way the young person will understand. If possible, engage the young person in considering different management options as this will more likely lead to a plan he or she agree with and will better adhere to. Let them know what you think is going well in their lives, as well as where the challenges seem to lie. Finally, negotiate with them about when they think would be a good time to come back to see you again to review how things are going.

Additional resources

- World Health Organization. Adolescent job aid: a handy desk reference tool for primary level health workers. Available at http://whqlibdoc.who.int/publications/2010/9789241599962_eng.pdf
- UNICEF. The State of the World's Children 2011. Adolescence: an age of opportunity. Available at http://www.unicef.org.au/downloads/Publications-(1)/SOWC-2011-Full-Report.aspx
- International Conference on Population and Development Beyond 2014. Bali Global Youth Forum Declaration. Available at http://unfpa.org/webdav/site/global/shared/documents/events/2012/Bali%20Global%20youth%20Forum%20Declaration%20FINAL-1.pdf
- USAID. Youth in Development Report: realizing the demographic opportunity. Washington DC, October 2012. Available at http://transition.usaid.gov/our_work/policy_planning_and_learning/documents/Youth_in_Development_Policy.pdf

REFERENCES

Ambresin AE, Bennett K, Patton GC, Sanci LA, Sawyer SM (2013) Assessment of youth-friendly health care: a systematic review of indicators drawn from young people's perspectives. *J Adolesc Health* 52:670–81.

Azzopardi P (2012) Adolescent health comes of age. *Lancet* 379:1583–4.

Azzopardi P, Brown AD, Zimmet P *et al.* (2012) Type 2 diabetes in young Indigenous Australians in rural and remote areas: diagnosis, screening, management and prevention. *Med J Aust* 197:32–6.

Beaglehole R, Bonita R, Alleyne G *et al.* (2011) UN high-level meeting on non-communicable diseases: addressing four questions. *Lancet* 378:449–55.

Black RE, Victora CG, Walker SP *et al.* (2013) Maternal and child undernutrition and overweight in low-income and middle-income countries. *Lancet* 382:427–51.

Broutet N, Lehnertz N, Mehl G *et al.* (2013) Effective health interventions for adolescents that could be integrated with human papillomavirus vaccination programs. *J Adolesc Health* 53:6–13.

Department of Health (2011) You're Welcome: quality criteria for young people friendly health services. https://www.gov.uk/government/uploads/system/uploads/attachment_data/file/216350/dh_127632.pdf

Ford C, English A, Sigman G (2004) Confidential health care for adolescents: position paper for the Society for Adolescent Medicine. *J Adolesc Health* 35:160–7.

Glasier A, Gulmezoglu AM, Schmid GP, Moreno CG, Van Look PF (2006) Sexual and reproductive health: a matter of life and death. *Lancet* 368:1595–607.

Gore FM, Bloem PJ, Patton GC *et al.* (2011) Global burden of disease in young people aged 10–24 years: a systematic analysis. *Lancet* 377:2093–102.

International Diabetes Federation (2011) *Global IDF/ISPAD Guideline for Diabetes in Childhood and Adolescence.* Brussels, Belgium: IDF.

Lansdown G (2011) Every child's right to be heard: a resource guide on the UN Committee on the Rights of the Child general comment no.12. Available at http://www.savethechildren.org.uk/resources/online-library/every-childs-right-be-heard

Mangiaterra V, Pendse R, McClure K, Rosen J (2008) Making pregnancy safer: adolescent pregnancy. Available at http://www.who.int/maternal_child_adolescent/documents/mpsnnotes_2_lr.pdf

Murray CJL, Vos T, Lozano R *et al.* (2013) Disability-adjusted life years (DALYs) for 291 diseases and injuries in 21 regions, 1990–2010: a systematic analysis for the Global Burden of Disease Study 2010. *Lancet* 380:2197–223.

Patton GC, Coffey C, Sawyer SM *et al.* (2009) Global patterns of mortality in young people: a systematic analysis of population health data. *Lancet* 374:881–92.

Patton GC, Coffey C, Cappa C *et al.* (2012) Health of the world's adolescents: a synthesis of internationally comparable data. *Lancet* 379:1665–75.

RACP (2008) Routine adolescent psychosocial health assessment: position statement. Sydney: Royal Australasian College of Physicians. Available at http://www.racp.edu.au/index.cfm?objectid=B56658DA-08B2-14E3-0EE26F1635D1314E

Sawyer SM, Afifi RA, Bearinger LH *et al.* (2012) Adolescence: a foundation for future health. *Lancet* 379:1630–40.

Sawyer SM, Ambresin AE, Bennett KE, Patton GC (2014) A measurement framework for quality health care for adolescents in hospital. *J Adolesc Health* 55(4):484–90.

Tylee A, Haller DM, Graham T, Churchill R, Sanci LA (2007) Youth-friendly primary-care services: how are we doing and what more needs to be done? *Lancet* 369:1565–73.

UNICEF (2011) The State of the World's Children 2011. Adolescence: an age of opportunity. Available at http://www.unicef.org.au/downloads/Publications-(1)/SOWC-2011-Full-Report.aspx

Viner RM, Ozer EM, Denny S *et al.* (2012) Adolescence and the social determinants of health. *Lancet* 379:1641–52.

Weithorn LA, Campbell SB (1982) The competency of children and adolescents to make informed treatment decisions. *Child Dev* 53:1589–98.

WHO (2002) Adolescent friendly health services: an agenda for change. Available at http://www.who.int/maternal_child_adolescent/documents/fch_cah_02_14/en/

WHO (2006) Quality of care: a process of making strategic choices in health systems. Available at http://apps.who.int/iris/handle/10665/43470

WHO (2007) Adolescent pregnancy: unmet needs and undone deeds: a review of the literature and programmes. Available at http://whqlibdoc.who.int/publications/2007/9789241595650_eng.pdf. Accessed 21 February 2012.

WHO (2010a) Monitoring the building blocks of health systems: a handbook of indicators and their measurement strategies. Available at http://www.who.int/healthinfo/systems/monitoring/en/

WHO (2010b) Adolescent job aid: a handy desk reference tool for primary health workers. Available at http://www.who.int/maternal_child_adolescent/documents/9789241599962/en/

World Bank (2007) WDR 2007: Development and the next generation. Available at http://web.worldbank.org/WBSITE/EXTERNAL/EXTDEC/EXTRESEARCH/EXTWDRS/0,,contentMDK:23062361~pagePK:478093~piPK:477627~theSitePK:477624,00.html

CHAPTER 15
Sexual and Reproductive Health and Rights

Elissa C. Kennedy[1], Alice G. Mark[2], Dalia Brahmi[2], Nathalie Dhont[3], and Els M.M. Leye[4]

[1]Burnet Institute and Monash University, Melbourne, Australia
[2]Ipas, Chapel Hill, NC, USA
[3]The Walking Egg Foundation and Ziekenhuis Oost-Limburg Hospital, Genk, Belgium
[4]International Centre for Reproductive Health, Ghent University, Ghent, Belgium

Key learning objectives

- Define sexual and reproductive health (SRH) and rights and outline the core principles of providing SRH services in resource-limited settings.

- Recognize the importance of contraception to women's and children's health and identify key clinical considerations regarding provision of contraception.

- Understand the factors that contribute to unsafe abortion and its associated morbidity and mortality, and articulate the principles of providing comprehensive safe abortion and post-abortion care.

- Appreciate the significance of infertility and an approach to its prevention, investigation, and management in resource-limited settings.

- Characterize the prevalence and impact of sexual violence and female genital mutilation, and summarize the essential components of prevention and management.

Abstract

Access to comprehensive sexual and reproductive health information and services is a fundamental right and has broad implications for the health of women and children, gender equality, poverty reduction, and sustainable development. Despite these imperatives, access to quality services is poor in many resource-limited settings, contributing to high unmet needs and preventable morbidity and mortality. This chapter discusses some important considerations and principles for sexual and reproductive healthcare providers, with a particular focus on contraception, comprehensive abortion care, infertility, sexual violence, and female genital mutilation.

Key words: sexual and reproductive health, sexual and reproductive rights, family planning, contraception, abortion, infertility, gender-based violence, sexual violence, female genital mutilation

Essential Clinical Global Health, First Edition. Edited by Brett D. Nelson.
© 2015 John Wiley & Sons, Ltd. Published 2015 by John Wiley & Sons, Ltd.
Companion website: www.essentialseries.com/globalhealth

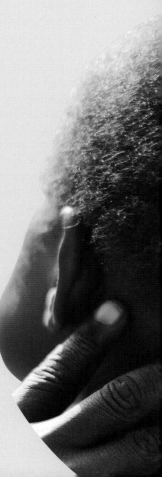

Introduction

Sexual and reproductive health (SRH) is a broad concept that encompasses all matters related to sexuality and relationships, pregnancy, and birth. Optimal SRH relies on people being able to have a responsible, satisfying, and safe sex life, free from discrimination, coercion, and violence, and having the capability to reproduce and the freedom to decide if, when, and how often to do so (United Nations, 1995). Central to achieving the highest standard of SRH are sexual and reproductive rights, many of which are recognized in national laws and international human rights agreements (Box 15.1). In addition to being critical for individual health and well-being, SRH is also essential for the achievement of many other population health and development goals including gender equality, poverty reduction, and environmental sustainability (UN Millennium Project, 2006).

Globally, sexual and reproductive ill-health accounts for around one-third of the total burden of disease for women of reproductive age, and unsafe sex is among the leading risk factors for poor health in low-income countries (Glasier *et al.*, 2006). Poor women and men are disproportionately affected, as are adolescents, particularly girls (Bearinger *et al.*, 2007). People living with HIV, people living with disability, people who buy or sell sex, migrant workers, men who have sex with men, and gender minorities also suffer an excess burden of poor SRH due to discrimination, violence, and inadequate access to information and services (Glasier *et al.*, 2006). Populations affected by complex emergencies are particularly vulnerable, and SRH services are an essential component of the immediate and ongoing humanitarian response in these settings (IWAG, 2010). While the burden of poor SRH predominantly affects women, men are an important target for services. In addition to their own SRH concerns, men also have a role as decision-makers in many settings with implications for the health and well-being of women and girls (Guttmacher, 2003; PMNCH, 2013).

The determinants of SRH are complex and often related to entrenched sociocultural norms, taboos, and practices. Important factors may include:

- cultural beliefs and norms regarding sexual behavior and discussion of sexual matters;
- gender inequality and women's lack of autonomy to make decisions regarding SRH;
- laws and policies that limit access to comprehensive information and services, discriminate against population groups or behaviors, or fail to address harmful practices (such as child marriage or sexual violence);
- poverty;
- limited access to information; and
- poor access to quality services (WHO, 2010a).

It is important that clinicians are familiar with these context-specific factors in order to provide sensitive and culturally appropriate care, while also recognizing that all individuals, regardless of age or marital status, have the right to SRH information and services (Box 15.2). These rights have been articulated in the International Conference on Population and Development Programme of Action, and adopted by 179 governments.

Despite these commitments, many people are denied access to comprehensive information and services. Clinicians' own judgmental attitudes, discomfort discussing sexual matters, and personal objections to providing information and/or services are major barriers to improving SRH. However, in keeping with international rights commitments and evidence-based practice, clinicians have a responsibility to provide comprehensive and high-quality care that is not limited by their own moral, religious, or other beliefs (Box 15.3). This is particularly important in resource-limited settings where there may be no or limited choice of provider. Where aspects of SRH cannot be provided, every effort should be made to enable clients to access alternative services.

Box 15.1 Sexual and reproductive rights (Newman & Helzner, 1999)

Sexual and reproductive rights include the right of all individuals, regardless of race, gender, age, marital status, sexual orientation, disability, religious, or political beliefs, and free of coercion, discrimination, and violence, to:

- the highest attainable standard of sexual and reproductive health, including access to sexual and reproductive healthcare services;
- information related to sexuality, reproduction, and the availability of services;
- confidentiality, privacy, and dignity;
- respect for bodily integrity;
- pursue a satisfying, safe, and pleasurable sex life free from the risk of sexually transmitted infections, HIV, and unintended pregnancy;

- choose their partner;
- decide whether or not to be sexually active;
- consensual sexual relations;
- consensual marriage;
- decide whether or not to have children and the number, timing, and spacing of children;
- access to safe, effective, affordable, and acceptable contraception methods of their choice, as well as other methods for regulation of fertility which are not against the law;
- access to appropriate healthcare services that will enable women to go safely through pregnancy and childbirth and provide couples with the best chance of having a healthy infant.

Box 15.2 Essential sexual and reproductive healthcare (UNFPA, 2008)

- Information, education, and counseling about sexuality and reproductive health.
- Contraception.
- Antenatal, safe delivery, and postnatal care.
- Prevention and appropriate treatment of infertility.
- Prevention of unsafe abortion, provision of safe abortion where legal, and management of post-abortion complications.

- Prevention, care, and treatment of reproductive tract infections, reproductive cancers, STIs, and HIV.
- Prevention and surveillance of violence against women, care for survivors of violence, and other actions to eliminate traditional harmful practices, such as female genital mutilation.

Box 15.3 Core principles for providers of SRH services

- Consider your own attitudes and beliefs and how these may impact your ability to provide comprehensive information and services. If you are not able to provide a service, it is essential to refer to an alternative provider.
- Be aware of relevant laws and regulations. These may relate to providing contraception to unmarried people, requirements for spousal or parental consent for services (such as sterilization or abortion), legal context of abortion, and processes for reporting sexual violence. While it is important to be familiar with these, you should endeavor to provide all clients with

comprehensive and confidential services to the fullest extent possible.
- Provide client-focused care:
  ◦ non-judgmental, respectful, and sensitive;
  ◦ confidential and private;
  ◦ supports and enables informed, voluntary decision-making;
  ◦ provides adequate, unbiased information and counseling;
  ◦ includes a range of options and referral where needed;
  ◦ ensures informed consent is obtained, free from coercion.

Contraception

Contraception, often referred to as "family planning", includes the range of methods (modern contraceptives and traditional methods) that enable individuals and couples to attain the desired number, timing, and spacing of their children. Around

61% of reproductive-age women in low- and middle-income countries are currently using some type of contraception and the majority are using a modern method (Darroch, 2013). However, there are significant disparities: in the least developed countries, only 28% of women are using a modern method, with the lowest contraceptive prevalence rates in sub-Saharan Africa.

In low- and middle-income countries, around 26% of women of reproductive age (some 222 million women) want to avoid pregnancy but are not using a modern method of contraception (Darroch, 2013). These women with unmet need for contraception account for around 80% of the 80 million unintended pregnancies every year. There are many reasons why women who want to avoid pregnancy are not using an effective method of contraception (Sedgh *et al.*, 2007):

- poor access to affordable services, particularly among adolescents, the poor, and unmarried people;
- limited choice of methods;
- poor quality of services;
- concerns about health risks or side effects;
- personal or partner objection for cultural or religious reasons;
- inadequate knowledge;
- perceived low risk of pregnancy.

Enabling women and adolescent girls to delay, space (>24 months between births), and limit the number of births has profound benefits for the health of women and children. Meeting the need for modern contraception would reduce maternal deaths by around 30% and child deaths by 20% and would avert 54 million unintended pregnancies and 26 million abortions each year (Cleland *et al.*, 2012). Improving access to contraception also has broader socioeconomic benefits such as prolonging girls' education, enabling women to participate in employment and economic activities, and contributing to women's empowerment (Cates, 2010).

Commonly available contraception methods are summarized in Table 15.1. Not all methods are widely available in every country so it is important to be familiar with local contraception and reproductive health programs. In general, modern contraceptives are highly effective and safe, and indeed are much safer than unintended pregnancy in resource-limited settings. Key contraindications are included in Table 15.1, with a more extensive list detailed in the World Health Organization (WHO) *Medical Eligibility Criteria for Contraceptive Use.* The full criteria as well as a simple tool and mobile application can be downloaded from WHO (2009a).

In general, healthy women can be provided with the method of their choice without requiring physical examination or laboratory testing. For women who wish to use intrauterine devices (IUDs), it is necessary to conduct a pelvic examination and risk assessment for sexually transmitted infections (STIs), with laboratory testing for STIs if available (see Chapter 16). If a risk assessment is negative, an IUD may be provided at the first visit while awaiting laboratory testing. Blood pressure screening is desirable for women using hormonal methods, but where this cannot be provided these methods should not be withheld. Contraception services are also an opportunity to provide breast examination and cervical cancer screening, where available. However, a woman's refusal to consent to these investigations should not prevent her from being provided with the method of her choice.

Immediate initiation of contraception on request improves user satisfaction and may overcome barriers associated with delayed provision. Hormonal methods and IUDs can be commenced at any time during the menstrual cycle if it is reasonably certain that the woman is not pregnant. Where pregnancy testing is not available or is cost-prohibitive, a provider can be reasonably sure that a women is not pregnant if she has no symptoms or signs of pregnancy and meets any one of the following:

- no intercourse since last normal menses;
- been correctly and consistently using a reliable method of contraception;
- within 7 days after last normal menses;
- within 7 days after abortion or miscarriage;
- within 4 weeks postpartum (non-lactating);
- fully or nearly fully breastfeeding, amenorrheic, and less than 6 months postpartum (WHO, 2004, 2011a).

The key to high-quality contraception services is providing counseling that enables informed voluntary decision-making. Clients should be provided with information regarding method effectiveness, correct use, mechanism of action, common side effects, benefits and risks, and advised when to seek help and follow-up. Concerns about side effects are a common reason for discontinuation, so adequate counseling and providing access to a wide range of methods are important. There are several guidelines and clinical tools available to assist with contraception counseling and method provision (see Additional resources section). Some clients, such as adolescents and women living with HIV, require special attention; key considerations are summarized in Table 15.2. To increase access, contraception services should be integrated with other health services, including maternal and child health, sexual health clinics, and HIV services. Information needs to be provided to all men and women of reproductive age who come into contact with health services.

Comprehensive abortion care

Of an estimated 43.8 million abortions that took place worldwide in 2008, 49% were unsafe (Sedgh *et al.*, 2012). The WHO defines unsafe abortion as a procedure to terminate an unwanted pregnancy by persons lacking the necessary skills, or in an environment lacking minimal medical standards, or both. Almost all unsafe abortions occur in developing countries, where legal restrictions and limited resources impede access to safe services. Worldwide, 5 million women are hospitalized or disabled and 47,000 women die because of unsafe abortion each year (WHO, 2011b). Replacing unsafe services with safe care can almost entirely prevent abortion-related death and disability.

Table 15.1 Overview of commonly available contraception methods.

Method	Mechanism of action	Effectiveness with common use (within first year of use)	Key benefits and indications[a]	Important considerations[b]
Modern methods				
Subdermal implant (progestogen-only)	Thickens cervical mucus; prevents ovulation in at least half of cycles	99.95%	Very effective Long-acting (3–5 years) Protection against pregnancy within 24 hours of insertion Reversible, with immediate return to fertility Does not rely on daily use or frequent access to supplies Not required to keep contraceptives at home (private) Can be used by lactating women Suitable for delaying, spacing and limiting births May help reduce anemia secondary to menorrhagia	Requires insertion and removal by a trained provider Changes in menstrual bleeding may be unacceptable to some clients Precautions and contraindications include: • Breast cancer • Thromboembolism • Liver disease • Unexplained vaginal bleeding • Some drug interactions (including some TB drugs)
Male sterilization (vasectomy)	Surgical occlusion of the vasa deferentia	99.85% after 3-month semen evaluation (97–98% without evaluation)	Highly effective, permanent method Suitable for limiting births Very safe, with few contraindications or complications Does not interfere with menstrual cycle	Permanent method so requires careful counseling Must ensure that voluntary, informed consent is obtained and documented free from coercion by relatives or service providers Small risk of complications Another form of contraception needed for at least 12 weeks post-vasectomy (or until no sperm present in ejaculate)
Intrauterine device (levonorgestrel-containing)	Inhibition of sperm migration; inhibition of ovum transport; inhibition of fertilization; thickening of cervical mucus	99.8%	Very effective Long-acting (5 years) Effective immediately (no back-up method required) Reversible, with immediate return to fertility Does not rely on daily use or frequent access to supplies Not required to keep contraceptives at home (private) Can be used by lactating women May reduce dysmenorrhea and anemia due to menorrhagia	Requires insertion and removal by a trained provider In addition to the precautions and contraindications for copper intrauterine devices: • Breast cancer • Liver disease • Thromboembolism
Female sterilization (tubal ligation)	Surgical occlusion of the fallopian tubes	99.5%	Highly effective, permanent method Suitable for limiting births Very safe, with few contraindications or complications Does not interfere with menstrual cycle	Permanent method so requires careful counseling Must ensure that voluntary, informed consent is obtained and documented free from coercion by relatives or service providers Small risk of complications

(Continued)

Table 15.1 Overview of commonly available contraception methods. (*Continued*)

Method	Mechanism of action	Effectiveness with common use (within first year of use)	Key benefits and indications[a]	Important considerations[b]
Intrauterine device (copper-containing)	Inhibition of sperm migration; inhibition of ovum transport; inhibition of fertilization	99.2%	Very effective Long-acting (up to 12 years) Effective immediately (no back-up method required) Reversible, with immediate return to fertility Does not rely on daily use or frequent access to supplies Not required to keep contraceptives at home (private) Can be used by lactating women Can be used as emergency contraception if inserted within 5 days of unprotected sex (or within 5 days of ovulation)	Requires insertion and removal by a trained provider Can cause menorrhagia, especially in the first 3–6 months, which may contribute to anemia Precautions and contraindications include: • Pelvic inflammatory disease • Puerperal or post-abortion sepsis • Current STI • Genital tract, cervical, endometrial or ovarian malignancy • Uterine abnormalities (e.g., fibroids) • Gestational trophoblastic disease • Unexplained vaginal bleeding • Advanced AIDS (unless clinically well on antiretroviral therapy)
Lactational amenorrhea method (LAM)	Frequent breastfeeding prevents ovulation	98% (in the first 6 months after childbirth)	Highly effective if: • Less than 6 months postpartum • Amenorrhea • Fully or near fully breastfeeding Safe with no side effects Encourages optimal infant nutrition	May not be advisable for women for whom unintended pregnancy carries an unacceptable risk, or when there are conditions that may affect breastfeeding
Progestogen-only injectable	Thickens cervical mucus; prevents ovulation in at least half of cycles	97%	Reversible Does not require daily use (injection every 2–3 months) Not required to keep contraceptives at home (private) Can be used by lactating women Can be used by women with contraindications to estrogen-containing contraceptives Reduces dysmenorrhea and anemia related to menorrhagia Reduces the risk of endometrial cancer and sickle cell crises	Delayed return to fertility (6–10 months) Changes in menstrual bleeding may be unacceptable to some clients Requires regular access to services and supplies Precautions and contraindications include: • Breast cancer • Liver disease • Cardiovascular disease • Unexplained vaginal bleeding • Some drug interactions (including some TB drugs)

Table 15.1 Overview of commonly available contraception methods. (*Continued*)

Method	Mechanism of action	Effectiveness with common use (within first year of use)	Key benefits and indications[a]	Important considerations[b]
Combined injectable	Prevents ovulation; thickens cervical mucus	97%	Reversible Does not require daily use (monthly injection) Not required to keep contraceptives at home (private) Less changes to menstrual bleeding compared with progestogen-only injectables May have additional health effects similar to combined oral contraceptives	May be a delayed return to fertility (1 month on average) Requires regular access to services and supplies Precautions, contraindications and drug interactions similar to combined oral contraceptives
Combined oral contraceptives ("the pill")	Prevents ovulation; thickens cervical mucus	92%	Reversible with immediate return to fertility Reduces dysmenorrhea and anemia associated with menorrhagia Reduces the risk of ovarian and endometrial cancer and acute pelvic inflammatory disease	Requires ability and motivation to take daily and access to reliable supplies Cannot be used by lactating women in the first 6 months postpartum Precautions and contraindications include: • Cardiovascular disease (including thromboembolism, hypertension) • Diabetes mellitus • Hyperlipidemia • Liver disease, gallbladder disease • Breast cancer • Migraine with aura • Smoking if aged >35 years • Drug interactions (including some TB and HIV drugs)
Progestogen-only pills ("minipill")	Thickens cervical mucus; prevents ovulation in at least half of cycles	92%	Reversible with immediate return to fertility Can be used by lactating women Can be used by women with contraindications to estrogen-containing contraceptives	Requires ability and motivation to take daily and access to reliable supplies Precautions and contraindications include: • Breast cancer • Liver disease • Some drug interactions (including some TB drugs)
Male condom	Barrier method (prevents sperm entering the uterine cavity)	85%	Very few side effects and contraindications Protects against STIs, HIV, and unintended pregnancy Can be used in conjunction with other methods (dual protection) Available without medical prescription and from non-health providers	Less effective than other methods Coital dependent Requires partner cooperation, which may be difficult for some women to negotiate Not advisable for women for whom unintended pregnancy carries a high risk

(*Continued*)

Table 15.1 Overview of commonly available contraception methods. (*Continued*)

Method	Mechanism of action	Effectiveness with common use (within first year of use)	Key benefits and indications[a]	Important considerations[b]
Female condom	Barrier method (prevents sperm entering the uterine cavity)	79%	Very few side effects and contraindications Protects against STIs, HIV, and unintended pregnancy Can be used in conjunction with other methods (dual protection) Can be inserted before sex	Less effective than other methods Coital dependent Requires partner cooperation, which may be difficult for some women to negotiate Not advisable for women for whom unintended pregnancy carries a high risk High cost compared with male condoms
Emergency contraceptive pill (levonorgestrel-only (LNG), combined, or single-dose ulipristal)	Inhibits or delays ovulation; may inhibit ovum and sperm transport and fertilization	60–90% (with each use)	Can be used up to 5 days after unprotected sexual intercourse, when: • No contraceptive method used • Contraceptive method misuse (missed pills, condom breakage, etc.) • Sexual violence *Note*: emergency contraception is not a form of abortion	More effective the sooner it is taken after intercourse (LNG most effective within 72 hours) Clients should be provided with counseling regarding regular contraception and initiated on other methods as appropriate
Traditional methods				
Fertility awareness methods (based on calendar or symptoms)	Avoid unprotected vaginal intercourse around the time of ovulation	75%	No side effects After initial instruction there are few costs and no need to access services frequently May be acceptable to clients with religious or other objections to modern methods	Less effective than modern methods Relies on women being able to determine when they are most fertile, which may be difficult for those with irregular cycles (including adolescents) and women who are breastfeeding Requires partner cooperation and high levels of motivation May require three or more cycles to learn the technique Not advisable for women for whom unintended pregnancy carries an unacceptable risk
Withdrawal (coitus interruptus)	Ejaculation outside the vagina	73%	No side effects No costs, not dependent on access to health services May be acceptable to clients with religious or other objections to modern methods	Less effective than modern methods Requires partner cooperation and a high level of awareness and motivation Not advisable for women for whom unintended pregnancy carries an unacceptable risk

[a] Clients should be provided with the method of their choice unless contraindications exist.
[b] Please refer to the WHO Medical Eligibility Criteria for a comprehensive description of precautions, contraindications and drug interactions.
Source: adapted from WHO (2010d, 2011a) and IPPF (2004).

Table 15.2 Key considerations for clients with special needs.

Client	Rationale	Contraceptive considerations	Other considerations
Adolescents	Increased risk of maternal and perinatal morbidity and mortality associated with early pregnancy (<18 years) Adolescents experience higher rates of contraceptive discontinuation, method failure, and are less tolerant of side effects, so careful counseling is required	All contraceptive methods can be used safely including IUDs and contraceptive implants Permanent methods are generally not appropriate, and traditional methods may be less effective among adolescents Emergency contraception can be safely used by adolescents Factors that may influence contraceptive choice include: • Frequency of sex • Ability and motivation to use a method regularly • Need for "private" methods • Costs • Adolescents may also be at risk of STIs, including HIV, so dual protection should be promoted	All young people should be provided with comprehensive, sensitive, non-judgmental care regardless of age or marital status. Privacy and confidentiality are essential. Be aware of local laws or regulations regarding informed consent, while providing comprehensive services to the fullest extent possible. Address other aspects of sexual and reproductive health (including puberty, sexuality, relationships, STIs) as well as other health concerns (see Chapter 14 on adolescent health).
Postpartum	Birth spacing <18 months increases the risk of maternal and perinatal morbidity and mortality	Sterilization can be provided within 7 days (or after 6 weeks) of delivery IUD can be inserted within 48 hours (or after 4 weeks) of delivery If breastfeeding: • LAM may be suitable • Non-hormonal methods can be used immediately • Progestogen-only methods can generally be used 6 weeks after delivery	Contraception counseling should be part of routine antenatal and postnatal care.
Post-abortion	Fertility can return as soon as 2 weeks post-abortion High risk of repeat unintended pregnancy	All methods are safe to use in a healthy woman • Fertility-based methods may be used after the return of the first menses in women with a history of regular cycles • IUD may be inserted immediately after vacuum aspiration or dilatation and evacuation and once it is reasonably certain a woman is no longer pregnant after medical abortion • The risk of IUD expulsion is slightly higher after second-trimester abortion • Caution should be used regarding immediate sterilization following abortion • Education about emergency contraception should be provided	Counseling and care should also be provided for STIs and HIV as appropriate.

(Continued)

Table 15.2 Key considerations for clients with special needs. (*Continued*)

Client	Rationale	Contraceptive considerations	Other considerations
People living with HIV	HIV-positive women have an increased risk of adverse pregnancy outcomes HIV is one of the leading contributors to maternal death in high-prevalence settings Without access to effective interventions, the risk of vertical transmission to the infant is around 20–45% (<5% with appropriate care) Voluntary use of contraception to prevent unintended pregnancy is an important component of preventing pediatric HIV infections	Clinically well women and those on antiretroviral therapy can use most methods safely IUD is not recommended for women with advanced, untreated AIDS Fertility-awareness methods may be less effective due to changes in the menstrual cycle Hormonal methods may interact with some antiretroviral and TB drugs	Dual protection should be promoted to protect against STIs and HIV transmission. In some settings, women living with HIV have reported coerced abortion or sterilization. Many women living with HIV want to have children, and they have the right to receive comprehensive, non-discriminatory information and services. While HIV-positive women require careful counseling regarding pregnancy, the aim of contraception services is to prevent *unintended* pregnancies and therefore should support informed voluntary choices.
People living with disability	Around 15% of the world's population are living with a disability, and they have the same SRH needs as others Many face significant barriers to accessing information and services and experience discriminatory or coercive practices (such as forced sterilization or forced abortion)	Many contraceptive methods can be used safely Factors that may influence choice of method include: • Individual preferences and fertility desires • Nature of the disability • Ease of use of the method • Access to regular supplies and services • Impact on menstrual hygiene • Specific medical eligibility criteria	Disability alone is not an indication for contraception. Women living with disability have the same reproductive rights (including the right to decide if and when to have children) as other women. Decisions regarding contraception should be informed, voluntary and made by the client to the fullest extent possible. Where competency to provide informed consent is compromised, decisions should be made in consultation with the client, guardian/family member/support person and other relevant agencies (depending on context). Decisions should be based on the client's needs and uphold their reproductive rights.
Older women	Women aged over 35 years have among the highest unmet need for contraception to limit births, and also have an increased risk of maternal mortality	In general, all methods are safe to use in healthy women Older women may be more likely to have a medical condition that may restrict the use of some hormonal methods Fertility-awareness methods may be less effective as women approach menopause Longer-acting or permanent methods may be appropriate among women who want to stop childbearing Reversible contraceptive methods should be stopped 12 months after the last menstruation	Advice and care related to menopause and screening for other reproductive health concerns should be provided. Sexually active older women may also be at risk of STIs and should be advised to use condoms, even if they no longer need contraception.
Men	Men are an important influence on women's contraceptive use, method choice, and continuation in many settings Men also have their own SRH needs and are users of important contraception methods	Vasectomy is simple, safe, and highly effective but uptake is low in many settings Barrier methods and traditional methods require a high level of male cooperation and motivation	Many contraception services are targeted at women; therefore, efforts may be needed to make services more male-friendly. Encourage couple counseling, but always provide an opportunity for individual counseling.

Source: adapted from WHO (2005, 2009c, 2011a).

When performed by skilled providers using appropriate technologies, abortion is extremely safe. For example, in the United States, where 1.2 million abortions occur per year, the mortality rate is 0.6 deaths per 100,000 abortions, and a woman's risk of dying in childbirth is 14 times higher (8.8 deaths per 100,000 live births) than during an abortion (Raymond & Grimes, 2012).

Legal status of abortion

Unsafe abortion is more likely in settings where abortion is legally restricted and where providers or health systems impose unnecessary barriers. Health workers can check a country's abortion laws at the Center for Reproductive Rights' The World's Abortion Laws Map at www.worldabortionlaws .com.

Almost all countries permit abortion in some circumstances, and most permit abortion to save a woman's life and preserve her health. Restricting legal access to abortion does not decrease the need for abortion or reduce the number of induced abortions, but leads to women seeking unsafe abortion and suffering the ensuing complications (Box 15.4) (WHO, 2012). Worldwide, abortion rates are lower where the law is most liberal (Sedgh *et al.*, 2012).

Regardless of the law regarding induced abortion, treating complications of spontaneous or unsafely induced abortion is permissible everywhere. Appropriate treatment of abortion complications is an effective strategy for reducing maternal morbidity and mortality in areas where safe services remain restricted (Box 15.5).

In addition to legal hurdles, women may face other social or cultural barriers that prevent them from accessing safe

---

Box 15.4 The impact of abortion legislation on maternal mortality in Romania
(Horga *et al.*, 2013)

Between 1966 and 1989, abortion was highly restricted in Romania and the pro-natalist regime banned modern contraceptives (Figure 15.1). This resulted in the dramatic increase in maternal mortality from 85 per 100,000 live births in 1965 to 169 per 100,000 live births in 1989. The vast majority of deaths, 87%, were related to complications of unsafe abortions. One year after the fall of the Ceaușescu regime and the reversal of the abortion

ban, maternal mortality fell by half. A network of contraception clinics developed in the 1990s and policies were implemented that provided free contraceptives to marginalized groups. The modern contraceptive prevalence rate is now 61% and abortion-related maternal mortality has dropped from 147 per 100,000 live births in 1989 to 5.2 per 100, 000 in 2012.

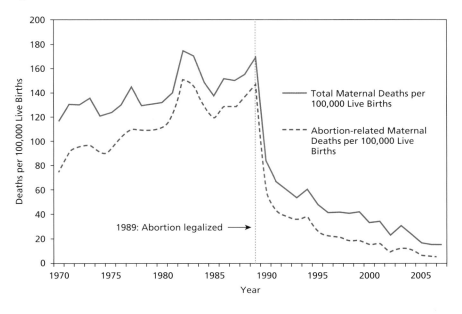

Figure 15.1 Total vs. abortion-related maternal deaths per 100,000 live births in Romania, 1970–2005. *Source*: Benson *et al.* (2011), figure 2, p. 5.

Box 15.5 Post-abortion care

Post-abortion care (PAC) is a strategy for treating complications of spontaneous and unsafely induced abortion in areas where access to legal, safe services is limited. Treating illness or injury after spontaneous or induced abortion is permitted everywhere. PAC reduces maternal morbidity and mortality from unsafe abortion in areas where introducing safe services is not possible. The PAC model includes the following features.

1. Mobilizing resources to prevent unwanted pregnancy and unsafe abortion.
2. Engagement with communities and service providers to increase women's access to timely care for abortion complications.
3. Counseling to identify and respond to women's emotional and physical health needs.
4. Treatment of complications (see Chapters 25 and 26 for management of trauma and critical illness):
   (a) Incomplete abortion
      (i) Uterine evacuation with misoprostol or vacuum aspiration
      (ii) Consider antibiotics
   (b) Bleeding
      (i) Manage as for shock if severe hemorrhage
      (ii) Identify and treat the cause (incomplete abortion, lacerations, uterine perforation, infection)
   (c) Intra-abdominal injury
      (i) Manage as for shock
      (ii) Refer for surgical care
   (d) Sepsis
      (i) Manage as for shock
      (ii) Identify and treat the source (incomplete abortion, injury, pelvic abscess, peritonitis, tetanus)
      (iii) Broad-spectrum intravenous antibiotics
      (iv) Consider tetanus vaccine and antitoxin if not immunized
   (e) Shock
      (i) Resuscitation (oxygen, intravenous fluids, broad-spectrum intravenous antibiotics, blood transfusion, consider tetanus vaccine).
5. Contraception counseling and services to prevent unwanted pregnancy.
6. Management of other SRH concerns as appropriate (e.g., STIs, HIV).

For more information refer to www.pac-consortium.org

Increasingly, reproductive health services, including safe abortion, have been framed as a human right. In 2011, the UN Special Rapporteur of the Human Rights Council reported that criminalizing abortion effectively restricts human rights as the right to SRH is a fundamental part of the right to health (Grover, 2011). The report recommended that where criminal or legal barriers to reproductive health exist, it is the obligation of the State to remove them.

A harm reduction strategy for women seeking abortion in restricted environments supports giving women information on safer self-use of medications for abortion (Box 15.6). This strategy focuses on reducing the risk of self-induced abortion rather than abortion's legal or moral status and supports women's right to health in any setting (Erdman, 2012). A number of global women's health organizations, such as Women on Web (see Additional resources section), use this strategy to assist women in need of safer care despite local legal restrictions.

Clinical care

The two WHO recommended methods for treating incomplete abortion, missed abortion, and induced abortion in the first trimester are vacuum aspiration or medications. Vacuum aspiration evacuates the contents of the uterus using suction provided by a hand-held portable aspirator (Figure 15.2) or an electric pump.

Medications stimulate uterine contractions and cause expulsion of the products of conception without instrumentation. For incomplete or missed abortion, misoprostol may be offered as an alternative to expectant management. For induced abortion, a combined regimen of mifepristone and misoprostol is the most effective medical method (Box 15.6). Where mifepristone is not available, misoprostol alone may be used.

The choice of vacuum aspiration or medical method depends on the woman's clinical presentation, eligibility, preferences, availability of equipment, and provider training (Table 15.3). Sharp curettage is not a WHO recommended method of uterine evacuation (WHO, 2012).

Women present for abortion less commonly in the second trimester but access to safe services is critical for these women. As gestational age increases, so does the complexity and potential complications of abortion. Women presenting in the second trimester have often encountered social, economic, and health system barriers before obtaining care (Gallo & Nghia, 2007; Harries *et al.*, 2007). On average, younger women access abortion at later gestational ages than older women (Lim *et al.*, 2012; Pazol *et al.*, 2012). Dilation and evacuation and medical methods are recommended at this gestational age and may be offered based on provider experience, facility capacity, and the woman's preference.

Counseling women and providing them with contraception is an integral part of comprehensive abortion care. For women who are medically eligible, all contraception, including IUDs and implants, may be started immediately after an

services. For example, even in areas where abortion is legal, adolescents and young women face particular barriers to accessing safe abortion because of stigma around youth sexuality, traditional gender roles, poverty, violence, poor knowledge of the law, lack of youth-friendly services, and negative provider attitudes.

uncomplicated vacuum aspiration (WHO, 2009b). Pills, injectables, and implants may be started with the first pill of medical abortion, and IUDs may be inserted when it is reasonably certain the woman is no longer pregnant (WHO, 2012).

Box 15.6 Protocols for medical abortion

Misoprostol for incomplete abortion, uterine size less than 13 weeks
- Misoprostol 400 μg sublingually *or* 600 μg orally × 1 dose

Mifepristone and misoprostol for induced abortion, gestational age up to 13 weeks from the last menstrual period
- Up to 10 weeks: mifepristone 200 mg orally × 1 dose, then wait 24–48 hours and give misoprostol 800 μg buccally. Misoprostol may also be given vaginally or sublingually before 9 weeks.
- 10–13 weeks: mifepristone 200 mg orally, followed 36–48 hours later by misoprostol 800 μg vaginally, then 400 μg vaginally or sublingually every 3 hours for a maximum of five doses of misoprostol or until the products of conception are expelled.

Misoprostol alone for induced abortion, gestational age up to 13 weeks from the last menstrual period
- Misoprostol 800 μg vaginally every 3–12 hours for a maximum of three doses *or* misoprostol 800 μg sublingually every 3 hours for a maximum of three doses.

Infertility

Infertility is defined as the inability to conceive after 1 year of regular and unprotected intercourse. Infertility in a couple who have never conceived is primary infertility; infertility after at least one conception (not necessarily a live birth) is secondary infertility. The reported international prevalence of infertility is estimated at approximately 8–10% of couples and is remarkably similar between high- and low-income countries (Boivin *et al.*, 2007).

The suffering caused by infertility in low- and middle-income countries is immense (van Balen & Bos, 2009). Childless couples, especially women, may suffer marital problems, often leading to abuse and/or divorce, and can face stigma and isolation from family and community. Additionally, infertile women may lose the social and financial security provided by marriage and children in old age (Dyer *et al.*, 2002, 2004; Dhont *et al.*, 2011a).

Causes of infertility

Both male and female factors can cause infertility (Figure 15.3). Female factors include ovulatory dysfunction (including polycystic ovarian syndrome), tubal and peritoneal pathology, and uterine pathology (e.g., submucous myoma, adhesions, uterine septum). In low-income countries, most infertility is acquired through reproductive tract infections (sexually transmitted, puerperal, and post-abortion infections) causing pelvic inflammatory disease (PID) and leading to tubal blockage. These infections are responsible for much of the high rates of secondary infertility in certain regions of Africa (up to 23%) (Cates *et al.*, 1985; Larsen, 2000). Overall, a tubal factor can be found in up to 75% of couples experiencing infertility in developing countries. Prevention of STIs (including HIV), safer childbirth, better access to contraception and

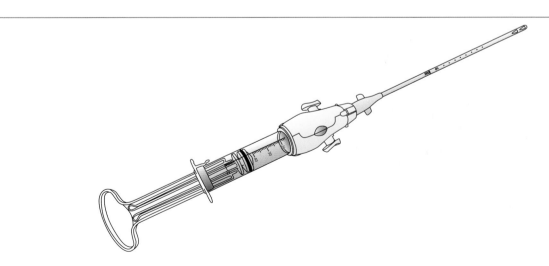

Figure 15.2 Manual vacuum aspirator. *Source*: Ipas/Stephen C. Edgerton, reproduced with permission of Ipas.

Table 15.3 Comparing methods of induced abortion in first trimester.

	Vacuum aspiration	Medical abortion with mifepristone and misoprostol	Medical abortion with misoprostol only
What is it?	A procedure that uses electric or manual suction instruments to evacuate the uterus to remove the pregnancy by suction	Medications taken together that cause the uterus to expel the pregnancy	A medication that causes the uterus to expel the pregnancy
How does it work?	The pregnancy is removed from the uterus through a cannula attached to an electric pump or hand-held aspirator	Mifepristone makes the pregnancy detach from the side of the uterus. Misoprostol causes contractions that expel the pregnancy	Misoprostol causes contractions that expel the pregnancy
When can it be used?	From detection of pregnancy to 13 weeks (throughout first trimester)	From detection of pregnancy to 13 weeks (throughout first trimester)	From detection of pregnancy to 13 weeks (throughout first trimester)
Where can it be used?	In a healthcare facility	Mifepristone (first pill) is usually given at the clinic Misoprostol (second set of pills) may be taken at clinic or home for women with pregnancies under 10 weeks. For pregnancies at 10–13 weeks, women should take misoprostol in the facility	Misoprostol may be taken at the clinic or home for women with pregnancies under 9 weeks. For pregnancies at 9–13 weeks, women should take misoprostol in the facility
How effective is it?	97–99.5%	95–98%	83–87%
Safe and effective for young women as for adults?	Yes	Yes	Yes
What are the side effects?	Bleeding and cramping	Bleeding and cramping are expected. Possible side effects are nausea, vomiting, diarrhea, fever/chills or dizziness	Bleeding and cramping are expected. Possible side effects are nausea, vomiting, diarrhea, fever/chills or dizziness
What are possible complications?	Rare complications include injury to the uterus or cervix, excessive bleeding, infection, blood collecting in the uterus, or incomplete abortion. Failed vacuum aspiration occurs in <1% of women, especially when performed by a skilled provider	Rare complications include excessive bleeding and infection Failed medical abortion occurs in 5%, and ongoing pregnancy occurs in less than 1% of women	Rare complications include excessive bleeding and infection Failed medical abortion occurs in 15%, and ongoing pregnancy occurs in 4–6% of women
How is it typically used?	The pregnancy is removed with suction through a tube inserted into an electric pump or hand-held aspirator. Procedure time is 2–10 min Completion of the procedure is immediately confirmed, requiring only one facility visit	Mifepristone is taken by mouth (swallowed) One or two days later, misoprostol is put under the tongue, inside the cheek, or in the vagina. The abortion usually occurs within 4–6 hours of misoprostol, but can take up to several days	Misoprostol is put either under the tongue or in the vagina and doses are repeated The abortion usually occurs within 24 hours, but can take up to several days
What if the abortion fails?	The procedure is repeated	The pregnancy is removed through vacuum aspiration. If aspiration services are not available, a second dose of misoprostol can be offered with close follow-up	The pregnancy is removed through vacuum aspiration

Source: Ipas (2013), reproduced with permission of Ipas.

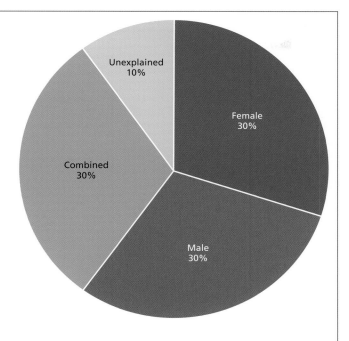

Figure 15.3 Causes of infertility.

comprehensive abortion care could substantially reduce the prevalence of infertility in such settings.

Investigations

Infertility investigations usually start after 1 year of trying to conceive, but they can start earlier if the history indicates abnormal menstrual cycles (periods not between 21 and 35 days) or any other elements predisposing to infertility (such as older age or past PID). One should always aim to include both female and male partners in the work-up. Testing for HIV is essential as prevalence is reportedly much higher in infertile (especially secondary infertile) couples (Dhont et al., 2011b). Most of the tests listed here can be performed at the district hospital level, with the exception of laparoscopy and hysteroscopy, which may be less accessible in resource-limited settings.

Female

Ovulation
- Regular menstrual cycle confirms ovulation.
- In case of amenorrhea (missed three cycles or 6 months without periods), a progestin challenge test can be performed and is based on the premise that progestin treatment (e.g., progesterone acetate 10 mg daily for 5–7 days) will induce menses only in those having anovulation and not in those with genital tract outflow abnormalities (e.g., transverse vaginal septum, hymen imperforatum) or in those with premature menopause.

Tubal patency
- Hysterosalpingography (HSG): after injection of radio-opaque material into cervical canal, radiography (or fluoroscopy when available) can visualize the shape of the uterine cavity and the patency of the tubes. Needs to be performed after menstruation and before ovulation, usually between day 4 and days 10–12. Prophylaxis with doxycycline 200 mg/day for 3 days is indicated.
- Laparoscopy if HSG abnormal.

Uterus
- Gynecological examination.
- Transvaginal ultrasound.
- Hysteroscopy.
- Cervical factor: post-coital test (Box 15.7).

Male

Sexual function
- Ask about erectile and ejaculatory function and frequency of intercourse.

Semen
- Semen analysis (goal concentration of at least 15 million/mL and at least 32% with progressive motility); if abnormal, repeat test after 1 month. For post-coital test refer to Box 15.7.

Box 15.8 Simple methods to determine the fertile period

The most fertile period is 1–2 days before ovulation. Menstruation usually occurs 14 days after ovulation. Therefore, in a 28-day cycle, the most fertile period is on day 12–13. At this time the cervical mucus is watery, clear, and can be stretched between the fingers up to 10 cm. By using a combination of calculation and cervical mucus assessment (done by woman or partner), the couple can have a fairly accurate idea about the fertile period.

Table 15.4 Treatment of infertility according to etiology.

Etiology	Treatment
Ovulatory factor	Clomiphene citrate 50 mg daily days 3–7; if no response, increase up to maximum dose of 150 mg daily plus ultrasound monitoring (cancel treatment if more than two follicles 15 mm) Gonadotropins (expensive) Ovarian drilling (laparoscopic puncturing of the ovaries) if no response
Tubal factor	Surgery (laparoscopic preferably) but low success rate IVF
Uterine factor	Surgery (hysteroscopic preferably): polypectomy, myomectomy, adhesiolysis
Cervical factor	IUI
Mild male factor	Clomiphene citrate 25 mg/day or IUI Ligation varicocele IUI
Severe male factor	IVF/ICSI

IUI, intrauterine insemination, sometimes associated with ovarian stimulation (clomiphene citrate or gonadotropins to increase success rate, but may have multiple pregnancies); IVF, in vitro fertilization; ICSI, intracytoplasmatic sperm injection.

If all investigations are normal, infertility is unexplained. If the female's age is below 35, conservative management can be advocated with instructions about how to identify her fertile period by calculating cycle length or by assessment of cervical mucus (Box 15.8).

Treatment

An overview of the treatment of infertility according to etiology is provided in Table 15.4. Intrauterine insemination (IUI), *in vitro* fertilization (IVF), and intracytoplasmic sperm injection (ICSI) are, unfortunately for most developing countries, only available in the private sector at a prohibitive cost (US$3000–8000 for one cycle) (Dyer *et al.*, 2013). Recently, low-cost IVF methods have been developed, are currently being tested in various settings, and might become available in the near future (Klerkx *et al.*, 2013). Regardless of the availability of infertility treatments, all individuals and couples require psychosocial support. Counseling should be provided to help couples gain an understanding of their realistic options (including exploring alternatives such as adoption, if appropriate) and how to deal with the disappointment, grief, and social consequences of infertility where services are not available.

Sexual violence and female genital mutilation

Sexual violence

Sexual violence is defined as:

> any sexual act, attempt to obtain a sexual act, unwanted sexual comments or advances, or acts to traffic, or otherwise directed against a person's sexuality using coercion, by any person regardless of their relationship to the victim, in any setting including, but not limited to, home and work (WHO, 2010b).

Globally, 36% of women have experienced physical and/or sexual violence, with intimate partners the major perpetrators

(WHO, 2013a). Many experience violence as children or adolescents, and many young women report their first sex was coerced or forced. Up to 21% of respondents in a multi-country study reported sexual abuse under the age of 15 years, and between 6 and 59% of women had experienced sexual coercion from an intimate partner in their lifetime (Dartnall & Jewkes, 2013).

Clinical management

Physical consequences can occur in the short or long term and include genital or non-genital injuries and, in some cases, death. Rape can result in unwanted pregnancies, unsafe abortions, STIs including HIV, sexual dysfunction, infertility, pelvic pain, PID, and urinary tract infections. Women who have experienced intimate-partner violence are also more likely to have a low-birthweight baby. Psychological consequences include rape trauma syndrome, post-traumatic stress disorder, depression, social phobias, anxiety, increased substance use, and suicidal behavior. Long term, these complications may include chronic headaches, fatigue, sleep disturbances, recurrent nausea, eating disorders, menstrual pain, and sexual difficulties (WHO, 2003, 2013a).

Individuals who have suffered sexual violence should be offered immediate care, which includes meeting the health needs of survivors and collecting evidence for medicolegal purposes (Table 15.5). No forensic examination should be done if there are no local capacities and/or requirements for testing forensic evidence (Jina & Thomas, 2013).

Comprehensive care should address physical injuries, pregnancy prevention and management, and risk of infection (STIs, HIV, hepatitis B) (Table 15.6). Social support and counseling are important for recovery, and all survivors should be offered emotional and social support. Follow-up services, including a medical check-up at 2 weeks, 3 months, and 6 months after the assault, and referral for counseling and other support services should also be provided. Comprehensive guidelines for identification and care for survivors of sexual violence are available from WHO (2003, 2013b).

Prevention

Health workers are ideally placed to recognize and intervene in sexual violence since they are frequently consulted by victims and are often confronted with its physical and mental health

Table 15.5 Components of a medical forensic examination.

Main component	What does it entail?
Initial assessment	Grant immediate access to a trained health worker Assess acute health needs Always give priority to safety, health, and well-being of patient Use sensitive language Do not re-victimize the patient (do not use judgmental language) Obtain informed consent
Medical history	Ensure compliance with national guidelines on clinical examinations, if any Cover any known health problems, immunization status, and medications Cover recent gynecological history in the case of sexual assault Obtain an account of the violent events, including details of actual or attempted sexual activity. Ensure use of non-judgmental language Note any use of condoms and lubricant and activities that may alter evidence (e.g., bathing) Note any symptoms developed after the assault
Physical examination	Note the patient's general appearance, demeanor, and mental functioning Note the patient's vital signs (blood pressure, temperature, pulse, respiration rate) Examine the patient from head to toe, after having explained all the procedures to your patient. Throughout the examination, inform the patient what you plan to do next and ask permission Note and describe any physical injuries Photograph any injuries Order diagnostic tests Draw blood samples for testing for HIV, hepatitis B, syphilis, and other STIs
Genito-anal examination	Try to make the patient as comfortable as possible Explain each step of the procedure Perform procedures of a routine genito-anal examination
Recording and classifying injuries	If health workers did not receive training or have skills to accurately document and interpret injuries, document the injuries using standard terminology and defer the interpretation to a forensic specialist Adopt a systematic approach to describe and record physical characteristics of wounds Use standard, universally accepted descriptive terms for classifying wounds
Diagnostic tests, specimen collection, and forensic issues	Check with your clinic, hospital or laboratory as to what medical specimens are required, when and how they should be collected, and how long each test takes to process For the benefit of the patient, collect any forensic evidence during the medical examination Health workers should have a good understanding of components and requirements of forensic examinations

Source: adapted from WHO (2003).

Table 15.6 Treatment and follow-up for survivors of sexual violence.

Condition	Key considerations
Physical injury	In the case of life-threatening injuries, refer to emergency treatment (see Chapter 25) In the case of less severe injuries: • Provide wound care (including antibiotics if appropriate) • Consider tetanus vaccination • Pain relief
Pregnancy prevention and management	Assess for current pregnancy (pregnancy test if available) If not currently pregnant, offer emergency contraception up to 5 days after the sexual assault Note that emergency contraceptive pills can be safely prescribed if pregnancy cannot be ruled out with certainty Return for pregnancy testing if the next menstrual period is missed In case of a confirmed pregnancy, discuss options (including safe abortion where available) and provide psychosocial support (clinicians must be aware of local laws related to induced abortion) Inform the woman of her rights and respect her decision at all times
Sexually transmitted infections	Offer prophylaxis/presumptive treatment for chlamydia, gonorrhea, trichomoniasis and syphilis (depending on local prevalence) based on local STI guidelines (see Chapter 16)
HIV/AIDS	Risk of HIV acquisition is increased with penetrative sexual assault, vaginal or anal trauma, multiple number of perpetrators and assaults, presence of STIs or other genital lesions, and local high HIV prevalence Offer baseline counseling and testing for HIV with repeat testing at 6, 12, and 24 weeks Consider post-exposure prophylaxis within 72 hours depending on the presence of risk factors and local guidelines and protocols
Hepatitis B	Offer baseline testing if available Offer immunization if never vaccinated or incomplete vaccination

Source: adapted from WHO (2003, 2013b).

consequences (van den Ameele *et al.*, 2013). They might also be the earliest point of contact for survivors of violence. The health professional's role concerns mainly the identification of persons in a violent situation and early intervention, as well as care for the individual after violence (secondary and tertiary prevention). Secondary prevention should be offered in a sensitive non-judgmental way (van den Ameele *et al.*, 2013), should not break confidentiality, and should not put women at risk of retribution, additional violence, or further victimization (USAID, IGWG, PRB, 2010).

Female genital mutilation

Female genital mutilation (FGM) comprises all procedures on the external female genitalia, whereby healthy tissue is altered for non-medical reasons. It is classified into four main types, depending on the degree of cutting (Figure 15.4).

FGM predominantly occurs in 27 African countries; 87 million girls and women aged 15 and older have undergone FGM in these African countries and Yemen (Yoder *et al.*, 2013). Each year, 3 million are at risk of being cut (UNICEF, 2013).

Clinical management

Short-term complications of FGM include bleeding, severe pain, damage to tissues, shock, infection, septicemia, and urinary retention. Long-term physical complications include keloid formation, cysts, clitoral neuroma, vulval abscess, reproductive tract infections, acute/chronic pelvic infection, infertility, fistulae and incontinence, vaginal obstruction, menstrual disorders, and ulcers. The management of most of the short-term complications will be the same as the management of trauma and infection due to other causes (see Chapter 25). For more details on the management of the long-term complications of FGM refer to the manual of the Kenyan Ministry of Health (see Additional resources section).

The type of FGM must be examined at first antenatal attendance to assess the type, degree of vulval and vaginal scarring, and the size of the vaginal opening. Problems during pregnancy and delivery are mainly observed in women with type III FGM and will depend on the size of the vaginal opening, the parity of the woman, and the elasticity of the scar (Federale Overheidsdienst Volksgezondheid, Veiligheid van de Voedselketen en Leefmilieu, GAMS Belgium, 2011). If the urinary opening can be observed or if two fingers can be passed

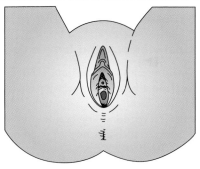

Normal anatomy

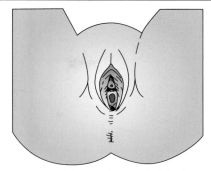

Type 1 - partial or total removal of the clitoris (clitoridectomy)

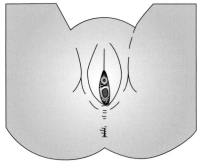

Type 2 - clitoridectomy plus partial or total removal of the labia minora (excision)

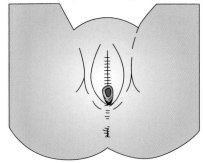

Type 3 - narrowing of the vaginal opening through cutting or repositioning of the labia with or without clitoridectomy (infibulation)

Figure 15.4 Types of female genital mutilation. *Source*: Clarice Illustrations, reproduced with permission of Clarice Illustrations.

into the vagina without discomfort, the mutilation is unlikely to cause major physical problems at delivery, whether in a clinic or at home (Kenya Ministry of Health, 2008). Ideally, infibulations, or surgical/sutured closures, should be opened during the second trimester and performed by an appropriately trained provider. The advantages of such de-infibulation during pregnancy, and the subsequent physiological changes affecting menstruation and urination, should be carefully explained to the woman and her partner.

Prevention

Healthcare providers are important advocates and well placed to inform patients of the devastating health consequences of FGM. Pregnancy provides a good opportunity to give women education and information about basic health, normal and cut genitals, childbirth, and postnatal care (Kenya Ministry of Health, 2008). Pregnancy is also an ideal time to counsel a woman and her partner about the dangers of repeated re-infibulations. Healthcare providers must not perform any FGM, be it a type I, type IV (incisions), or a re-infibulation. Performing FGM constitutes a breach of medical professionalism and ethical responsibility, is likely to contribute to legitimization and institutionalization of the

practice, and thus contributes to upholding the practice (WHO, 2010c).

Additional resources

Contraception

- World Health Organization (2010) Medical eligibility criteria for contraceptive use, 4th edn. http://www.who.int/reproductivehealth/publications/family_planning/9789241563888/en/index.html
- World Health Organization and Johns Hopkins Bloomberg School of Public Health/Center for Communication Programs (2011) Family planning. A global handbook for providers, 2011 update. http://www.who.int/reproductivehealth/publications/family_planning/9780978856304/en/index.html
- World Health Organization and John Hopkins Bloomberg School of Public Health / Center for Communication Programs (2007) Decision-making tool for family planning clients and providers. http://www.who.int/reproductivehealth/publications/family_planning/dmt_cdrom/en/index.html

Comprehensive abortion care

- World Health Organization (2012) Safe abortion: technical and policy guidance for health systems, 2nd edn. http://www.who.int/reproductivehealth/publications/unsafe_abortion/9789241548434/en/
- Women on Web. https://www.womenonweb.org/
- Ipas (2013) Clinical updates in reproductive health. http://www.ipas.org/clinicalupdates
- Gynuity (2009) Misoprostol for treatment of incomplete abortion: an introductory guidebook. http://gynuity.org/resources/info/guidebook-on-misoprostol-for-treatment-of-incomplete-abortion/
- Ipas (2013) Woman-centered comprehensive abortion care: a reference manual, 2nd edn. http://www.ipas.org/~/media/Files/Ipas%20Publications/ACREFE13.ashx?utm_source=resource&utm_medium=meta&utm_campaign=ACREFE13

Infertility

- The Walking Egg Foundation: www.thewalkingegg.com
- Biomedical infertility care in poor resource countries. Barrier, access and ethics: http://www.fvvo.be/monographs/biomedical-infertility-care-in-poor-resource-countries-barriers-access-and-ethics/

Sexual violence and female genital mutilation

- World Health Organization (2003) Guidelines for medico-legal care for victims of sexual violence. Gender and Women's Health, Family and Community Health, Injuries and Violence Prevention, Non-communicable Diseases and Mental Health. Available at http://whqlibdoc.who.int/publications/2004/924154628X.pdf
- Ministry of Health, Republic of Kenya. Management of complications, pregnancy, childbirth and the postpartum period in the presence of FGM/C. A reference manual for health service providers. Available at http://www.popcouncil.org/pdfs/frontiers/reports/Kenya_FGC_Pregnancy.pdf
- Bott S, Guedes A, Claramunt MC, Guezmes A (2004) Improving the health sector response to gender-based violence: a resource manual for health care professionals in developing countries. http://www.ippfwhr.org/sites/default/files/GBV_cdbookletANDmanual_FA_FINAL.pdf

REFERENCES

Bearinger LH, Sieving RE, Ferguson J, Sharma V (2007) Global perspectives on the sexual and reproductive health of adolescents: patterns, prevention, and potential. *Lancet* 369:1220–31.

Benson J, Andersen K, Samandari G (2011) Reductions in abortion-related mortality following policy reform: evidence from Romania, South Africa and Bangladesh. *Reprod Health* 8:39.

Boivin J, Bunting L, Collins JA, Nygren KG (2007) International estimates of infertility prevalence and treatment-seeking: potential need and demand for infertility medical care. *Hum Reprod* 22:1506–12.

Cates W, Farley TM, Rowe PJ (1985) Worldwide patterns of infertility: is Africa different? *Lancet* ii:596–8.

Cates W Jr (2010) Family planning: the essential link to all eight Millennium Development Goals. *Contraception* 81:460–1.

Cleland J, Conde-Agudelo A, Peterson H, Ross J, Tsui A (2012) Contraception and health. *Lancet* 380:149–56.

Darroch JE (2013; Trends in contraceptive use. *Contraception* 87:259–63.

Dartnall E, Jewkes R (2013) Sexual violence against women: the scope of the problem. *Best Pract Res Clin Obstet Gynaecol* 27:3–13.

Dhont N, van deWijgert J, Coene G, Gasarabwe A, Temmerman M (2011a) "Mama and papa nothing": living with infertility among an urban population in Kigali, Rwanda. *Hum Reprod* 26:623–9.

Dhont N, Muvunyi C, Luchters S et al. (2011b) HIV infection and sexual behaviour in primary and secondary infertile relationships: a case-control study in Kigali, Rwanda. *Sex Transm Infect* 87:28–34.

Dyer SJ, Abrahams N, Hoffman M, van der Spuy ZM (2002) "Men leave me as I cannot have children": women's experiences with involuntary childlessness. *Hum Reprod* 17:1663–8.

Dyer SJ, Abrahams N, Mokoena NE, van der Spuy ZM (2004) "You are a man because you have children": experiences, reproductive health knowledge and treatment-seeking behaviour among men suffering from couple infertility in South Africa. *Hum Reprod* 19:960–7.

Dyer SJ, Sherwood K, McIntyre D, Ataguba JE (2013) Catastrophic payment for assisted reproduction techniques with conventional ovarian stimulation in the public health sector of South Africa: frequency and coping strategies. *Hum Reprod* 28:2755–64.

Erdman JN (2012) Harm reduction, human rights, and access to information on safer abortion. *Int J Gynaecol Obstet* 118:83–6.

Federale Overheidsdienst Volksgezondheid, Veiligheid van de Voedselketen en Leefmilieu, GAMS Belgium (2011) *Vrouwelijke genitale verminking. Handleiding voor de betrokken beroepssectoren*. Brussels: FOD Volksgezondheid.

Gallo MF, Nghia NC (2007) Real life is different: a qualitative study of why women delay abortion until the second trimester in Vietnam. *Soc Sci Med* 64:1812–22.

Glasier A, Gülmezoglu AM, Schmid GP, Moreno CG, Van Look PF (2006) Sexual and reproductive health: a matter of life and death. *Lancet* 368:1595–607.

Grover A (2011) *Interim Report of the Special Rapporteur on the Right of Everyone to the Enjoyment of the Highest Attainable Standard of Physical and Mental Health*. New York: United Nations.

Guttmacher A (2003) *In Their Own Right: Addressing the Sexual and Reproductive Health Needs of Men Worldwide*. New York: Alan Guttmacher Institute.

Harries J, Orner P, Gabriel M, Mitchell E (2007) Delays in seeking an abortion until the second trimester: a qualitative study in South Africa. *Reprod Health* 4:7.

Horga M, Gerdts C, Potts M (2013) The remarkable story of Romanian women's struggle to manage their fertility. *J Fam Plann Reprod Health Care* 39:2–4.

Ipas (2013) *Women-Centered, Comprehensive Abortion Care: Reference Manual*, 2nd edn. Chapel Hill, NC: Ipas.

IPPF (2004) *Medical and Service Delivery Guidelines for Sexual and Reproductive Health Services*, 3rd edn. London: International Planned Parenthood Federation.

IWAG (2010) *Inter-Agency Field Manual on Reproductive Health in Humanitarian Settings*. New York: Inter-agency Working Group on Reproductive Health in Crises.

Jina R, Thomas LS (2013) Health consequences of sexual violence against women. *Best Pract Res Clin Obstet Gynaecol* 27:15–26.

Kenya Ministry of Health (2008) Management of complications, pregnancy, childbirth and the postpartum period in the presence of FGM/C. A reference manual for health service providers. Nairobi: Ministry of Health, Republic of Kenya.

Klerkx E, Janssen M, van Blerkom J, Campo R, Ombelet W (2013) IVF for 200 Euro per cycle. European Society of Human Reproduction and Embryology Annual Meeting, London.

Larsen U (2000) Primary and secondary infertility in sub-Saharan Africa. *Int J Epidemiol* 29:285–91.

Lim L, Wong H, Yong E, Singh K (2012) Profiles of women presenting for abortions in Singapore: focus on teenage abortions and late abortions. *Eur J Obstet Gynecol Reprod Biol* 160:219–22.

Newman K, Helzner JF (1999) IPPF charter on sexual and reproductive rights. *J Womens Health Gend Based Med* 8:459–63.

Pazol K, Creanga AA, Zane SB, Burley KB, Jamieson DJ (2012) Abortion surveillance: United States, 2009. *MMWR Surveill Summ* 61:1–44.

PMNCH (2013) *Engaging Men and Boys in RMNCH. Knowledge Summary: Women's and Children's Health*. New York: Promundo, United Nations Population Fund, World Health Organization.

Raymond EG, Grimes DA (2012) The comparative safety of legal induced abortion and childbirth in the United States. *Obstet Gynecol* 119:215–19.

Sedgh G, Hussain R, Bankole A, Singh S (2007) Women with unmet need for contraception in developing countries and their reasons for not using a method. Occasional Report No. 37. New York: Alan Guttmacher Institute.

Sedgh G, Singh S, Shah IH, Åhman E, Henshaw SK, Bankole A (2012) Induced abortion: incidence and trends worldwide from 1995 to 2008. *Lancet* 379:625–32.

United Nations (1995) Report of the International Conference on Population and Development, Cairo, 5–13 September, 1994. New York: United Nations.

UN Millennium Project (2006) Public Choices, Private Decisions: Sexual and Reproductive Health and the Millennium Development Goals. New York: United Nations Development Programme.

UNFPA (2008) *Making Reproductive Rights and Sexual and Reproductive Health a Reality for All. Reproductive Rights and Sexual And Reproductive Health Framework*. New York: United Nations Population Fund.

UNICEF (2013) Female Genital Mutilation/Cutting: A Statistical Overview and Exploration of the Dynamics of Change. New York: United Nations Children's Fund.

USAID, IGWG, PRB (2010) The crucial role of health services in responding to gender based violence. Available at http://www.prb.org/igwg_media/crucial-role-hlth-srvices.pdf

van Balen F, Bos HM (2009) The social and cultural consequences of being childless in poor-resource areas. *Facts Views Vision ObGyn* 1:106–21.

van den Ameele S, Keygnaert I, Rachidi A, Roelens K, Temmerman M (2013) The role of the healthcare sector in the prevention of sexual violence against sub-Saharan transmigrants in Morocco: a study of knowledge, attitudes and practices of healthcare workers. *BMC Health Serv Res* 13:77.

WHO (2003) *Guidelines for Medico-Legal Care for Victims of Sexual Violence*. Geneva: Gender and Women's Health, Family and Community Health, Injuries and Violence Prevention, Non-Communicable Disease and Mental Health, World Health Organization.

WHO (2004) *Selected Practice Recommendations for Contraceptive Use*, 2nd edn. Geneva: World Health Organization.

WHO (2005) *Decision-Making Tool for Family Planning Clients and Providers*. Baltimore and Geneva: World Health Organization and Johns Hopkins Bloomberg School of Public Health/Centre for Communication Programs Information and Knowledge for Optimal Health.

WHO (2009a) Medical eligibility criteria wheel for contraceptive use, 2008 update. Available at http://www.who.int/reproductivehealth/publications/family_planning/9789241547710/en/

WHO (2009b) Medical Eligibility Criteria for Contraceptive Use. Geneva: Department of Reproductive Health and Research, World Health Organization.

WHO (2009c) Promoting sexual and reproductive health for persons with disabilities. WHO/UNFPA guidance note. Geneva: Department of Reproductive Health and Research, World Health Organization.

WHO (2010a) Social Determinants of Sexual and Reproductive Health. Informing Future Research and Programme Implementation. Geneva: World Health Organization.

WHO (2010b) Preventing Intimate Partner and Sexual Violence Against Women. Taking Action and Generating Evidence. Geneva: World Health Organization and London School of Hygiene and Tropical Medicine.

WHO (2010c) *Global Strategy to Stop Health-care Providers from Performing Female Genital Mutilation*. Geneva: World Health Organization.

WHO (2010d) *Medical Eligibility Criteria for Contraceptive Use*, 4th edn. Geneva: World Health Organization.

WHO (2011a) *Family Planning. A Global Handbook for Providers, 2011 update*. Geneva: Department of Reproductive Health and Research World Health Organization, Johns Hopkins Bloomberg School of Public Health Center for Communication Programs Knowledge for Health Project.

WHO (2011b) *Unsafe Abortion: Global and Regional Estimates of the Incidence of Unsafe Abortion and Associated Mortality in 2008*. Geneva: World Health Organization.

WHO (2012) *Safe Abortion: Technical and Policy Guidance for Health Systems*, 2nd edn. Geneva: World Health Organization.

WHO (2013a) *Global and Regional Estimates of Violence Against Women: Prevalence and Health Effects of Intimate Partner Violence and Non-Partner Sexual Violence*. Geneva: World Health Organization, London School of Hygiene and Tropical Medicine, South African Medical Research Council.

WHO (2013b) *Responding to Intimate Partner Violence and Sexual Violence Against Women: WHO Clinical and Policy Guidelines*. Geneva: World Health Organization.

Yoder SP, Wang S, Johansen E (2013) Estimates of female genital mutilation/cutting in 27 African countries and Yemen. *Stud Fam Plann* 44:189–204.

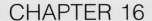

CHAPTER 16

Sexually Transmitted Infections

Susanna E. Winston[1], Hillary Mabeya[2], and Susan Cu-Uvin[3]

[1]Hasbro Children's Hospital, Providence, RI, USA
[2]Moi University, Eldoret, Kenya
[3]Brown University, Providence, RI, USA

Key learning objectives

- Understand the global burden of sexually transmitted infections (STIs).
- Become familiar with common presentations of STIs.
- Learn about available diagnostics and current treatment recommendations.
- Become familiar with preventive strategies for STIs.

Abstract

Sexually transmitted infections (STIs) are bacterial, viral, and parasitic pathogens that are transmitted through sexual contact. They are a major and growing cause of global morbidity, with approximately 500 million new cases of the four curable STIs each year. STIs are often grouped by clinical presentation or syndrome as infections causing (i) genital ulcer disease and buboes, (ii) vaginal discharge, (iii) urethritis in men and cervicitis in women, (iv) lower abdominal pain in women, and (v) other STIs. Specific STI syndromic management guidelines, which provide diagnostic and treatment guidelines through easy-to-follow flowcharts, have been developed by the World Health Organization (WHO) to help practitioners in resource-limited settings when laboratory evaluation for confirming a diagnosis is limited. This chapter reviews the syndromic categories of STIs, common presentations of specific causative organisms, various testing modalities, and typical treatment options, including the WHO syndromic management flowcharts.

Key words: sexually transmitted infection, STI, STD, reproductive health, syndromic management, chlamydia, gonorrhea, syphilis, HSV, pelvic inflammatory disease

Essential Clinical Global Health, First Edition. Edited by Brett D. Nelson.
© 2015 John Wiley & Sons, Ltd. Published 2015 by John Wiley & Sons, Ltd.
Companion website: www.essentialseries.com/globalhealth

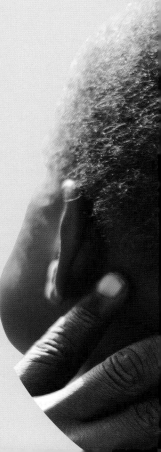

Introduction

Sexually transmitted infections (STIs) are bacterial, viral, and parasitic pathogens that are transmitted through sexual contact. While sexual transmission is most common, many can also be transmitted from mother to child during pregnancy and birth, through human tissue or blood products, and occasionally through non-sexual contact (WHO, 2007a).

STIs are a major and growing cause of global morbidity. The WHO estimates that there are approximately 500 million new cases each year of the four curable STIs (*Chlamydia trachomatis*, *Neisseria gonorrhoeae*, syphilis, and *Trichomonas vaginalis*), which represents a significant increase from previous years (WHO, 2012a). STIs can have serious complications, including decreased fertility, adverse outcomes in pregnancy for mother and newborn, cervical cancer, and increased transmission of HIV (WHO, 2007a).

Risk factors for acquiring STIs include behaviors that increase potential exposure (e.g., having multiple concurrent sexual partners, inconsistent condom use, alcohol and drug use) and biological risk factors such as cervical ectopy (Burstein, 2011). STIs are preventable, although mitigating these risk factors is challenging. Specific groups at particularly high risk due to their biological and social vulnerability include adolescents, men who have sex with men, people living with HIV/AIDS, and pregnant women.

STIs by clinical presentation

STIs are often grouped by clinical presentation, or syndrome. Specific STI syndromic management guidelines, which provide diagnostic and treatment guidelines through easy-to-follow flowcharts, have been developed by the WHO to help practitioners in resource-limited settings. Importantly, these guidelines recommend treatment empirically at the first visit, decreasing loss to follow-up, and cover the most important causes of STIs. Integration of local epidemiology into these guidelines maximizes their effectiveness (WHO, 2005). STIs can be grouped in the following categories, as infections causing (i) genital ulcer disease (GUD) and buboes, (ii) vaginal discharge, (iii) urethritis in men and cervicitis in women, (iv) lower abdominal pain in women, and (v) other STIs. HIV is an important STI that is covered in Chapter 18, and it is critical to incorporate HIV testing as part of care for any individual presenting with STI symptoms.

Infections causing genital ulcer disease and buboes

Anogenital ulcerative lesions can be painful, non-painful, pruritic, and vary in size. They may be associated with discharge, buboes (localized swelling in the groin due to inguinal lymphadenopathy), and/or systemic symptoms. Herpes simplex virus (HSV) and syphilis are the most common causes of GUD, although this varies by region. Less common etiologies include chancroid, granuloma inguinale, and lymphogranuloma venereum (LGV) (Centers for Disease Control and Prevention, 2010).

While each infection has hallmark symptoms, history and physical examination do not always distinguish between causative organisms. Therefore, when possible, diagnostic testing should be performed. Important non-infectious causes of genital ulcers include aphthous ulcers, cancerous lesions, and drug reactions.

Herpes simplex virus

HSV is the most common cause of GUD globally. Prevalence is highest in sub-Saharan Africa, followed by eastern Asia (Looker *et al.*, 2008). The classic presentation is multiple painful vesicular lesions that evolve to ulcers. It can cause more severe disease, including meningitis or encephalitis. Two types exist, HSV-1 and HSV-2. Globally, HSV-2 causes most cases of recurrent genital herpes, although most people infected are asymptomatic. Congenital HSV can cause severe morbidity and mortality in neonates.

Diagnosis

Presumptive diagnosis is generally based on the presence of typical painful lesions. Laboratory testing can be performed in cases where diagnosis is questioned, in which case serologic testing is most common. Virologic testing using polymerase chain reaction (PCR) is the test of choice in cerobrospinal fluid (CSF) when evaluating for central nervous system infection (Centers for Disease Control and Prevention, 2010).

Treatment

HSV is not curable. The goals of treatment are to decrease the severity and duration of symptoms, frequency of recurrences, and transmission risk to partners. Treatment should be provided to individuals with an initial outbreak, as primary HSV-2 can have prolonged and severe symptoms, including neurological involvement. Subsequent episodic or suppressive therapy can be offered based on severity and frequency of outbreaks. The natural history is for recurrences to become less frequent.

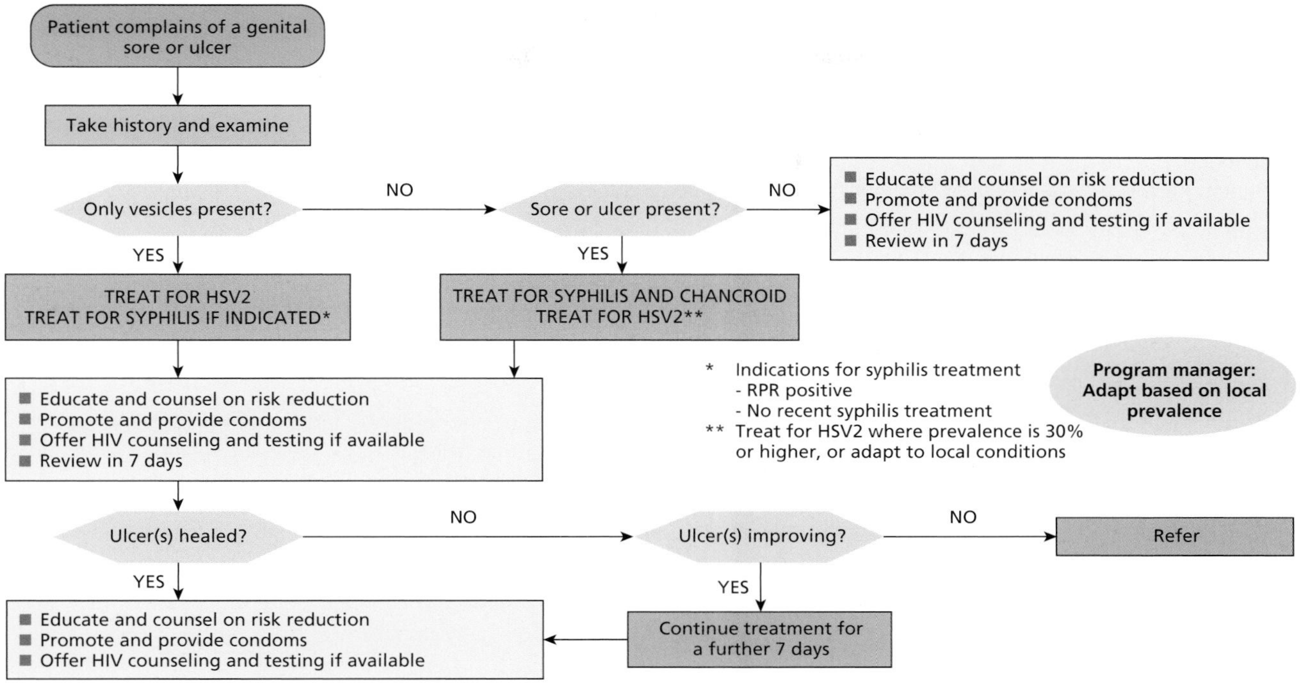

Figure 16.1 Flowchart for genital ulcer disease, male or female. *Source*: WHO (2005), flowchart 3, p. 109. Reproduced with permission of the World Health Organization.

Patients on suppressive therapy should be periodically reassessed for the need to continue. See Figure 16.1 and Table 16.1 for specifics of management.

Syphilis

Although curable, syphilis, caused by *Treponema pallidum*, remains a major cause of GUD worldwide, second to HSV. Prevalence is highest in sub-Saharan Africa (WHO, 2012a). It is a systemic infection, divided into overlapping stages that correspond with clinical symptoms. Primary syphilis is characterized by a painless ulcer or chancre. Symptoms of secondary syphilis include primarily skin rash, mucocutaneous lesions, and lymphadenopathy. Gummatous lesions – soft rubbery granulomas with necrotic centers found in the liver, skin, brain, or other tissue – are characteristic of tertiary syphilis. Neurosyphilis can be manifested as meningitis, altered mental state, stroke, or loss of vibratory sensation. Latent, or asymptomatic, infection is divided into early latent (known acquisition in the last year), late latent (acquisition beyond 1 year earlier), and latent syphilis of unknown duration. Infection during pregnancy can lead to perinatal complications, including high rates of stillbirth and significant morbidity and mortality in the newborn. Congenital syphilis can present with blister-like rashes often on the palms and soles, watery nasal discharge, pneumonia, sharp-edged and anteriorly bowed tibias, bridgeless nose, notched teeth, hearing loss, and blindness.

Diagnosis

Diagnosis of primary syphilitic chancre is made clinically – classically, a non-painful ulcer. Darkfield microscopy to visualize spirochetes in the ulcer tissue requires a well-trained technician. To diagnose later-stage infection, a combination of two types of serologic test is used: non-treponemal tests such as VDRL (Venereal Disease Research Laboratory) and RPR (rapid plasma reagin) and treponemal tests such as fluorescent treponemal antibody absorbed (FTA-ABS) and the *T. pallidum* passive particle agglutination (TP-PA) assay. These two types of tests are used in combination to improve specificity. Non-treponemal titers correlate to disease activity; a fourfold or greater change in titer is considered significant, and titers should decline with treatment. Treponemal tests, on the other hand, do not correlate with disease activity and are not used as a test of response to treatment. In cases where there is concern for neurosyphilis, analysis of CSF is needed. Increased number of nucleated cells and protein in the CSF are suggestive, and a positive non-treponemal test in the CSF is considered diagnostic.

Treatment

Figure 16.1 illustrates syndromic management of GUD. First-line therapy is penicillin administered parenterally (i.v./i.m.) as outlined in Table 16.1. In cases of infection in pregnancy and neurosyphilis, alternative therapy to penicillin should not be

Table 16.1 Treatment recommendations for genital ulcer disease, by infectious etiology.

Etiology	Preferred	Alternative	If pregnant, breastfeeding, or <16 years old
Syndromic treatment principles: if vesicles present, treat for HSV and syphilis (if positive test for syphilis or no recent treatment). For ulcers, treat with single-dose therapy for syphilis *plus* single or multi-dose therapy for chancroid; if HSV common (>30% prevalence), add treatment for HSV. Add treatment for granuloma inguinale or LGV where prevalence is high			
HSV2			
Initial episode	Aciclovir: 400 mg p.o. three times daily for 7–10 days or 200 mg p.o. five times daily for 7–10 days	Famciclovir: 250 mg p.o. three times daily for 7–10 days Valaciclovir: 1 g p.o. twice daily for 7–10 days	Use when risk outweighs benefit. Dosage is same for primary infection
Recurrent episode	Aciclovir: 400 mg p.o. three times daily for 5 days or 800 mg p.o. twice daily for 5 days. For PLWH: 400 mg p.o. three times daily for 5–10 days	Famciclovir: 125 mg p.o. twice daily for 5 days; 1 g p.o. twice daily for 1 day; 500 mg p.o. once, then 250 mg p.o. twice daily for two subsequent days. For PLWH: 500 mg p.o. twice daily for 5–10 days Valaciclovir: 1 g p.o. once daily for 5 days. For PLWH: 1 g p.o. twice daily for 5–10 days	Use when risk outweighs benefit. Dosage is same for primary infection
Suppressive therapy	Aciclovir: 400 mg p.o. twice daily. For PLWH: 400–800 mg p.o. two to three times daily	Famciclovir: 250 mg p.o. twice daily (for PLWH, 500 mg p.o. twice daily) *or* 500 mg or 1 g p.o. once daily (for PLWH, 500 mg p.o. twice daily) Valaciclovir: 500 mg to 1 g p.o. once daily (for PLWH, 500 mg p.o. twice daily)	Use when risk outweighs benefit
Syphilis			
Primary, secondary, or early latent	Benzathine penicillin: 2.4 million units i.m. once	Doxycycline: 100 mg p.o. twice daily for 14 days Tetracycline: 500 mg p.o. four times daily for 14 days	Benzathine penicillin 2.4 million units i.m. once *Alternative should not be used in pregnancy*
Latent >1 year or unknown	Benzathine penicillin: 2.4 million units i.m. once weekly for 3 weeks	Doxycycline: 100 mg twice daily for 28 days Tetracycline: 500 mg p.o. four times daily for 28 days	Benzathine penicillin 2.4 million units i.m. weekly for 3 weeks *Alternative should not be used in pregnancy*
Neurosyphilis	Aqueous crystalline penicillin G: 3–4 million units i.v. every 4 hours for 10–14 days	Procaine penicillin G: 2.4 million units i.m. once daily for 10–14 days *and* Probenecid: 500 mg p.o. four times daily for 10–14 days	Aqueous crystalline penicillin G 3–4 million units i.v. every 4 hours for 10–14 days *Alternative should not be used in pregnancy*
Chancroid			
	Azithromycin: 1 g p.o. once	Ciprofloxacin: 500 mg p.o. twice daily for 3 days	Azithromycin, ceftriaxone, or erythromycin
	Ceftriaxone: 250 mg i.m. once	Erythromycin base: 500 mg p.o. three times daily for 7 days	
Treatment of partners: partners with sexual contact within 10 days prior to symptoms should be evaluated and offered treatment regardless of symptoms			

Table 16.1 Treatment recommendations for genital ulcer disease, by infectious etiology. (*Continued*)

Etiology	Preferred	Alternative	If pregnant, breastfeeding, or <16 years old
Granuloma inguinale (Note: all treatment should be for at least 3 weeks, until all lesions resolved)	Doxycycline: 100 mg p.o. twice daily	Azithromycin: 1 g p.o. once weekly or 1 g p.o. once, then 500 mg p.o. once daily Ciprofloxacin: 750 mg p.o. twice daily Erythromycin: 500 mg p.o. four times daily Trimethoprim/sulfamethoxazole: 1 DS tablet p.o. twice daily	Azithromycin or erythromycin
	Treatment of partners: partners with sexual contact within 60 days prior to symptoms should be evaluated and offered treatment. Unknown if there is benefit to treatment in the absence of symptoms		
Lymphogranuloma venereum	Doxycycline: 100 mg p.o. twice daily for 21 days	Erythromycin base: 500 mg p.o. four times daily for 21 days Tetracycline: 500 mg p.o. four times daily for 14 days	Erythromycin base
	Treatment of partners: partners with sexual contact within 60 days prior to symptoms should be evaluated, tested (if available), and treated for chlamydia (azithromycin 1 g p.o. once, or doxycycline 100 mg p.o. twice daily for 7 days)		

PLWH, people living with HIV/AIDS.

used even in patients with penicillin allergies; instead, penicillin desensitization should be carried out.

Chancroid

Chancroid is caused by *Haemophilus ducreyi*. The classic clinical presentation is of painful, deep, necrotizing genital ulcer(s) with tender inguinal lymphadenopathy (buboes), which can drain spontaneously if left untreated. Rates of chancroid are declining globally, although it is still prevalent in eastern and southern Africa and parts of Asia and should be included in syndromic treatment in those areas (Steen, 2001).

Diagnosis

Diagnosis is largely clinical; culturing *H. ducreyi* requires special media that are not widely available, and the sensitivity is below 80%. Established CDC criteria used for surveillance are shown in Box 16.1. These criteria must be used with caution clinically, as co-infection with *T. pallidum* and HSV does occur (Centers for Disease Control and Prevention, 2010).

Treatment

The preferred regimens are single-dose treatments. Resistance to ciprofloxacin and erythromycin has been reported but is not

---

Box 16.1 CDC surveillance criteria for chancroid

- Painful genital ulcer.
- Negative syphilis testing (darkfield microscopy, or serological tests after 7 days of ulcers).
- Clinical presentation typical for chancroid.
- Negative HSV testing.

---

known to be widespread (Ison *et al.*, 1998; Lewis, 2003). Follow-up examination within a week of treatment is important. Lack of clinical improvement suggests inaccurate diagnosis, co-infection with another STI, insufficient treatment due to HIV (may require longer treatment), or antibiotic resistance (Centers for Disease Control and Prevention, 2010). See Figures 16.1 and 16.2 and Table 16.1 for syndromic management and treatment recommendations.

Granuloma inguinale (donovanosis)

Granuloma inguinale is caused by *Klebsiella granulomatis*. Granuloma inguinale is rare in developed countries but endemic in some tropical areas, including parts of India, the

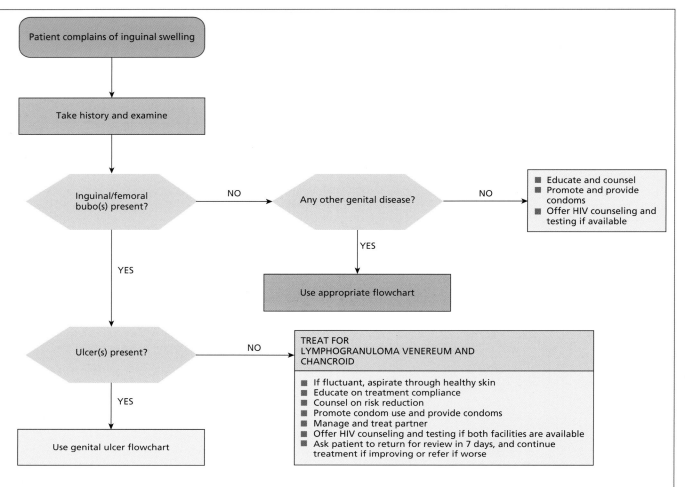

Figure 16.2 Flowsheet for inguinal bubo, male or female. *Source*: WHO (2005), flowchart 4, p. 114. Reproduced with permission of the World Health Organization.

Caribbean, and southern Africa (O'Farrell, 2002). Typical presentation is a painless, slowly progressive, ulcerative lesion on the genitals or perineum that bleeds easily. Pseudo-buboes (subcutaneous granulomas) can occur. Extragenital infection can occur with direct extension of infection to the pelvis or by dissemination to intra-abdominal organs, bones, or the mouth.

Diagnosis

Diagnosis is largely clinical. Culture of this fastidious organism is difficult and not a sensitive test. Definitive diagnosis requires visualization of Donovan bodies (purple rod-shaped 0.5- to 1-μm organisms within monocytes on Geimsa stain) on biopsy or crush preparation.

Treatment

Treatment is curative, although it takes time, often weeks to months (Table 16.1).

Lymphogranuloma venereum

LGV is a less common cause of anogenital ulcers, caused by *Chlamydia trachomatis* serotypes L1, L2, or L3. The most common manifestation is a self-limited ulcer or papule at the site of inoculation, followed by tender, unilateral, inguinal and/or femoral lymphadenopathy. Proctocolitis can occur after rectal exposure and, without treatment, can lead to colorectal fistulas and strictures (Centers for Disease Control and Prevention, 2010).

Diagnosis

Diagnosis is based on having appropriate clinical findings without an alternate diagnosis in a region with known LGV. *Chlamydia trachomatis* testing should be conducted, if available. This can be done by culture, direct immunofluorescence, or nucleic acid amplification tests (NAAT), the latter being the most sensitive and specific but not widely available in resource-limited settings.

Treatment

See Figures 16.1 and 16.2 for syndromic management and Table 16.1 for treatment recommendations.

Infections causing vaginal discharge

Vaginitis is extremely common and can be due to both infectious and non-infectious causes. Infectious vaginitis can be associated with pruritus, vaginal soreness, dyspareunia (painful sexual intercourse), and dysuria (painful urination). When available, laboratory testing should be done in conjunction with careful history and examination to determine the specific etiology of vaginal complaints.

Bacterial vaginosis

Bacterial vaginosis (BV) is a polymicrobial clinical syndrome resulting from a change in the vaginal flora, with replacement of *Lactobacillus* species with other organisms, particularly anaerobic Gram-negative rods. *Gardnerella vaginalis* is commonly detected and implicated, although the mechanism by which BV occurs is not clear. Multiple sexual partners and lack of condom use are risk factors, although BV also occurs in women who have never had sex. BV is the most common cause of vaginitis in women presenting to care, although most cases of BV are asymptomatic. Infection with BV is associated with increased acquisition of other STIs, including HIV.

Diagnosis

Clinically, BV is usually diagnosed by Amsel's criteria (Box 16.2). The gold standard diagnosis is a Gram stain of vaginal fluid and assigning a Nugent score based on quantification of *Lactobacillus*, *Gardnerella/Bacteroides*, and curved Gram-variable rods. This method requires trained personnel and time, and is thus not commonly used clinically. Strict use of Amsel's criteria is considered to be over 90% sensitive with a specificity of 77% (Landers *et al.*, 2004). Newer testing methods now exist, including DNA hybridization and chromogenic enzyme detection, although they may not be available in resource-limited areas.

Box 16.2 Amsel's criteria

At least three of the four criteria should be present for a confirmed diagnosis:

1. Thin, white, yellow, homogeneous discharge.
2. Clue cells on microscopy (epithelial cells with adherent bacteria).
3. pH of vaginal fluid >4.5.
4. Fishy odor with 10% potassium hydroxide (KOH) solution ("whiff test").

Treatment

Treatment is recommended for women with symptoms and pregnant women (Figure 16.3 and Table 16.2).

Trichomonas vaginalis

Trichomoniasis is caused by the protozoan *T. vaginalis*. It is the most prevalent non-viral STI globally, the vast majority of cases occurring in resource-limited settings (Johnston & Mabey, 2008). Infection is often asymptomatic (Sutton *et al.*, 2007; Johnston & Mabey, 2008). When symptomatic in men, it can present with urethritis. In women, it presents with yellow-green, frothy, foul-smelling vaginal discharge and vulvar irritation. Because of its high prevalence, testing is recommend for all women seeking care for vaginal discharge, and screening should be considered in those at high risk for infection.

Diagnosis

Microscopy of a wet preparation slide of vaginal secretions is typically used for the diagnosis of vaginal trichomoniasis, determined by visualization of motile trichomonads. However, this method has a sensitivity of only approximately 70%, and even less so for infections in men (Nye *et al.*, 2009; Centers for Disease Control and Prevention, 2010). Culture is sensitive and highly specific, but rarely available. Several newer tests include immunochromatographic capillary flow dipstick technology, nucleic acid hybridization testing, and NAATs. Reported sensitivities and specificities for these tests vary, but are generally in excess of 80% and 90% respectively, and even higher (>88% and >98%) for NAAT-based testing (Nye *et al.*, 2009; Centers for Disease Control and Prevention, 2010).

Treatment

Syndromic management of vaginal discharge includes treatment for trichomoniasis (Figure 16.3). Treatment options are listed in Table 16.2. Topically applied antimicrobials are considerably less efficacious (<50%) and not recommended (Centers for Disease Control and Prevention, 2010).

Candida

Vulvovaginal candidiasis is usually caused by *Candida albicans*. An estimated 75% of women will have at least one episode in their lifetime. Classically, thick white "curdy" vaginal discharge and vulvar erythema, edema, and pruritus are present. The majority of cases will be uncomplicated, but 10–20% of women will have complicated infections, including recurrent infections (more than four per year), severe infections (fissure formation, extensive vulvar erythema, excoriations), or non-albicans *Candida*. Candidal infection can occur concomitantly with STIs.

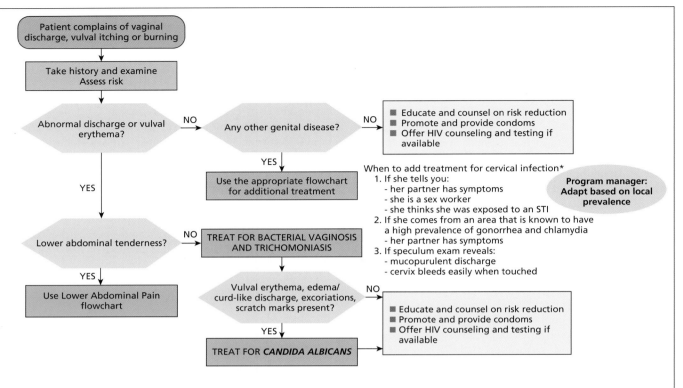

Figure 16.3 Flowsheet for vaginal discharge. *Source*: WHO (2005), flowchart 1, p. 101. Reproduced with permission of the World Health Organization.

Diagnosis

Diagnosis of candidal vaginitis is based on symptoms of vaginitis, hallmark thick discharge and pruritus, and detection of yeast or hyphae/pseudohyphae in vaginal secretions. Yeast can be detected either by wet preparation or Gram stain. Culture is less frequently used, but if available should be considered in severe cases, particularly if there is a concern for non-albicans yeast. Nucleic acid hybridization testing may be available in some locations but is not widely available in resource-limited settings.

Treatment

Empiric treatment should be considered for symptomatic women with any sign of yeast infection by examination. Both topical and systemic antifungals can be used to treat vulvovaginal *Candida* infection, depending on severity of infection (Figure 16.3 and Table 16.2).

Infections causing urethritis or cervicitis and pelvic inflammatory disease

Symptoms of urethritis include purulent discharge, dysuria, or pruritis. Asymptomatic infections are common. Cervicitis is characterized by the presence of purulent endocervical exudate and/or endocervical bleeding on examination. Symptoms are commonly absent but can include abnormal vaginal discharge and intermenstrual vaginal bleeding. Infectious causes are most notoriously *N. gonorrhoeae* and *C. trachomatis*. *Mycoplasma genitalium* has also been associated with urethritis. HSV and *T. vaginalis* are associated with cervicitis as well. Complications of urethritis and cervicitis include pelvic inflammatory disease (PID), which can lead to scarring in the female upper genital tract, pregnancy complications, and infertility. Different testing methods can help distinguish causative organisms. In the absence of diagnostics, empiric treatment should cover gonorrhea and chlamydia (Tables 16.3 and 16.4 and Figures 16.4 and 16.5).

Gonorrhea

Gonorrhea is the second most commonly reported bacterial STI globally (Sutton *et al.*, 2007). Regional prevalence varies widely. Infection with *N. gonorrhoeae* can be localized or systemic. The majority of cases are uncomplicated urethritis or cervicitis. Pharyngitis and proctitis occur. Acute male urethral infections typically cause sufficiently significant symptoms to lead men to seek treatment. Women may be asymptomatic or have minimal symptoms until complications (e.g., PID) have

Table 16.2 Treatment recommendations for vaginal discharge, by infectious etiology.

Etiology	Preferred	Alternative	If pregnant or breastfeeding
Syndromic treatment principles: Treat for bacterial vaginosis and *Trichomonas vaginalis*; if specific symptoms (Box 16.1), add treatment for *Candida albicans*; if specific risk factors or signs (Box 16.1), add treatment for cervicitis, treating both *N. gonorrhoeae* and *C. trachomatis* (Table 16.3)			
Bacterial vaginosis	Metronidazole: 2 g p.o. once, 500 mg p.o. four times daily for 7 days, *or* 0.75% gel (5 g applicator intravaginally once daily for 5 days)	Tinidazole: 2 g p.o. once daily for 2 days; 1 g p.o. once daily for 5 days Clindamycin: 300 mg p.o. three times daily for 7 days *or* 2% cream (5 g applicator intravaginally once daily for 7 days) *or* 100 mg ovule (one intravaginally once daily for 3 days)	*Preferably after first trimester* Metronidazole 200–300 mg p.o. three times daily for 7 days *or* 0.75% gel (5 g applicator intravaginally once daily for 5 days) *or* clindamycin 300 mg p.o. three times daily for 7 days
Trichomonas vaginalis	Metronidazole: 2 g p.o. once	Tinidazole: 2 g p.o. once *or* 500 mg twice daily for 5 days Metronidazole: 500 mg p.o. four times daily for 7 days	*Preferably after first trimester* Metronidazole 200–300 mg p.o. three times daily for 7 days *or* 0.75% gel (5 g applicator intravaginally once daily for 5 days) *or* clindamycin 300 mg p.o. three times daily for 7 days

Candida albicans	Fluconazole: 150 mg p.o. once
	Miconazole vaginal suppository (one of the following):
	  Vaginal suppository 100 mg once daily for 7 days
	  Vaginal suppository 200 mg once daily 3 days
	  Vaginal suppository 1.2 g once
	  Vaginal cream 2% (5 g for 7 days)
	  Vaginal cream 4% (5 g for 3 days)
	
	Clotrimazole (one of the following):
	  Vaginal tablet 100 mg twice daily for 3 days
	  Vaginal cream 1% (5 g for 7–14 days)
	  Vaginal cream 2% (5 g for 3 days)
		Nystatin: 100,000-unit vaginal tablet once daily for 14 days
		Terconazole (one of the following):
		  Vaginal cream 0.4% (5 g for 7 days
		  Vaginal cream 0.8% (5 g for 3 days)
		  Vaginal suppository 80 mg once daily for 3 days
		Tioconazole: 6.5% ointment (5 g once)
		Butoconazole cream: vaginal cream 5 g for 3 days
			Miconazole 200 mg vaginal suppository, once daily for 3 days *or* clotrimazole 100 mg vaginal tablet twice daily for 3 days *or* nystatin 100,000 unit vaginal tablet once daily for 14 days

occurred. Infection during pregnancy can be transmitted to the neonate and cause blindness. Disseminated gonorrhea occurs in 0.5–3% of infections. Clinical manifestations include petechial or pustular skin lesions, asymmetrical arthralgia, tenosynovitis, or septic arthritis. Rarely does it cause endocarditis or meningitis (Centers for Disease Control and Prevention, 2010).

Diagnosis

A Gram stain demonstrating polymorphonuclear leukocytes with intracellular Gram-negative diplococci is highly specific (>99%) and sensitive (>95%) in symptomatic males. However, a negative Gram stain cannot rule out infection in asymptomatic cases nor is it adequate testing in specimens

from other sites. Other detection methods include culture, nucleic acid hybridization tests, and NAATs. NAATs can be performed on the widest variety of specimen types (most commonly endocervical and urine) when appropriate laboratory validation tests have been done (Centers for Disease Control and Prevention, 2010). The sensitivity of NAATs is superior to culture. When no diagnostics are available, clinical diagnosis is made when symptoms of urethritis or cervicitis are present.

Treatment

See Table 16.3 for recommended treatment. Currently, cephalosporins remain first choice, although resistance is a concern. Resistance to fluoroquinolones and macrolides is well established. Treatment failure with oral cefixime has occurred in

Table 16.3 Treatment for cervicitis and urethritis.

Etiology	Preferred	Alternative	If pregnant, breastfeeding, or <16 years old
Syndromic treatment principles: if vaginal discharge and if specific risk factors or signs (Box 16.1) add treatment for cervicitis, treating both *N. gonorrhoeae* and *C. trachomatis*. If male urethral discharge, treat for *N. gonorrhoeae* and *C. trachomatis*. One-time dose regimens are usually best for adherence			
Neisseria gonorrhoeae			
Uncomplicated urethritis, cervicitis	Ceftriaxone 250 mg i.m. once *and* Azithromycin 1 g p.o. once *or* Doxycycline 100 mg p.o. twice daily for 7 days	Cefixime 400 mg p.o. once (only if ceftriaxone not available) *and* Azithromycin 1 g p.o. once *or* Doxycycline 100 mg p.o. twice daily for 7 days	Ceftriaxone 250 mg i.m. once (125 mg if <45 kg) *and* azithromycin 1 g p.o. once
Pharyngitis	Ceftriaxone 250 mg i.m. once *and* Azithromycin 1 g p.o. once *or* Doxycycline 100 mg p.o. twice daily for 7 days		Ceftriaxone 250 mg i.m. once (125 mg if <45 kg) *and* azithromycin 1 g p.o. once
Disseminated gonorrhea	Ceftriaxone 1–2 g i.v. every 24 hours (length depends on extent of infection). Consultation with infectious disease expert recommended		Ceftriaxone
Conjunctivitis (adult)	Ceftriaxone 1 g i.m. once, eye irrigation with saline		Ceftriaxone
Treatment of partners	Partners with sexual contact within 60 days prior to symptoms should be evaluated, tested (if available), and treated for gonorrhea and chlamydia		
Chlamydia trachomatis			
	Azithromycin 1 g p.o. once *or* Doxycycline 100 mg p.o. twice daily for 7 days	Erythromycin base 500 mg, erythromycin ethylsuccinate 800 mg p.o. four times daily for 7 days Levofloxacin 500 mg once daily for 7 days Ofloxacin 300 mg twice daily for 7 days Tetracycline 500 mg p.o. four times daily for 7 days	Azithromycin 1 g p.o. once *or* amoxicillin 500 mg p.o. three times daily for 7 days *or* erythromycin base 500 mg p.o. four times daily for 7 days
Treatment of partners	Partners with sexual contact within 60 days prior to symptoms should be evaluated, tested (if available), and treated for chlamydia		
Non-gonococcal urethritis			
	Azithromycin 1 g p.o. once *or* Doxycycline 100 mg p.o. twice daily for 7 days	Erythromycin base 500 mg, erythromycin ethylsuccinate 800 mg p.o. four times daily for 7 days Levofloxacin 500 mg once daily for 7 days Ofloxacin 300 mg twice daily for 7 days	
Recurrent	Metronidazole 2 g p.o. once *or* Tinidazole 2 g p.o. once		
Treatment of partners	Partners with sexual contact within 60 days prior to symptoms should be evaluated, tested (if available), and treated with a regimen effective against chlamydia		

Table 16.4 Treatment regimen for PID.

Etiology	Ambulatory treatment	Inpatient treatment #1	Inpatient treatment #2
Syndromic treatment principles: empiric treatment for *N. gonorrhoeae*, *C. trachomatis*, and anaerobic organisms. All regimens should complete 14 days, but can transition to p.o./i.m regimen			
N. gonorrhoeae (ambulatory)	Ceftriaxone 250 mg i.m./i.v. daily *or* Cefoxitin 2 g i.m. once *and* Probenecid 1 g p.o.	Cefoxitin 2 g i.v. every 6 hours *or* Cefotetan 2 g i.v. every 12 hours	Clindamycin 900 mg i.v. every 8 hours
C. trachomatis	Doxycycline 100 mg p.o./i.v. twice daily *or* Tetracycline 500 mg orally four times a day	Doxycycline 100 mg p.o./i.v. every 12 hours	Gentamicin: load with 2 mg/kg once, then 1.5 mg/kg every 8 hours (or 3–5 mg/kg once daily)
Anaerobes	Metronidazole 400–500 mg p.o./i.v. twice daily *or* Chloramphenicol 500 mg p.o./i.v. four times daily	Covered by cefoxitin/cefotetan	

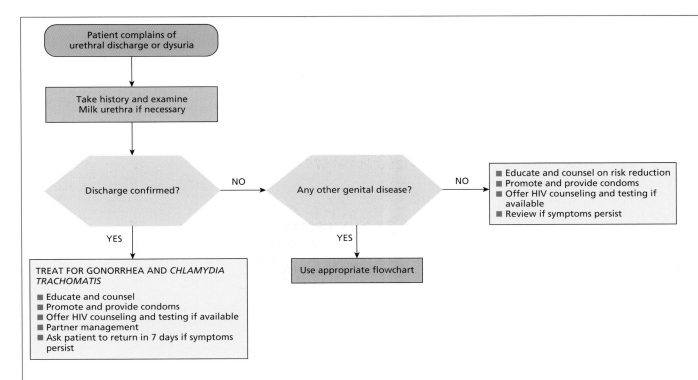

Figure 16.4 Flowsheet for urethritis in males. *Source*: WHO (2005), flowchart 5, p. 116. Reproduced with permission of the World Health Organization.

Japan, Norway, and the UK (WHO, 2012b). Resistance to parenteral ceftriaxone has been reported as well (Ohnishi *et al.*, 2011). The WHO has additional guidelines for cases with suspected resistance (WHO, 2012b).

Chlamydia

Chlamydial genital infection is one of the most common STIs (WHO, 2012a). Prevalence is highest in persons aged 25 years or older. Asymptomatic infection is common. *Chlamydia* can cause urethritis, cervicitis, or rectal and oropharyngeal infec-

tion. Women are particularly at risk from sequelae of *C. trachomatis*, including PID, ectopic pregnancy, and infertility. Subclinical upper-reproductive-tract infection can be present with uncomplicated cervical infection. Infection during pregnancy can lead to neonatal infection, causing conjunctivitis and pneumonia.

Diagnosis

In the absence of diagnostics, infection is assumed with symptoms of urethritis or cervicitis. Cell culture, direct

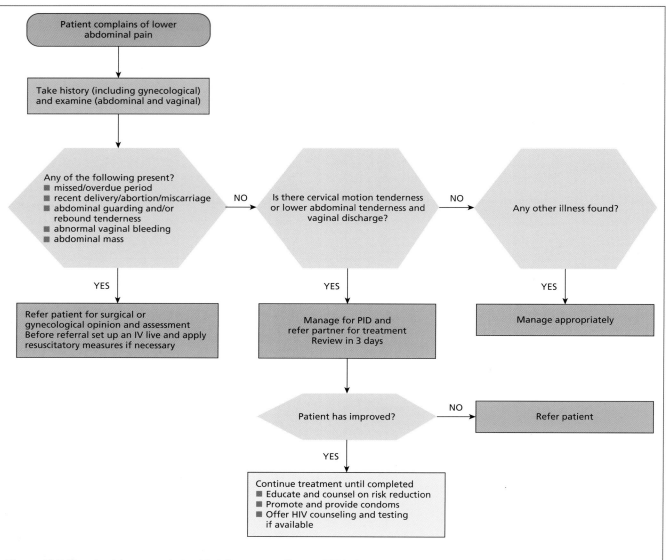

Figure 16.5 Flowsheet for suspected pelvic inflammatory disease (PID). *Source*: WHO (2005), flowchart 2, p. 105. Reproduced with permission of the World Health Organization.

immunofluorescence, enzyme immunoassay, nucleic acid hybridization tests, and NAATs are all methods used to detect *C. trachomatis* on endocervical specimens and male urethral swabs, with NAATs performing the best. Vaginal, rectal, and oropharyngeal swabs can be used with NAAT testing, depending on the commercial test used and/or when laboratory validation tests have been performed (Centers for Disease Control and Prevention, 2010).

Treatment

Macrolides are the preferred treatment (Table 16.3).

Non-chlamydial non-gonoccocal urethritis

In most cases of non-chlamydial, non-gonococcal urethritis (NGU), no organism is found. *Mycoplasma genitalium* is thought to account for 15–25% of NGU in the United States. *Trichomonas vaginalis* and HSV can also cause urethritis (Centers for Disease Control and Prevention, 2010).

Diagnosis

Confirmation of urethritis is by evaluating for non-specific findings such as pyuria and more than five cells per high-power field on urethral discharge. Gram stain can be helpful if the symptoms are not clear or in cases of failed empiric treatment (Centers for Disease Control and Prevention, 2010). Testing for *N. gonorrhoeae*, *C. trachomatis*, *T. vaginalis*, and HSV should be performed, if available, to rule out other causes.

Treatment

Treatment should be based on testing when available (Table 16.3).

Pelvic inflammatory disease

PID is inflammation in the female upper genital tract, including endometritis, salpingitis, tubo-ovarian abscess, and pelvic peritonitis. *Neisseria gonorrhoeae* and *C. trachomatis* are most often implicated, but infection is often polymicrobial. PID can be a sequela of untreated cervical infection and can result in scarring and infertility.

Diagnosis

Clinical diagnosis is based on lower abdominal pain with cervical motion, uterine, or adnexal tenderness (Figure 16.5). This diagnosis is imprecise, with the positive predictive value depending heavily on the epidemiologic characteristics of the population (i.e., increased risk for exposure to STIs). Additional supportive data include fever, many leukocytes on wet mount preparation, and increased acute-phase reactants such as C-reactive protein and white blood cell count (Centers for Disease Control and Prevention, 2010). Where available, testing for *N. gonorrhoeae* and *C. trachomatis* should be done.

Treatment

Treatment should be started as soon as presumed diagnosis is made. Treatment must include coverage for *N. gonorrhoeae*, *C. trachomatis*, and anaerobic organisms. Recommended regimens are shown in Table 16.4. Sexual partners should be referred for testing and/or treatment for *N. gonorrhoeae* and *C. trachomatis*.

Human papillomavirus infection

There are more than 100 types of human papillomavirus (HPV), over 40 of which can infect the genital area. Most HPV infections go unrecognized as either subclinical or asymptomatic infections and self-resolve. Low-risk HPV types, such as 6 and 11, cause genital warts. Genital warts are generally asymptomatic but can be painful or pruritic. High-risk oncogenic types, most notably 16 and 18, are associated with cervical cancer (70% due to 16 and 18) and other anogenital cancers (WHO, 2007b). Symptoms occur only late in the disease course, and therefore screening for cervical lesions is encouraged where possible.

Diagnosis

Genital warts are diagnosed clinically by visual inspection but can be confirmed by pathology if the diagnosis is uncertain, particularly if they appear unusual or show lack of response to therapy.

Cervical cancer screening programs utilize Pap tests and colposcopy or VIA (visual inspection with acetic acid with or without Lugol's iodine) for the detection of precancerous/cancerous lesions. HPV tests that detect viral nucleic acid or capsid protein can be used in conjunction with Pap tests and are recommended when available for women aged over 30 years undergoing cervical cancer screening and in women over 21 years with abnormal Pap test results (Centers for Disease Control and Prevention, 2010).

Treatment

Subclinical HPV infection typically resolves spontaneously, so no treatment is necessary. Treatment for genital warts depends on provider and patient preference. Some lesions will spontaneously resolve, so time itself is one option. Patient- and provider-administered treatment options are listed in Table 16.5. No one treatment is superior, and therefore choice of regimen used should be based on availability, patient preference, and provider experience. Genital warts typically respond to therapy in a time frame of 3 months.

For cervical lesions, treatment depends on the results of cytopathology with appropriate follow-up and rescreening, colposcopy, or other intervention (see Additional resources section). Two HPV vaccines exist and are becoming increasingly available globally.

Table 16.5 Treatment for genital warts.
Patient-applied
Podofilox 0.5%: apply to warts twice daily for 3 days, rest 4 days then repeat. Up to four treatments
Imiquimod 5% cream: apply at bedtime for 6–10 hours, then wash off. Can be applied three times in a week for a maximum of 1 week
Sinecatechins 15% ointment: apply three times daily, 16 weeks maximum
Provider-applied
Cryotherapy
Podophyllin resin 10–25%: apply small amount, dry, wash off in 1–4 hours. Weekly application
Trichloroacetic acid 80–90%: apply small amount, dry. Weekly application
Surgical removal

Prevention

The mainstay of prevention of STIs is limiting exposure. Education about abstinence, limiting the number of sexual partners, and utilization of condoms are the most widely employed measures in campaigns targeting reduction of STIs. Although effective, implementation of these public health measures can be challenging. In many circumstances, at-risk populations often do not have the power to refuse sex or control whom they have as partners, and use of condoms may not be considered acceptable for various reasons, including suggesting that the user has HIV.

Contraception methods other than condoms should not be considered to have significant activity against STIs. Male circumcision has been demonstrated to reduce rates of STIs, and particular attention has been given to this in light of an association with reduced HIV rates (Weiss et al., 2006; Mehta et al., 2012).

Vaccine-preventable STIs

Currently, vaccine-preventable STIs include hepatitis A, hepatitis B, and HPV. Two types of HPV vaccine exist, covering types 6, 11, 16, and 18 or only types 16 and 18. These vaccines are becoming more widely available globally through active campaigns to decrease cost and aid in broader distribution in resource-limited settings.

Post-exposure prophylaxis for STIs

In cases of known exposure with an infected sexual partner or unknown exposure in the context of sexual assault, post-exposure prophylaxis (or preemptive treatment) should be offered for gonorrhea, chlamydia, and trichomoniasis. HIV post-exposure prophylaxis is discussed in Chapter 18.

Additional resources

- CDC website: http://www.cdc.gov/STD/
- WHO website: http://www.who.int/topics/sexually _transmitted_infections/en/index.html
- WHO STI-specific publications: http://www.who.int/ reproductivehealth/publications/en/
- WHO cervical cancer specific publications: http://www .who.int/maternal_child_adolescent/documents/cervical _cancer_prevention/en/

REFERENCES

Burstein GR (2011) Sexually transmitted infections. In: Kliegman RM, Stanton BMD, St Geme J, Schor NF, Behrman RE (eds) Nelson Textbook of Pediatrics, 19th edn. Philadelphia: Elsevier, pp. 705–13.

Centers for Disease Control and Prevention (2010) Sexually transmitted diseases treatment guidelines, 2010. MMWR Morb Mortal Wkly Rep 59(RR-12):1–110.

Ison CA, Dillon J-AR, Tapsall JW (1998) The epidemiology and global antibiotic resistance of Neisseria gonorrhoeae and Haemophilus ducreyi. Lancet 351(Suppl. III):8–11.

Johnston VJ, Mabey DC (2008) Global epidemiology and control of Trichomonas vaginalis. Curr Opin Infect Dis 21:56–64.

Landers DV, Wiesenfeld HC, Heine RP, Krohn MA,Hillier SL (2004) Predictive value of the clinical diagnosis of lower genital tract infection in women. Am J Obstet Gynecol 190:1004–10.

Lewis DA (2003) Chancroid: clinical manifestations, diagnosis and management. Sex Transm Infect 79:68–71.

Looker KJ, Garnett GP, Schmid GP (2008) An estimate of the global prevalence and incidence of herpes simplex virus type 2 infection. Bull WHO 86:805–12.

Mehta SD, Moses S, Parker CB, Agot K, MacClean I, Bailey RC (2012) Circumcision status and incident herpes simplex virus type 2 infection, genital ulcer disease, and HIV infection. AIDS 26:1141–9.

Nye MB, Schwebke JR, Body BA (2009) Comparison of APTIMA Trichomonas vaginalis transcription-mediated amplification to wet mount microscopy, culture, and polymerase chain reaction for diagnosis of trichomoniasis in men and women. Am J Obstet Gynecol 200:188e1–7.

O'Farrell N (2002) Donovanosis. Sex Transm Infect 78:452–7.

Ohnishi M, Golparian D, Shimuta K et al. (2011) Is Neisseria gonorrhoeae initiating a future era of untreatable gonorrhea? Detailed characterization of the first strain with high-level resistance to ceftriaxone. Antimicrob Agents Chemother 55:3538–45.

Steen R (2001) Eradicating chancroid. Bull WHO 79:818–26.

Sutton M, Sternberg M, Koumans EH, McQuillan G, Berman S, Markowitz I (2007) The prevalence of Trichomonas vaginalis infection among reproductive-age women in the United States, 2001–2004. Clin Infect Dis 45:1319–26.

Weiss HA, Thomas SL, Munabi SK, Hayes RJ (2006) Male circumcision and risk of syphilis, chancroid, and genital herpes: a systematic review and meta-analysis. Sex Transm Infect 82:101–9.

WHO (2005) Integrating STI/RTI Care for Reproductive Health. Sexually Transmitted and Other Reproductive Tract Infections: A Guide to Essential Practice. Geneva: World Health Organization.

WHO (2007a) *Global Strategy for the Prevention and Control of Sexually Transmitted Infections, 2006–2015: Breaking the Chain of Transmission.* Geneva: World Health Organization.

WHO (2007b) Cervical Cancer, Human Papillomavirus (HPV), and HPV Vaccines: Key Points for Policy-Makers and Health Professionals. Geneva: World Health Organization.

WHO (2012a) *Global Incidence and Prevalence of Selected Curable Sexually Transmitted Infections, 2008.* Geneva: World Health Organization.

WHO (2012b) Global Action Plan to Control the Spread and Impact of Antimicrobial Resistance in Neisseria Gonorrhoeae. Geneva: World Health Organization.

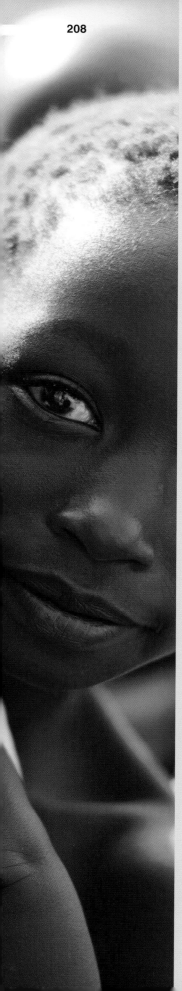

CHAPTER 17
Maternal Health

Melody Eckardt[1,2], Roy Ahn[1,3], and Marisa Nádas[4]
[1]Massachusetts General Hospital, Boston, MA, USA
[2]Boston University School of Medicine, Boston, MA, USA
[3]Harvard Medical School, Boston, MA, USA
[4]Albert Einstein College of Medicine, Bronx, NY, USA

Key learning objectives

- Know the main components of antenatal care.
- Understand the normal progression of labor and delivery.
- Identify the critical opportunities for family planning in the pregnancy and postpartum period.
- Understand the management of the most common complications of labor and delivery.

Abstract

Approximately 800 women die from preventable causes related to pregnancy and childbirth every day, and 99% of these deaths occur in developing countries. The leading causes of maternal mortality worldwide are hemorrhage, hypertensive diseases, sepsis, and unsafe abortion. Cost-effective interventions exist for each of these conditions. However, a leading challenge facing developing countries is lack of access to proper maternal healthcare. This chapter provides an overview of evidence-based solutions for the prevention and management of maternal mortality and morbidity. These interventions include quality antenatal care, labor monitoring and management, emergency obstetric care, postpartum care, and family planning and contraception.

Key words: maternal health, maternal mortality, antenatal care, labor management, birth attendant, family planning, postpartum hemorrhage, puerperal sepsis, preeclampsia

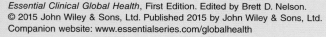

Introduction

According to the World Health Organization (WHO), approximately 800 women die from preventable causes related to pregnancy and childbirth every day, and 99% of these deaths occur in developing countries (Figure 17.1) (WHO, 2012a). More than half of maternal deaths are due to just two causes: hemorrhage and hypertensive diseases in pregnancy. When sepsis and unsafe abortion are added, more than three-quarters of maternal deaths are accounted for. Cost-effective interventions exist for each of these conditions. By ensuring access to effective treatment of these diseases for women in the developing world, more than 200,000 lives could be saved each year (WHO *et al.*, 2012).

One of the main health challenges facing developing countries is the lack of access to proper maternal healthcare. Two-thirds of women in low- and lower-middle-income countries attend only one prenatal care visit. Only one-third of women in low-income countries and only half of women in lower-middle-income countries will receive at least four prenatal care visits (WHO, 2013). Furthermore, only 47% of births in low-income countries and 60% of births in lower-middle-income countries are attended by skilled birth attendants. Finally, access to emergency cesarean section, which can be life-saving to mothers and newborns, is also severely limited in the developing world.

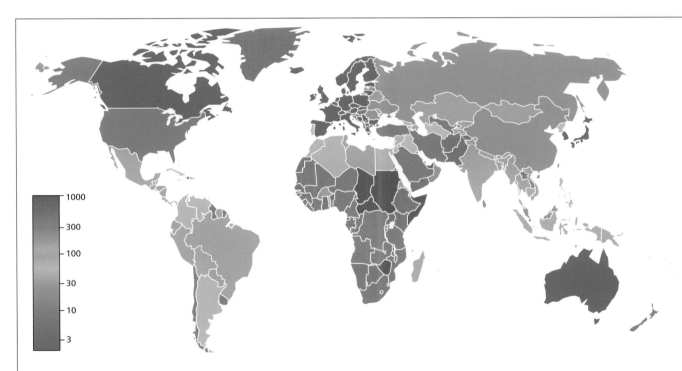

Figure 17.1 Maternal mortality ratio worldwide, 2010. The maternal mortality ratio is the annual number of female deaths per 100,000 live births from any cause related to or aggravated by pregnancy or its management (excluding accidental or incidental causes). The MMR includes deaths during pregnancy, childbirth, or within 42 days of termination of pregnancy, irrespective of the duration and site of the pregnancy, for a specified year. *Source*: Wikimedia © Mikael Häggström. Reproduced under the Creative Commons license.

Antenatal care

Antenatal care serves many purposes in promoting the health of the pregnant woman and her newborn during pregnancy, birth, and after birth (Box 17.1). The frequency of antenatal care visits during pregnancy varies significantly. In many high-income countries, for instance, antenatal care starts early in the first trimester, and pregnant women have monthly visits until 28 weeks of pregnancy, then biweekly visits until 36 weeks of pregnancy when visits become weekly. This generally results in an average of about 13 antenatal care visits during a 9-month pregnancy. Box 17.2 summarizes how the length of a pregnancy is measured.

In the developing world, however, the WHO considers four antenatal visits to be complete antenatal care. These visits usually occur during the fourth, sixth, eighth, and ninth

---

Box 17.1 Antenatal care

- Promote good health habits in pregnancy and after birth including diet, breastfeeding, and infant care.
- Check for viability and appropriate growth of the fetus.
- Identify high-risk pregnancies to allow for additional surveillance and birth planning.
- Provide medications and vaccines to promote maximum health for the mother and infant.
- Educate regarding warning signs and emergency planning during pregnancy and birth.

---

months of pregnancy. In practice, women often begin their visits after quickening (maternal sensation of fetal movement) around 20 weeks. Only 50% of women in resource-limited settings attend all four prenatal visits, and one-quarter of women in these regions receive no antenatal care at all. Table 17.1 shows the recommended tasks at each of the four WHO antenatal visits.

At each antenatal visit, a basic assessment is performed that includes the following.

- Maternal weight check
  - To assess maternal nutrition and appropriate growth
  - A rapid increase in weight gain may be due to fluid retention and edema and therefore may be a sign of preeclampsia.
- Fundal height: measured in centimeters from the upper rim of the public symphysis. This should be equal to the number of weeks of pregnancy beginning at 20 weeks.
- Fetal heart rate measurement: normal range is 110–160 beats per minute (bpm).
- Assessment of fetal position (e.g., vertex or breech presentation): clinically significant after 36 weeks and as labor nears.

Signs and symptoms are also reviewed at each visit. The pregnant woman is asked several questions regarding the presence of any vaginal bleeding, leaking of amniotic fluid, uterine contractions, and whether she feels the baby moving. It is important to inquire about fever and dysuria, as urinary tract infections (UTIs) can lead to preterm delivery and serious pyelonephritis if not treated. However, UTIs during pregnancy can also be asymptomatic. Additionally, persistent headache, visual changes, and non-dependent swelling may be evidence of preeclampsia.

Antenatal care visits can help anticipate pregnancy-related health conditions. For instance, preeclampsia is a potentially life-threatening condition of pregnancy. Early signs may include elevated blood pressure, swelling, and proteinuria. Each visit also includes assessment of blood pressure, physi-

cal assessment for swelling and, if testing is available, assessment of urine for protein. Use of portable ultrasound during visits can also provide much information about the baby (Box 17.3).

Vitamin supplementation is recommended for all pregnant women and should include a daily minimum of 400 μg folic acid for the prevention of neural tube defects and 60 mg or more of elemental iron for the prevention of iron-deficiency anemia. Supplementation should ideally start prior to conception and be continued while breastfeeding.

Laboratory testing, where available, is an important part of antepartum care. This includes testing for syphilis and HIV, and hemoglobin testing for anemia. Both syphilis and HIV must be treated to avoid maternal-to-child transmission. In cases of severe anemia, iron supplementation should be increased. Antenatal blood typing, including Rh antigen testing, is rarely done in resource-limited settings; although Rh-negative women require injections of anti-D antibody to prevent Rh sensitization, this is seldom available. Similarly, hepatitis B immunoglobulin and serum genetic screening for aneuploidy, or an abnormal number of chromosomes, are generally not available.

Finally, treatment and prevention of infectious diseases is an important part of antenatal care, especially in the developing world (Table 17.2). Where malaria is endemic, pregnant women should receive intermittent preventive treatment for malaria. This is given as three tablets of sulfadoxine–pyrimethamine (500/25 mg) to all pregnant women in both the second and third trimesters (regardless of peripheral blood smear or result of rapid testing). Pregnancy is also an opportune time to encourage the use of insecticide-treated bednets for malaria prevention by all members of a household, especially pregnant women and young children. If helminths are endemic, treatment should be considered for all pregnant women. Pregnant women should also be carefully immunized against tetanus, both for her own protection and to provide passive immunity to her infant at birth.

Pregnancy causes significant changes in physiology that may affect the course of other diseases in pregnant mothers. These changes include an increase in cardiac output, blood volume expansion, decreased systemic vascular resistance, and changes in the immune system and clotting cascade. Pregnant women with cardiac conditions, such as rheumatic heart disease, may experience a significant worsening of their symptoms. Asthma may be more dangerous. Pregnant women with influenza or chickenpox are more likely to become seriously ill. Therefore, pregnant women should be assessed for underlying communicable and non-communicable diseases and managed carefully during pregnancy.

Peripartum care

The intrapartum period – from the onset of labor until delivery is complete – is a critical time for ensuring safe delivery and

Table 17.1 Recommended tasks at each of the four WHO antenatal visits.

	4 months (18–24 weeks)	6 months (24–32 weeks)	8 months (32–36 weeks)	9 months (36–40 weeks)
General				
Complete physical and pelvic examination	✓			
Basic assessment of pregnancy	✓	✓	✓	✓
Determine estimated due date and if multiple gestation	✓			
Review past obstetric history	✓			
Ask about signs and symptoms	✓	✓	✓	✓
Discuss a birth and emergency plan	✓	✓	✓	✓
Disease screening				
Check for preeclampsia	✓	✓	✓	✓
Syphilis testing	✓			
Check for anemia	✓	✓	✓	✓
HIV testing	✓			(✓)[a]
Preventive measures				
Tetanus toxoid immunization	✓	✓		
Multivitamin or iron with folic acid	✓	✓	✓	✓
Deworming		✓		
Intermittent preventive treatment for malaria		✓	✓	✓
Encourage sleeping under an insecticide-treated bednet	✓	✓	✓	✓
Counseling				
Family planning counseling			✓	✓
Counseling on cessation of smoking, alcohol, and drug use (if applicable)	✓	✓	✓	✓
Counseling on nutrition and selfcare	✓	✓	✓	✓
Domestic violence screening	✓	✓	✓	✓

[a] Repeat HIV testing in high-HIV settings.
Source: adapted from Gupta N, Nelson BD, Kasper J, Hibberd PL (eds) *MassGeneral Hospital for Children Handbook of Pediatric Global Health*. New York: Springer, 2014.

Box 17.2 Length of a pregnancy

Pregnancy for medical providers is documented in weeks. The estimated delivery date of any given pregnancy in a woman with a normal menstrual cycle is 40 weeks from the first day of the last menstrual period. However, any pregnancy delivering between 37 and 42 weeks of gestation is considered a full-term pregnancy. Pregnancy is generally divided into trimesters. The first is up through 12 weeks, the second is up through 23 weeks, and the third begins at 24 weeks continuing through the end of pregnancy.

Thus, estimated delivery date = first day of last menstrual period + 9 months + 7 days.

Box 17.3 Assessment using ultrasound

Basic assessment with portable ultrasound can be very helpful in pregnancy. Simple point-of-care ultrasound should include the following (Figure 17.2).

- Assessment of viability: does the baby have a heartbeat?
- Fetal position: is the baby in the normal and safer cephalic position?
- Placental location: does the placenta cross the cervical os?

- Amniotic fluid levels: usually a good sign of placental function.
- Fetal size and dates

Using a vaginal ultrasound probe, it is also possible to determine whether there is an intrauterine or ectopic pregnancy and to assess pregnancy dating and viability early and with better accuracy.

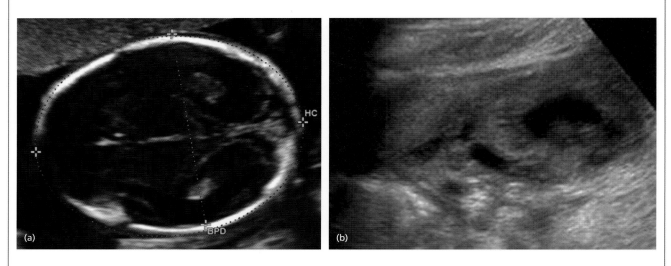

Figure 17.2 Maternal ultrasound images. (a) The fetal head is easily identified by the smooth, bright, fetal skull. The markings show the measurement of the obstetric biparietal diameter. (b) The dark central area is a fetal sac in the fallopian tube with a small fetus inside, consistent with an ectopic pregnancy.

Table 17.2 Antenatal care: infectious disease treatments and prophylaxis.

Malaria IPT	Three tablets sulfadoxine–pyrimethamine (500/25 mg) in two doses of three tablets each in the second and third trimesters to all pregnant women in endemic areas
Helminths	Treat in third or late second trimester (avoid first trimester when able) with one of the following regimens: • Albendazole 400 mg × 1 • Mebendazole 500 mg × 1 or 100 mg twice daily for 3 days • Pyrantel 10 mg/kg × 1 Repeat dose in third trimester if prevalence in population is >50%
Syphilis	For primary infection, treat with benzathine penicillin G 2.4 million units i.m. in a single dose (usually administered as 1.2 million units in each buttock)
HIV	Begin maternal antiretroviral treatment and dose to prevent maternal-to-child transmission (see Chapter 18 on HIV/AIDS)
Tetanus toxoid immunization	If previously vaccinated as a child, one dose of 0.5 mL is sufficient. If not vaccinated as a child, give the first dose at the first antenatal visit, with subsequent doses at 4 weeks, 6 months, and then two more at yearly intervals

IPT, intermittent preventive treatment.

should occur within an appropriate healthcare facility. The maternal survival series in *The Lancet* (Campbell & Graham, 2006) states:

> Evidence shows that the best intrapartum-care strategy is likely to be one in which women routinely choose to deliver in a health centre, with midwives as the main providers, but with other attendants working with them in a team.

A minority (15%) of deliveries will require emergency medical intervention, most of which will be among low-risk women with no risk factors for complications. The vast majority of these complications will be due to one of the five most common causes of maternal mortality: hemorrhage, obstructed labor, infection, unsafe abortion, and eclampsia (UNFPA, 2002). Therefore, choosing to deliver in a healthcare center with trained providers is the safest option for all women.

Contributing significantly to these causes of maternal mortality are barriers to quality care. Thaddeus and Maine (1994) have proposed the model of the "three delays of care" to conceptualize the barriers to adequate and timely obstetric care (Figure 17.3). A key approach to maternal morbidity and mortality reduction is labor planning. Healthcare providers should discuss a birth plan prior to labor and delivery and should strongly recommend a facility-based delivery. The first delay, the decision to seek care, can be targeted by educating pregant women about the danger signs during and after birth that require medical intervention at a healthcare facility with trained providers. Additionally, the discussion should include a clear plan for accessing care (e.g., means of transportation to appropriate facility, travel costs), thereby targeting the second delay of care in Thaddeus and Maine's model.

A well-equipped healthcare facility is one that is prepared to handle all the common and major complications of childbirth. The United Nations Population Fund (UNFPA) has defined the services necessary for a facility to qualify as appropriate for peripartum care, and these services are termed "emergency obstetric care" (EmOC). UNFPA clearly states that the goal is for **all** women to deliver in an EmOC-capable facility (UNFPA, 2012).

There are two levels of EmOC services: (i) basic EmOC (BEmOC) and (ii) comprehensive EmOC (CEmOC) (Table 17.3). Women with low-risk uncomplicated pregnancies can deliver at BEmOC-capable facilities but, in case it is needed, there should be a CEmOC-capable facility nearby with adequate transportation available to reach it. CEmOC facilities can serve as referral centers for many surrounding BEmOC sites, in addition to serving as a site of delivery for higher-risk pregnancies. Joint guidelines from UNFPA, WHO, and UNICEF recommend four BEmOC facilities and one CEmOC facility for every 500,000 people (UNFPA, 2008).

The basics of labor

Labor is defined as the presence of regular contractions with cervical change. Labor is divided into three stages (Table 17.4); the first stage of labor is subdivided into latent and active phases based on the rate of cervical dilation (Figure 17.4). The active phase of labor is generally considered to start at a dilation of between 3 and 6 cm but is determined by the rate of cervical change (1 cm or more per hour).

The partograph (Figure 17.5) is a tool used to monitor labor progress, as well as maternal and fetal well-being. Studies have demonstrated that use of the partograph results in fewer interventions in labor and increased rates of vaginal delivery (WHO, 1994). The modified WHO partograph should be initiated with every woman as she enters the active phase of labor. All sections, excluding the cervical examination which is performed approximately every 4 hours, should be filled out with each evaluation every 30 minutes. There is no consensus on the frequency of fetal heart auscultation during labor and delivery. An NIH consensus conference in 1979 recommended auscultation every 15 minutes in the first stage of labor and every 5 minutes in the second stage, although this near-continuous monitoring is not practical in most resource-limited settings (Young, 2013). An abnormal fetal heart rate, as defined by a frequency of less than 110 bpm or greater than 160 bpm, is an indication for consultation with an

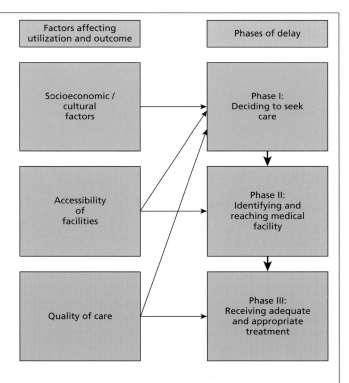

Figure 17.3 The three delays of care. This model describes three key activities in the process of accessing obstetric care: deciding to seek care, reaching a health facility, and receiving adequate care at the facility. Reprinted from Thaddeus S & Maine D. Too far to walk: maternal mortality in context, *Soc Sci Med* 38, 1091–1110, 1994 with permission from Elsevier.

Table 17.3 Signal functions of EmOC facilities.

Facility signal functions	Basic EmOC	Comprehensive EmOC
Administer parenteral antibiotics	✓	✓
Administer parenteral oxytocics	✓	✓
Administer parenteral anticonvulsants	✓	✓
Perform manual removal of placenta	✓	✓
Perform removal of retained products (e.g., suction or sharp uterine curettage)	✓	✓
Perform operative vaginal delivery (e.g., vacuum or forceps delivery)	✓	✓
Perform blood transfusion		✓
Perform cesarean delivery		✓

Source: Lawn & Kerber (2006).

Table 17.4 Stages of labor.

First	From onset of labor to full cervical dilation
Second	From full dilation of the cervix to expulsion of the fetus
Third	From expulsion of the fetus to expulsion of the placenta

appropriately trained clinician to evaluate for expedited delivery. The "alert" and "action" lines on the partograph are markers of an abnormal labor curve; when one of these lines is crossed in the graph, an evaluation should be undertaken for labor dystocia (slow or absent labor progress), and an intervention such as labor augmentation or cesarean delivery should be considered. Figure 17.5 shows a sample partograph for a labor that was augmented with oxytocin and resulted in a vaginal delivery.

Another situation requiring careful evaluation is malposition or malpresentation of the newborn. Malposition refers to a vertex presentation other than occiput anterior (the newborn coming out head first and facing toward the mother's coccyx). Malpositioning is a common reason for labor dystocia. Malpresentation refers to a presenting part other than the vertex or top of the newborn's head. Possibilities include breech presentation, face presentation, brow presentation, shoulder presentation, and compound presentation (in which an extremity presents along with the presenting part). Of these, the face presentation with the chin anterior is the only malpresentation where proceeding with a vaginal delivery is recommended. For all other malpresentations, an appropriately trained clinician should be consulted for probable cesarean delivery.

Shoulder dystocia is a complication of vaginal delivery for which providers should be prepared at every delivery. Shoulder dystocia describes the situation where the fetal head has delivered but the shoulders cannot be delivered with the usual maneuvers of childbirth. Risk factors for shoulder dystocia include fetal macrosomia and maternal diabetes; however, shoulder dystocia cannot usually be predicted (American College of Obstetricians and Gynecologists, 2002). Signs of shoulder dystocia include a delivered fetal head that remains tightly applied to the vulva, a retracted chin that depresses the perineum, and a failure to deliver the anterior shoulder with gentle downward traction on the head (WHO, 2003). Panel 17.1 provides basic maneuvers to resolve shoulder dystocia. Concurrent to the application of these maneuvers, the delivering provider should immediately call for assistance. If maneuvers cannot be performed due to inadequate vaginal space, an episiotomy (an incision made at the vaginal introitus) may be performed. In addition to the maneuvers in the figure, higher morbidity procedures such as symphysiotomy and the Zavanelli maneuver have been described (Sandberg, 1985).

The role of birth attendants

It is widely recommended that all women deliver with a skilled birth attendant, defined as:

> [an] accredited health professional – such as a midwife, doctor or nurse – who has been educated and trained to proficiency in the skills needed to manage normal (uncomplicated) pregnancies, childbirth and the immediate postnatal period, and in the identification, management and referral of complications in women and newborns (WHO, 2004).

The role of the traditional birth attendant (TBA), which refers to any birth attendant who is not accredited as a health professional or who has not been trained to proficiency in what is considered to be safe birth practices, has evolved over time. In a WHO document addressing newborn care in Africa, a new progressive role is described with the TBA as an advocate for mothers obtaining skilled care during delivery, emphasizing the

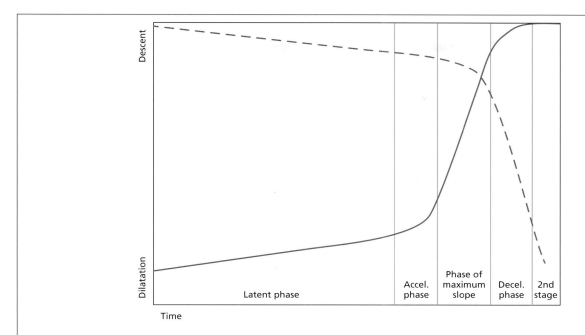

Figure 17.4 Phases of labor. *Source*: Cohen & Friedman (2011), figure 3.9, p. 43. Reproduced with permission from John Wiley & Sons, Inc., Hoboken, NJ.

importance of good working relations between the healthcare system and the TBAs (Lawn & Kerber, 2006).

The role of a skilled birth attendant is to monitor labor and delivery for signs of complications. In addition to this trained provider, a 2011 Cochrane review found that the presence of a continuous intrapartum support person is associated with improved labor outcomes, namely shorter labors, higher rates of spontaneous vaginal delivery, decreased use of intrapartum analgesia, and higher rates of satisfaction with the birthing experience. This support person may be trained or untrained, but subgroup analyses demonstrated greater efficacy when the woman was not part of the hospital staff or the patient's social network. This low-technology intervention of having an intra-partum support person present during labor is notable for its potential implementation and benefit in any setting (Hodnett *et al.*, 2011).

For births that are unable to take place in an appropriate facility, the WHO describes health behaviors to be promoted and implemented in all settings. The WHO emphasizes good hygiene and refers to the six "cleans" of a clean delivery (see Chapter 6). For births unattended by skilled birth attendants, danger signs (Table 17.5) should push women to immediately seek care.

Treatment for, and prevention of, leading causes of maternal mortality

Maternal mortality is defined as any maternal death related to pregnancy that occurs during pregnancy, birth, or within 42 days (6 weeks) of the termination of pregnancy. The leading causes of maternal mortality include hemorrhage, hypertension, sepsis, and abortion, which together account for more than three-quarters of all maternal deaths.

Hemorrhage that occurs before birth is called antenatal hemorrhage and may be caused by placenta previa, placental abruption, or a ruptured ectopic pregnancy. In placenta previa, the placenta overlies the cervix and therefore blocks the birth canal. Cervical dilation or mild trauma to the cervix such as what occurs with intercourse or a speculum examination can cause significant bleeding when placenta previa is present. Delivery requires cesarean section. Placental abruption involves the placenta becoming detached prematurely from the uterine wall. Causes of abruption include trauma, abnormal implantation of the placenta into the uterine wall, and hypertension. Ectopic pregnancy is a pregnancy that develops outside the uterus, often in the fallopian tube. An ectopic pregnancy can cause significant internal hemorrhage if it ruptures. Treatment before rupture can include methotrexate injection, which inhibits growth of the embryo, but treatment often requires surgical removal of the affected fallopian tube.

The most common type of fatal hemorrhage in pregnancy is postpartum hemorrhage, or hemorrhage occurring after birth. A common mnemonic used to help remember the causes of postpartum hemorrhage is the four Ts: Tone, Trauma, Tissue, and Thrombin. Bleeding can occur from lacerations of the cervix, vagina, or perineum incurred through the birth process (Trauma) or due to retained products of conception or clots within the uterus (Tissue). Coagulation abnormalities,

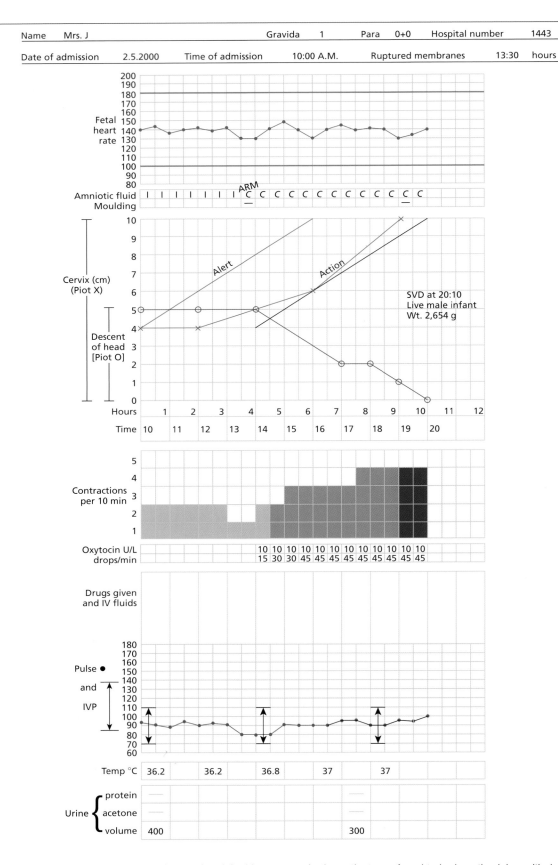

Figure 17.5 A sample partograph, properly completed. In this partograph, the patient was found to be in active labor with 4 cm of cervical dilation at 10:00. She had no cervical change 2 hours later. At 13:00 her contraction frequency decreased. At 14:00 she was started on oxytocin, with subsequent labor progress and a vaginal delivery. *Source*: WHO (2003), figure S-7, p. S-61. Reproduced with permission of the World Health Organization.

Panel 17.1: Maneuvers for management of shoulder dystocia. Note that delivery of the posterior arm is associated with the highest rate of delivery compared with the other maneuvers (Hoffman *et al.*, 2011). Adapted from Rodis (2013)

Maneuver	Description
McRoberts maneuver	Hyperflexion and abduction of the hips
McRoberts maneuver and suprapubic pressure	An assistant applies pressure suprapubically (just superior to the pubic bone) with a palm or fist. The pressure is directed downward (toward a point below the pubic bone) and laterally (toward the baby's face or sternum) in conjunction with McRoberts maneuver. The goal of this action is to bring the shoulders into an oblique plane because this plane has the widest diameter of the maternal pelvis.
Delivery of the posterior arm	Flexion of the elbow, sweep of the posterior arm across the fetal chest, and delivery of the arm out of the vagina.
Rubin maneuver	The clinician places one hand in the vagina behind the posterior fetal shoulder and applies pressure in the direction of the fetal face, rotating it anteriorly. If the fetal spine is on the maternal left, the clinician's right hand is used, and vice-versa. Alternatively, this maneuver can be attempted by placing the hand behind the anterior shoulder, if it is more accessible, and rotating it posteriorly.
Woods screw maneuver	The clinician places one hand in the vagina in front of the posterior shoulder and applies pressure in the direction of the fetal spine, rotating it 180 degrees until it becomes the anterior shoulder. The anterior shoulder dislodges during this process.
Gaskin all-fours	Placement of woman on hands and knees, with subsequent gentle downward traction on fetal head to deliver the shoulder
Clavicular fracture	Intentional fracture of the clavicle to shorten the biacromial diameter

both inherited and acquired, such as hemophilia or dissemi-nated intravascular coagulopathy, can cause postpartum hem-orrhage (Thrombin). However, the most common cause is uterine atony, or failure of the uterine muscle to contract after birth (Tone). Blood vessels that feed the placental bed run through the uterine muscle tissue. Failure of the muscle to contract after birth results in failure of these blood vessels to constrict and leads to hemorrhage. Risk factors for uterine atony include multiple gestation, multiparity, polyhydramnios, macrosomia, prolonged or rapid labor, infection, or labor aug-mented with medications.

Panel 17.2 gives a detailed outline of treatment for post-partum hemorrhage at the bedside. If none of these maneuvers succeed in controlling the postpartum hemorrhage, the mother will need surgery and potentially a hysterectomy. She should be taken to a surgical center immediately (Box 17.4).

Hypertensive disorders of pregnancy

The spectrum of hypertensive disorders in pregnancy include chronic hypertension, gestational hypertension, preeclampsia, and eclampsia. A pregnant woman is diagnosed with a hyper-tensive disorder if her blood pressure is more than 140 mmHg systolic or more than 90 mmHg diastolic on two occasions 4–6 hours apart or if diastolic blood pressure is more than 110 mmHg on one occasion. Hypertension is classified as pregnancy-induced if it occurs for the first time after 20 weeks of gestation or up to 12 weeks after delivery. If it occurs before 20 weeks of gestation, it is classified as chronic hypertension. When the blood pressure prior to 20 weeks of gestation is unknown, differentiation between chronic and pregnancy-induced hypertension may be impossible. In this case, the high blood pressure is managed as gestational hypertension.

Table 17.5 Danger signs during and immediately after childbirth (Lawn & Kerber, 2006). If any of these danger signs are present, mother and newborn should be immediately brought for care at a hospital or health center.

Mother

- If water breaks but she is not in labor after 6 hours
- Labor pains continue for more than 12 hours
- Heavy bleeding (soaks more than two or three pads in 15 minutes)
- Placenta not expelled 1 hour after birth of newborn
- Fits or convulsions

Newborn

- Difficulty breathing (no cry at birth)
- Not able to feed
- Fever (>38.0°C) or feels cold (<35.5°C)
- Very small (<1500 g or born earlier than 32 weeks)
- Fits or convulsions

  Panel 17.2 Treatment of postpartum hemorrhage at the bedside

Prevention: active management of the third stage of labor

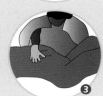

Once the baby is born and before the placenta is delivered, a prophylactic dose of medication is given to help the uterus contract. This is usually oxytocin 10 mg i.m. or oral misoprostol 600 mg. Before giving the medication, the clinician must be sure there is not another baby inside the mother's uterus waiting to be delivered

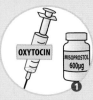

Next, once the cord has been cut between the placenta and newborn, the placenta is delivered with gentle traction on the umbilical cord. This is performed while supporting the uterus with a hand on the abdomen pushing upward above the pubic symphysis to prevent inversion of the uterus

The provider then massages the fundus of the uterus until adequate uterine tone can be felt. This maneuver can be repeated any time postpartum bleeding returns

Panel 17.2 Treatment of postpartum hemorrhage at the bedside (*Continued*)

Initial treatment of postpartum hemorrhage

Early breastfeeding is good for both the baby and the mother. It causes the release of natural oxytocin, a potent uterotonic

It is essential that the clinician checks the mother for any tears to the perineum, vagina, or cervix and sutures tears when needed

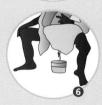

The new mother should be encouraged to urinate or, if necessary, a Foley catheter can be used to empty the bladder. A full bladder may mechanically prevent normal uterine contraction

Advanced treatment of postpartum hemorrhage (required when bleeding is acute and severe or when initial maneuvers fail)

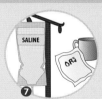

When the mother's bleeding is very heavy after birth she may quickly become hemodynamically unstable. Intravenous fluid resuscitation is started promptly with normal saline. A blood transfusion may be needed

Uterotonic medications can be given in treatment doses. Oxytocin can be given as 20–40 IU in the intravenous bag and run rapidly, and misoprostol 800–1000 µg p.r. or p.o. can be given. Methergine is contraindicated if the patient has elevated blood pressure but otherwise can be given as 0.2 mg i.m.

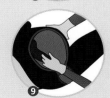

Placenta or blood clots that are still inside the uterus can keep the uterus from contracting completely. Using clean gloves, these products of conception can be removed manually while massaging the uterus

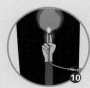

Uterine bleeding can also be stopped with compression. An intrauterine balloon can be used to apply pressure to the bleeding placental bed and create tamponade. If surgical therapies are not immediately available and the patient will have to be transferred, the uterine balloon can prevent excessive blood loss during transport (Box 17.4)

Box 17.4 Intrauterine balloon tamponade

Using a urinary catheter, string, condom, syringe, and one-way valve, a uterine balloon can be easily constructed (Figure 17.6) (Nelson *et al.*, 2013). Using the string, tie the condom onto the bladder end of the catheter and insert into the uterus. Inflate the catheter balloon with 15 mL of water. Then place the one-way valve on to the other end of the catheter. Inflate the condom with water inside the uterus until the bleeding stops. Usually this will require 300–500 mL of water. Clamp the catheter to prevent leakage of fluid, and leave the balloon in place 6–24 hours. A prophylactic dose of a broad-spectrum antibiotic at time of placement is recommended to prevent puerperal infection.

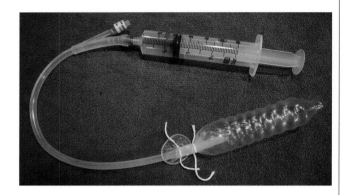

Figure 17.6 Equipment for intrauterine balloon tamponade.

Box 17.5 Signs of preeclampsia

Preeclampsia can be classified as mild or severe. Severe preeclampsia is noted when one or more of the following signs is present.

- Resting systolic blood pressure ≥160 mmHg or diastolic ≥110 mmHg on two occasions at least 6 hours apart.
- Proteinuria of ≥5 g in a 24-hour urine collection, or 3+ urine dip collected on two occasions at least 4 hours apart.
- Oliguria with urine output <500 mL per 24 hours.
- Pulmonary edema.
- Epigastric or right upper-quadrant pain.
- Impaired liver function.
- Thrombocytopenia.
- Fetal growth restriction.
- Cerebral or visual disturbances, including persistent severe headache.

Box 17.6 Management of eclamptic seizures

- Ensure the mother is in a safe place away from sharp objects and not at risk of falling from the bed.
- Place her in the lateral decubitus position.
- Suction oral secretions and vomitus.
- Administer oxygen.
- Give magnesium sulfate 10 g i.m. and 4 g bolus i.v. over 5 minutes. Give a maintenance dose of 5 g i.m. every 4 hours. Continue treatment for 24 hours after delivery or the last convulsion, whichever occurs last.
- If eclampsia, and no magnesium is available, give diazepam 10 mg i.v. slowly over 2 minutes.

Gestational hypertension is more common among women who are pregnant for the first time. Women with diabetes, underlying vascular problems, or multiple pregnancies (e.g., twins) are also at higher risk of developing gestational hypertension. Both chronic hypertension and gestational hypertension must be controlled during pregnancy, with a blood pressure less than 140/90 mmHg. Elevated blood pressure may result in poor placental perfusion, leading to complications such as fetal growth restriction, fetal demise, and placental abruption.

Women with gestational and chronic hypertension are at high risk of developing preeclampsia or eclampsia. Signs of preeclampsia include elevated blood pressure, edema, and protein in the urine (>0.3 g in 24 hours) (Box 17.5). In resource-limited settings without laboratory quantification of protein in the urine, urine dipsticks at or above 2+ or foamy urine may be signs of significant protein in the urine. Women may experience persistent headaches, visual changes, hyper-reflexia, and epigastric pain. Preeclampsia may quickly develop into eclampsia, which is the presence of seizures. Eclampsia greatly increases the risk of adverse outcomes.

Eclamptic seizures may occur regardless of the severity of the hypertension, are difficult to predict, and can often occur in the absence of hyperreflexia, headache, or visual changes. Convulsions are tonic–clonic and resemble grand mal seizures of epilepsy. They may recur in rapid sequence, as in status epilepticus, and end in death. Approximately 25% of eclamptic seizures occur after delivery of the newborn. Box 17.6 summarizes how to manage eclamptic seizures.

HELLP syndrome is a subset of severe preeclampsia. It is noted on laboratory evaluation and includes hemolysis (H), elevated liver enzymes (EL), and low platelets (LP). Where

Box 17.7 Antihypertensive therapy in preeclampsia

- Hydralazine is the drug of choice.
- Give hydralazine 5–10 mg i.v. slowly every 10 minutes until blood pressure is lowered (goal diastolic blood pressure 90–100 mmHg). Repeat every 3 hours as needed or give hydralazine 12.5 mg i.m. every 2 hours as needed.
- If hydralazine is not available or effective, give labetalol or nifedipine.
  - Labetalol 10 mg i.v. If response to labetalol is inadequate (diastolic blood pressure remains >110 mmHg) after 10 minutes, give labetalol 20 mg i.v. Dose can be increased every 10 minutes by doubling, up to 80 mg in two doses. Maximum total dosing is 220 mg. Avoid in asthma or congestive heart failure.
  - Nifedipine 10 mg orally. Repeat in 30 minutes if necessary.

available, laboratory evaluation in preeclampsia should include hemoglobin, platelet count, serum creatinine, and transaminase levels. Uric acid is also frequently elevated in preeclampsia. In HELLP, lactic acid dehydrogenase may be elevated due to hemolysis, and a peripheral blood smear may show direct evidence of hemolysis.

The only cure for preeclampsia or eclampsia is delivery of the newborn. Magnesium sulfate is given immediately on diagnosis to prevent seizures and labetalol, hydralazine, or nifedipine are given to lower blood pressure. This may provide enough time for the addition of antenatal steroids in prematurity (to help with fetal lung maturity) and for induction of labor to allow for vaginal birth. Magnesium should be continued for 24 hours after delivery or the last convulsion, whichever occurs last. Antihypertensive therapy should be continued as long as the diastolic blood pressure is 110 mmHg or more (Box 17.7). Continue to monitor urine output and check for pulmonary edema and HELLP.

Puerperal sepsis

Puerperal sepsis is bacteremia caused by infection around the time of birth. Infection during pregnancy and the postpartum period may be caused by a combination of organisms, including aerobic and anaerobic cocci and bacilli. The source is most frequently ascending infection from the vaginal area into the uterus, resulting in endomyometritis. This often is a result of unclean practices by birth attendants and clinicians. Again, see Chapter 6 for the six recommended "cleans" for the clean management of birth. Symptoms of endomyometritis include fever and abdominal pain with fundal tenderness. If untreated, these infections are often fatal.

Other causes of postpartum fever must be considered as well. These include pneumonia, atelectasis, UTI, wound or episiotomy infection, breast engorgement, mastitis, drug fever, deep venous thrombosis, and pulmonary embolus. A physical examination, including a pelvic examination, is necessary to rule out hematoma or retained membranes. Urinalysis and, when clinically indicated, a chest X-ray should be performed.

Treatment for puerperal fever caused by endomyometritis includes intravenous antibiotics until 14–48 hours afebrile and improved physical examination findings:

- ampicillin 2 g i.v. every 6 hours;
- *plus* gentamicin 5 mg/kg i.v. every 24 hours;
- *plus* metronidazole 500 mg i.v. every 8 hours.

If the patient is unresponsive to intravenous antibiotics after 48–72 hours of treatment, consider septic pelvic thrombophlebitis, drug fever, or abscess.

Obstetric fistula

A devastating morbidity resulting from childbirth around the globe is obstetric fistula. Obstetric fistula is an opening between the vagina and bladder and/or between the vagina and rectum that results from prolonged labor, often from labor lasting for days. The fistula leaves women leaking urine or feces continuously and often results in social isolation, worsening poverty, and depression.

Fistula affects about 2 million women worldwide, with 50,000–100,000 new cases each year (UNFPA, 2013). It is most common in resource-poor communities in Asia and sub-Saharan Africa where obstetric care and access to cesarean section is limited. Prevention involves timely diagnosis of obstructed labor and delivery via cesarean section, as well as good maternal nutrition. The treatment is surgical repair, which is often expensive and of limited availability.

Women in resource-limited settings who have previously had children should be asked about continuous urinary leaking or poor fecal control and be evaluated for fistula. Appropriate referrals should be made for surgical repair.

Family planning and contraception

Prevention of maternal deaths starts with providing women and families with the ability to control the number of pregnancies and optimize their timing. The inter-pregnancy interval is defined as the time period from the birth of one child to the conception of the next. Studies have demonstrated increased risk of adverse fetal and maternal outcomes with an inter-pregnancy interval of less than 18 months. From the fetal perspective, studies have found a significantly increased risk of low birthweight and preterm delivery for pregnancies conceived less than 18 months after the last pregnancy (Conde-Agudelo *et al.*, 2006). Inter-pregnancy intervals less than 6 months are associated with increased risk of maternal death,

Box 17.8 The WHO four key activities to sustain exclusive breastfeeding

1. Initiation of breastfeeding within the first hour of life.
2. Exclusive breastfeeding, which means the infant only receives breast milk without any additional food or drink, not even water.
3. Breastfeeding on demand, which means as often as the child wants, day or night.
4. No use of bottles, teats, or pacifiers.

months, WHO (2012b) recommends four key activities (Box 17.8).

Postpartum contraception is critical for prevention of unplanned pregnancies. In non-breastfeeding women, ovulation returns on average 6 weeks postpartum, with ovulation documented as early as 3–4 weeks postpartum (Jackson & Glasier, 2011). Therefore, initiation of contraception soon after delivery is essential for pregnancy planning. Ideally, a contraceptive plan is formulated during prenatal care, confirmed prior to postpartum discharge from the hospital, and initiated prior to postpartum discharge or within the first few weeks of the postpartum period. Most forms of contraception can be started after obtaining a medical history and blood pressure measurement; they require no laboratory evaluation, and only intrauterine devices require a pelvic examination.

third trimester bleeding, premature rupture of membranes, and puerperal infection (Conde-Agudelo & Belizán, 2000). Suspected contributors to these findings include maternal nutritional depletion, increased psychosocial stressors, and later initiation of prenatal care (Klerman et al., 1998). Increased risk of adverse outcomes has also been noted with an inter-pregnancy interval in excess of 59 months.

Interventions to promote optimal inter-pregnancy intervals include encouragement of exclusive breastfeeding for the first 6 months, patient education surrounding birth spacing, and postpartum contraception. In order to support women in establishing and sustaining exclusive breastfeeding for 6

Additional resources

- World Health Organization (2003) Managing complications in pregnancy and childbirth. http://www.who.int/reproductivehealth/publications/maternal_perinatal_health/9241545879/en/
- World Health Organization (2009) *Medical Eligibility Criteria for Contraceptive Use*, 4th edn. http://www.who.int/reproductivehealth/publications/family_planning/9789241563888/en/

REFERENCES

American College of Obstetricians and Gynecologists (2002) Shoulder dystocia. ACOG Practice Bulletin No. 40. *Obstet Gynecol* 100:1045–50.

Campbell OM, Graham WJ (2006) Strategies for reducing maternal mortality: getting on with what works. *Lancet* 368:1284–99.

Cohen W, Friedman E (2011) *Labor and Delivery Care: A Practical Guide.* Hoboken, NJ: Wiley-Blackwell.

Conde-Agudelo A, Belizán JM (2000) Maternal morbidity and mortality associated with interpregnancy interval: cross sectional study. *BMJ* 321:1255–9.

Conde-Agudelo A, Rosas-Bermúdez A, Kafury-Goeta AC (2006) Birth spacing and risk of adverse perinatal outcomes: a meta-analysis. *JAMA* 295:1809–23.

Hodnett ED, Gates S, Hofmeyr GJ, Sakala C, Weston J (2011) Continuous support for women during childbirth. *Cochrane Database Syst Rev* (2):CD003766.

Hoffman MK, Bailit JL, Branch DW et al. (2011) A comparison of obstetric maneuvers for the acute management of shoulder dystocia. *Obstet Gynecol* 117:1272–8.

Jackson E, Glasier A (2011) Return of ovulation and menses in postpartum nonlactating women: a systematic review. *Obstet Gynecol* 117:657–62.

Klerman L, Cliver S, Goldenberg R (1998) The impact of short interpregnancy intervals on pregnancy outcomes in a low-income population. *Am J Public Health* 88:1182–5.

Lawn J, Kerber K (eds) (2006) *Opportunities for Africa's Newborns: Practical Data, Policy and Programmatic Support for Newborn Care in Africa.* Geneva: WHO on behalf of The Partnership for Maternal, Newborn and Child Health.

Nelson BD, Stoklosa H, Ahn R et al. (2013) Uterine balloon tamponade for postpartum hemorrhage control among community-based health providers in South Sudan. *Int J Gynecol Obstet* 122:27–32.

Rodis JF (2013) Shoulder dystocia: intrapartum diagnosis, management and outcome. Available at http://www.uptodate.com/contents/shoulder-dystocia-intrapartum-diagnosis-management-and-outcome

Sandberg EC (1985) The Zavanelli maneuver: a potentially revolutionary method for the resolution of shoulder dystocia. *Am J Obstet Gynecol* 152:479–84.

Thaddeus S, Maine D (1994) Too far to walk: maternal mortality in context. *Soc Sci Med* 38:1091–110.

UNFPA (2002) Maternal mortality update 2002: a focus on emergency obstetric care. Available at unfpa.org/

webdav/site/global/shared/documents/ publications/2003/mmupdate-2002_eng.pdf

UNFPA (2008) Providing emergency obstetric and neonatal care to all in need. Available at http:// www.unfpa.org/public/mothers/pid/4385

UNFPA (2012) Urgent report: Providing emergency obstetric and newborn care. Available at http:// www.unfpa.org/webdav/site/global/shared/factsheets/srh/ EN-SRH%20fact%20sheet-Urgent.pdf

UNFPA (2013) Campaign to end fistula. Available at www.endfistula.org

WHO (1994) World Health Organization partograph in management of labor. *Lancet* 343:1399–404.

WHO (2003) *Managing Complications in Pregnancy and Childbirth: A Guide for Midwives and Doctors.* Geneva: World Health Organization.

WHO (2004) Making pregnancy safer: the critical role of the skilled attendant: A joint statement by WHO, ICM and FIGO. Available at http://whqlibdoc.who.int/ publications/2004/9241591692.pdf

WHO (2012a) Maternal mortality. Fact Sheet No. 348, May 2012. Available at http://www.who.int/ mediacentre/factsheets/fs348/en/index.html

WHO (2012b) Exclusive breastfeeding. Available at http://www.who.int/nutrition/topics/exclusive _breastfeeding/en/

WHO (2013) Global health observatory data repository. Available at http://apps.who.int/gho/data/view.main

WHO, UNICEF, UNFPA, The World Bank (2012) Trends in maternal mortality: 1990 to 2010. Available at http://www.unfpa.org/webdav/site/global/shared/ documents/publications/2012/Trends_in_maternal _mortality_A4-1.pdf >

Young BK (2013) Intrapartum fetal heart rate assessment. Available at http://www.uptodate.com/contents/ intrapartum-fetal-heart-rate-assessment

Part 4
Infectious Diseases

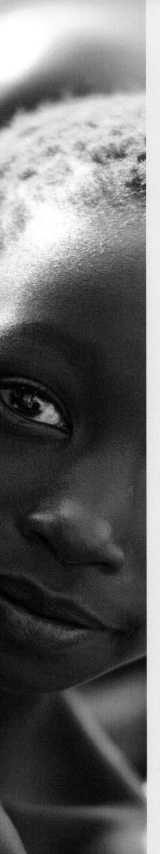

CHAPTER 18
HIV/AIDS

Jeff A. Robison[1], Sahera Dirajlal-Fargo[2], and Carrie M. Cox[3]
[1]University of Utah, Salt Lake City, UT, USA
[2]Case Western Reserve University and Rainbow Babies & Children's Hospital, Cleveland, OH, USA
[3]Loyola University Chicago and Stritch School of Medicine, Maywood, IL, USA

Key learning objectives

■ Understand that HIV prevalence, diagnosis, and treatment protocols vary among different regions of the world and healthcare providers should consult local guidelines for care.

■ Recognize the signs, symptoms, and demographics that warrant HIV testing.

■ Understand how to make an accurate and definitive diagnosis of HIV in adults, children, and infants and when to initiate antiretroviral therapy.

■ Be familiar with what constitutes treatment failure, including an emphasis to ensure adherence.

■ Recognize that transmission of HIV can be prevented using a public health approach.

Abstract

An estimated 34 million people worldwide are living with HIV, and each year 2.5 million people become newly infected and 1.7 million people die from AIDS-related causes. HIV can be transmitted via sexual intercourse, contact with infected blood, or vertically from mother to child. Infants and children are almost exclusively infected through vertical transmission from an HIV-infected mother. Prevention of mother-to-child transmission (PMTCT) is possible, and the WHO has developed PMTCT guidelines for resource-limited settings that aim to decrease maternal-to-child transmission rates to less than 5%. The clinical presentation of HIV/AIDS is variable. Clinical staging conditions are used to guide treatment decisions. Antiretroviral therapy (ART) is a lifelong treatment, and criteria used to guide ART initiation include the age, pregnancy status, clinical stage, and immunological status (CD4 count) of an individual. Prevention measures, such as infant feeding practices, use of condoms, male circumcision, and use of prophylactic therapy in discordant couples, all play an important role in decreasing transmission.

Key words: HIV, AIDS, antiretroviral therapy, prevention of mother-to-child transmission (PMTCT), clinical staging, prevention, pre-exposure prophylaxis, post-exposure prophylaxis

Essential Clinical Global Health, First Edition. Edited by Brett D. Nelson.
© 2015 John Wiley & Sons, Ltd. Published 2015 by John Wiley & Sons, Ltd.
Companion website: www.essentialseries.com/globalhealth

Introduction

Infection with the human immunodeficiency virus (HIV) remains a prominent contributor to morbidity and mortality in the developing world despite progress in recent years. The consequences of the pandemic are particularly evident in the African region (Figure 18.1). An estimated 34 million people worldwide are living with HIV, and each year 2.5 million people become newly infected and 1.7 million people die from AIDS-related causes. The number of people living with HIV with access to antiretroviral therapy (ART) is only approximately 8 million (WHO, 2012a).

Prevention of HIV/AIDS should be a primary goal of healthcare providers, and the ability to recognize, diagnose, and treat patients with HIV infection is important for any provider practicing within areas of moderate to high prevalence. Further, it is important to understand that while international diagnostic and treatment guidelines for resource-limited settings have been established, specific guidelines for individual countries should be consulted in management decisions.

Basic HIV biology

HIV targets, infects, disables, and ultimately kills the human CD4 cell. CD4 cells are a critical component of the immune system, making hosts susceptible to disease on their demise. The ultimate resulting condition suffered by untreated individuals infected with HIV is the acquired immunodeficiency syndrome (AIDS).

HIV is a retrovirus: after infecting a CD4 cell, viral RNA genetic material is reverse transcribed into DNA by means of an enzyme called reverse transcriptase, after which this HIV DNA is integrated into the host's DNA (Figure 18.2). Viral components are then replicated using the host's cellular mechanisms. Final assembly precedes the release of the next generation of viruses, which then go on to infect more CD4 cells. As this process gains momentum, the host's viral load becomes ever higher as the CD4 count becomes lower (Figure 18.3).

There are two distinct HIV serotypes: types 1 and 2. HIV-2 is endemic in West Africa, Mozambique, and parts of India (Campbell-Yesufu & Gandhi, 2011). Common HIV antibody tests can detect both HIV-1 and HIV-2 but cannot distinguish between the two viruses. HIV-2 is typically associated with a slower decline of CD4 and lower viral load (Marlink *et al.*, 1994; Andersson *et al.*, 2000) but may not respond as predictably to certain treatment options. Healthcare providers should be familiar with local HIV serotypes (Tuaillon *et al.*, 2004).

Transmission

HIV can be transmitted via the following routes.

- Sexual intercourse (horizontal transmission)
  - Vaginal
  - Anal
- Contact with infected blood
  - Intravenous drug use or needle sharing
  - Contaminated blood transfusion
  - Occupational exposure
  - Traditional cutting with infected instruments

- Mother-to-child transmission (vertical transmission)
  - During pregnancy
  - At delivery
  - Post partum/breastfeeding.

Presentation and clinical diagnosis

The clinical presentation of HIV/AIDS is variable. Healthcare providers should be familiar with conditions associated with HIV/AIDS, which can be considered broadly as common non-HIV-specific conditions that happen more frequently or more severely and/or as conditions specific to persons with HIV/AIDS.

The presentation of HIV/AIDS is not only variable among individuals, but general characteristics of the disease may vary between infants and children compared with adults. For example, the **latency period** – or time between infection and progression of disease – can be rapid in infants, often leading to death if untreated within the first 1–2 years of life (Whitescarter *et al.*, 2008). However, in adults the latency period can last up to 10 years or more, and progression of disease is generally slower. Early detection and recognition of infection in infants is therefore especially critical.

Diagnosis and testing

Voluntary counseling and testing principles

Testing should be strongly recommended to patients in whom HIV/AIDS is suspected; however, testing must be voluntary. It is critical to have appropriate counseling available for the testing and care of patients. Before testing occurs, informed consent must be obtained from patients after a trained staff member performs a formal counseling session. When a young child is tested, staff should obtain consent from and provide counseling to a parent, understanding that an HIV-infected child was most likely vertically infected from the mother. For this reason, testing should also be offered to the mother, father, and other children when possible. When testing school-aged

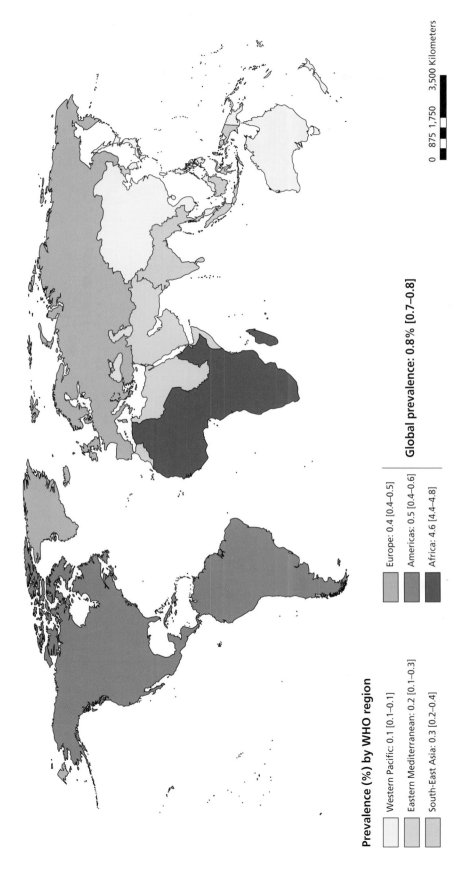

Prevalence (%) by WHO region

Western Pacific: 0.1 [0.1–0.1]

Eastern Mediterranean: 0.2 [0.1–0.3]

South-East Asia: 0.3 [0.2–0.4]

Europe: 0.4 [0.4–0.5]

Americas: 0.5 [0.4–0.6]

Africa: 4.6 [4.4–4.8]

Global prevalence: 0.8% [0.7–0.8]

0   875 1,750   3,500 Kilometers

Figure 18.1 HIV prevalence by country. *Source:* WHO (2013c). Reproduced with permission of the World Health Organization.

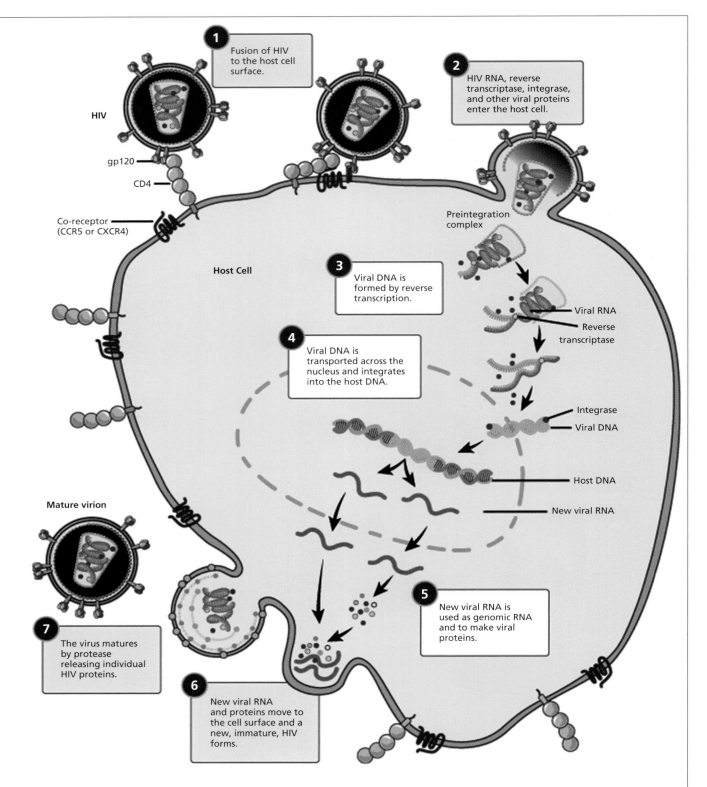

Figure 18.2 Steps in the HIV replication cycle. *Source*: reproduced courtesy of the National Institute of Allergy and Infectious Diseases.

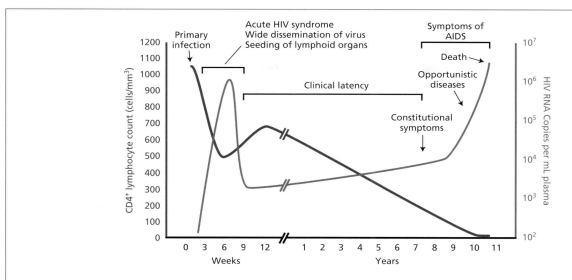

Figure 18.3 Clinical course of HIV/AIDS. *Source*: Pantaleo *et al.* (1993). Reproduced with permission of *The New England Journal of Medicine*.

children, parental consent and child assent with age-appropriate disclosure counseling should be done. Adolescents can and should provide their own consent for testing, and parental consent is typically not required according to national guidelines.

HIV/AIDS continues to carry significant stigma. Strict confidentiality must be maintained for individuals receiving testing and care. It is wholly up to the individual who is tested and/or infected with HIV to decide who knows about their condition. Healthcare providers should not disclose health information without the consent of the individual.

Pre-test counseling should include appropriate methods of disclosure for both positive and negative results in order to maximize adherence and future prevention. Counseling should emphasize HIV prevention strategies and that HIV/AIDS is not curable but treatable, and that careful adherence and follow-up are necessary for the rest of the individual's life.

Testing modalities

HIV testing has recently become much more readily available in resource-limited settings. Modalities include tests for HIV antibodies, HIV virus, and HIV-associated proteins (Table 18.1 and Figure 18.4).

The period between infection and the ability of an HIV test to reliably diagnose infection is known as the **window period**. Within the window period, an individual is infected with the virus but the test may be negative. This is of particular importance when considering the timing of initial testing and subsequent testing of infants born to HIV-infected mothers and/or in whom ongoing exposure to HIV may be occurring

through breastfeeding. Virologic testing has a 6-week window period while HIV antibody tests have a window period of approximately 3 months.

Establishing the diagnosis

Testing for HIV antibodies can occur rapidly and efficiently with results available at the same clinic visit. Rapid HIV antibody testing has become the standard in resource-limited settings. Testing should occur in any patient with signs, symptoms, or conditions associated with HIV. Programs for universal population screening should be considered in countries with high prevalence. Specific populations with increased risk for HIV should be particularly targeted for testing:

- individuals with active tuberculosis (Corbett *et al.*, 2003);
- commercial sex workers;
- men who have sex with men (MSM);
- hospitalized patients (Colvin *et al.*, 2001);
- malnourished individuals;
- intravenous drug users;
- pregnant women;
- children born to HIV-infected women.

International standards require a confirmatory test with different antigens (i.e., two different brands of antibody tests) or "relying on different operating characteristics" in order to confirm a positive test (WHO, 2007). This confirmatory test can be done, per national guidelines, either in series (i.e., second test only after one positive result) or in tandem (i.e., perform two tests at the same time).

Table 18.1 HIV testing modalities.

Test	Mode of detection	Characteristic	Limitations and use
Serologic			
HIV rapid test	Detects antibody	Rapid Inexpensive Highly sensitive	May be negative during window period and severe immunosuppression Two types of rapid tests often used to confirm diagnosis (see national guidelines)
HIV ELISA	Detects antibody	Highly sensitive	May be negative during window period and severe immunosuppression Requires serum A positive test requires confirmation by Western blot
HIV Western blot	Detects antibodies to protein p24, gp41, gp120, gp160		Used to confirm ELISA A positive test confirms the diagnosis An indeterminate result could mean early infection and should be repeated on the same sample and again 2 weeks later
Virologic			
HIV DNA PCR	*Qualitative test* Detects HIV DNA material inside replicating and non-replicating cells	Can be run on serum or dried blood spots (DBS) High sensitivity and specificity	Gold standard for infant diagnosis Highly sensitive even with infants on ARVs HIV can be detected 6 weeks after last exposure
HIV RNA PCR	*Quantitative test* Also known as viral load (no. of copies per mL)	Highly sensitive and specific	Expensive Can also be used for infant diagnosis ($>10,000$ copies/mL)
Ultrasensitive p24 antigen	Detects p24 antigen	Highly sensitive and specific	Laboratory equipment not available on a large scale
HIV culture	Detects presence of HIV virus in blood		Expensive and requires time

Establishing the diagnosis in infants and children

Infants and children are almost exclusively infected through vertical transmission from an HIV-infected mother. For this reason, and since maternal HIV antibodies can persist in an infant for up to 18 months, it can be difficult to accurately distinguish true HIV infection in infants and children compared with persistence of maternal antibodies if antibody testing alone is employed. Additionally, breastfeeding infants continue to be exposed to HIV and therefore a child cannot be considered definitively uninfected until breastfeeding has ceased and the window period has passed. Therefore, infants and children born to HIV-infected mothers can be categorized as uninfected, infected, or exposed. Prompt diagnosis of HIV/AIDS in infants and children is important because the disease can progress rapidly (Rouet *et al.*, 2003).

Recommendations for testing of infants and children have been established by the World Health Organization (WHO) (Table 18.2). They are based on a public health approach in resource-limited settings. Individual countries may have modifications to these guidelines based on HIV prevalence and availability of testing (WHO, 2010a, 2013a).

HIV-associated conditions and clinical staging

Certain conditions associated with HIV/AIDS are used as a measure of disease severity. This is known as **clinical staging**. Clinical staging conditions guide treatment decisions and often determine ART eligibility. Familiarity with these conditions is critical in both the diagnosis and care of persons with HIV/AIDS (Table 18.3).

Treatment

Antiretroviral therapy

ART describes the use of antiretroviral (ARV) drug combinations whose actions inhibit viral replication at different stages of the HIV life cycle (Table 18.4 and Figure 18.2). HIV can develop resistance to ARVs, so ART regimens generally involve the combined use of three different ARVs. Fixed-dose combinations of common ART regimens have become more readily available for use in resource-limited settings. International recommendations exist for appropriate ARV combinations (WHO, 2013a) (Table 18.5); however, individual countries have guidelines for first-line therapy, second-line therapy, and recommendations for special circumstances, such as use during pregnancy, use in infants previously exposed to ARVs through the mother, or use while on concomitant tuberculosis therapy. Regimens may be partly based on which fixed-dose combinations are available and feasible to procure. It is critical for healthcare providers to be familiar with national guidelines for ART.

Initiation of ART

ART should only be initiated after a patient has been screened and treated for any concurrent infections and has undergone counseling with a trained staff member. Individuals starting ART should understand that strict adherence is critical, that ART is a lifelong treatment, and that continued follow-up is necessary. Criteria to consider for ART initiation eligibility include the age, pregnancy status, clinical stage, and immunological status (CD4 count) of an individual. The WHO has outlined criteria for initiating ART in resource-limited settings for specific populations (WHO, 2013a) (Table 18.6).

Emerging literature indicates that earlier initiation of ART improves outcomes in both adults and infants/children; however, international and national guidelines are developed within a public health framework and reflect the feasible treatment strategies within different country situations. National guidelines are updated regularly to reflect current recommendations within the country context, and local ART guidelines should be frequently consulted.

Monitoring and modification of treatment

Healthcare providers should follow all HIV-infected and exposed individuals regularly. An initial thorough examination and history allows the healthcare provider to establish the clinical stage at the time of diagnosis and initiation of ART if indicated. Healthcare providers must make every attempt to support strict adherence and work with patients to identify and address barriers to adherence through continuous, lifelong counseling.

Modification of treatment may be necessary due to serious adverse medication reactions (Table 18.4) or treatment failure. Viral load monitoring is the preferred method to diagnose treatment failure. Treatment failure must be considered if viral load remains greater than 1000 copies/mL on two consecutive measurements after 3 months (virologic failure), if new or recurrent WHO stage 4 conditions occur (clinical failure), or if CD4 count suddenly or gradually drops below the CD4 at initiation of treatment or to less than 200 cells/mm³ in children

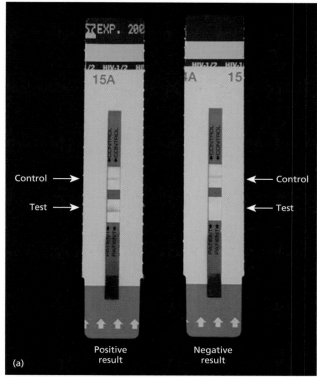
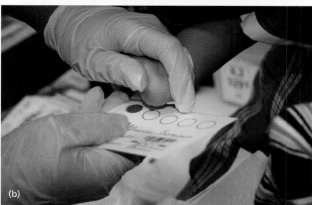

Figure 18.4 HIV tests commonly available in resource-limited settings. (a) Rapid test for HIV antibody. Immediate results are available and can be delivered at the initial visit. (b) Dried blood spot (DBS) for HIV DNA PCR. DBS is highly portable and stable at room temperature, making it ideal for resource-limited settings where on-site virologic testing may not be available. Logistical arrangements must be made for rapid transmission of results to patients (e.g., via SMS messaging) if the DBS is sent to another laboratory. *Source*: J. Kim, Johns Hopkins University, Baltimore, USA. Reproduced with permission of J. Kim.

Table 18.2 WHO recommended testing approach for infants.

Category	Test required	Purpose	Action
Well, HIV-exposed infant	Virologic testing at 4–6 weeks of age	To diagnose HIV	Start ART if HIV-infected
Infant: unknown HIV exposure	Maternal HIV serologic test or infant HIV serologic test	To identify or confirm HIV exposure	Need virologic test if HIV-exposed
Well, HIV-exposed infant at 9 months	HIV serologic test (at last immunization, usually 9 months)	To identify infants who have persisting HIV antibody or who have seroreverted	Those HIV seropositive need virologic test and continued follow-up; those HIV negative, assume uninfected, repeat testing required if still breastfeeding
Infant or child with signs and symptoms suggestive of HIV infection	HIV serologic test	To confirm exposure	Perform virologic test if <18 months of age
Well or sick child seropositive >9 months and <18 months	Virologic testing	To diagnose HIV	Reactive: start HIV care and ART
Infant or child who has completely discontinued breastfeeding	Repeat testing 6 weeks or more after breastfeeding cessation: usually initial HIV serologic testing followed by virologic testing for HIV-positive child and <18 months of age	To exclude HIV infection after exposure cases	Infected infants and children <5 years of age need to start HIV care, including ART

Source: WHO (2013a), table 5.1, p. 74. Reproduced with permission of the World Health Organization.

younger than 5 years or 100 cells/mm^3 in persons older than 5 years (immunologic failure). When possible, a CD4 count should be checked at treatment initiation and followed every 6 months, and viral load should be checked 6 months after initiation of ART and every 12 months thereafter. When treatment failure is recognized, counseling to ensure strict ART adherence is performed first, and then, if possible, follow-up confirmatory testing with CD4 or viral load is conducted. Confirmed failure of first-line ART requires change to second-line ART regimens per national guidelines (WHO, 2013a) (Table 18.7).

Common HIV-associated conditions

Malnutrition

HIV is frequently associated with malnutrition because of a combination of decreased intake, increased loss of nutrients, and increased metabolic demand. Infection, fever, gastrointestinal illness, and poverty are common to both malnutrition and HIV/AIDS. Malnutrition impairs the already suppressed immune system of HIV-infected people, increasing the risk of opportunistic infections and mortality, and may be predictive of disease progression and other comorbidities. Monitoring

and treating nutritional needs in HIV-infected individuals is a critical aspect of care.

Tuberculosis

Tuberculosis is the most common presenting illness among people living with HIV. One-third of HIV-infected individuals are co-infected with tuberculosis. Tuberculosis is the leading cause of death among people living with HIV and accounts for one in four HIV-related deaths (WHO, 2013b).

All patients with tuberculosis should be offered HIV testing. An HIV-infected individual may not be capable of mounting an appropriate immunologic response, so a negative tuberculosis skin test does not rule out tuberculosis. Sputum-smear microscopy for acid-fast bacilli (AFB) is the simplest available diagnostic method and is the mainstay of tuberculosis diagnosis in resource-limited settings since culture isolation is difficult. It is a highly specific, fast, and inexpensive method; however, the sensitivity of sputum-smear microscopy is lower in patients co-infected with HIV so multiple specimens should be collected. HIV-infected patients, especially infants and children, are more likely to have extrapulmonary tuberculosis or smear-negative pulmonary tuberculosis; consequently, clinical presentation, together with suggestive radiography findings, are most

Table 18.3 HIV clinical staging conditions.

	Clinical staging events seen in all ages	Clinical staging events unique to infants/children (<15 years old)	Clinical staging events unique to adolescents and adults (≥15 years old)
Clinical stage 1	Asymptomatic Persistent generalized lymphadenopathy		
Clinical stage 2	Papular pruritic eruptions Fungal nail infection Angular cheilitis Herpes zoster Recurrent or chronic upper respiratory tract infections (otitis media, otorrhea, sinusitis, tonsillitis, or pharyngitis) Recurrent oral ulcerations	Unexplained persistent hepatosplenomegaly Linear gingival erythema Extensive wart virus infection Extensive molluscum contagiosum Unexplained persistent parotid enlargement	Moderate unexplained weight loss (<10% of presumed or measured body weight) Seborrheic dermatitis
Clinical stage 3	Unexplained persistent diarrhea (14 days in children or 1 month in adults) Unexplained persistent fever (>37.5°C intermittent or constant, for longer than 1 month) Persistent oral candidiasis (after first 6–8 weeks of life) Oral hairy leukoplakia Pulmonary tuberculosis (currently) Acute necrotizing ulcerative gingivitis or periodontitis	Unexplained moderate malnutrition or wasting not adequately responding to standard therapy Lymph node tuberculosis Severe recurrent bacterial pneumonia Symptomatic lymphoid interstitial pneumonitis Chronic HIV-associated lung disease including bronchiectasis Unexplained anemia (<8 g/dL), neutropenia (<1000/mm³), or thrombocytopenia (<50,000/mm³) for more than 1 month	Unexplained severe weight loss (>10% of presumed or measured body weight) Severe bacterial infections (e.g., pneumonia, empyema, pyomyositis, bone or joint infection, meningitis or bacteremia) Unexplained anemia (<8 g/dL), neutropenia (<500/mm³), or thrombocytopenia (<50,000/mm³) for more than 1 month
Clinical stage 4	*Pneumocystis* pneumonia Chronic herpes simplex infection (orolabial or cutaneous of more than 1-month duration or visceral at any site) Esophageal candidiasis (or candidiasis of trachea, bronchi, or lungs) Extrapulmonary tuberculosis Kaposi sarcoma Cytomegalovirus infection: retinitis or affecting another organ, with onset at age older than 1 month Central nervous system toxoplasmosis (after 1 month of life) HIV encephalopathy Extrapulmonary cryptococcosis Disseminated endemic mycosis (coccidiomycosis or histoplasmosis) Progressive multifocal leukoencephalopathy Symptomatic HIV-associated nephropathy or cardiomyopathy Chronic cryptosporidiosis (with diarrhea) Disseminated non-tuberculous mycobacterial infection Chronic isosporiasis	Unexplained severe wasting, stunting, or severe malnutrition not responding to standard therapy Recurrent severe bacterial infections (e.g., empyema, pyomyositis, bone or joint infection, or meningitis but excluding pneumonia) Cerebral or B-cell non-Hodgkin lymphoma	HIV-wasting syndrome Recurrent severe bacterial pneumonia Recurrent non-typhoidal *Salmonella* bacteremia Lymphoma (cerebral or B-cell non-Hodgkin) or other solid HIV-associated tumors Invasive cervical carcinoma Atypical disseminated leishmaniasis

Source: adapted from WHO (2007).

Table 18.4 Commonly used ARVs.

Drug	Class	Serious side effects
Abacavir (ABC)	NRTI	Hypersensitivity reaction may be fatal: if available, test patients for HLA B5701 allele prior to initiation
Didanosine (DDI)	NRTI	Peripheral neuropathy, lactic acidosis, pancreatitis
Emtricitabine (FTC)	NRTI	Minimal toxicity
Lamivudine (3TC)	NRTI	Minimal toxicity
Stavudine (d4T)	NRTI	Peripheral neuropathy, lactic acidosis, lipoatrophy, mitochondrial toxicity, pancreatitis
Tenofovir (TDF)	NRTI*	Proximal renal tubular dysfunction including Fanconi syndrome, decreased bone mineral density
Zidovudine (AZT)	NRTI	Bone marrow suppression (macrocytic anemia, neutropenia), lactic acidosis, hyperperlipidemia, insulin resistance, lipoatrophy
Efavirenz (EFV)	NNRTI	Rash, CNS symptoms (dizziness, insomnia, seizures), increased transaminases, potentially teratogenic
Nevirapine (NVP)	NNRTI	Rash (including Stevens–Johnson syndrome), hepatitis, severe systemic hypersensitivity syndrome
Atazanavir (ATV)	PI	Indirect hyperbilirubinemia, first-degree AV block, hyperglycemia, inreased transaminases, nephrolithiasis, fat maldistribution
Darunavir (DRV)	PI	Rash (including Stevens–Johnson syndrome and erythema multiforme), hepatotoxicity, diarrhea, hyperlipidemia, fat maldistribution
Lopinavir/ritonavir (LPV/r)	PI	Gastrointestinal intolerance, asthenia, hyperlipidemia, fat maldistribution, PR and QT prolongation, risk of cardiotoxicity in infants
Nelfinavir (NFV)	PI	Diarrhea, hyperlipidemia, hyperglycemia, fat maldistribution
Ritonavir (r)	PI	Gastrointestinal intolerance, paresthesias, hyperlipidemia, hepatitis, asthenia, hyperglycemia, fat maldistribution, toxic epidermal necrolysis and Stevens–Johnson syndrome

Note that this table does not include all licensed ARVs but ARVs recommended by the WHO for first- and second-line therapy.
NRTI, nucleoside reverse transcriptase inhibitor; NRTI*, nucleotide reverse transcriptase inhibitor; NNRTI, non-nucleoside reverse transcriptase inhibitor; PI, protease inhibitor.
Source: National Institutes of Health: Panel on Antiretroviral Therapy and Medical Management of HIV-Infected Children (2012) and WHO (2010a).

Table 18.5 First-line ART regimens for adults, adolescents, pregnant and breastfeeding women, and children.

First-line ART	Preferred first-line regimens	Alternative first-line regimens
Adults (including pregnant and breastfeeding women and adults with TB and HBV co-infection)	TDF + 3TC (or FTC) + EFV	AZT + 3TC + EFV AZT + 3TC + NVP TDF + 3TC (or FTC) + NVP
Adolescents (10–19 years) ≥35 kg	TDF + 3TC (or FTC) + EFV	AZT + 3TC + EFV AZT + 3TC + NVP TDF + 3TC (or FTC) + NVP ABC + 3TC + EFV (or NVP)
Children 3 years to <10 years and adolescents <35 kg	ABC + 3TC + EFV	ABC + 3TC + NVP AZT + 3TC + EFV AZT + 3TC + NVP TDF + 3TC (or FTC) + EFV TDF + 3TC (or FTC) + NVP
Children <3 years	ABC or ABC + 3TC + LPV/r	ABC + 3TC + NVP AZT + 3TC + NVP

See Table 18.4 for definition of drug abbreviations. HBV, Hepatitis B virus.
Source: WHO (2013a), table 7.5, p. 112. Reproduced with permission of the World Health Organization.

Table 18.6 WHO guidelines for initiation of ART for adults, adolescents, children, and infants.

Population	Recommendation
Adults and adolescents (≥10 years)	Initiate ART if CD4 cell count ≤500 cells/mm³ • **As a priority**, initiate ART in all individuals with severe/advanced HIV disease (WHO clinical stage 3 or 4) or CD4 count ≤300 cells/mm³ Initiate ART regardless of WHO clinical stage and CD4 cell count • Active tuberculosis • HBV co-infection with severe chronic liver disease • Pregnant and breastfeeding women with HIV • HIV-positive individual in a serodiscordant partnership (to reduce HIV transmission risk)
Children ≥5 years old	Initiate ART if CD4 cell count ≤500 cells/mm³ • **As a priority**, initiate ART in all children with severe/advanced HIV disease (WHO clinical stage 3 or 4) or CD4 count ≤350 cells/mm³ Initiate ART regardless of CD4 cell count • WHO clinical stage 3 or 4 • Active tuberculosis
Children 1–5 years old[a]	Initiate ART in all infants regardless of WHO clinical stage and CD4 cell count • **As a priority**, initiate ART in all HIV-infected children 1–2 years old or with severe/advanced HIV disease (WHO clinical stage 3 or 4) or with CD4 count ≤750 cells/mm³ or <25%, whichever is lower
Infants <1 year old[a]	Initiate ART in all infants regardless of WHO clinical stage and CD4 cell count

[a] Initiate ART in all HIV-infected children below 18 months of age with presumptive clinical diagnosis of HIV infection.
Source: WHO (2013a), table 7.1, p. 92. Reproduced with permission of the World Health Organization.

Table 18.7 WHO recommended second-line ART regimens.

Second-line ART			Preferred regimens	Alternative regimens
Adults and adolescents (≥10 years) including pregnant and breastfeeding women			AZT + 3TC + LPV/r AZT + 3TC + ATV/r	TDF + 3TC (or FTC) + ATV/r TDF + 3TC (or FTC) + LPV/r
Children	If NNRTI-based first-line regimen used		ABC + 3TC + LPV/r	ABC + 3TC + LPV/r TDF + 3TC (or FTC) + LPV/r
	If PI-based first-line regimen used	<3 years	No change from first-line regimen use	AZT (or ABC) + 3TC + NVP
		3 years to <10 years	AZT (or ABC) + 3TC + EFV	ABC (or TDF) + 3TC + NVP

Source: WHO (2013a), table 7.17, p. 146. Reproduced with permission of the World Health Organization.

often used as criteria in diagnostic decisions. When a child is diagnosed with tuberculosis, efforts should be made to treat the source case (usually an AFB smear-positive adult). Principles of treating tuberculosis in HIV-infected patients are the same as in uninfected individuals, although strict attention to drug interactions is needed as many tuberculosis medications interact with ARVs, particularly rifampin with non-nucleoside reverse transcriptase inhibitors or protease inhibitors.

The WHO recommends starting ART in all HIV-infected individuals with active tuberculosis, regardless of CD4 count. Current recommendations advise starting ART as soon as possible, usually after at least 2 weeks but within 8 weeks of initiating antituberculosis medications (WHO, 2013b) (see Chapter 19). Recommendations regarding tuberculosis treatment with ART can be complex, and care providers are encouraged to consult local guidelines.

Pneumocystis pneumonia

Pneumocystis jirovecii is a parasite that can cause severe *Pneumocystis* pneumonia (PCP) in individuals with HIV/AIDS. PCP usually presents with cough, tachypnea, and shortness of breath. Lung examination may be normal, although patients are typically hypoxic and chest radiography may be remarkable for bilateral interstitial infiltrates (Figure 18.5). PCP is often the first AIDS-defining illness in children. PCP is best treated with trimethoprim–sulfamethoxazole, also known as co-trimoxazole. HIV-exposed infants should begin co-trimoxazole prophylaxis therapy (CPT) at 4–6 weeks of age until the risk of HIV transmission ends and the diagnosis of HIV has been definitively ruled out. All HIV-infected infants should take CPT until 5 years of age regardless of clinical symptoms or CD4 count. HIV-infected children over 5 years and adults should start CPT if symptomatic (WHO clinical stage 2, 3, or 4) or CD4 count below 350 cells/mm³. In settings with high HIV prevalence and infant mortality, all HIV-infected individuals should start on CPT regardless of CD4 or clinical stage (WHO, 2013a). Consult country-specific guidelines.

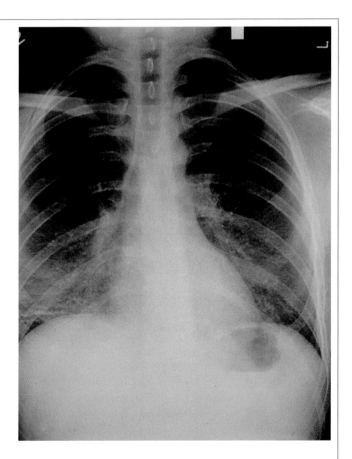

Figure 18.5 Chest radiograph in a patient with *Pneumocystis* pneumonia, showing bilateral interstitial infiltrates. *Source*: CDC Public Health Image Libary/Jonathan W.M. Gold.

Prevention

Prevention of mother-to-child transmission

HIV can be transmitted from an infected mother to a newborn during pregnancy, at birth, or through breast milk. Prevention of mother-to-child transmission (PMTCT) is possible, and broad prevention strategies have been very successful, making cases of new pediatric HIV/AIDS very rare in high-income countries. Significant strides have also been made to scale up PMTCT in high-burden, low- and middle-income countries. PMTCT strategies require significant coordination of care across many different sectors of the healthcare system from pregnancy through the first 2 years of life of the child. Promotion of the health of both the mother and child should be prioritized.

The WHO has released PMTCT guidelines in resource-limited settings, the implementation of which can decrease maternal-to-child transmission rates to less than 5% from an estimated baseline risk of 35% in a breastfeeding population (WHO, 2010b).

The latest WHO guidelines recommend that all HIV-infected pregnant and/or breastfeeding women initiate ART regardless of clinical stage or CD4 count and newborns should be started on once-daily nevirapine for 6 weeks while exposed through breast milk (WHO, 2013a). The decision to maintain women on lifelong ART after the cessation of breastfeeding may depend on individual eligibility for treatment (if CD4 count ≤500 cells/mm³ or clinical stage 3 or 4) per national guidelines, yet many advocate for lifelong ART for women even after cessation of breastfeeding.

Infant feeding

Despite the well-understood risks of HIV transmission through breast milk, exclusive breastfeeding for the first 6 months of life is recommended for all infants in resource-limited settings, with continuation of breastfeeding up to at least 12 months of age for HIV-exposed infants. Complementary feeding with age-appropriate food can be introduced at 6 months of age while breastfeeding continues. Breastfeeding should stop only once a nutritionally adequate and safe diet can be provided without breast milk. Studies have shown that replacement feeding (use of formula) increases the mortality risks associated with malnutrition and diarrheal illness and outweighs the potential benefits of decreased HIV transmission (Coutsoudis *et al.*, 2001; Iliff *et al.*, 2005). Mixed feeding – providing formula or any other food in addition to breast milk in infants less than 6 months of age – is strongly discouraged as it increases both mortality and rates of HIV transmission.

Prevention of sexual transmission

Efforts to prevent horizontal HIV transmission among sexual partners are multifaceted and include both biomedical and behavioral interventions.

Condoms

Correct and consistent use of male condoms reduce the risk of heterosexual transmission by 80% and offer 64% protection in anal intercourse for MSM (Weller & Davis-Beaty, 2009). Condom use is particularly important as co-infection with other sexually transmitted infections (STIs) increases the risk of HIV transmission. Unfortunately, young people, who are among the highest risk groups, often have limited access to accurate information and tools for HIV prevention, including condoms, HIV and STI testing, and healthcare services.

Medical male circumcision

Male circumcision, the surgical removal of the foreskin of the penis, is an evidence-based strategy that partially reduces the risk of sexual HIV acquisition by 66% in men (Siegfried *et al.*, 2009). Programs to provide adult men with voluntary circumcision are becoming routine components of HIV prevention programs in high-burden countries of southern and eastern Africa.

Discordant couples

Discordant couples, in which one person is HIV-infected and one is HIV-uninfected, are common. Strategies to decrease transmission between discordant couples include counseling services that support knowledge of HIV status, consistent and correct condom use, and treatment of eligible HIV-infected partners since ART of an infected partner decreases transmission to an uninfected partner (Gray *et al.*, 2001; Cohen *et al.*, 2011; WHO, 2013a).

Pre-exposure prophylaxis

Pre-exposure prophylaxis is a new HIV prevention method in which HIV-uninfected people at high risk of becoming HIV-infected (discordant couples, commercial sex workers, MSM) take a daily pill to reduce their risk of becoming infected. Efficacy studies have demonstrated that a once-daily pill containing tenofovir and emtricitabine was safe and provided additional protection against HIV infection among MSM and heterosexual couples when provided with comprehensive care (Peterson *et al.*, 2007; Grant *et al.*, 2010; Baeten *et al.*, 2012; Thigpen *et al.*, 2012; Van Damme *et al.*, 2012). The WHO offers guidance and recommendations for daily oral pre-exposure prophylaxis (WHO, 2012b).

Post-exposure prophylaxis

Post-exposure prophylaxis (PEP) refers to the medical treatment provided after exposure to prevent infection by a blood-borne pathogen, such as hepatitis or HIV.

Occupational exposures occur in healthcare settings with needlesticks or body fluid splash but may also occur among law enforcement workers, emergency rescue services, or waste collectors. PEP is the only way to prevent transmission of HIV

after exposure has occurred. The efficacy of PEP has been demonstrated (Cardo *et al.*, 1997) and generally includes combination ART. However, PEP is not 100% effective, and primary prevention with standard precautions and safe injection procedures are critical.

After an occupational exposure, assess HIV transmission risk and administer the first dose of PEP within 72 hours of exposure. Baseline HIV testing should be performed but should not delay starting PEP. PEP is continued for 28 days, with strict adherence and with follow-up HIV testing at 3 and 6 months.

In the setting of sexual assault, PEP should be included in the comprehensive services provided to victims, which may include preventive treatment for other STIs, pregnancy prevention, counseling, and support services. The risk of HIV transmission with sexual assault may be higher than with consensual sex.

Community-based approach to HIV prevention and care

Community-based interventions are an integral element in preventing HIV and improving access to care. Community mobilization programs can increase knowledge about HIV and provide improved access to testing, prevention, and care services. Community-based care, including home-based testing, community follow-up, and home-based palliative care services, provides support for hospital-based services. Programs to engage influential members of the community, including village chiefs, church leaders, traditional healers, teachers, schools, and traditional birth attendants, are an important component in the response to HIV.

Stigma and discrimination

Stigma and discrimination toward people living with HIV remains common and discourages people from seeking HIV

Clinical experience

"The health aspect of my work with migrant populations in Israel remains integrally intertwined with their daily struggle to forge a new life in their host country. While we as global health practitioners may see hoards of HIV and TB cases, it is the social determinants of health that take precedence when attempting to improve their lives. The challenging pursuit of employment and social and political inclusion as well as the battle against racism and xenophobia manifests in poor access to quality living conditions, medical care, and public health education. This context is critical to formulating an approach and producing quality services to improve health and well-being."

Jonah, physician working in Israel

testing services and complicates adherence to treatment. Community-wide efforts to educate people about HIV aim to decrease fear, stigma, and discrimination and are critical to prevention efforts and to the quality of life for people and communities living with HIV.

Additional resources

Manuals and e-books

- World Health Organization (2013) Consolidated guidelines on the use of antiretroviral drugs for treating and preventing HIV infection: recommendations for a public health approach. http://issuu.com/whohivaids/docs/who_consolidated_guidelines_full_ju/1?e=8844348/4087885
- World Health Organization (2013) *Pocket Book of Hospital Care for Children*, 2nd edn. http://who.int/maternal_child_adolescent/documents/child_hospital_care/en/index.html
- HIV Curriculum for the Health Care Provider, Baylor College of Medicine International Pediatric HIV Initiative, 4th edn. http://bipai.org/HIV-curriculum/

Websites

- Partners in Health Knowledge Center: http://www.pih.org/knowledge-center
- Columbia ICAP HIV resources: http://icap.columbia.edu/resources/
- Johns Hopkins HIV resources: http://main.ccghe.net/CCG/resources/HIV-AIDS_Resources
- Women, Children, and HIV. UCSF Center for HIV information: http://www.womenchildrenhiv.org/
- AIDS Images Library: searchable free online library of AIDS-related images, illustrations, and tables for medical professionals organized by disease. Available at http://www.aids-images.ch/

Mobile resources

- AIDSinfo from the NIH: http://www.aidsinfo.nih.gov/mobile-resources

Scientific articles and country specific guidelines

- UCSF care of HIV in the developing world: http://www.hivinsite.com/InSite?page=kbr-03-01-17 http://www.hivinsite.com/global?page=cr-00-04

REFERENCES

Andersson S, Norrgren H, da Silva Z et al. (2000) Plasma viral load in HIV-1 and HIV-2 singly and dually infected individuals in Guinea-Bissau, West Africa: Significantly lower plasma virus set point in HIV-2 infection than in HIV-1 infections. *Arch Intern Med* 160:3286–93.

Baeten JM, Donnell D, Ndase P et al. (2012) Antiretroviral prophylaxis for HIV prevention in heterosexual men and women. *N Engl J Med* 367:399–410.

Campbell-Yesufu OT, Gandhi RT (2011) Update on human immunodeficiency virus (HIV)-2 infection. *Clin Infect Dis* 52:780–7.

Cardo DM, Culver DH, Ciesielski CA et al. (1997) A case-control study of HIV seroconversion in health care workers after percutaneous exposure. *N Engl J Med* 337:1485–90.

Cohen MS, Chen YQ, McCauley M et al. (2011) Prevention of HIV-1 infection with early antiretroviral therapy. *N Engl J Med* 365:493–505.

Colvin M, Dawood S, Kleinschmidt I, Mullick S, Lallo U (2001) Prevalence of HIV and HIV-related diseases in the adult medical wards of a tertiary hospital in Durban, South Africa. *Int J STD AIDS* 12:386–9.

Corbett EL, Watt CJ, Walker N et al. (2003) The growing burden of tuberculosis: global trends and interactions with the HIV epidemic. *Arch Intern Med* 163:1009–21.

Coutsoudis A, Pillay K, Kuhn L et al. (2001) Method of feeding and transmission of HIV-1 from mothers to children by 15 months of age: prospective cohort study from Durban, South Africa. *AIDS* 15:379–87.

Grant RM, Lama JR, Anderson PL et al. (2010) Preexposure chemoprophylaxis for HIV prevention in men who have sex with men. *N Engl J Med* 363:2587–99.

Gray RH, Wawer MJ, Brookmeyer R et al. (2001) Probability of HIV-1 transmission per coital act in monogamous, heterosexual, HIV-1-discordant couples in Rakai, Uganda. *Lancet* 357:1149–53.

Iliff PJ, Piwoz EG, Tavengwa NV et al. (2005) Early exclusive breastfeeding reduces HIV-transmission and increases HIV-free survival. *AIDS* 19:699–708.

Marlink R, Kanki P, Thior I et al. (1994) Reduced rate of disease development after HIV-2 infection as compared to HIV-1. *Science* 265:1587–90.

National Institutes of Health: Panel on Antiretroviral Therapy and Medical Management of HIV-Infected Children (2012) Guidelines for the use of antiretroviral agents in pediatric HIV infection. Available at http://aidsinfo.nih.gov/contentfiles/lvguidelines/pediatricguidelines.pdf

Pantaleo G, Graziosi C, Fauci AS (1993) New concepts in the immunopathogenesis of human immunodeficiency virus infection. *N Engl J Med* 328:327–35.

Peterson L, Taylor D, Roddy R *et al.* (2007) Tenofovir disoproxil fumarate for prevention of HIV infection in women: a phase 2, double-blind, randomized, placebo-controlled trial. *PLoS Clin Trials* 2(5):e27.

Rouet F, Sakarovitch C, Msellati P *et al.* (2003) Pediatric viral human immunodeficiency virus Type 1 RNA levels, timing of infection, and disease progression in African HIV-1-infected children. *Pediatrics* 112:e289.

Siegfried N, Muller M, Deeks JJ, Volmink J (2009) Male circumcision for prevention of heterosexual acquisition of HIV in men. *Cochrane Database Syst Rev* (2):CD003362.

Thigpen MC, Kebaabetswe PM, Paxton LA *et al.* (2012) Antiretroviral preexposure prophylaxis for heterosexual HIV transmission in Botswana. *N Engl J Med* 367:423–34.

Tuaillon E, Gueudin M, Lemée V *et al.* (2004) Phenotypic susceptibility to nonnucleoside inhibitors of virion-associated reverse transcriptase from different HIV types and groups. *J Acquir Immune Defic Syndr* 37:1543–449.

Van Damme L, Corneli A, Ahmed K *et al.* (2012) Preexposure prophylaxis for HIV infection among African women. *N Engl J Med* 367:411–22.

Weller S, Davis-Beaty K (2009) Condom effectiveness in reducing heterosexual HIV transmission. *Cochrane Database Syst Rev* (1):CD003255.

Whitescarter J, Miotti P, Bazin B *et al.* (2008) KIDS-ART-LINC Collaboration. Low risk of death, but substantial program attrition, in pediatric HIV treatment cohorts in Sub-Saharan Africa. *J Acquir Immune Defic Syndr* 49:523–31.

WHO (2007) WHO Case Definitions of HIV for Surveillance and Revised Clinical Staging and Immunological Classification of HIV-Related Disease in Adults and Children. Geneva: World Health Organization.

WHO (2010a) Antiretroviral Therapy of HIV Infection in Infants and Children: Towards Universal Access: Recommendations for a Public Health Approach, 2010 Revision. Geneva: World Health Organization.

WHO (2010b) Antiretroviral Drugs for Treating Pregnant Women and Preventing HIV Infection in Infants: Foundations for a Public Health Approach, 2010 Revision. Geneva: World Health Organization.

WHO (2012a) Global fact sheet: World AIDS Day 2012. http://www.unaids.org/en/media/unaids/contentassets/documents/epidemiology/2012/gr2012/20121120_FactSheet_Global_en.pdf

WHO (2012b) Guidance on pre-exposure oral prophylaxis (PrEP) for serodiscordant couples, men and transgender women who have sex with men at high risk of HIV: recommendations for use in the context of demonstrative projects. http://apps.who.int/iris/bitstream/10665/75188/1/9789241503884_eng.pdf

WHO (2013a) Consolidated guidelines on the use of antiretroviral drugs for treating and preventing HIV infection: recommendations for a public health approach. Available at http://apps.who.int/iris/bitstream/10665/85321/1/9789241505727_eng.pdf

WHO (2013b) TB/HIV facts, 2012–2013. http://www.who.int/hiv/topics/tb/tbhiv_facts_2013/en/index.html

WHO (2013c) Global Health Observatory (GHO). Available at http://www.who.int/gho/hiv/en/

CHAPTER 19
Tuberculosis

Paul K. Drain
Massachusetts General Hospital and Harvard Medical School, Boston, MA, USA

Key learning objectives

- Understand the epidemiology and clinical manifestations of tuberculosis.
- Understand the diagnosis of latent and active tuberculosis, especially among HIV-infected individuals.
- Learn the treatment of latent and active tuberculosis in resource-limited settings.

Abstract

Tuberculosis has been a scourge of humankind for thousands of years (Box 19.1), but the global incidence of disease has been declining since 2004. Tuberculosis incidence remains highest in sub-Saharan Africa, Eastern Europe, and regions of Latin America. Most people who acquire tuberculosis will not develop symptoms or active disease, and HIV-infected people have greater risk for developing active tuberculosis. The classic clinical features of active pulmonary tuberculosis include chronic cough, fever, weight loss, and night sweats, but symptoms may not be present in all patients. Active tuberculosis is often diagnosed on clinical suspicion alone, and sputum-smear microscopy, mycobacterial culture, and the new Xpert MTB/RIF assay can be helpful. Standard treatment for drug-susceptible tuberculosis is a combination of four medications for at least 6 months. Patients with drug-resistant tuberculosis and HIV-infected individuals require unique treatment strategies. The BCG vaccine is administered in most resource-limited settings and has some efficacy in preventing miliary disease and tuberculosis meningitis among children. Large-scale global efforts aim to reduce tuberculosis mortality by investing in better diagnostic technologies, new medications, and a more efficacious vaccine.

Key words: tuberculosis, latent tuberculosis, active tuberculosis, pulmonary tuberculosis, multidrug-resistant tuberculosis, extremely drug-resistant tuberculosis, HIV/AIDS, diagnosis, treatment, prevention

Essential Clinical Global Health, First Edition. Edited by Brett D. Nelson.
© 2015 John Wiley & Sons, Ltd. Published 2015 by John Wiley & Sons, Ltd.
Companion website: www.essentialseries.com/globalhealth

Introduction and epidemiology

Despite the availability of effective medications, there are nearly 9 million new cases of active tuberculosis and 1.4 million tuberculosis-related deaths each year (World Health Organization, 2012a). After decades of worsening tuberculosis rates, the World Health Organization (WHO) estimates that tuberculosis incidence likely peaked in 2004 and has decreased at less than 1% per year ever since. Although this positive turn in the tuberculosis epidemic has sparked optimism, the current rate of decline will not come close to reaching a target of eliminating tuberculosis by the year 2050 (Lawn & Zumla, 2011).

The global distribution of tuberculosis is primarily concentrated in low- and middle-income countries (Figure 19.1). Twenty-two countries account for more than 80% of the cases of active tuberculosis in the world. Sub-Saharan Africa has the highest rate of tuberculosis per capita (262 new cases per 100,000 per year), which is driven in part by the HIV epidemic (World Health Organization, 2012a). The five countries with the highest incidence of tuberculosis are India, China, South Africa, Nigeria, and Indonesia. India and China have the highest absolute number of cases. In the United States and western European countries, the majority of cases occur in foreign-born residents and recent immigrants from tuberculosis-endemic countries.

The HIV/AIDS epidemic has had a profound impact on tuberculosis. About 13% of the cases of active tuberculosis worldwide involve co-infection with HIV (World Health Organization, 2012a). In some countries, such as South Africa, Swaziland, and Lesotho, roughly 60–70% of new tuberculosis infections are co-infected with HIV. Tuberculosis leads to an increase in HIV replication and accelerated progression of disease, and therefore HIV-infected people also have higher rates of death from tuberculosis compared with HIV-uninfected people. While immunocompetent individuals have a 10% lifetime risk of tuberculosis activation, HIV-infected individuals have a 10% annual risk of tuberculosis activation. Roughly 31% of the total annual tuberculosis deaths (or 430,000 deaths) occur among HIV-infected people, and an outbreak of a highly fatal drug-resistant strain of tuberculosis has been reported among HIV-infected persons in South Africa (Gandhi et al., 2006).

Box 19.1 Brief history of tuberculosis

The oldest tuberculosis bacilli were recovered from Egyptian mummies dating back to 2400 BCE. Around 460 BCE, Hippocrates described "phthisis," or consumption, as the most widespread disease of the times. During the 19th century, tuberculosis accounted for up to 25% of all deaths in Europe. In 1882, Robert Koch presented his discovery of the infectious cause of tuberculosis at the Berlin Physiological Society on March 24, a date that now marks World Tuberculosis Day. The first antibiotic for tuberculosis (streptomycin) was developed in 1943.

Pathogenesis

The *Mycobacterium tuberculosis* complex of organisms, all of which can cause human disease, consists of *M. tuberculosis, M. africanum, M. bovis, M. microti,* and *M. canetti. Mycobacterium tuberculosis* is an intracellular, aerobic, acid-fast, non-spore-forming bacillus. Despite popular belief, *M. tuberculosis* is not as highly contagious as the seasonal influenza virus, nor is tuberculosis likely to cause an active infection among those who become infected. The pathogen is almost always acquired

through the inhalation of small respiratory droplets that have been aerosolized from the cough of a tuberculosis-infected person (Figure 19.2). In more than 90% of persons with acute pulmonary infection, *M. tuberculosis* does not cause tissue damage or symptoms of disease. Thus, the vast majority of people who inhale tuberculosis will either eliminate or contain *M. tuberculosis* and not develop active disease.

Containment of *M. tuberculosis* infection will result in latent tuberculosis, a clinical condition in which the host immune system retains sufficient control over bacterial replication such that the individual does not develop signs or symptoms of disease. An estimated 2–3 billion people worldwide are believed to have latent infection, and they are at risk for reactivation of tuberculosis. Roughly 10% of latent tuberculosis infections will reactivate to become an active infection, which produces signs and symptoms of disease. The risk of reactivation is approximately 5% in the first 18 months after initial infection, and 5% for the person's remaining lifetime. Reactivation of tuberculosis typically occurs within the lungs, but it can appear at almost any site or organ in the body. Knowledge of the interaction between the host and latent tuberculosis is limited, and much research is focused on developing a better understanding of the protective immune responses to tuberculosis infections.

Cell-mediated immunity, primarily T lymphocytes and macrophages, plays a dominant role in the protective

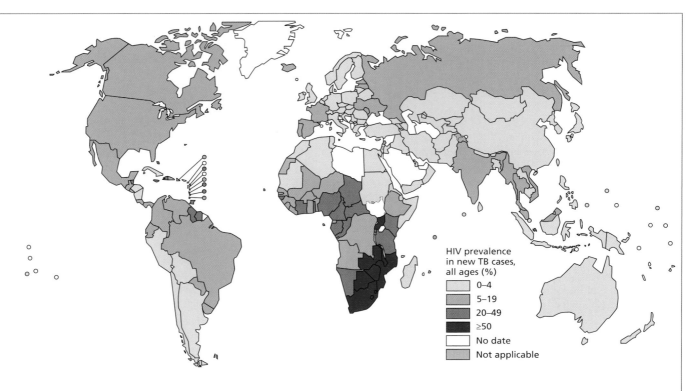

Figure 19.1 Estimated HIV prevalence in new tuberculosis cases, 2012. *Source*: World Health Organization (2013), figure 2.4, p. 14. Reproduced with permission of the World Health Organization.

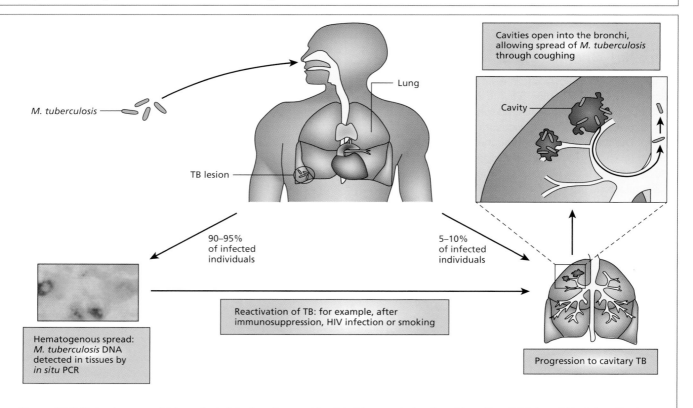

Figure 19.2 Natural course of tuberculosis infection. Source: Reprinted by permission from Macmillan Publishers Ltd: *Nature Reviews Immunology* 2005;5:661–67.

immunity to *M. tuberculosis*. Among people with an impaired immune system, such as people living with HIV/AIDS, granulomas are generally either absent or poorly formed. HIV causes both a functional and absolute depletion of CD4 T lymphocytes and cytokine production. As a result, people living with HIV generally have uncontrolled *M. tuberculosis* replication with little evidence of a host cellular response. The diminished host cellular response is the primary reason why HIV-infected people are 20–30 times more likely to have reactivation from a latent to an active tuberculosis infection.

Drug resistance

Drug-resistant tuberculosis has become a global problem. Recent estimates suggest that over 300,000 incident cases of multidrug-resistant tuberculosis (MDR-TB), defined as organisms resistant to at least isoniazid and rifampin, occur each year worldwide (World Health Organization, 2012a). MDR-TB cases occur in 4% of all new cases of active tuberculosis and in 20% of people diagnosed with a previously treated case of active tuberculosis. More than half of MDR-TB cases occur in five countries: China, India, the Russian Federation, Pakistan, and South Africa (Zignol *et al.*, 2012).

In recent years, there has been an emergence of extensively drug-resistant tuberculosis (XDR-TB). XDR-TB is resistant to both isoniazid and rifampin, as with MDR-TB, but is also resistant to fluoroquinolones (e.g., moxifloxacin, levofloxacin) and at least one injectable agent (e.g., amikacin, capreomycin, or kanamycin) (World Health Organization, 2011a). At least 84 countries have reported a case of XDR-TB. Recent reports have suggested the detection of totally drug-resistant tuberculosis, in which the strain is resistant to all known antituberculosis medications. Although a WHO-commissioned independent review found these strains to be more similar to XDR-TB than to a new totally drug-resistant strain, they may be a preview of future problems (World Health Organization, 2012b).

Drug-resistant strains of *M. tuberculosis* arise from spontaneous chromosomal mutations at a low frequency. Selection pressure caused by the misuse of antituberculosis drugs, such as monotherapy, results in the emergence of resistant mutations and drug-resistant organisms. This is called acquired resistance. The transmission of drug-resistant strains to another person, called primary resistance, can then result in infection and disease with MDR-TB and XDR-TB. The failure to promptly detect drug-resistant strains of tuberculosis can result in the prescribing of inappropriate regimens, treatment failures, increased mortality, and the emergence of more drug-resistant strains of tuberculosis.

Clinical presentation

The clinical features of active tuberculosis depend on the site of infection, and the lungs are the most common site for an

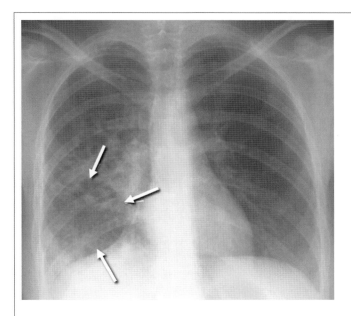

Figure 19.3 Chest radiograph showing a cavitary lesion in the right lower lobe from tuberculosis. *Source*: CDC Core Curriculum on Tuberculosis.

active infection (Figure 19.3). The classic clinical features of pulmonary tuberculosis include chronic cough ($\geq$3 weeks), fever, weight loss, and night sweats (Lawn & Zumla, 2011). Unlike most other bacterial infections, these symptoms occur gradually over a course of weeks to months due to the slow-growing nature of *M. tuberculosis*. A small minority of patients (10%) with active tuberculosis do not have any symptoms. The primary clinical risk factors for developing active pulmonary tuberculosis include poor nutrition, diabetes, smoking, alcohol, male gender, end-stage renal failure, malignancy, immunodeficiency, and living in an overcrowded area (Lawn & Zumla, 2011).

Extrapulmonary tuberculosis occurs in roughly 10–42% of patients with active tuberculosis infections, depending on ethnic background, age, comorbidities, genotype of the tuberculosis strain, and immune status (Caws *et al.*, 2008). The clinical features of extrapulmonary tuberculosis depend on the organ(s) infected. Common extrapulmonary sites include the pericardial sac (TB pericarditis), peritoneal lining (TB peritonitis), brain and meninges (TB meningitis), lumbar spine (Pott disease), and lymph nodes (TB lymphadenitis). TB pericarditis leads to signs and symptoms similar to heart failure, including dyspnea on exertion, distended neck veins, and presence of a pericardial effusion. TB meningitis causes headaches, altered mental status, and a lymphocyte-predominant leukocytosis in cerebrospinal fluid analysis. Additional sites may include the liver (TB hepatitis), as well as skin and soft tissue.

HIV co-infection may cause an atypical presentation of active tuberculosis. At CD4 T-cell counts below 200/mm^3

(Gandhi *et al.*, 2006), the presentation of pulmonary tuberculosis may include small pulmonary infiltrates, pleural effusions, or hilar lymphadenopathy. In contrast to immunocompetent patients, up to 50% of HIV-infected immunocompromised patients may have extrapulmonary manifestations. At CD4 T-cell counts below $100/mm^3$ (Gandhi *et al.*, 2006), there may be no radiographic changes on chest radiography, pulmonary findings may be absent, and tuberculosis may present as a disseminated infection with a non-specific chronic febrile illness.

🔍 Clinical pearl

Febrile illness in an HIV-infected immunocompromised patient should prompt consideration of active tuberculosis.

Tuberculosis-related immune reconstitution inflammatory syndrome (TB-IRIS) is an inflammatory reaction to tuberculosis antigens by the host immune system while receiving antiretroviral therapy (ART) for HIV. TB-IRIS occurs in at least 10% of HIV-infected patients who start ART in tuberculosis-endemic regions. TB-IRIS is most common among people with a CD4 T-cell nadir below $50 \, cells/mm^3$ (Gandhi *et al.*, 2006) but can occur at any CD4 T-cell count. TB-IRIS may occur from a previously undiagnosed tuberculosis infection, called "unmasking IRIS," or from a clinical worsening of existing tuberculosis while receiving antituberculosis medications, called "paradoxical IRIS." The common manifestations of TB-IRIS are worsening respiratory symptoms and increased lymphadenopathy. TB-IRIS can occur any time after the start of ART for HIV, but typically occurs within the initial 6 months of treatment.

Diagnosis

Latent tuberculosis

The Mantoux test, or tuberculin skin test, was developed in 1908 and has remained the mainstay of testing for latent tuberculosis infection. In this test, a small amount of purified protein derivative (PPD), obtained from *M. tuberculosis*, is injected intradermally into the forearm (Figure 19.4). People previously exposed to tuberculosis will mount an immune response to the mycobacterial proteins at the site of injection. The test result is read by measuring in millimeters the diameter of induration (palpable raised, hardened area), not erythema, 48–72 hours after inoculation (Figure 19.5). An interpretation of the test result is shown in Table 19.1.

A newer test for latent tuberculosis is the interferon-gamma release assay (IGRA) (Horsburgh & Rubin, 2011). IGRAs measure cytokine release when immune cells are exposed to tuberculosis antigens. IGRAs are as sensitive as the tuberculin skin test but have fewer false-positive results (McNerney *et al.*, 2012). There are advantages and disadvantages to both the Mantoux test and IGRAs. Although the Mantoux test requires

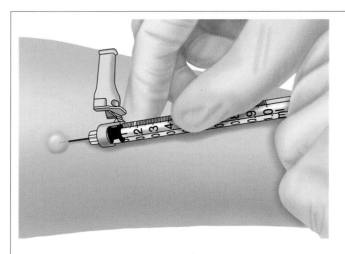

Figure 19.4 Placing a Mantoux test involves intradermally injecting a small amount of purified protein derivative obtained from *M. tuberculosis*. *Source*: CDC Core Curriculum on Tuberculosis.

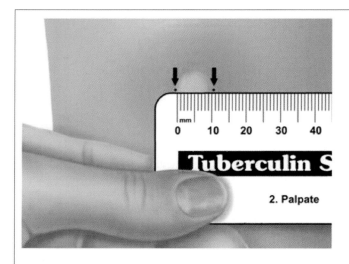

Figure 19.5 Interpreting a Mantoux test by measuring the diameter in millimeters of any induration (raised hardened area), but not the area of erythema. *Source*: CDC Core Curriculum on Tuberculosis.

a repeat visit, it is less expensive than IGRAs and is therefore preferred in resource-limited settings. However, since neither test is ideal, they are both underutilized in most tuberculosis-endemic regions.

Active tuberculosis

Sputum-smear microscopy for acid-fast bacilli (Figure 19.6) and culture in liquid medium with subsequent drug-susceptibility testing are recommended for diagnosing active

Table 19.1 Interpretation of the tuberculin skin test (TST).

TST induration	Considered positive in:
≥5 mm	Recent contact with an active TB case HIV-infected people Transplant recipients People with chronic liver or renal failure Persons receiving TNF-α inhibitors or who are otherwise immunosuppressed
≥10 mm	Foreign-born persons from high TB-endemic region Laboratory or health personnel Intravenous drug user Staff or residents of high congregate settings (e.g., nursing homes, prisons) Children <5 years old with active TB case in the family
≥15 mm	All people

TNF, tumor necrosis factor.
Source: adapted from Zumla *et al.* (2013).

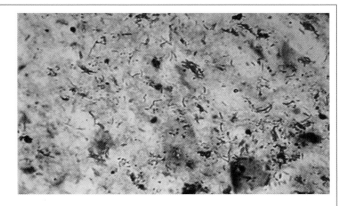

Figure 19.6 Acid-fast bacilli (stained red) on smear microscopy.
Source: CDC Core Curriculum on Tuberculosis.

tuberculosis. In children less than 5 years old, a gastric aspirate should be obtained in place of sputum. The use of solid culture medium, which can take weeks longer than using liquid medium, is less expensive and often used in resource-limited settings. However, liquid and solid culture methods are both time- and labor-intensive and therefore are not accessible to all clinics in tuberculosis-endemic regions (Keeler *et al.*, 2006). In sub-Saharan Africa, roughly 50% of clinics have access to a laboratory capable of performing sputum culture for tuberculosis (Saito *et al.*, 2012). Diagnostic testing for extrapulmonary tuberculosis may include fine needle aspiration or biopsy but depends on the location of the suspected infection. The

Mantoux test and IGRAs have no role in diagnosing active tuberculosis infections because they are negative in approximately 30% of active tuberculosis cases and do not distinguish between latent and active infections.

Additional diagnostics that overcome some of the limitations of previous testing are becoming available. The Xpert MTB/RIF assay is a new molecular diagnostic test that can detect pulmonary tuberculosis within 2 hours of sputum sample collection, is more sensitive than smear microscopy for acid-fast bacilli, and provides information on rifampin resistance, a marker of MDR-TB (Boehme *et al.*, 2010). The assay represents a substantial advancement in tuberculosis diagnostics, has been endorsed by the WHO, and will be introduced in over 20 tuberculosis-endemic countries within the next several years (World Health Organization, 2011b). However, the assay's high costs, operator time, and reliance on electricity may render it impractical for use at the clinical point-of-care in many resource-limited settings (Boehme *et al.*, 2011). The WHO still identifies research and development of novel rapid diagnostics as a research priority, and several new diagnostic modalities are anticipated in the coming years (World Health Organization, 2010a; Stop TB Partnership, 2011).

In the setting of increasing drug resistance, susceptibility testing is critical. Drug-susceptibility testing is generally performed with an automated liquid culture system, which requires 4–13 days for results. Newer molecular line-probe assays can yield drug-susceptibility results within 24 hours. Even if the Xpert MTB/RIF assay is performed, the WHO recommends standard drug-susceptibility testing to confirm rifampin resistance and susceptibility to other antituberculosis medications (World Health Organization, 2011b). Unfortunately, drug-susceptibility testing is not available in many tuberculosis-endemic countries. Consequently, only 10% of MDR-TB cases are being diagnosed worldwide, and just half of those are receiving appropriate treatment (World Health Organization, 2011a, 2012a).

Since 25% of newly diagnosed HIV-infected patients in tuberculosis-endemic regions have undiagnosed active tuberculosis, all HIV-infected patients should be screened for tuberculosis (Lawn & Zumla, 2011). Among HIV-infected patients, sputum-smear microscopy for acid-fast bacilli and chest radiography commonly provide false-negative results. A high index of clinical suspicion in a tuberculosis-endemic region must be maintained, and use of a clinical algorithm for signs and symptoms is sufficient to make the diagnosis (Cain *et al.*, 2010). Presence of a cough lasting 2–3 weeks has a diagnostic sensitivity of less than 50% for active tuberculosis (Getahun *et al.*, 2011). Screening for any of cough, fever, night sweats, or weight loss has a sensitivity of 79% and specificity of 50%, which should prompt a clinician to pursue additional tests for tuberculosis (World Health Organization, 2010b). Conversely, the absence of cough, fever, night sweats, and weight loss has a high negative predictive value for excluding active tuberculosis, and WHO guidelines recommend this screening method to exclude active tuberculosis among people living with HIV in resource-limited settings.

Treatment

Latent tuberculosis

Persons identified with a latent tuberculosis infection are at risk for reactivation and require preventive treatment. The preferred regimen is isoniazid alone for 9 months, which is about 70–90% effective for preventing conversion to active tuberculosis. Persons taking isoniazid should minimize alcohol intake to prevent hepatotoxicity. A recent study has shown that weekly administration of isoniazid and rifapentine for 12 weeks, which was directly observed in a clinic, was as effective as daily self-dosing of isoniazid for 9 months among HIV-uninfected adults (Sterling *et al.*, 2011).

HIV-infected people with a latent tuberculosis infection may benefit from a longer duration of isoniazid prophylaxis. However, the WHO recommends daily isoniazid therapy for at least 6 months for all newly diagnosed HIV-infected adults without active tuberculosis in a tuberculosis-endemic region, regardless of testing for a latent tuberculosis infection. Since a benefit has only been shown among patients with a positive Mantoux test, and clinicians lack confidence in existing diagnostic modalities to exclude active tuberculosis, the adoption of this recommendation has been slow.

Active tuberculosis

The standard regimen for drug-sensitive tuberculosis consists of rifampin, isoniazid, pyrazinamide, and ethambutol, often referred to as RHZE (Table 19.2). Most tuberculosis-endemic regions have these four antituberculosis medications in one pill, called a fixed drug concentration pill, which is then dosed by weight. This regimen achieves cure rates of over 90% in treatment programs that provide directly observed therapy (World Health Organization, 2012a). Treatment is given as a 2-month induction/intensive phase with all four medications, followed by a 4-month continuation phase with isoniazid and rifampin. Risk factors for relapse include pulmonary cavitations, extensive disease, immunosuppression, and sputum culture positive after 2 months of antituberculosis therapy. The presence of any of these factors generally warrants extending therapy to 9 months total. In addition, persons being retreated for a subsequent occurrence of tuberculosis should receive some second-line medications and have drug-susceptibility testing, when possible. Clinicians must pay particular attention to possible drug–drug interactions, particularly with rifampin (a potent cytochrome P450 inducer) and ART. Any regimen for the retreatment or recurrence of tuberculosis should be guided by drug-susceptibility testing, if possible.

Treating drug-resistant tuberculosis is complicated and should be guided by drug-susceptibility testing. Treatment for

Table 19.2 Tuberculosis medications.

First-line oral therapy
Rifampin/rifampicin (R)   Isoniazid (H)   Pyrazinamide (Z)   Ethambutol (E)
Second-line options
Fluoroquinolones (levofloxacin, moxifloxacin, gatifloxacin, ofloxacin)   Parenteral agents (amikacin, kanamycin, capreomycin)   Thioamides (ethionamide, prothionamide)   Cycloserine   Terizidone   Para-aminosalicylic acid   Group 5 agents[a] (clofazimine, linezolid, amoxicillin/clavulanate, imipenem/cilastatin, clarithromycin)
Newer medications
Bedaquiline (TMC-207)   Delamanid (OPC-67683)   PA-824   Sutezolid (PNU 100480)   AZD 5847   SQ-109
[a] Group 5 agents have an unclear role for use in MDR-TB treatment.

MDR-TB is administered for at least 20 months and should include at least four second-line medications, preferably with a fluoroquinolone, an injectable agent, as well as pyrazinamide. These treatment regimens are complex, with different toxicities and drug–drug interactions, and they should be provided in consultation with an infectious disease physician. Several new promising antituberculosis medications are in various stages of development and clinical trials, so better options may be available soon.

For HIV co-infected patients, antituberculosis mediations should be initiated at least 2 weeks before ART. The WHO recommends starting ART within 8 weeks of antituberculosis therapy for all patients, and within 2 weeks for those with a CD4 count below $50\,cell/mm^3$ (Gandhi *et al.*, 2006; World Health Organization, 2012c). This does not apply to patients with TB meningitis, since they appear to fare worse with early initiation of ART, due to the risk of IRIS causing severe neurological inflammation.

Tuberculosis control and vaccination

The primary mode of tuberculosis prevention is through adequate case detection, providing effective treatment, and decreasing person-to-person transmission. The goal of decreasing person-to-person transmission is achieved through containment and contact tracing, which has often proved challenging in resource-limited settings. One of the Millennium Development Goals is to reverse the incidence of tuberculosis by 2015, so progress toward this goal is being monitored against certain targets (World Health Organization, 2012d). The worldwide case detection rate has increased substantially but appears to have plateaued at 60%, which is substantially lower than the 70% target. A major impediment to achieving control of tuberculosis is the lack of resources to effectively implement the Global Plan to Stop TB, a broad international collaboration of governments and organizations that aims to eradicate tuberculosis (World Health Organization, 2010a). The estimated funding needed for the period 2006–2015 was US$60 billion, which is much higher than what has been made available thus far (Lawn & Zumla, 2011).

The Bacillus Calmette–Guérin (BCG) vaccine, which is derived from *M. bovis* and was first administered to humans in 1921, is the only licensed vaccine for tuberculosis. The BCG vaccine has an estimated overall 50% efficacy for preventing childhood TB meningitis and miliary tuberculosis, which are the most deadly forms of tuberculosis in children, but the effect of BCG vaccination wanes over time and the efficacy against adult pulmonary tuberculosis is variable (Colditz *et al.*, 1994). BCG vaccination has been given to 4 billion people and to more than 90% of children in the world today, making it the most widely used vaccine in the world (Lawn & Zumla, 2011). The WHO recommends BCG vaccination to infants at birth in tuberculosis-endemic regions around the globe. However, the BCG vaccine should not be administered to HIV-infected newborns, since it can cause a fatal disseminated infection in immunosuppressed people. Individuals who have received BCG vaccination in childhood can still be screened with the Mantoux test, although prior BCG may result in a false positive; in this case, if the test is positive, additional testing is recommended, such as with IGRAs. Positive skin tests more than 15 years since vaccination or with more than 15 mm of induration are most likely not a result of BCG vaccination.

There is a critical need for a universally effective vaccine for the control of tuberculosis. A major international effort has reinvigorated the development of a more effective and sustainable vaccine. There are currently more than 30 possible vaccine candidates in the pipeline, and 12 vaccines have already entered clinical trials (World Health Organization, 2012d). The mechanisms for these vaccines are broad and include primary immunogens, which could either replace the BCG vaccine or serve as immunogenic boosters for the BCG vaccine.

Future directions

Tuberculosis remains a major cause of morbidity and mortality worldwide, and the HIV/AIDS epidemic has posed difficult diagnostic and treatment challenges that threaten the global efforts to control tuberculosis. Newer molecular diagnostic tests allow for easier and more rapid diagnosis, but efforts are still needed to expand the reach of those tests to resource-limited settings. Meanwhile, there still remains a critical need for a simple inexpensive test that can be used at the clinical point-of-care. The emergence of drug-resistant tuberculosis has reduced the efficacy of existing antituberculosis medications, but new antituberculosis medications may soon provide shorter treatment regimens for drug-sensitive infections and more effective treatments for both latent and multidrug-resistant infections. A rich pipeline of new vaccine candidates offers hope for accelerating tuberculosis control by reducing new infections.

As a result of large-scale global efforts, the world is on track to halve tuberculosis mortality from 1990 levels by 2015, which will be a major achievement. Although there appears to be much promise in reducing the global burden of tuberculosis, there must be a strong and sustained political and financial commitment among policy-makers and funders. Greater investments in new technologies, basic science, and translational and applied research will lead to progress in the development of improved tuberculosis diagnostics, drugs, treatment regimens, biomarkers of disease activity, and vaccines.

Additional resources

- World Health Organization. Global tuberculosis report 2013. Available at http://www.who.int/tb/publications/global_report/en/
- World Health Organization. Treatment of tuberculosis: guidelines for national programmes. Available at http://www.who.int/tb/publications/tb_treatmentguidelines/en/index.html
- US Centers for Disease Control and Prevention. Tuberculosis guidelines. Available at http://www.cdc.gov/tb/publications/guidelines/HIV_AIDS.htm

REFERENCES

Boehme CC, Nabeta P, Hillemann D *et al.* (2010) Rapid molecular detection of tuberculosis and rifampin resistance. *N Engl J Med* 363:1005–15.

Boehme CC, Nicol MP, Nabeta P *et al.* (2011) Feasibility, diagnostic accuracy, and effectiveness of decentralized use of the Xpert MTB/RIF test for diagnosis of tuberculosis and multidrug resistance: a multicentre implementation study. *Lancet* 377:1495–505.

Cain KP, McCarthy KD, Heilig CM *et al.* (2010) An algorithm for tuberculosis screening and diagnosis in people with HIV. *N Engl J Med* 362:707–16.

Caws M, Thwaites G, Dunstan S *et al.* (2008) The influence of host and bacterial genotype on the development of disseminated disease with *Mycobacterium tuberculosis. PLoS Pathog* 4(3):e1000034.

Colditz GA, Brewer TF, Berkey CS *et al.* (1994) Efficacy of BCG vaccine in the prevention of tuberculosis: meta-analysis of the published literature. *JAMA* 271:698–702.

Gandhi NR, Moll A, Sturm AW *et al.* (2006) Extensively drug-resistant tuberculosis as a cause of death in patients co-infected with tuberculosis and HIV in a rural area of South Africa. *Lancet* 368:1575–80.

Getahun H, Kittikraisak W, Heilig CM *et al.* (2011) Development of a standardized screening rule for tuberculosis in people living with HIV in resource-constrained settings: individual participant data meta-analysis of observational studies. *PLoS Med* 8(1):e1000391.

Horsburgh CR, Rubin EJ (2011) Latent tuberculosis infection in the United States. *N Engl J Med* 364:1441–8.

Keeler E, Perkins MD, Small P *et al.* (2006) Reducing the global burden of tuberculosis: the contribution of improved diagnostics. *Nature* 444(Suppl. 1):49–57.

Lawn SD, Zumla AI (2011) Tuberculosis. *Lancet* 378:57–72.

McNerney R, Maeurer M, Abubaker I *et al.* (2012) Tuberculosis diagnostics and biomarkers: needs, challenges, recent advances, and opportunities. *J Infect Dis* 205(Suppl. 2):S147–58.

Saito S, Howard AA, Reid MJ *et al.* (2012) TB diagnostic capacity in sub-Saharan African health care settings. *J Acquir Immune Defic Syndr* 61:216–20.

Sterling TR, Villarino ME, Borisov AS *et al.* (2011) Three months of rifapentine and isoniazid for latent tuberculosis infection. *N Engl J Med* 365:2155–66.

Stop TB Partnership (2011) An international roadmap for tuberculosis research: towards a world free of tuberculosis. www.stoptb.org/assets/documents/resources/publications/technical/tbresearchroadmap.pdf

World Health Organization (2010a) *Global Plan to Stop TB 2011–2015.* Geneva: World Health Organization.

World Health Organization (2010b) *Treatment of Tuberculosis: Guidelines*, 4th edn. Geneva: World Health Organization.

World Health Organization (2011a) *Tuberculosis MDR-TB and XDR-TB: 2011 progress report.* Geneva: World Health Organization.

World Health Organization (2011b) *Rapid implementation of the Xpert MTB/RIF diagnostic test: technical and operational "how-to": practical considerations.* Geneva: World Health Organization.

World Health Organization (2012a) Global Tuberculosis Report 2012. Geneva: World Health Organization.

World Health Organization (2012b) *Totally Drug-resistant TB: A WHO Consultation on the Diagnostic Definition and Treatment Options.* Geneva: World Health Organization.

World Health Organization (2012c) WHO Policy on Collaborative TB/HIV Activities. Geneva: World Health Organization.

World Health Organization (2012d) *Stop TB Partnership. Tuberculosis Vaccine Candidates, 2011.* Geneva: World Health Organization.

World Health Organization (2013) Global tuberculosis report 2013. Geneva: World Health Organization. Available from: http://www.who.int/tb/publications/global_report/gtbr13_main_text.pdf

Zignol M, van Gemert W, Falzon D *et al.* (2012) Surveillance of anti-tuberculosis drug resistance in the world: an updated analysis, 2007–2010. *Bull WHO* 90:111D–119D.

Zumla A, Raviglione M, Hafner R, Fordham von Reyn C (2013) Tuberculosis. *N Engl J Med* 368:745–55.

CHAPTER 20
Neglected and Other Tropical Diseases

Cordelia E.M. Coltart[1], Ranu S. Dhillon[2], and Christopher J.M. Whitty[3]

[1]The Hospital for Tropical Diseases, University College London Hospitals, and The London School of Hygiene and Tropical Medicine, London, UK

[2]Brigham and Women's Hospital, Boston, and Harvard Medical School, Boston, MA, USA

[3]Earth Institute and School of International and Public Affairs, Columbia University, New York, NY, USA

Key learning objectives

- Understand what is meant by the term "neglected tropical diseases" and which diseases this term incorporates.
- Learn the epidemiology and geographical distribution of the neglected tropical diseases.
- Understand the basic disease processes, including transmission mechanisms, for the major neglected tropical diseases.
- Recognize the common clinical features and diagnostic patterns of the major neglected tropical diseases.
- Understand generic treatment and prevention options for the major neglected tropical diseases and be able to apply these principles in combination with more specific local guidelines.

Abstract

Neglected tropical diseases (NTDs) are a major cause of morbidity and mortality for the poorest populations. NTDs include helminth infections, filariasis, leishmaniasis, schistosomiasis, trypanosomiasis, arboviruses, rickettsiae, and other conditions found in developing countries. NTDs are termed "neglected" as they attract little funding and are a relatively low priority on the global research agenda. However, NTDs affect more than 1 billion people worldwide, particularly those living in remote areas without access to safe water, sanitation, and healthcare infrastructure. The challenge for global health professionals is to access these communities and establish the capacity for treatment, prevention and, when possible, elimination. This chapter provides an overview of the major NTDs and reviews their epidemiology, natural history, clinical features, diagnosis, treatment, and prevention. The goal is to provide global health professionals with an understanding of the basic disease processes and the appropriate insight to search out further information.

Key words: neglected tropical diseases, parasitic diseases, soil-transmitted helminths, *Strongyloides*, schistosomiasis, filariasis, leishmaniasis, trypanosomiasis, rickettsia, arbovirus

Essential Clinical Global Health, First Edition. Edited by Brett D. Nelson.
© 2015 John Wiley & Sons, Ltd. Published 2015 by John Wiley & Sons, Ltd.
Companion website: www.essentialseries.com/globalhealth

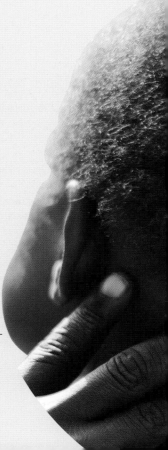

Introduction

Neglected tropical diseases (NTDs) are communicable diseases typically found among the poorest communities in 149 endemic countries. Many NTDs produce debilitating infections that cause significant morbidity and mortality. Worldwide, these conditions affect over 1 billion people and pose a threat to many more (Hotez *et al.*, 2007), although given the current lack of information, the actual number is likely to be far higher.

The term "neglected tropical diseases" is applied variably, ranging from the 17 infectious disease entities defined by the World Health Organization (WHO) (Box 20.1) to any tropical disease other than HIV, tuberculosis, and malaria, including even non-infectious conditions. Some of the diseases are due to poverty and poor sanitation and do not require tropical conditions (e.g. soil-transmitted helminths), while others do require tropical conditions (e.g., lymphatic filariasis). NTDs are termed "neglected" as they attract little funding and are a relatively low priority on the global research agenda. Historically, this resulted in a lack of data for forming evidence-based approaches for diagnosis, management, and prevention.

As NTDs are often found in remote areas without access to safe water, sanitation, and healthcare infrastructure, the challenge for global health professionals is to access these communities and establish the potential to apply interventions for treatment, prevention and, when possible, elimination. As globalization leads to increasingly mobile populations that carry diseases across borders and continents, health professionals in all settings must recognize and manage these conditions.

The clinical picture caused by NTDs is diverse, ranging from asymptomatic infections with parasitic worms to the fulminant presentation of hemorrhagic fever. Many NTDs present with non-specific symptoms, making diagnosis difficult in settings with limited laboratory capacity. The geographic distribution and risk factors for NTDs are similarly varied, requiring location-specific knowledge of endemic disease patterns (Table 20.1).

This chapter provides an overview of the major NTDs and reviews the epidemiology, natural history, and clinical features of these diseases. General approaches for diagnosis and treatment are also summarized, although these may vary by setting, and the reader should consult country-specific guidelines. The goal is to provide an understanding of the basic disease processes and the appropriate insight for global health professionals to seek out further information.

Box 20.1 Neglected tropical diseases

Buruli ulcer disease (*Mycobacterium ulcerans* infection)
Chagas disease (American trypanosomiasis)
Cysticercosis
Dengue
Dracunculiasis (guinea-worm disease)
Echinococcosis
Food-borne trematode infections
Human African trypanosomiasis (sleeping sickness)
Leishmaniasis
Leprosy
Lymphatic filariasis (elephantiasis)
Onchocerciasis (river blindness)
Rabies
Schistosomiasis (bilharziasis)
Soil-transmitted helminth infections
Trachoma
Yaws

Table 20.1 Selected tropical diseases by exposure risk factor.

Risk factor	Diseases
Freshwater exposure	Schistosomiasis Leptospirosis
Specific rural locations, hospitals	Viral hemorrhagic fever
Safari/game parks	Tick typhus Trypanosomiasis
Animal exposure	Rabies (bite from infected animals, often stray dogs) Anthrax (exposure to infected hides)
Caves	Histoplasmosis

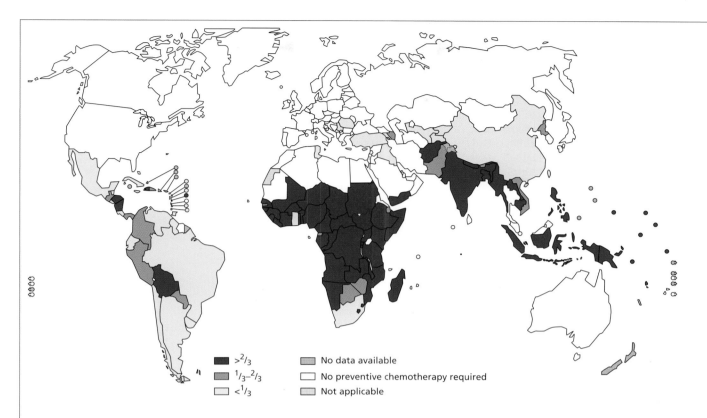

Figure 20.1 Proportion of children 1–14 years of age in the country requiring mass drug administration for soil-transmitted helminths, 2011. *Source*: WHO (2011). Reproduced with permission of the World Health Organization.

Parasitic diseases

Helminth infections

Helminth infections are caused by parasitic worms and affect approximately 2 billion people globally. These diseases are the most common parasitic cause of infection in developing countries and are thought to be one of the most important causes of chronic disease worldwide. Indeed, approximately 85% of the NTD-related disease burden results from helminth infections (Bethony *et al.*, 2006; Hotez *et al.*, 2007). The exact burden of disease is difficult to determine as these infections are often asymptomatic and thus undiagnosed.

Helminth infections are categorized into three groups.

1. Nematodes (roundworms): *Ascaris lumbricoides*, *Trichuris trichiura* (whipworm), hookworms, *Toxocara* spp., *Enterobius vermicularis* (threadworm), *Trichinella spiralis*, *Strongyloides stercoralis*, the filarias.
2. Trematodes (flukes): *Schistosoma* spp. (blood flukes); *Clonorchis sinensis*, *Fasciola* spp. and *Opisthorchis* spp. (liver flukes); *Paragonimus* spp. (lung flukes).
3. Cestodes (tapeworms or flatworms): *Taenia solium* (pork tapeworm causing cysticercosis), *Taenia saginata* (beef tape-

worm), *Diphyllobothrium* spp. (fish tapeworm), *Echinococcus* spp. (causing hydatid disease).

The most common helminths to infect humans are those transmitted by fecal contamination in or on the soil (soil-transmitted helminths), predominantly roundworm (*A. lumbricoides*), whipworm (*T. trichiura*), and hookworms (*Necator americanus*, *Ancylostoma duodenale*) (Table 20.2). More than 1.5 billion people (approximately 24% of the world's population) are infected with soil-transmitted helminth infections worldwide. *Ascaris lumbricoides* alone affects upwards of 1 billion people. Figure 20.1 shows the proportion of children by country who require preventive chemotherapy for soil-transmitted helminths. These infections are ubiquitous in communities without access to proper sanitation.

Strongyloidiasis

Epidemiology

Infection with *Strongyloides stercoralis* occurs throughout the world, most commonly in tropical/subtropical regions. The prevalence is unclear, with estimates ranging from 3 million to 100 million persons infected globally (Centers for Disease Control and Prevention, 2012). Once acquired, infection is

Table 20.2 Common helminth infections in humans.

Diseases/infection	Parasite life cycle	Clinical features	Diagnosis	Treatment
Overview of soil-transmitted helminth infections				
Soil-transmitted helminths	Transmitted via eggs in feces of infected person. Adult worms live in human intestine and produce thousands of eggs per day that are passed out in the stool. Once defecated, eggs mature to infective stage in the soil. Fresh feces do not cause infection, and there is no direct person-to-person spread. Infection occurs when infective eggs are either ingested (e.g., oral contact with contaminated unwashed hands or consumption of unwashed vegetables and fruit) or when eggs hatch in the soil and produce larvae that penetrate skin to cause infection.	Usually determined by intensity of infection *Light infections*: Asymptomatic or minor gastrointestinal symptoms *Heavy infections*: Anemia and protein deficiencies due to blood loss and malabsorption, especially in pregnancy *Children*: Often heavily infected from a young age with constant reexposure, so more severe manifestations. Present with abdominal pain, malaise, poor appetite, diarrhea and, in severe cases, intestinal obstruction. Consequences of infection include anemia, growth retardation, and impaired cognitive development (Bleakley, 2003; Miguel & Kremer, 2003).	Microscopic identification of eggs in the stool. The intensity of infection is determined with quantification methods (e.g., Kato–Katz technique).	Albendazole or mebendazole (see below) *Prevention*: In endemic areas (Figure 20.1), the WHO recommends mass drug administration (MDA) for at-risk populations to decrease overall worm burden: children, pregnant women, people with increased nutritional needs and in high-risk occupations (tea-pickers, miners). Albendazole or mebendazole is used. The frequency of MDA depends on prevalence in the target population: once a year if prevalence is 20–49% and twice a year if >50%. Note that women in the first trimester of pregnancy should not be treated due to concern of fetal harm.
Nematodes (roundworms)				
Ascaris lumbricoides	Adult worm is 20–35 cm long and lives in the small intestine. Produces up to 200,000 eggs per day, which mature in excreted feces in soil. On ingestion, mature eggs release larvae in the stomach that invade intestinal mucosa, travel to the pulmonary circulation, into alveoli and up bronchus before swallowed back into the small intestine. Mature into adult worms during this migration.	Usually asymptomatic Growth retardation Cognitive impairment Mechanical obstruction Loeffler syndrome and allergic effects (Figure 20.2)	Microscopic identification of eggs in stool. Kato–Katz method used to quantify burden.	Albendazole 400 mg single dose or mebendazole 500 mg single dose or mebendazole 100 mg twice daily for 3 days

Table 20.2 Common helminth infections in humans. (*Continued*)

Diseases/infection	Parasite life cycle	Clinical features	Diagnosis	Treatment
Hookworms (*Ancylostoma duodenale*, *Necator americanus*)	Adult worm is approximately 1 cm long and attaches to intestinal mucosa. Females produce up to 30,000 eggs per day. Humans infected by walking barefoot on contaminated soil. (*A. duodenale* can be acquired by ingestion of larvae.) Larvae penetrate skin and are carried by the circulation to the lungs, across the alveoli and up the trachea, where they are swallowed into the small intestine.	Usually asymptomatic Growth retardation Cognitive impairment Zinc, Vitamin A, or folate deficiency Anemia (secondary to blood loss from mucosa): this can be severe when combined with coexisting infections such as malaria or other nutritional deficiencies, occasionally leading to cardiac failure Loeffler syndrome (Figure 20.2).	Microscopic identification of eggs in stool. Kato–Katz method used to quantify burden.	Albendazole 400 mg single dose or mebendazole 100 mg twice daily for 3 days (mebendazole 500 mg single dose is not as effective)
Cutaneous larva migrans (*Ancylostoma braziliense*, *A. caninum*)	Animal hookworms that infect humans via penetration of the epidermis. Cannot penetrate the dermis and thus only affect the skin.	Intensely itchy, serpiginous track under the skin	Clinical	Ivermectin 200 µg single dose or once daily for 2 days or albendazole 400 mg once daily for 3 days
Whipworm (*Trichuris trichiura*)	Adult worm is 4 cm long and whip-shaped. One end of the worm tunnels into the colonic mucosa, with the other end free in the lumen. Female worms produce up to 20,000 eggs per day, which embryonate in soil. Infection occurs when eggs are ingested. Larvae are released into the stomach and move into the intestine, where they develop into adults.	Painful diarrhea Rectal prolapse Inflammatory colitis in reaction to infection, leading to colonic bleeding and nutritional deficiencies Children can get dysenteric syndrome with massive worm burden	Microscopic identification of eggs in stool. Kato–Katz method used to quantify burden. Worms are visible on anoscopy, colonoscopy, or sigmoidoscopy.	Mebendazole 100 mg twice daily for 3 days or albendazole 400 mg once daily for 3 days
Guinea worm (dracunculiasis)	Adult worms live in the subcutaneous tissues. Females emerge from the skin and release larvae when in contact with water. Small crustaceans (copepods) ingest larvae. Humans are infected by drinking water contaminated by infected copepods. Larvae released in the gastrointestinal tract and penetrate into the abdominal cavity where they develop into adults.	Skin papule or blister at site where female adult emerges from skin to release larvae Non-specific symptoms (fever, nausea, diarrhea)	Clinical recognition of papule and related history	Slow extraction of the worm using a stick to wind out over weeks to months (Figure 20.3) Targeted for elimination by WHO by 2015

(*Continued*)

Table 20.2 Common helminth infections in humans. (*Continued*)

Diseases/infection	Parasite life cycle	Clinical features	Diagnosis	Treatment
Trematodes (flukes)				
Liver flukes (*Clonorchis sinensis*, *Fasciola* spp., *Opisthorchis* spp.)	Adults reside in the biliary ducts, from whence they release eggs into the stool. Eggs are ingested by snails, wherein they develop before being released into the water. *Clonorchis* and *Opisthorchis* species penetrate into the flesh of freshwater fish and infect humans when they eat these fish. *Fasciola* species encyst on aquatic vegetation and cause infection when vegetation is eaten, e.g., watercress. Geographical distribution is widespread across the globe for *Fasciola*, whereas *Clonorchis* is found across Asia and *Opisthorchis* primarily in southeast Asia.	Fever, right upper quadrant pain, jaundice, hepatomegaly Increased risk for cholangiopathies including cholangiocarcinoma	Microscopic identification of eggs in the stool. Biliary imaging with ultrasound, CT, MRI, or ERCP can also make diagnosis.	*Clonorchis* and *Opisthorchis*: praziquantel 75 mg/kg three times daily for 3 days *Fasciola*: triclabendazole 10 mg/kg single dose or once daily for 2 days
Cestodes (tapeworms or flatworms)				
Tape worm (*Taenia solium* [pork tapeworm and cysticercosis/neurocysticercosis], *T. saginata* [beef tape worm])	Humans infected by eating meat (beef for *T. saginata* or pork for *T. solium*) containing cysticerci. However, infection can occur via ingestion of feces from an infected human carrier and, therefore, can occur in populations that do not eat pork or meat. Pigs (*T. solium*) and cattle (*T. saginata*) are infected by eating infested vegetation. Eggs hatch in these animals and evolve into cysticerci in the muscle. In *T. solium*, humans ingesting eggs can develop Cysticercosis. *T. solium* grow 2–7 m in length and are found in Central and South America, Africa, India, and Asia. *T. saginata* is usually <5 m in length and primarily found in Eastern Europe, Russia, East Africa, and Latin America.	Mostly asymptomatic Weight loss, colic, nausea, increased appetite Neurocysticercosis: headache, seizures, mental status changes, focal symptoms	Identification of proglottids or eggs in the stool. CT/MRI and serology aid diagnosis of neurocysticercosis.	Intestinal disease: praziquantel 5–10 mg/kg single dose Neurocysticercosis: antiepileptic treatment, antiparasitic treatment with albendazole or praziquantel, usually with corticosteroids and surgical intervention based on case-specific characteristics.
Hydatid disease (*Echinococcus granulosus*)	Life cycle usually involves dogs and sheep. Dogs eat cysts contained in sheep organs. Cysts develop into intestinal worms in dogs and release eggs in stool that are ingested by sheep, thereby continuing the cycle. Humans are infected by ingesting eggs in food or water contaminated with dog feces. The eggs hatch and infection takes hold in liver or other organs where hyatid cysts are formed.	Liver and occasionally lung cysts grow slowly (1 cm/year) and are usually asymptomatic. Enlarging cysts can cause abdominal pain, hepatomegaly, or jaundice. Cyst rupture leads to anaphylaxis.	Cysts are seen on ultrasound, CT, or MRI. Serology may aid diagnosis.	Determined based on case-specific characteristics and may include PAIR (percutaneous needle aspiration–injection–reaspiration) and albendazole. Some cysts require surgical excision.

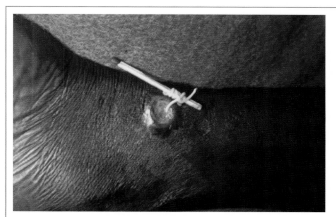

Figure 20.3 A guinea worm is slowly extracted from where it emerged in a lower extremity. *Source*: CDC Public Health Image Library.

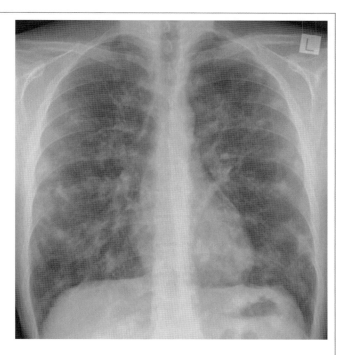

Figure 20.2 Loeffler syndrome is a pneumonitis caused by inflammatory response to helminth larval migration through the lungs. It classically occurs with *Ascaris*, *Strongyloides*, and *Schistosoma* infections. If diagnosis is uncertain, treatment with albendazole is given empirically. *Source*: Pasricha *et al.* (2011), figure 3, p. 206. Reproduced with permission from Oxford University Press.

often lifelong as *Strongyloides*, unlike other helminths, can complete its entire life cycle in humans. Disseminated infection is primarily seen in immunosuppressed states, including co-infection with human T-cell lymphotropic virus (HTLV)-1, hematologic malignancies, corticosteroid therapy, or chemotherapy. There is limited evidence of increased prevalence or severity of infection among people with HIV (Viney *et al.*, 2004).

Transmission

Infective larvae are released in the stool of an infected person. These larvae penetrate the skin of people who come in direct contact with soil or sewage contaminated by these feces. The larvae enter the bloodstream and travel to the lungs where they enter the alveoli. They then migrate up the trachea and are swallowed into the small intestine where they develop into adults. Adult worms release eggs that hatch into non-infective larvae before release in the stool. The larvae mature into an infective stage in the soil and repeat the cycle. In some people, the larvae become infective before being defecated and instead penetrate through the intestinal or perianal mucosa to cause autoinfection and potentially lifelong infection if untreated. Autoinfection can also lead to a massively increased parasite burden, known as hyperinfection.

Presentation

Infections are usually asymptomatic or cause mild non-specific symptoms such as fatigue and weight loss. Symptomatic cases exhibit localized manifestations including an itchy, fast-moving, recurrent, serpiginous rash (larva currens) from the migrating autoinfective larvae; Loeffler syndrome from larvae in the lungs (Figure 20.3); or gastrointestinal symptoms such as diarrhea and abdominal pain.

Disseminated strongyloidiasis occurs in immunosuppressed patients or those with hyperinfection. This syndrome produces life-threatening multiorgan dysfunction and is commonly complicated by Gram-negative sepsis. Patients may exhibit fever, respiratory distress, diarrhea, jaundice, shock, disseminated intravascular coagulation, and coma.

Diagnosis

Diagnosis is made by microscopic identification of larvae in the stool. Infections take 2–4 weeks after transmission for larvae to be present in the feces. Microscopy has low sensitivity except in disseminated disease when the larval burden is high in stool and sputum. Serologic testing has over 80% sensitivity, but cannot be used to monitor treatment since it does not revert to a negative result after recovery. Another option for diagnosis is the duodenal string test where mucus collected from a partially swallowed capsule of string is examined for larvae.

Treatment

The treatment of choice for strongyloidiasis in the immunocompetent patient is a stat dose of ivermectin 200 μg/kg. For disseminated strongyloidiasis, immunosuppression should be reduced or stopped if possible. Daily ivermectin is given until symptoms resolve and stool microscopy is negative for 2 weeks.

Schistosomiasis

Schistosomiasis is an important public health problem caused by trematodes from the genus *Schistosoma*.

Epidemiology

More than 240 million people in over 70 countries are infected, with over 90% of these cases in Africa. Infection also occurs in the Middle East, South America, the Caribbean, and Southeast Asia. The prevalence of schistosomiasis is highest in 15–20 year olds. The intensity of infection also peaks during this age before declining in adults (King *et al.*, 1988; Gryseels *et al.*, 2006). Intensity of infection tends to be heavy in fewer than 10% of people in endemic communities, most likely in those having regular contact with infected fresh water (Kabatereine *et al.*, 2004; Clements *et al.*, 2006).

Transmission

Infection occurs when larval cercariae penetrate the skin of people swimming, fishing, or bathing in infected fresh waters. The cercariae travel via the blood and lymphatics to the lungs where they migrate through the pulmonary capillaries into the heart. They travel via the circulation to the liver, where they mature into adult worms. These adult worms settle permanently in the venous vasculature near different organs depending on the species: *S. mansoni* and *S. intercalatum* near the colon, *S. haemotobium* near the urinary bladder, and *S. japonicum* and *S. mekongi* near the small intestine.

Adult worms mate, and the eggs produced by the female travel via the blood to either the intestine, where they penetrate the intestinal wall and are released into the stool, or, in the case of *S. haemotobium* infection, to the urinary bladder, where they penetrate the bladder wall and are excreted in the urine. The eggs hatch on contact with fresh water and infect freshwater snails. After maturation within these snails, infectious cercariae are released into fresh water and infect humans to continue the cycle.

Presentation

Most cases are asymptomatic. However, Swimmer's itch, a pruritic rash at the site of larval penetration (see Chapter 28, Figure 28.7), can develop a day after exposure. Acute schistosomiais, Katayama fever, typically occurs 4–6 weeks after initial infection, and is due to an immune complex-mediated phenomenon which is marked by fever, urticarial rash, cough, wheeze, diarrhea, hepatosplenomegaly, and eosinophilia. This syndrome is more common among non-immune people from non-endemic areas (Bottieau *et al.*, 2006). Acute schistosomiasis is usually self-limiting.

Chronic infection can develop causing intestinal disease with diarrhea, abdominal pain, and intestinal polyps (all species); urogenital diseases such as bladder carcinoma, ureteric obstruction, and genital or placental lesions (*S. haemotobium*); or hepatic pathology complicated by portal hypertension and splenomegaly (*S. mansoni, S. japonicum, S. mekongi*). Rare complications include transverse myelitis, pulmonary disease, or cutaneous lesions.

Diagnosis

Diagnosis is made by microscopic detection of eggs in the stool, urine, semen, or tissue from other sites of infection. Serologic testing of antibodies against schistosome eggs is also available. While these diagnostics are appropriate for chronic disease, both are negative in acute infection where immature schistosomes have yet to produce eggs.

Treatment

Acute or chronic infection with *S. mansoni, S. haemotobium*, and *S. intercalatum* is treated with praziquantel 40 mg/kg in two divided doses, while infection with *S. japonicum* and *S. mekongi* is treated with praziquantel 60 mg/kg in three divided doses. For acute cases, the same treatment should be repeated 6–8 weeks later as praziquantel does not effectively treat immature schistosomes. Steroids can also be given during Katayama fever to alleviate symptoms.

Prevention

Prevention is pursued through education, sanitation programs, and mass drug administration (MDA). Education strategies encourage avoidance of infected fresh waters and the use of protective clothing and footwear for high-risk professions (e.g., fisherman). Sanitation efforts seek to establish proper sanitation facilities and limit defecation and urination into fresh waters. The WHO recommends MDA for at-risk populations residing in endemic areas, including school-aged children, people in professions requiring freshwater contact (e.g., farmers, irrigation workers), and entire communities in highly endemic areas. MDA uses a single dose of praziquantel 40 mg/kg and can be integrated into other community-based NTD initiatives, such as annual MDAs for onchocerciasis and lymphatic filariasis.

Filarias

The filarias are caused by nematodes transmitted via insect vectors. The causative organisms are grouped into three categories.

1. Lymphatic filariasis: *Wuchereria bancrofti, Brugia malayi, Brugia timori*.
2. Subcutaneous filariasis: *Loa loa, Onchocerca volvulus, Mansonella streptocerca*.
3. Serous cavity filariasis: *Mansonella perstans, Mansonella ozzardi*.

The treatment of some filarial infections are complicated by co-infection with other filarial infections of the same geographical distribution (see Table 20.3 for precautions and cross reactions).

Leishmaniasis

Leishmaniasis is a spectrum of diseases caused by *Leishmania* protozoa. Cases are found in more than 90 countries across

Table 20.3 Common filarial infections.

Diseases/infection	Epidemiology	Vector	Clinical features	Diagnosis	Treatment	Prevention
Lymphatic filariasis (*W. bancrofti, B. malayi, B. timori*)	Affects more than 120 million worldwide, with >90% caused by *W. bancrofti*. Two-thirds of cases occur in Asia, also endemic in parts of sub-Saharan Africa, Latin America, the Caribbean, and the Pacific Islands.	*Culex, Anopheles, Aedes, Mansonia,* and *Coquillettidia* mosquitoes	*Acute infection:* fever, tender lymphadenopathy, lymphangitis (legs, testicles, and breasts). Episodic recurrence and complicated by bacterial infection. Night-time wheezing caused by hyperreactivity to microfilariae in the lungs *Chronic infection:* lymphedema (elephantiasis; Figure 20.4), hydrocele, and chyluria due to lymphatic rupture into renal pelvis	Microscopic identification of microfilariae on peripheral blood smear. Blood collection must be done at night because of nocturnal periodicity. Serologic testing available.	*No co-infection:* DEC 6 mg/kg for 12 days *Co-infection with onchocerciasis:* ivermectin 150 µg/kg single dose followed 1 month later with DEC 6 mg/kg for 12 days or doxycycline 200 mg once daily for 4–6 weeks followed by ivermectin 150 µg/kg single dose *Co-infection with low-level Loa loa microfilaremia:* DEC 8–10 mg/kg for 21 days *Co-infection with high-level L. loa microfilaremia:* doxycycline 200 mg daily for 4–6 weeks or albendazole 200–400 mg twice daily for 21 days *Chronic lymphedema:* skin care; exercise, massage, and elevation for lymph flow	Insecticide-treated nets, topical repellents MDA: albendazole 400 mg single dose and DEC 6 mg/kg single dose If also endemic with onchocerciasis or loiasis: albendazole 400 mg single dose and ivermectin 150 µg/kg single dose Targeted for elimination by WHO by 2020
Onchocerciasis (*O. volvulus*), also known as river blindness	Second leading cause of blindness worldwide (~500,000 cases); 37 million cases in 30 sub-Saharan African countries. Pockets of infection in Yemen and six countries in Latin America. Transmission greatest in riverine areas.	*Simulium* blackfly	*Eye:* dying microfilariae cause reversible inflammation in cornea but damage becomes permanent without treatment, leading to blindness *Subcutaneous nodules:* contain adult worms, itchy, predominantly over bony prominences (e.g., iliac crests) *Skin:* itchy lesions over trunk and limbs, may be pigmented	*Skin snip:* shavings from six sites examined for microfilariae *Slit-lamp:* visualize microfilariae or typical lesions in the eye *Surgical resection:* remove nodule and examine for adult worm	Ivermectin 150 µg/kg single dose, repeated monthly for 2 months, and then at 3–6 month intervals until asymptomatic. May take over 10 years	*MDA:* ivermectin 150 µg/kg single dose annually *Global control initiatives:* African Program for Onchocerciasis Control has goal of elimination in 23 countries by 2015; Onchocerciasis Control Programme does aerial larviciding in 11 West African countries
Loiasis (*Loa loa*), also known as African eye worm	Affects 3–13 million people in 11 countries in West and Central Africa.	Female *Chrysops* fly (also known as deer fly or mango fly); day biting	Most are asymptomatic. If symptoms, itching and localized subcutaneous "Calabar" swellings (see Chapter 28, Figure 28.9). Visible crawling of worm beneath conjunctiva and local inflammation but without significant ocular damage (see Chapter 28, Figure 28.10).	Microscopic identification of microfilariae on peripheral blood smear. Blood collection must be done during day because of diurnal periodicity. Serologic testing if not from endemic area. Identification of adult worms in resected subcutaneous tissue also possible.	*Low-level microfilaremia:* DEC 8–10 mg/kg daily for 21 days *High-level microfilaremia:* apheresis or albendazole 200 mg twice daily for 21 days prior to DEC 8–10 mg/kg daily for 21 days *Co-infection with onchocerciasis:* ivermectin 150 µg/kg single dose followed 1 month later with DEC 8–10 mg/kg daily for 21 days	Protective clothing, topical repellents

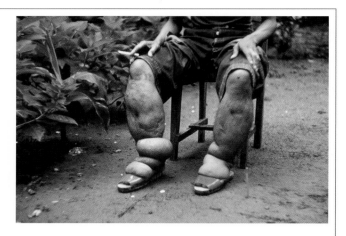

Figure 20.4 Advanced elephantiasis caused by lymphatic filariasis. *Source*: CDC Public Health Image Library.

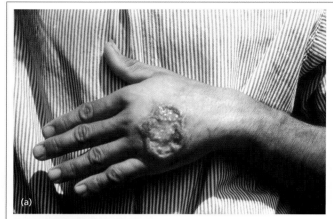

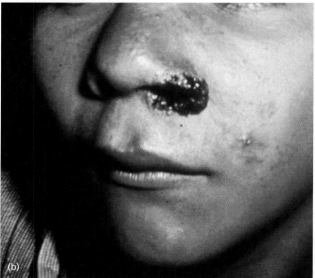

Figure 20.5 (a) Cutaneous leishmaniasis. *Source*: CDC Public Health Image Library/D.S. Martin. (b) Mucocutaneous leishmaniasis. *Source*: CDC Public Health Image Library/Mae Melvin.

five continents (WHO, 2010a). Clinical manifestations range from cutaneous disease to disfiguring mucocutaneous involvement to visceral systemic disseminated disease.

Cutaneous leishmaniasis

Cutaneous leishmaniasis typically involves a single local skin ulcer, but can occasionally cause more widespread disease.

Epidemiology

Approximately 1 million new cases of cutaneous leishmaniasis occur each year. Cases are categorized as Old World or New World according to the *Leishmania* species, which are usually isolated to specific geographic locations. Old World disease is predominantly found in Africa and the Middle East, while New World disease is mainly seen in Central and South America.

Transmission

Humans are infected when *Leishmania* promastigotes are injected into the skin via the bite of an infected female sandfly. The promastigotes are phagocytosed and become intracellular amastigotes within host macrophages. These macrophages are subsequently ingested by a feeding sandfly within which amastigotes mature into promastigotes. The promastigotes are transmitted to another host (human or other mammal) when the sandfly takes a blood meal, thus restarting the cycle.

Rare cases of blood-borne transmission through intravenous drug use, transfusions, organ transplantation, and congenital infection have been reported (Meinecke *et al.*, 1999; Cruz *et al.*, 2002; Dey & Singh, 2006; Antinori *et al.*, 2008).

Presentation

A skin papule appears weeks to months after the initial bite. The papule evolves into a nodule or plaque-like lesion before

progressing to form a painless ulcer with an indurated border (Figure 20.5a). The ulcer may be dry or wet, depending on the infecting species, and ultimately heals over the course of years. More severe disease may occur, particularly in the setting of immunosuppression. Patients may develop multiple or larger lesions, subcutaneous nodules, or regional lymphadenopathy.

Patients infected by species found in New World settings (especially Brazil, Peru, or Bolivia) are at risk for mucocutaneous disease (Figure 20.5b), where local cutaneous infection occurs first but then metastasizes to widespread mucocutaneous involvement, leading to significant disfigurement and possibly death.

Diagnosis

The diagnosis of cutaneous leishmaniasis should be considered in anyone with chronic non-healing skin lesions and a history of travel to endemic areas. Diagnosis is often clinical, but it can be confirmed by identification of the parasite on full-thickness skin biopsy from the edge of an active ulcer. Amastigotes can be detected in these samples by smears, culture, or polymerase chain reaction (PCR). Speciation is useful for guiding treatment.

Treatment

Treatment varies according to the species and clinical presentation. Lesions can resolve spontaneously, but the mainstay of treatment for uncomplicated Old World cutaneous leishmaniasis is with local topical medications. Systemic therapy may be needed for New World cases caused by species with the potential for mucocutaneous disease or those with "complicated disease" (e.g., four or more lesions, lesions >5 cm, regional lymphadenopathy, failure of local therapy, immunosuppression).

Local treatment is with intralesional pentavalent antimony (e.g., sodium stibogluconate) repeated as necessary for healing. Alternatives include topical paromomycin or, for small isolated lesions, cryotherapy or radiotherapy. Systemic treatment is with intravenous sodium stibogluconate. Alternative agents are miltefosine, amphotericin, and pentamidine.

Prevention

Wearing clothing, using topical repellents, and avoiding areas with sandflies are the key tenets to preventing leishmaniasis. Vector and reservoir control strategies such as insecticide spraying and clearing of rodent burrows can also reduce transmission.

Visceral leishmaniasis

Visceral leishmaniasis is a severe disease associated with about 10% mortality (WHO, 2008).

Epidemiology

There are approximately half a million cases of visceral leishmaniasis reported annually, about 60,000 of which result in death. Visceral leishmaniasis is mainly caused by *L. donovani* (found in South Asia and the Horn of Africa) and *L. infantum* (found in the Mediterranean, Middle East, Central Asia, and Brazil).

Transmission

Transmission is the same as for the cutaneous form.

Presentation

While many infections are asymptomatic, others produce symptoms after a 2–6 month incubation period. These cases present with fever, night sweats, malaise, weight loss, and progressive abdominal distension due to massive splenomegaly. Pancytopenia results from bone marrow suppression, splenic sequestration, and hemolysis and can lead to immunosuppression and bacterial superinfection. Other findings include lymphadenopathy and moderate hepatomegaly. Visceral leishmaniasis is also known as kala-azar, Hindi for "black fever," due to hyperpigmentation of the skin that is occasionally seen among cases in South Asia (Bern *et al.*, 2000).

Diagnosis

Diagnosis is confirmed with identification of the parasite on a smear or culture of tissue from the bone marrow or spleen. Splenic aspiration is risky and should be undertaken with precautions. Serology and molecular testing are available in specialized laboratories.

Treatment

Visceral leishmaniasis is almost always fatal without treatment. This is particularly true for patients with HIV co-infection, and treatment for this group should be aggressive (van Griensven *et al.*, 2013). Treatment options vary by setting and include amphotericin B, pentavalent antimonial drugs (e.g., sodium stibogluconate), paromomycin, and miltefosine. As regimens vary extensively, providers should consult local guidelines.

Prevention

Preventive approaches are the same as for cutaneous disease.

Trypanosomiasis

Trypanosomiasis is caused by protozoa of the genus *Trypanosoma*. Trypanosomes lead to two distinct diseases: human African trypanosomiasis (known as sleeping sickness) and American trypanosomiasis (known as Chagas disease).

Human African trypanosomiasis (sleeping sickness)

Human African trypanosomiasis appears in two variations, East and West African trypanosomiasis, both of which are fatal without treatment.

Epidemiology

Human African trypanosomiasis occurs in approximately 30 countries in sub-Saharan Africa. The incidence and prevalence is difficult to determine as many cases occur in remote areas without healthcare infrastructure and go unreported. Incidence may increase in war-torn areas due to lapses in control programs involving active case finding and early treatment (Barrett *et al.*, 2003). WHO has targeted this infection for elimination by 2020.

The two variants of African trypanosomiasis are caused by different species of *Trypanosoma brucei*. East African trypanosomiasis is caused by *Trypanosoma brucei rhodesiense* and occurs predominantly in East Africa, including Tanzania, Uganda, Malawi, and Zambia. Humans are incidental hosts, and game animals are the main reservoir. West African trypanosomiasis is caused by *Trypanosoma brucei gambiense* and is found in West and Central Africa, including Angola, South Sudan, and the Democratic Republic of Congo. Humans are the primary reservoir.

Transmission

Transmission is the same for both variants. Humans are infected when a tsetse fly of the genus *Glossina* introduces infective trypomastigotes into the skin during feeding. Trypomastigotes pass into the bloodstream, lymphatics, and connective tissues, and can also penetrate into the cerebrospinal fluid (CSF), infecting the brain. A tsetse fly taking a blood meal will ingest circulating trypomastigotes. Inside the fly, parasites undergo several transformations before becoming trypomastigotes ready for injection into another human host.

Presentation

East African trypanosomiasis causes an acute painful chancre at the bite wound. This is followed by a severe febrile illness with headaches, weight loss, myalgia, arthralgia, and rash. Central nervous system (CNS) infection causes meningoencephalitis and rapid deterioration of mental status and neurologic function. If untreated, patients develop multiorgan failure and die within 1–3 months of infection.

West African trypanosomiasis leads to a more insidious picture. A chancre is rarely seen and, during early disease, patients remain asymptomatic or experience intermittent fevers, fatigue, arthralgia, myalgia, itching, and headaches. Painless posterior cervical lymphadenopathy (Winterbottom's sign) and splenomegaly are classic findings in West African trypanosomiasis. CNS invasion occurs months to years later and causes sleep disturbances, forgetfulness, abnormal behavior, psychosis, and focal motor symptoms including tremor. These symptoms progress to daytime somnolence, seizures, coma, and death.

Diagnosis

Diagnosis of West African trypanosomiasis relies on a card agglutination test that can be performed in the field. There is no similar test for East African trypanosomiasis, which requires microscopic identification of parasites in blood, lymph node aspirates, or CSF to confirm diagnosis. Microscopy has higher yield in East African trypanosomiasis due to greater numbers of circulating trypanosomes. In patients who undergo lumbar puncture, CSF examination reveals leukocytosis and elevated IgM (Lejon & Büscher, 2005).

Treatment

Treatment options are highly toxic and should therefore be informed by local guidelines. East African trypanosomiasis is treated with suramin during early disease and melarsoprol during late (CNS) disease. West African trypanosomiasis is now mainly treated with nifurtimox-eflornithine (NECT), although pentamidine can be used in early (non-CNS) disease.

Chagas disease (American trypanosomiasis)

Chagas disease is caused by *Trypanosoma cruzi* and is is a major parasitic cause of morbidity and mortality in the western hemisphere (WHO, 2004).

Epidemiology

Chagas disease affects 8–10 million people, most of whom reside in Latin America, and is a major cause of heart disease in the region.

Transmission

Humans are infected via contact with triatomine bug feces that contain infective trypomastigotes. Trypomastigotes enter through the bite wound or via mucous membranes after the triatomine bug has taken a blood meal and defecated on the skin. The trypomastigotes invade human cells where they transform into intracellular amastigotes that ultimately develop into trypomastigotes. They burst out of the cell and enter the bloodstream where they go on to invade other cells or are taken up by a feeding triatomine bug. Within the bug, the trypomastigotes undergo further transformations before being defecated onto a human or other mammalian host to repeat the cycle.

As vector-control efforts have succeeded, other routes of transmission have become increasingly important for the spread of Chagas disease. Congenital infection now causes one-quarter of all new cases (Organización Panamericana de la Salud, 2006). Transmission also occurs via blood transfusion, organ transplantation, and ingestion of food or drink contaminated with triatomine bug feces.

Presentation

Acute Chagas disease is often subclinical. Swelling and inflammation at the bite site, known as a chagoma, may be seen with associated lymphadenopathy. If infection takes place via the conjunctiva, unilateral eye swelling (Romaña's sign) can occur (Figure 20.6). Fever may occur 2–4 weeks after infection, correlating with initial parasitemia. Rarely, patients can develop myocarditis or meningoencephalitis during the acute phase.

The chronic phase of the infection begins when parasitemia becomes undetectable. In the "indeterminate" form, patients have serologic evidence of infection but no clinical manifestations. Of such patients, 30% go on to develop cardiac and gastrointestinal findings consistent with chronic disease. Parasitic invasion of the heart muscle can cause dilated cardiomyopathy, arrhythmias, aneurysm, thromboembolic events, and sudden death. Parasitic destruction of the autonomic ganglia of the gastrointestinal tract causes megaesophagus, achalasia, and megacolon.

Diagnosis

During the acute phase, Chagas disease can be diagnosed by microscopic identification of trypomastigotes on blood smear. Where available, PCR can also be used during this period. For chronic infection, parasites will not be found in the blood and diagnosis is made by serology. Since no single assay has sufficient sensitivity and specificity, two different serologic tests are used in combination.

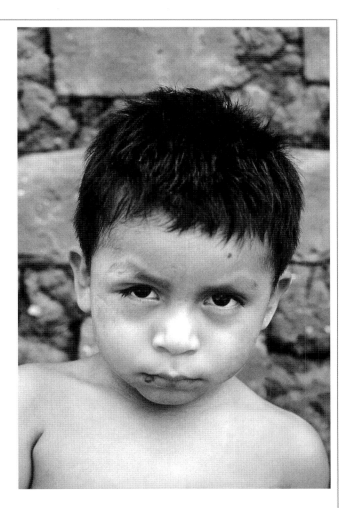

Figure 20.6 Unilateral eye swelling, or Romaña's sign, in a young boy in Panama with acute Chagas infection. *Source*: CDC Public Health Image Library/Mae Melvin.

Treatment

Benznidazole or nifurtimox can be used in the early acute phase before symptoms appear. Benznidazole can also be used in the chronic phase, but with less effect. Cardiac and gastrointestinal manifestations require management as indicated for these complications.

Arthropod-borne infections

Several groups of NTDs are transmitted by arthropod vectors, including arboviruses and rickettsiae.

Arboviruses

There are over 500 arboviruses, only some of which cause human disease. Each virus is usually limited to specific geographic locations based on the distribution of its transmitting vector. Arboviruses typically have a short incubation period followed by a systemic, usually self-limiting, febrile illness. However, more severe patterns can be seen including encephalitis (e.g., Rift Valley fever, West Nile virus) and arthralgias (e.g., chikungunya, dengue). Table 20.4 describes select diseases caused by arboviruses.

Rickettsial infections

Rickettsiae are intracellular bacilli transmitted by ticks, fleas, lice, and mites. These infections are subdivided into three categories:

1. typhus group;
2. spotted fever group;
3. "other group" consisting of pathogenic bacteria that were previously classified as rickettsiae, including *Bartonella* spp., *Coxiella burnetii*, *Ehrlichia*, and *Anaplasma*.

Table 20.5 provides an overview of rickettsial infections and details on specific diseases.

Other tropical diseases

Table 20.6 provides a brief summary of other important tropical diseases.

Traveler-related illness

With populations around the world being more mobile than ever before, infectious disease epidemiology is changing. Healthcare practitioners must maintain vigilance for NTDs across all settings and especially among travelers and migrants in non-endemic settings. Table 20.7 summarizes common tropical diseases (other than HIV, tuberculosis, and malaria) that cause fever with or without rash by their relative frequency in different geographic regions. For a full discussion of traveler-related illness, beyond just neglected tropical diseases, see Chapter 36.

Additional resources

- World Health Organization. Neglected tropical diseases. Available at http://www.who.int/neglected_diseases/en/
- Centers for Disease Control and Prevention (CDC): http://www.cdc.gov/
- The Cochrane Library. Neglected Tropical Diseases Collection. Available at http://www.thecochranelibrary.com/details/collection/805883/Neglected-tropical-diseases.html

Table 20.4 Select arbovirus infections in humans.

Diseases/ infection	Epidemiology	Vector	Incubation	Clinical features	Diagnosis	Treatment
Dengue	Widespread throughout tropics, and particularly in Asia (Southeast Asia), Latin America, and the Pacific Islands	*Aedes* mosquito; day biting	Usually 4–8 days (range 3–14 days)	*Dengue fever (DF)*: mild febrile illness often associated with retro-orbital pain, headache, myalgia, arthralgia (lower back usually), and a blanching rash *Dengue hemorrhagic fever (DHF)*: severe erythrodermic rash with petechiae, bleeding gums, epistaxis, and gastrointestinal hemorrhage. Defined by hemorrhagic findings, platelets <100/mm³, evidence of plasma leakage, and fevers *Dengue shock syndrome (DSS)*: the above DHF signs and symptoms, plus with pulse pressure <20mmHg or systolic blood pressure <90mmHg. Mortality of up to 40%	Clinical. PCR and serology possible at specialized laboratories. High cross-reaction with other flaviviruses.	Supportive treatment. Identify those at risk of shock and monitor carefully. Aggressive fluid resuscitation may be needed.
Chikungunya	Outbreaks have occurred in countries in Africa, Asia, Europe (Italy and France), India, and Pacific Ocean	*Aedes* mosquito; day biting	Usually 2–3 days (range 1–12 days)	Febrile illness, headache, with arthralgia as prominent feature. Fever resolves within 5–7 days, but some patients continue to have chronic arthralgia with joint stiffness and swelling.	Clinical. Serology possible at specialized laboratories.	Supportive care. NSAIDs may be helpful.
Yellow fever	Present in most of sub-Saharan Africa (32 countries), Asia and South America	*Aedes* mosquito; day biting	3–6 days	Most cases are with mild 3–4 days of fever, headache, chills, back pain, loss of appetite, nausea, and vomiting. Severe cases exhibit liver failure with jaundice and gastrointestinal bleeding and have up to 20% mortality.	Clinical. Where possible, PCR and serology with comparison of repeat measurements to demonstrate change in titer.	No treatment available. Effective vaccination is mainstay to prevent infection and limit outbreaks. Many countries require proof of vaccination for entry.

Table 20.5 Rickettsial infections.

Diseases/ infection	Epidemiology	Vector	Clinical features	Diagnosis	Treatment	Prevention
Overview of rickettsial disease	Found throughout the world with highest transmission in settings where people are outdoors and exposed to vectors.	Fleas, lice, ticks, or mites	Incubate over 5–14 days and most produce non-specific symptoms of variable severity including fever, headaches, myalgia, rash, lymphadenopathy, and, occasionally, a classic inoculation eschar.	Clinical (history and examination). Serology generally requires comparison of initial and convalescent measurements, so only useful for confirmation during the recovery. In severe cases, findings include thrombocytopenia, leukocytosis, anemia, and abnormal liver tests.	Doxycycline 100 mg twice daily or 200 mg once daily with duration dependent on the specific infection, although a 5–7 day course is appropriate in most situations. Alternatives include azithromycin, chloramphenicol, fluoroquinolones, and rifampin.	*Lice and flea-borne:* treat clothes with insecticide (e.g., DDT, malathion, permethrin), topical repellents). Rodent control and avoidance of dogs and cats in endemic areas. *Tick-borne:* protective clothing, rapid removal of ticks.
Typhus group						
Murine typhus (*R. typhi*)	Occurs episodically in environments with rats and humans in close proximity. Worldwide distribution, but rare.	Flea-borne: rat flea *Xenopsylla cheopis* is the main vector. Rats are the main reservoir. Humans are infected by contamination of broken skin with infected flea feces.	Fever, headaches, myalgia, and rash. Gastrointestinal symptoms common in children.	Clinical history suggestive of possible exposure	Usually self-limiting. Doxycycline 100 mg twice daily for 5 days or until 48 hours after fever subsides.	Hygiene and rat control efforts
Epidemic typhus (*R. prowazekii*)	Not routinely monitored, but problematic in times of war, conflict, famine, and natural disasters when body lice thrive. Recently seen in refugee camps in cooler mountainous areas in Africa, Mexico, Asia, and Central and South America.	Louse-borne: transmitted to humans by infected lice feces rubbed into skin injuries (including lice bites) or mucous membranes. Inhalation of infected feces may also play a role. Humans are the reservoir, and lice become infected by feeding on infected humans.	Most patients develop a rash starting on the trunk and spreading to limbs. Rash can be macular, maculopapular, or petechial. CNS symptoms with cerebral vasculitis often occur and diarrhea, pulmonary involvement, myocarditis, splenomegaly, and conjunctivitis may occur. Mortality rate of 10–40% without treatment.	Serology: fourfold antibody response seen 10–21 days after onset of symptoms.	Doxycycline	Treat clothes and sheets with insecticide (e.g., DDT, malathion, lindane). Antibiotic prophylaxis with doxycycline 200 mg once weekly may be used, particularly during outbreaks.

(Continued)

Table 20.5 Rickettsial infections. (*Continued*)

Diseases/infection	Epidemiology	Vector	Clinical features	Diagnosis	Treatment	Prevention
Spotted fever group						
African tick bite fever/African tick typhus (*R. africae*)	Endemic in sub-Saharan Africa, especially in rural areas and game parks in southern Africa.	Tick-borne: *Amblyomma hebraeum* tick of large ruminants and wildlife species in rural areas	Eschar and rash with fever are strongly suggestive. Resolves quickly with doxycycline; if it does not, reconsider diagnosis.	Clinical	Doxycycline	Protective clothing, rapid removal of ticks
Mediterranean spotted fever (*R. conorii*)	Endemic in sub-Saharan Africa, North Africa, Mediterranean (late spring and summer), Indian subcontinent, Europe, and Middle East.	Tick-borne: brown dog tick *Rhipicephalus sanguineus*	Eschar and rash (papular or purpuric) more common. Most patients have a mild illness, but it can rarely be fatal with pneumonitis, meningoencephalitis, disseminated intravascular coagulation, and renal failure.	Clinical	Doxycycline	Protective clothing, rapid removal of ticks
Rocky mountain spotted fever (*R. rickettsii*)	USA, Canada, Mexico, Central America, and parts of South America.	Tick borne: *Dermacentor* spp., *Rhipicephalus sanguineus*	Fever, headache, and rash that evolves from maculopapular to petechial. High mortality if untreated.	Clinical; serology requires comparison of initial and convalescent measurements, so only useful for confirmation during the recovery. Thrombocytopenia that worsens with disease progression can be a clue.	Doxycycline 100 mg twice daily until at least 3 days after fever subsides (5–7 days total in most cases)	Protective clothing, rapid removal of ticks, topical repellents
Scrub typhus (*Orientia tsutsugamushi*)	Central, East, and Southeast Asia; northern Australia.	Trombiculid mite	High fevers, severe headache, and diffuse myalgias frequently accompanied by rash and eschar. Pneumonitis is common. Some cases progress to multiorgan failure.	Clinical, with serologic confirmation using multiple measurements to demonstrate change in titer.	Doxycycline 100 mg twice daily; duration of treatment is unclear but likely requires 5 or more days	Topical repellents (e.g., DEET) and treating clothing and sheets (e.g., permethrin). Antibiotic prophylaxis with doxycycline 200 mg once weekly may be used in endemic areas.

Diseases/ infection	Epidemiology	Vector	Clinical features	Diagnosis	Treatment	Prevention
Other infections						
Trench fever (*Bartonella quintana*)	Other infections (previously classified as rickettsial infections): Gram-negative intracellular bacteria transmitted via arthropod vectors.	Human body louse (*Pediculus humanus* var. *corporis*) transmitting bacterium *Bartonella quintana*.	Acute "5-day cyclical fever," headache, dizziness, and shin pain. Mainly self-limiting. Chronic infection with bacteremia, endocarditis, or bacillary angiomatosis in immunocompromised.	Culture is definitive. Serology variable and PCR still being validated, although both can contribute to diagnosis while awaiting culture	Doxycycline 200 mg once daily for 4 weeks and gentamicin 3 mg/kg i.v. overlapping during the first 2 weeks	Hygiene and proper shelter
Cat scratch fever (*Bartonella henselae*)	Worldwide; in North America, peaks during fall/early winter.	*Bartonella henselae* bacterium transmitted between cats by the cat flea vector, but to humans via cat scratch or bite or by a flea bite.	Tender, self-limiting lymphadenopathy without fever. Can cause infective endocarditis (often culture negative), bacteremia, bacillary angiomatosis, or peliosis hepatitis in immunocompromised.	Serology. Biopsy and PCR may be used to confirm diagnosis	Some experts propose only treating if severe. Others recommend azithromycin for 5 days with 500 mg once on day 1 and 250 mg once daily for days 2–5.	Treat cats for fleas, immediately wash bites and scratches
Q fever (*Coxiella burnetii*)	Worldwide; often in dry arid areas associated with animal excrement.	*Coxiella burnetii* infection via inhalation of contaminated aerosols from urine, feces, milk, and amniotic fluids of infected animals (most commonly cattle, sheep, goats).	*Acute disease*: can be asymptomatic in 50% of cases and causes self-limiting febrile illness in others. Occasionally may lead to hepatitis or pneumonitis *Chronic disease*: can present with endocarditis, valve disease, vascular aneurysms, or bone infection	Serology	*Acute disease*: doxycycline 100 mg twice daily for 14 days *Chronic disease*: doxycycline 100 mg twice daily and hydroxychloroquine daily for 18–24 months	Occupational safety standards in dealing with animals and their products. Vaccine available but rarely and selectively used.

Source: adapted from Cowan (2000).

Table 20.6 Overview of other notable tropical diseases.

Diseases/infection	Summary	Diagnosis	Treatment
Leprosy/Hansen's disease (*Mycobacterium leprae*)	Chronic inflammatory disease of the skin and peripheral nerves. Once a major public health problem, prevalence has declined since the 1980s (WHO, 2010b). Greatest number of new cases seen in India, Brazil, Indonesia, Bangladesh, and Nigeria. Infection occurs in 5% of those exposed. Produces a wide variety of clinical findings including nodular skin lesions, hypopigmented or reddened spots, dysesthesias, paralysis, muscle wasting, ulcers, and tender thickening of the nerves. Cases are categorized based on immune response and pattern of skin findings.	Clinical. Confirmation by identifying acid-fast bacilli in the cutaneous nerve on skin biopsy.	Multidrug regimen that includes rifampicin, dapsone, and clofazimine. Length of treatment, monitoring, and adjunctive steroid treatment depends on the type of disease. Targetted for elimination by WHO by 2020.
Amebiasis/amebic liver abscess (ALA) (*Entamoeba histolytica*)	Caused by protozoan parasite. Fecal–oral transmission of amebic cysts. Most infections are largely asymptomatic. When symptoms occur, patients experience intestinal disease ranging from non-specific gastrointestinal symptoms to fulminant dysentery, marked by fever, bloody diarrhea, and abdominal pain. May present with disseminated disease including abscess formation in the liver or, rarely, ectopic sites. Occasionally, amebomas (amebic granulomas) seen in the wall of the colon, mimicking malignancy. ALA most often seen in men aged 18–50. Up to 20% of ALA is complicated by rupture, commonly through the diaphragm.	*Intestinal*: microscopic identification of trophozoites in the stool, antigen testing, or serology. *Extraintestinal/ALA*: antigen testing or serology.	*Intestinal*: metronidazole 500–750 mg three times daily for 7–10 days (or tinidazole 2 g once daily for 3 days) followed by a luminal agent (paromomycin, diiodohydroxyquin, *or* diloxanide furoate). *Extraintestinal/ALA*: same as for intestinal disease.
Rabies (rabies virus)	Rare but fatal viral infection transmitted by the bite of infected animals, most commonly dogs. Kills up to 70,000 people annually. Leads to a progressive encephalomyelitis. Early symptoms include apprehension, headache, fever, malaise, and tingling at the bite wound. Symptoms progress to hydrophobia and spasm of swallowing muscles. Two-thirds of cases develop frothing of the mouth. Advances to delirium, convulsions, and paralysis of the limbs and respiratory muscles. Prognosis is grim and coma and death, often due to cardiac failure, occur within 1–2 weeks.	Clinical. Because of low sensitivity of testing, multiple modalities used on multiple specimen types.	Vigorous cleaning and flushing of bite wounds. Urgent administration of immunoglobulin and vaccine. Once symptoms start, recovery is very unlikely.
Leptospirosis (*Leptospira* spp.)	Caused by bacteria excreted in the urine of wild and domestic animals (especially rats, cattle). Humans infected by contact of the skin or mucous membranes with contaminated water or, occasionally, food or soil. Greatest risk for veterinarians, sewage workers, and others in close contact with animals or waste. Outbreaks of leptospirosis caused by widespread exposure to infected water (e.g., floods). Occurs worldwide, but most common in temperate or tropical climates. After incubation of 2 days to 4 weeks, presents with sudden onset fever, headache, muscle aches, vomiting, or diarrhea. Can be biphasic with a brief period of improvement before symptoms recur. Without treatment, can last from a few days to months. In severe disease, known as Weil's disease, patients may experience renal failure, liver failure, or meningitis.	Serology with microscopic agglutination test	Acute infection is self-limiting but treatment with doxycycline (or penicillin) may reduce duration and shedding. Weil's disease is probably largely immunologically mediated; treatment, especially of renal failure, is supportive.

Table 20.6 Overview of other notable tropical diseases. (*Continued*)

Diseases/infection	Summary	Diagnosis	Treatment
Brucellosis (*Brucella* spp.)	Chronic granulomatous disease caused by Gram-negative bacteria. Transmission through contact with infected fluids from animals (e.g., sheep, cattle, goats, pigs) or their products including unpasteurized cheese and milk. After a 2–4 week incubation period, patients experience an insidious febrile illness with constitutional symptoms and lymphadenopathy. Systemic involvement of almost any organ system can occur including bone (spondylitis), cardiac (endocarditis), reproductive (spontaneous abortion), gastrointestinal (hepatitis, peritonitis), and CNS (meningitis, encephalitis).	Serology	*Uncomplicated*: doxycycline 100 mg twice daily for 6 weeks with streptomycin 1 g i.m. once daily for 14–21 days or with rifampin 600–900 mg once daily for 6 weeks. *Complicated disease*: requires tailored treatment depending on organs involved.
Melioidosis (*Burkholderia pseudomallei*)	Endemic in Southeast Asia, northern Australia, and the Caribbean. Caused by bacteria found in the mud and surface water of endemic areas (e.g., rice paddies); patients with diabetes and renal failure at greatest risk. Can be asymptomatic, but often fatal – presents with septicemia, bone disease, parotid gland involvement, and lung pathology including pneumonia or cavitary disease.	Culture	Ceftazidime *or* imipenem i.v. for >2 weeks followed by high-dose trimethoprim/ sulfamethoxazole for 3–6 months.
Plague (*Yersinia pestis*)	Found in Africa, Southeast Asia, and the Americas. Transmitted via the bite of an infected rodent flea. After 2–6 day incubation, can present in three patterns *Bubonic plague*: local tender lymphadenitis that subsequently develops into a "bubo" (swollen lymph node). Accompanied by sudden onset of fever, headache, and weakness. May lead to sepsis *Septicemia plague*: sepsis without preceding bubo *Pneumonic plague*: sudden-onset dyspnea, cough, pleurisy, and fever.	Clinical suspicion confirmed by culture from lymph node, blood, or sputum or serology with comparison of repeat measurements to demonstrate change in titer.	Gentamicin 5 mg/kg daily for 10 days *or* until 2 days after fever stops
Viral hemorrhagic fevers (VHF) (Lassa, Ebola, Marburg, Crimean-Congo)	Until the recent Ebola epidemic that began in West Africa in December 2013, this group of VHFs had been relatively uncommon. Nevertheless, they have always had significant public health importance due to their potential to cause epidemics. Most of these viruses are found in sub-Saharan Africa. Crimean-Congo hemorrhagic fever is also seen in former Soviet Union and East and South Asia. VHFs cause a spectrum of disease ranging from asymptomatic infections to rapidly fatal infection. They typically cause sore throat and conjunctivitis and progress to bleeding tendencies, fever, and shock. Liver involvement and jaundice is common.	Clinical	Isolation of suspected cases due to risk of direct spread

Table 20.7 Neglected tropical diseases causing fever in travelers by geographic location. See Chapter 36 for full discussion of illnesses in returning travelers.

Region	Occurrence	Undifferentiated fever	Fever and rash
Sub-Saharan Africa	Common	Rickettsiae	Rickettsiae Acute schistosomiasis (Katayama)
	Occasional	Brucellosis Enteric fever Leptospirosis Acute schistosomiasis Amebic liver abscess Visceral leishmaniasis	Dengue Other arboviruses (Rift Valley fever, West Nile fever, yellow fever) Meningococcus
	Rare	Histoplasmosis Trypanosomiasis Viral hemorrhagic fevers	Viral hemorrhagic fevers
Southeast Asia	Common	Chikungunya Dengue Enteric fever Leptospirosis	Dengue
	Occasional	Amebic liver abscess	
	Rare	Brucellosis Rickettsiae Acute schistosomiasis Hantavirus Japanese encephalitis Scrub typhus	Rickettsiae Acute schistosomiasis (Katayama)
South/Central Asia	Common	Enteric fever Chikungunya Dengue Leptospirosis	Dengue
	Occasional	Amebic liver abscess Leptospirosis	
	Rare	Brucellosis Rickettsiae Crimean-Congo hemorrhagic fever	Rickettsiae
Middle East/ North Africa	Common	Brucellosis Enteric fever	
	Occasional	Leptospirosis *Coxiella*	Dengue Rickettsiae
	Rare	Amebic liver abscess Chikungunya Dengue Visceral leishmaniasis	Acute schistosomiasis (Katayama)
South/Latin America	Common		Dengue
	Occasional	Enteric fever Leptospirosis Dengue Histoplasmosis Coccidioidomycosis	
	Rare	Rickettsiae	

Source: adapted from Johnston *et al.*, 2009.

REFERENCES

Antinori S, Cascio A, Parravicini C, Bianchi R, Corbellino M (2008) Leishmaniasis among organ transplant recipients. *Lancet Infect Dis* 8:191–9.

Barrett MP, Burchmore RJ, Stich A *et al.* (2003) The trypanosomiases. *Lancet* 362:1469–80.

Bern C, Joshi AB, Jha SN *et al.* (2000) Factors associated with visceral leishmaniasis in Nepal: bed-net use is strongly protective. *Am J Trop Med Hyg* 63:184–8.

Bethony J, Brooker S, Albonico M *et al.* (2006) Soil-transmitted helminth infections: ascariasis, trichuriasis, and hookworm. *Lancet* 367:1521–32.

Bleakley H (2003) Disease and development: evidence from hookworm eradication in American South. *J Eur Econ Assoc* 1:376–86.

Bottieau E, Clerinx J, de Vega MR *et al.* (2006) Imported Katayama fever: clinical and biological features at presentation and during treatment. *J Infect* 52: 339–45.

Centers for Disease Control and Prevention (2012) *Strongyloides*: epidemiology and risk factors. Available at http://www.cdc.gov/parasites/strongyloides/epi.html

Clements AC, Moyeed R, Brooker S (2006) Bayesian geostatistical prediction of the intensity of infection with *Schistosoma mansoni* in East Africa. *Parasitology* 133:711–19.

Cowan G (2000) Rickettsial diseases: the typhus groups of fevers: a review. *Postgrad Med J* 76:269–72.

Cruz I, Morales MA, Noguer I, Rodríguez A, Alvar J (2002) Leishmania in discarded syringes from intravenous drug users. *Lancet* 359:1124–5.

Dey A, Singh S (2006) Transfusion transmitted leishmaniasis: a case report and review of literature. *Indian J Med Microbiol* 24:165–70.

Gryseels B, Polman K, Clerinx J, Kestens L (2006) Human schistosomiasis. *Lancet* 368:1106–18.

Hotez PJ, Molyneux DH, Fenwick A *et al.* (2007) Control of neglected tropical diseases. *N Engl J Med* 357:1018–27.

Johnston V, Stockley JM, Dockrell D *et al.* (2009) Fever in returned travellers presenting in the United Kingdom: recommendations for investigation and initial management. *J Infect* 59(1):1–18.

Kabatereine NB, Brooker S, Tukahebwa EM, Kazibwe F, Onapa AW (2004) Epidemiology and geography of *Schistosoma mansoni* in Uganda: implications for planning control. *Trop Med Int Health* 9:372–80.

King CH, Keating CE, Muruka JF *et al.* (1988) Urinary tract morbidity in schistosomiasis haematobia: associations with age and intensity of infection in an endemic area of Coast Province, Kenya. *Am J Trop Med Hyg* 39:361–8.

Lejon V, Büscher P (2005) Cerebrospinal fluid in human African trypanosomiasis: a key to diagnosis, therapeutic decision and post-treatment follow-up. *Trop Med Int Health* 10:395–403.

Meinecke CK, Schottelius J, Oskam L, Fleischer B (1999) Congenital transmission of visceral leishmaniasis (Kala Azar) from an asymptomatic mother to her child. *Pediatrics* 104:e65.

Miguel EA, Kremer M (2003) Worms: identifying impacts on education and health in the presence of treatment externalities. *Econometrica* 72:159–217.

Organización Panamericana de la Salud (2006) *Estimación cuantitativa de la enfermedad de Chagas en las Americas.* Montevideo: Organización Panamericana de la Salud.

Pasricha JM, Street AC, Leder K (2011) A rash and cough in a traveler. *Clin Infect Dis* 53:205–6.

van Griensven J, Diro E, Lopez-Velez R *et al.* (2013) HIV-1 protease inhibitors for treatment of visceral leishmaniasis in HIV-co-infected individuals. *Lancet Infect Dis* 13:251–9.

Viney ME, Brown M, Omoding NE *et al.* (2004) Why does HIV infection not lead to disseminated strongyloidiasis? *J Infect Dis* 190:2175–80.

WHO (2004) *The World Health Report 2004: Changing History.* Geneva: World Health Organization.

WHO (2008) *The Global Burden of Disease: 2004 Update.* Geneva: World Health Organization.

WHO (2010a) Essential leishmaniasis maps. http://www.who.int/leishmaniasis/leishmaniasis_maps/en/

WHO (2010b) Leprosy fact sheet. *Wkly Epidemiol Rec* 85:46–8.

WHO (2011) Distribution of soil-transmitted helminthiases and proportion of children (aged 1–14 years) in each endemic country requiring preventive chemotherapy for the diseases. Available at http://www.who.int/intestinal_worms/epidemiology/Soil _transmitted_helminthiases_2011.jpg

Part 5
Non-Communicable
Diseases

CHAPTER 21

Cardiovascular Disease

Robert N. Peck[1,2,3], Johannes Kataraihya[2,3], and Luke R. Smart[1,2]

[1]Weill Cornell Medical College, New York, NY, USA
[2]Catholic University of Health and Allied Sciences, Mwanza, Tanzania
[3]Weill Bugando School of Medicine, and Bugando Medical Centre, Mwanza, Tanzania

Key learning objectives

- Understand the variable epidemiology of cardiovascular disease in different regions.
- Learn how and why the presentations of cardiovascular disease may differ.
- Understand the importance of history and physical examination for cardiovascular medicine in resource-limited settings.
- Recognize the utility of bedside cardiac ultrasound.
- Learn to identify local resource limitations and find local cardiovascular guidelines.
- Appreciate the importance of community education, screening, and primary care in cardiovascular public health.

Abstract

The burgeoning epidemic of non-communicable diseases in global health has been well recognized and documented. Cardiovascular disease is at the top of the list. Diagnosis and treatment of cardiovascular disease in the global health setting requires knowledge of local epidemiology, careful history-taking, and excellent physical examination skills. In addition, one needs to become proficient with locally available diagnostic modalities, medications, and treatment protocols while remaining cognizant of local resource limitations.

Key words: cardiovascular disease, ischemic heart disease, rheumatic heart disease, infective endocarditis, endomyocardial fibrosis, hypertension, Chagas disease, heart failure, peripartum cardiomyopathy, HIV cardiomyopathy

Essential Clinical Global Health, First Edition. Edited by Brett D. Nelson.
© 2015 John Wiley & Sons, Ltd. Published 2015 by John Wiley & Sons, Ltd.
Companion website: www.essentialseries.com/globalhealth

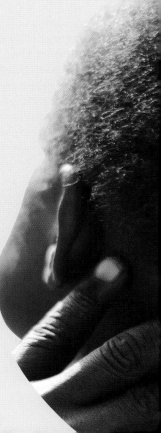

Introduction and epidemiology

Non-communicable diseases (NCDs) have overtaken communicable diseases as the most common cause of premature death in low- and middle-income countries (LMICs) within regions such as sub-Saharan Africa (Figure 21.1). This epidemic of NCDs is largely driven by four factors: obesity, increased salt intake, smoking, and excessive alcohol. Underlying these four drivers of the NCD epidemic are the rapid urbanization and industrialization of LMICs and resultant changes in patterns of diet and exercise. In the Moscow Declaration of 2011, the World Health Organization (WHO) recognized this epidemic of NCDs – particularly cardiovascular disease (CVD), diabetes mellitus, chronic lung disease, and cancer – as one of the greatest barriers to health worldwide (World Health Organization, 2011a). Among NCDs, CVD is the leading cause of premature mortality and accounts for nearly 40% of all NCD deaths in people less than 70 years of age. Three-quarters of CVD-related deaths occur in LMICs.

The category of CVD encompasses a variety of diseases that affect the heart and/or the vasculature. The pattern of specific CVDs differs regionally. Some conditions, such as ischemic heart disease and aortic aneurysm, occur more frequently in high-income countries (HICs) but are now becoming more common in LMICs. Others, such as congestive heart failure, are a common endpoint for several etiologies that differ according to region (e.g., ischemic heart disease, cardiomyopathy, rheumatic heart disease). Still others, such as Chagas or endomyocardial fibrosis, are endemic only in certain regions.

Figure 21.2 illustrates how the age-adjusted mortality rates of two common CVDs (ischemic heart disease and stroke) vary between countries. Ischemic heart disease mortality is generally higher in Asia, Eastern Europe, and North Africa, whereas, stroke mortality is generally higher in sub-Saharan Africa and Asia. HICs such as the United States and Europe have lower age-adjusted mortality rates because ischemic heart disease and stroke usually cause death in older people in these countries.

The regional distribution of risk factors is a major contributor to the variability of CVD epidemiology (Avezum et al., 2009; Dalal et al., 2011). Hypertension is a prime example. One-quarter of the world's adult population has hypertension, likely increasing to 30% by 2025 (Mittal & Singh, 2010). The most recent Global Burden of Disease study reported that hypertension is now the leading risk factor for disability-adjusted life years (DALYs) worldwide (Lim et al., 2012). In some regions of the world, such as sub-Saharan Africa, hypertension was previously considered rare but is now nearing epidemic proportions. Studies from Tanzania, Nigeria, and South Africa consistently report that 15–20% of all adult hospital admissions in Africa are due to hypertension-related diagnoses. In addition, these patients are admitted to the hospital (and dying) at younger ages (Peck et al., 2013). As communicable diseases are controlled, the morbidity and mortality attributable to hypertension-related diseases will continue to swell in LMICs (Ibrahim & Damasceno, 2012). Figure 21.2c illustrates the age-adjusted prevalence of hypertension in different countries worldwide, with the highest rates being seen in Africa and Eastern Europe.

Other CVD risk factors also vary according to region. Rates of smoking, for example, are generally low in sub-Saharan Africa, moderate in South America, and high in China and Eastern Europe. The prevalence of obesity has a similar distribution: low in sub-Saharan Africa, moderate in South America, and high in the United States and Europe. Data regarding the distribution of CVDs and risk factors are available from the WHO website (http://www.who.int/topics/cardiovascular_diseases/en/).

The distribution of CVDs is partly explained by the impact of economic development. Table 21.1 describes the relationship between stages of development and types of CVD observed in different regions. Of note, many regions contain countries in different stages of development. In sub-Saharan Africa, for example, urban centers in South Africa or Botswana may be at stage 3 or 4, while rural areas of Chad or the Democratic Republic of Congo may still be in stage 1. In addition, many regions of the world are currently in transition between different stages of economic development.

Red flag

In whatever region of the world you will be working, find a review article or meta-analysis that describes the distribution of CVDs in that region, such as the examples provided in the Additional resources section (Avezum et al., 2009; Dalal et al., 2011).

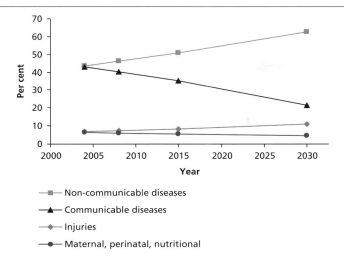

Figure 21.1 Estimated proportions of age-standardized mortality rates by cause in sub-Saharan Africa. Mortality estimates were standardized to the WHO World Standard Population. *Source*: Dalal *et al.* (2011), figure 1, p. 887. Reproduced with permission of Oxford University Press, from data sourced from World Health Organization. Global Burden of Disease. Projections of mortality and burden of disease, 2002–2030.

Clinical experience

"The regional variation of cardiovascular disease epidemiology has important implications for clinical medicine. Common things are common. One of the keys to being a good global health clinician is learning what diseases are common in your region by talking to local clinicians and reading the medical literature, particularly research done in your region. For example, in Tanzania, when I see an adult with a massive pericardial effusion, I can be relatively confident that this is due to TB, and I might even start treatment for TB immediately. Why? Local data and local experience teach me that TB is by far the most common cause of massive pericardial effusion in my region."

Robert, physician working in Tanzania

Presentation

CVDs in LMICs often present differently than in HICs due to a number of factors: distribution of disease, stage of presentation, tolerance to discomfort, and linguistic descriptions of symptoms. Patients frequently present at a later stage of disease and report only a short period of illness even though milder symptoms were present for a lengthy period of time. Also, similar words (when translated) may be used to describe different symptoms. In Kiswahili, for example, the word for "fever" can be used to describe any discomfort and may not

specifically refer to symptoms of elevated body temperature. Understanding these types of differences is critical in every context. The following are a few common differences in the presentation of CVDs in LMICs.

- *Younger age of onset.* CVDs often present at younger ages in LMICs. Heart failure, for example, commonly presents in the second to fourth generations of life compared with HICs where heart failure is typically a disease of the elderly. This early presentation is due to the higher prevalence of rheumatic heart disease, undiagnosed congenital heart disease, and dilated cardiomyopathies secondary to HIV and pregnancy, all conditions that tend to present in late childhood and young adulthood. Hypertension and hypertension-related complications also often present at a younger age in LMICs due to uncontrolled essential hypertension and higher rates of secondary hypertension (mostly renal).
- *Later presentation.* As a result of limited community awareness efforts and deficiencies in primary care, CVDs also often present at very late stages in LMICs. The diagnosis of hypertension, for example, might be delayed until a patient presents with severe complications such as stroke or hypertensive emergency. Late presentation complicates clinical diagnosis since the late-stage manifestations of these diseases are often different from the early stages. In "burnt-out" hypertensive heart disease, for example, patients can present with severe biventricular heart failure due to chronic hypertension but with normal or even low blood pressures since the left ventricle is no longer able to exert sufficient force to maintain high blood pressures.

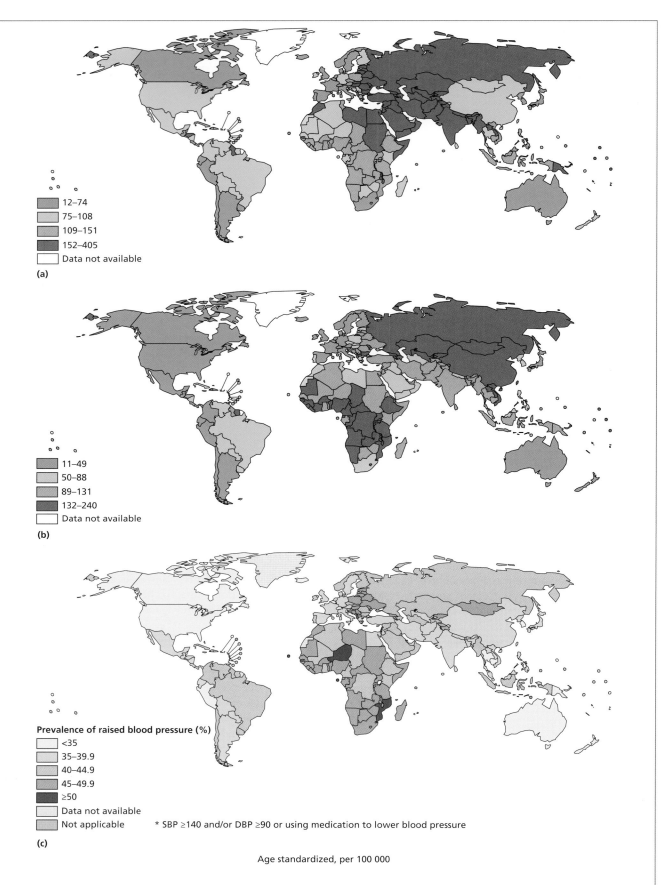

(a)

- 12–74
- 75–108
- 109–151
- 152–405
- Data not available

(b)

- 11–49
- 50–88
- 89–131
- 132–240
- Data not available

(c)

Prevalence of raised blood pressure (%)

- <35
- 35–39.9
- 40–44.9
- 45–49.9
- ≥50
- Data not available
- Not applicable   * SBP ≥140 and/or DBP ≥90 or using medication to lower blood pressure

Age standardized, per 100 000

Figure 21.2 (a) Age-standardized mortality rates from ischemic heart disease. (b) Age-standardized mortality rates from cerebrovascular disease. *Source*: World Health Organization, 2013 (World Health Organization, 2011b, 2013), figures 1 and 2, p. 9. Reproduced with permission of the World Health Organization. (c) Prevalence of high blood pressure, one of the major risk factors for CVD. *Source*: World Health Organization (2011a,b). Reproduced with permission of the World Health Organization.

Table 21.1 Relationship between cardiovascular disease (CVD) and stages of development.

Stages of development	Deaths from CVD	Predominant risk factors	Predominant CVDs	Regional examples
1. "Age of pestilence and famine" (low-income countries)	5–10%	Infections, nutritional deficiencies	Rheumatic heart disease, HIV and peripartum cardiomyopathies, TB pericardial disease	Central, Eastern and Western sub-Saharan Africa
2. "Age of receding pandemics" (low- and middle-income countries)	10–35%	Infections, nutritional deficiencies and excess, hypertension	As above, plus hypertensive heart disease, hemorrhagic stroke, hypertensive emergencies	Southeast and South Asia, Andean, Tropical and Central Latin America, Caribbean, southern sub-Saharan Africa, Oceania
3. "Age of degenerative and man-made diseases" (middle- and high-income countries)	35–60%	Nutritional excess, diabetes, hypertension, tobacco use, alcohol abuse, physical inactivity	Hypertensive heart disease, stroke (in the young), ischemic heart disease (in the young)	Eastern and Central Europe, Central and East Asia, North Africa, Middle East, Southern Latin America
4. "Age of delayed degenerative diseases" (high-income countries)	<40%	Hypertension, nutritional excess, diabetes	Stroke and ischemic heart disease (in the old), hypertensive heart disease	Western Europe, North America, Australasia, high-income Asia Pacific

Source: adapted from Yusuf *et al.* (2001a).

Clinical experience

"As a trainee traveling to work in a hospital in sub-Saharan Africa, I incorrectly assumed that my experience with cardiovascular disease at home would more than suffice for the "few" cases that I might see. The number of cases far surpassed my expectations. Without advanced imaging and laboratory tests to fall back on, my meager experience in relying on physical exam alone for diagnosis was all too obvious. Local colleagues taught me to exam the cardiovascular system carefully and thoroughly, from the wrist, to the neck veins, to the precordium. I found myself thinking carefully about each aspect of the exam. Bedside ultrasound suddenly became a crucial confirmatory tool for determining the source of heart failure or hypotension. Most importantly, I learned that my relationship with local physicians enabled me to get up to speed in common etiologies, diagnostic techniques, treatment protocols, and medication availability. I realized that experience at home does not always translate to experience abroad, and strong local relationships help bridge that gap."

Luke, global health fellow working in Tanzania

- *Interactions with traditional medicine.* Many people in LMICs prefer traditional herbal and spiritual medicine to modern Western medicine. Patients with CVD have frequently attended at least one traditional healer before attending a clinic or hospital. This can affect the presentation of CVDs in several ways. First, it can further delay presentation. Second, traditional herbal remedies can cause adverse effects (such as acute kidney or liver injury) or may interact with cardiovascular medications through the cytochrome P450 system. Lastly, continued traditional medicine utilization after discharge may interfere with regular clinic attendance or adherence to medications. For these reasons, a detailed, tactful, and non-judgmental history of attendance to traditional healers and treatments received is essential.
- *Causes of chest pain.* Chest pain is extremely common in LMICs, but its causes vary in different regions. In countries where ischemic heart disease is still uncommon, pulmonary, infectious, gastrointestinal, and musculoskeletal causes of chest pain are more prevalent. In some regions, chest pain is also a frequent symptom of psychiatric somatization, whereas in other regions abdominal pain is more common.
- *Heart failure.* While left heart failure remains the leading cause of right heart failure worldwide, cor pulmonale (right

heart failure due to lung disease) is more prevalent in LMICs than in HICs. Higher rates of cor pulmonale in LMICs are due to chronic untreated lung diseases (e.g., tuberculosis) or pulmonary hypertension from recurrent pulmonary emboli, HIV, or schistosomiasis. When evaluating a patient with heart failure, it is important to determine if it is right heart failure, left heart failure, or both, since the differential diagnosis and treatment of these syndromes is different. Pure right heart failure generally presents with leg and abdominal swelling but generally without orthopnea and paroxysmal nocturnal dyspnea.

Diagnosis

Diagnostic laboratory and radiographic tests are often lacking in LMICs. In order to diagnose and treat CVDs, skill and creativity are often required in the utilization of limited diagnostic resources. See Panel 21.1 for critical diagnostic resources for LMICs. Panel 21.2 discusses how to complete a systematic and thorough cardiovascular examination.

Bedside cardiac ultrasound is another useful tool for the diagnosis and management of CVD in resource-limited settings. Even in LMICs, many hospitals are equipped with

Panel 21.1: Rather than left-justifying all of the illustrations in this Panel (on this page and subsequent pages), would it look better to center the illustrations within the left-hand column? Or perhaps simply shrink the images slightly (and make them all similar sizes) so that there's a little more space and all of the images in this Panel don't look as crowded?

History and physical examination resources

History
The importance of taking a careful history in resource-limited settings cannot be overestimated. The clinical answer is usually in the history. This is why it is critical that if you are working across a language barrier, you either learn some of the local language or find a reliable translator or, ideally, both

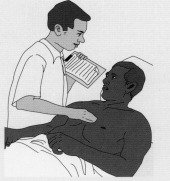

Physical examination
Learn to be systematic and rigorous in your physical examination so that you do not miss important clues

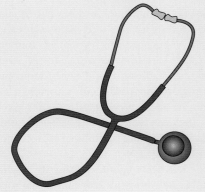

Stethoscope
Learn to hear normal heart sounds, murmurs, rubs, and gallops by listening carefully to every patient

Panel 21.1 (Continued)

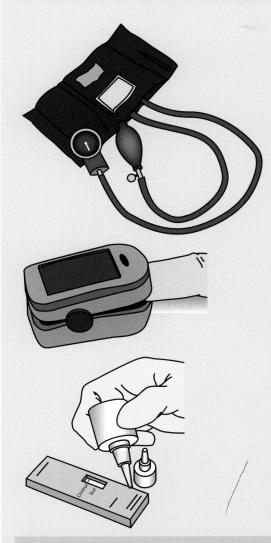

Blood pressure cuff
Do not assume that a functional cuff will be available for you in the wards or clinics

Portable pulse-oximeter
Oximetry is often not available on the wards, and hypoxia is very common among patients in resource-limited settings due to late presentation. Therefore, try to carry your own pulse oximeter. Compact affordable oximeters can be purchased ahead of time within most pharmacies in high-income countries

HIV test
Provider-initiated counseling and testing (PICT) for HIV should ideally be performed at every patient encounter in LMICs where HIV is endemic. There are many important interactions between HIV and CVDs. HIV is related to an increased incidence of pericardial disease (particularly TB pericarditis), dilated cardiomyopathy, and vasculopathy (Ntsekhe & Hakim, 2005)

Essential diagnostic tests with variable availability

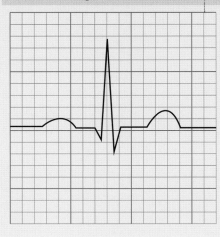

Electrocardiogram (ECG)
ECGs are obviously important for the diagnosis of ischemic heart disease and arrhythmias but may not be available in some settings. Many arrhythmias can be diagnosed by physical examination alone

(Continued)

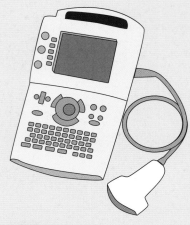

Echocardiogram
Echocardiography is important for the diagnosis of structural heart disease but is not available at many health facilities in LMICs. With some basic training, doctors can use bedside ultrasonography to determine the presence of pericardial effusion, the size of heart chambers, and the general contractility of the left ventricle. See Figure 21.3 for details

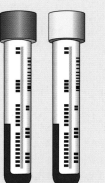

Modern cardiac biomarkers (troponins, CK-MB)
Modern cardiac biomarkers may not be available. In the absence of these, older cardiac enzymes such as LDH and ALT can be used

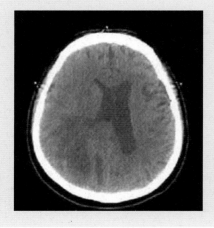

CT/MRI
CT scanners are not available in most health facilities in LMICs. In these facilities, the diagnosis of stroke is usually made on the basis of history, physical examination, and clinical scores. The visualization of cardiopulmonary pathology largely depends on chest radiography in different views (PA, lateral, decubitus, etc.) plus cardiac ultrasound

Panel 21.2

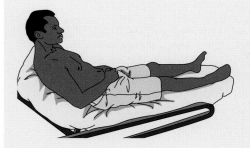

Position
The cardiovascular examination should always be performed in the cardiac position with the patient sitting up at 45°

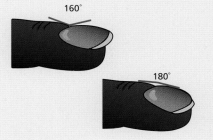

160°

180°

Hands
Start with examination of the hands for warmth, cyanosis, clubbing or signs of infective endocarditis (such as Janeway lesions, Oslers nodes, or splinter hemorrhages)

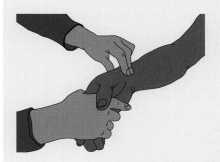

Pulse
The right radial pulse is examined for (i) rate, (ii) regularity (if irregular, categorize as irregularly irregular, regularly irregular, or regular with occasional irregularities), and (iii) synchronicity with the femoral and left radial pulses. If the pulse is irregularly irregular, calculate the pulse deficit (heart rate – pulse rate) as this can be used to confirm the diagnosis of atrial fibrillation

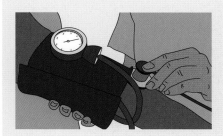

Blood pressure
Should be measured in both arms. Pulsus paradoxicus should be assessed if there is any concern for cardiac tamponade

(Continued)

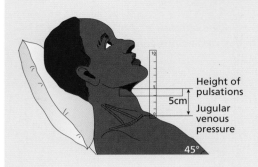

Jugular vein

Jugular venous pressure is measured as the number of vertical centimeters above the sternal angle (3–5 cm is normal). Kussmaul's sign should be assessed if restrictive pericarditis or constrictive cardiomyopathy are on the differential diagnosis

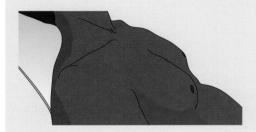

Precordial inspection

The precordium should be inspected for any bulging of the left side of the chest cage (which may indicate massive cardiomegaly) as well as for any visible apical or precordial hyperactivity

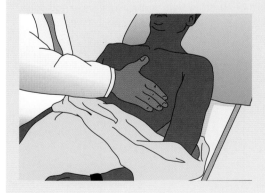

Precordial palpation

The apex of the heartbeat should be located and described as normal, unpalpable, heaving, or tapping. The apex beat is normally located at the fifth intercostal space in the mid-clavicular line. Any parasternal heave should be noted as evidence of right ventricular hypertrophy

👁 **Panel 21.2 (*Continued*)**

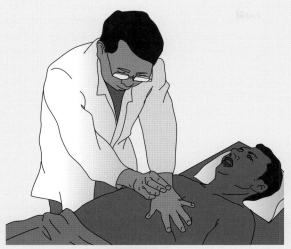

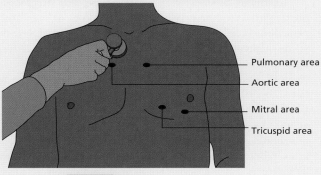

Pulmonary area

Aortic area

Mitral area

Tricuspid area

Precordial percussion

Percussion is not generally performed on cardiovascular examination but may be useful in detecting cardiomegaly in cases where the apex beat cannot be palpated

Precordial auscultation

Auscultation should be performed with both the bell and the diaphragm of the stethoscope in all four auscultatory areas. Listen to both S1 and S2 before listening to any added sounds such as murmurs, rubs, gallops (S3 or S4), clicks, or snaps. Any murmurs should be described carefully in terms of their location, timing (systolic, diastolic, or both), intensity (grades 1–5), quality (high- or low-pitched), pattern (crescendo–decrescendo, holosystolic, etc.), and whether there is any radiation to the neck or axilla

Other

The bases of the lungs should be examined for any crackles, the abdomen should be examined for tender hepatomegaly or hepatojugular reflux, and the ankles should be examined for any pitting edema an ultrasound machine. Learning the basics of cardiac ultrasound takes daily practice and supervision but can usually be achieved in 2–3 months. Bedside cardiac ultrasound can be used to rapidly identify pericardial and pleural effusions, cardiac chamber sizes, left ventricular contractility, and inferior vena cava diameter and variability (proxies for right atrial pressure). Although bedside cardiac ultrasound cannot replace formal echocardiography, simplified echocardiographic strategies for cardiac ultrasound have been shown to be useful in the diagnosis and management of heart failure (Kwan *et al.*, 2013). Bedside cardiac ultrasound is also useful in quickly determining the etiology of shock (e.g., cardiogenic, hypovolemic, septic) as well as in guiding procedures such as pericardial and pleural tapping. Figure 21.3 illustrates some of the findings that can be demonstrated with bedside cardiac ultrasound.

A few of the interesting endemic CVDs that may be relatively exclusive to working in LMICs are described below.

Rheumatic heart disease

Rheumatic fever and rheumatic heart disease (RHD) remain common in LMICs (Remenyi *et al.*, 2013). RHD is strongly associated with poverty and is one of the leading causes of heart failure in many LMICs. In HICs, the incidence of RHD began to decline before the invention of penicillin, likely due to improvements in housing and hygiene. Similar declines are occurring in many LMICs.

Acute rheumatic fever is caused by untreated pharyngitis with rheumatogenic strains of group A *Streptococcus pyogenes*, typically occurring between 5 and 15 years of age. In LMICs, acute streptococcal pharyngitis often goes undiagnosed and untreated due to the high frequency of sore throat in childhood and the cost of care. If a rheumatogenic strain infects a susceptible host, an autoimmune reaction occurs 2–3 weeks later, and antibodies cross-react with joint synovium, heart, brain, and skin tissue. This cross-reactivity leads to the symptoms of acute rheumatic fever that are described in the Jones criteria. On examination, patients may have signs of arthritis in one or more large joints, tachycardia, mitral regurgitation, or pericardial friction rubs.

RHD is a subsequent complication of recurrent acute rheumatic fever. Symptoms typically begin between 15 and 25 years of age (sometimes as early as 6 years). Recurrent carditis causes fibrosis and calcification of the heart valves, leading to stenosis and/or regurgitation. The mitral valve is the most commonly affected valve, followed by the aortic and rarely the tricuspid valves. If not diagnosed and corrected early, these valvular lesions will lead to ventricular hypertrophy, dilation, and failure. Because of mitral valve involvement, the left atria are often massively enlarged, leading to atrial arrhythmias and atrial thrombi that can embolize. RHD is also a major risk factor for infectious endocarditis. In LMICs, patients with RHD often present to health facilities only after developing symptoms of heart failure. Echocardiography can be used to confirm the diagnosis by demonstrating valvular stenosis and/or regurgitation with thickening or "clubbing" of the valves (Figure 21.3).

Treatment depends on stage of disease. For streptococcal pharyngitis, treatment with a single dose of benzathine penicillin is effective in preventing rheumatic fever. For acute rheumatic fever, the recommended treatment is high-dose aspirin, penicillin V, and, if severe carditis is present, steroids. Treatment for acute rheumatic fever should be followed by 10 years of prophylaxis with monthly benzathine penicillin injections to prevent recurrent streptococcal pharyngitis. In patients with RHD, monthly benzathine penicillin should be given for life, together with treatment for heart failure. Infective endocarditis prophylaxis should also be given. A consultation for potential cardiothoracic surgery should be obtained early to evaluate for possible valve replacement or repair.

Chagas disease

Chagas disease, caused by the parasite *Trypanosoma cruzi*, is confined to endemic areas of Central and South America. The distribution of Chagas disease, as with many parasitic infections, is related to the distribution of its vector (the reduviid bug) in combination with socioeconomic factors such as housing. The reduviid bug transmits *T. cruzi* to humans through infected feces that come into direct contact with the skin, mucous membranes, or conjunctiva. During the acute phase, non-specific symptoms predominate, including swelling at the site of the bite (chagoma), lymphadenopathy, rash, hepatosplenomegaly, or meningoencephalitis. Romaña's sign, periorbital swelling caused by irritation of the conjunctiva when the initial infection occurs very close to the eye, is a classic but rare finding (see Chapter 20, Figure 20.6). On entering the bloodstream (usually after 2–4 weeks) fevers may be present. The parasite is deposited in the tissue of the heart and gastrointestinal tract, where it can have either a benign course (75%) or cause persistent infection and severe cardiac or gastrointestinal symptoms (25%). Cardiovascular

---

▌ Red flag

Simplified JONES criteria for the diagnosis of rheumatic fever

- **J**oints: migratory, oligoarthritis of large joints
- **O**bvious: pericarditis, myocarditis, and/or valvular regurgitation due to inflammatory pancarditis
- **N**odules
- **E**rythema marginatum (erythematous macules with serpiginous well-demarcated edges and central clearing)
- **S**ydenham's chorea (rapid involuntary muscle movements)

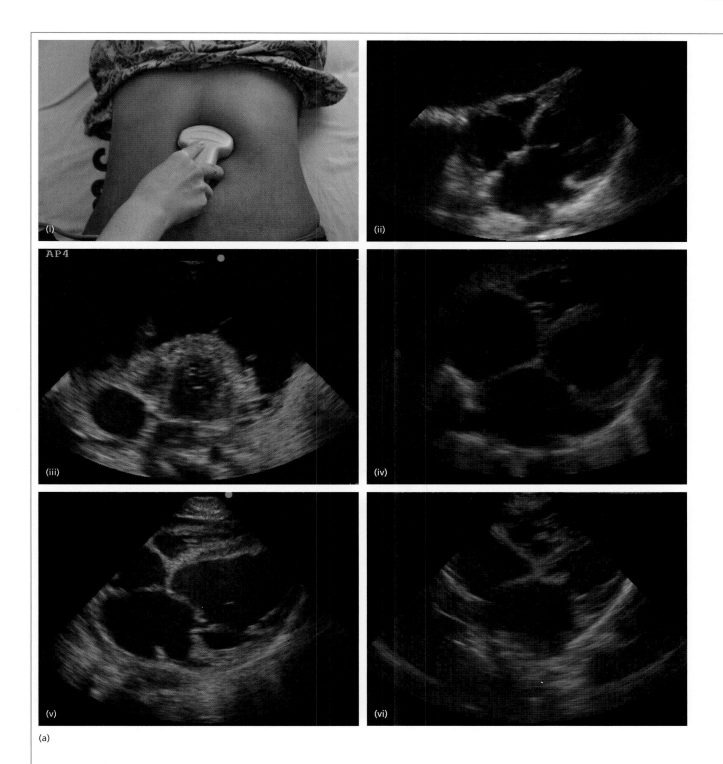

Figure 21.3 (a) Cardiac ultrasound images demonstrating (i) subxiphoid or subcostal probe placement; (ii) normal subxiphoid view of the heart; (iii) large tuberculosis pericardial effusion with fibrinous strands; (iv) dilated cardiomyopathy with four-chamber dilation (note how all four chambers appear dilated compared with normal subxiphoid view); (v) isolated dilation of the left ventricle and atrium with normal-sized right atrium and ventricle; (vi) rheumatic heart disease with mitral valve thickening.

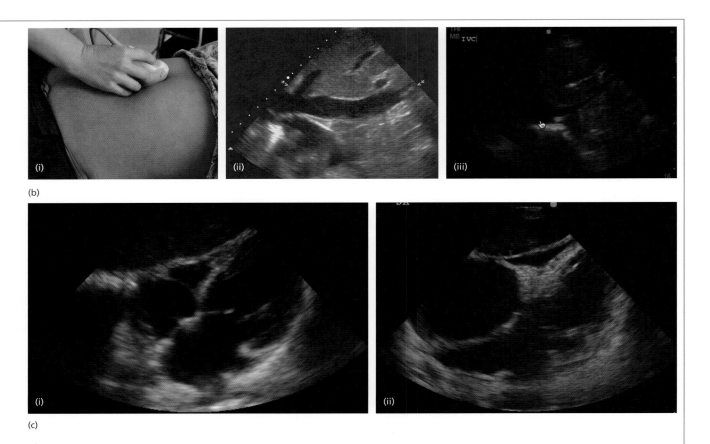

Figure 21.3 (*Continued*) (b) Inferior vena cava (IVC) ultrasound demonstrating (i) probe placement for IVC imaging; (ii) dilated IVC; and (iii) collapsed IVC. (c) Endomyocardial fibrosis (EMF): (i) normal heart in subxiphoid view compared with (ii) heart with EMF (note small fibrosed right ventricle and massively dilated right atrium).

manifestations include arrhythmia, conduction disorders, ventricular aneurysm, thromboembolic events, progressive dilated cardiomyopathy, cardiac failure, and sudden death. The parasite can be identified by microscopy of blood or cerebrospinal fluid (wet mount or Giemsa stain), PCR for parasite DNA, or serology for anti-*T. cruzi* IgG. The acute infection should be treated with either benznidazole or nifurtimox. The chronic phase can be treated with benznidazole, but treatment is seldom effective. Cardiac and gastrointestinal manifestations are managed symptomatically according to presentation. In resource-rich settings, a pacemaker may be placed for the management of arrhythmias or high-grade atrioventricular blocks, and cardiac surgery or even cardiac transplantation is considered as needed.

Endomyocardial fibrosis

Endomyocardial fibrosis (EMF) is a disease found primarily in wet, tropical, rural regions mostly in sub-Saharan Africa but also in Southeast Asia and Latin America. Patients usually present between 10 and 15 years of age, although late presentation (around 30 years) can occur. The pathophysiology of EMF seems to be similar to that of hypereosinophilic syndrome, with eosinophilic infiltration of the myocardium leading to the cardiac fibrosis. The trigger for EMF is not known, but infections (such as filariasis) or nutritional causes seem most likely to explain the geographic distribution. Myocardial fibrosis leads to both restrictive filling of the ventricles and to tethering of the atrioventricular valves, leading to mitral and/or tricuspid regurgitation. Early in the disease, patients may experience non-specific symptoms such as fevers, chills, night sweats, facial swelling, itching, cough, dyspnea, and abdominal swelling. The disease usually progresses slowly to right and/or left heart failure. Patients can have associated massive tense ascites as well as pleural and/or pericardial effusions. On examination, regurgitant mitral/tricuspid murmurs are sometimes present, although an S3 gallop and diminished S1/S2 are more common. Patients may also have atrial fibrillation, finger clubbing, and/or cyanosis. The typical distribution of edema in patients with right-sided EMF is sometimes described as "a potato on toothpicks," with massive ascites but very little edema of the extremities. Diagnosis is usually made by echocardiogram. The use of corticosteroids early in the course of the disease has been suggested as a way to prevent progression to cardiac fibrosis but most patients present only after fibrosis has occurred. Medical therapy for heart failure is the mainstay of treatment, although surgery to remove endomyocardial fibrosis (stripping) or cardiac transplantation may be considered where available. Patients with right-sided EMF can often live for many years with dual diuretic therapy (furosemide plus spironolactone) plus regular therapeutic ascitic tapping. Patients with left-sided EMF often die at an early age due to either arrhythmia or severe intractable left heart failure.

Treatment

Treatment of CVDs in LMICs is often complicated by (i) lack of certain drugs and treatments, (ii) high cost of long-term care for chronic CVDs, and (iii) resultant non-compliance. Understanding local drug supply and the socioeconomic status of the local patient population is critical to providing good care. Learn what drugs are regularly available and how much they cost by visiting local pharmacies and talking to local providers. Ask patients what they can (and cannot) afford. Learn local and international guidelines for the management of CVDs in resource-limited settings. Many LMICs are currently in the process of developing national guidelines for the management of CVDs. Local guidelines exist in many large hospitals. Some organizations like Médecins Sans Frontières and the World Heart Federation have clinical guidelines that are available online (see Additional resources section).

In 2007, the WHO published guidelines for primary and secondary prevention of CVDs, including tables for calculating 10-year cardiovascular risk (World Health Organization, 2007). Table 21.2 provides primary prevention recommendations.

The treatment of hypertension in LMICs is similar to that in HICs except for the notable differences outlined in the WHO recommendations in Figure 21.4, plus any differences necessitated by local resource limitations. Since cost and availability are often major barriers to treatment in resource-limited settings, inexpensive once-daily thiazide diuretics are often a good choice for first-line therapy of mild hypertension. Moderate hypertension often requires at least two antihypertensive drugs, and combination pills are preferable in order to minimize the pill burden. If the blood pressure is not controlled with concurrent use of three different classes of antihypertensive drugs, secondary causes of hypertension should be investigated.

The main difference in treatment of ischemic heart disease in LMICs is the availability of revascularization therapy. If cardiac catheterization is not available, as in many LMICs,

emergent intravenous thrombolytic therapy should be considered in the setting of acute myocardial infarction if within 6–12 hours of the onset of chest pain. In some LMICs, even thrombolytic drugs are not available. In these settings, intravenous heparin infusions may be given for the first 48–72 hours. In all settings, in the absence of contraindications, aspirin 300 mg and/or clopidogrel 300 mg should be given immediately, and patients should then be continued indefinitely on aspirin 75 mg. A beta-blocker should be given to reduce the heart rate into the range of 50–80 bpm (if blood pressure allows). Nitrates and morphine should be given for pain, together with oxygen therapy.

Medical treatment of heart failure in LMICs is similar to that in HICs. Patients presenting with decompensated heart failure should be treated with LMNOP: **l**asix, **m**orphine (for dyspnea), **n**itrates, **o**xygen therapy, and **p**ositioning (sitting cardiac posture). Patients with cardiogenic shock are usually given dopamine and/or dobutamine infusions. Epinephrine infusions can be used in settings where other inotropes are not available. Beta-blockers should be avoided in patients with severe valvular heart disease and severe anemia.

Prevention

Prevention of CVDs is, of course, better than awaiting the need for treatment. Efforts to prevent CVDs in global health need to focus on culturally appropriate community education and disease screening, as well as development of infrastructure for primary care. HIV primary care infrastructure in LMICs may serve as both a foundation and a model for such efforts (Harries *et al.*, 2009). Health education messages should focus on increasing exercise, decreasing salt intake, cessation or prevention of smoking, and moderation of alcohol intake. Political interventions are needed to reduce smoking and improve diet.

Figure 21.4 portrays the three major strategies for reducing the burden of CVDs: population-based socioeconomic approaches, individualized strategy (primary prevention), and clinical strategy (secondary prevention). Socioeconomic and political population-based interventions have the greatest potential for preventing CVDs in the general population but also require the greatest political will. The integration of these three strategies has already proven to be successful in HICs where the burden of CVDs has been declining for the past 20 years.

Additional resources

- Parry E, Godfrey R, Mabey D, Gill G (eds) (2004) *Principles of Medicine in Africa*, 3rd edn. Cambridge, UK: Cambridge University Press. See especially the sections on NCDs and the heart.
- World Health Organization. Moscow Declaration. The First Global Ministerial Conference on Healthy Lifestyles

Table 21.2 Primary prevention of cardiovascular disease stratified by risk of future disease. Treatment is adjusted based on the patient's risk of having a fatal or non-fatal vascular event in the next 10 years.

Risk of having a vascular event in the next 10 years	<10%	10–20%	20–30%	>30%
Risk	Low	Moderate	High	Very high
Strategy	Conservative management. Lifestyle changes	Monitor risk profile every 6–12 months	Monitor risk profile every 3–6 months	Monitor risk profile every 3–6 months
Smoking	Discourage non-smokers from starting Encourage smokers to quit and support their efforts Advise users of other forms of tobacco to stop		Provide nicotine replacement therapy, nortriptyline, and/or amfebutamone (bupropion) to those who fail to quit with counseling.	
Diet	Encourage all to reduce total fat and saturated fat intake Goal: total fat <30% of calories, saturated fat <10% of calories (no *trans* fatty acids), polyunsaturated <10% of calories, monounsaturated 10–15% Reduce salt intake by one-third, goal <5 g (90 mmol) per day Eat 400 g per day of fruits, vegetables, whole grains, and pulses			
Physical activity	Encourage all to engage in 30 min of moderate physical activity per day			
Weight control	Encourage overweight and obese to lose weight with reduced calorie diet and increased physical activity			
Alcohol	Encourage all to reduce alcohol consumption to <3 units per day			
Blood pressure	Provide treatment and lifestyle advice to all with BP >160/100 mmHg *or* <160/100 mmHg with target organ damage			
	If BP persistently >140/90 mmHg, provide lifestyle strategies. Check BP and CVD risks every 2–5 years.	If BP persistently >140/90 mmHg, provide lifestyle strategies. Check BP and CVD risks every year.	If BP persistently >140/90 mmHg despite lifestyle strategies for 4–6 months, start medication. Low-dose thiazide diuretic, ACE inhibitor, or calcium-channel blocker are first-line. A beta-blocker is also an option.	If BP persistently >130/80 mmHg, start/add medication. Thiazide, ACE inhibitor, or calcium-channel blocker are first-line. A beta-blocker is also an option.
Lipid	If total cholesterol >8 mmol/L (320 mg/dL), start lipid-lowering diet and give a statin			
		Follow lipid-lowering diet	If >40 years old and high cholesterol (>5.0 mmol/L) and/or LDL >3.0 mmol/l despite diet, start statin	Follow lipid-lowering diet and start statin. At a minimum, goal total cholesterol is <5.0 mmol/L and LDL <3.0 mmol/L *or* a reduction of total cholesterol by 25% and LDL by 30%, whichever approach results in greater reduction.
Glucose	As per moderate risk if resources permit.	If fasting blood glucose >6 mmol/L (>108 mg/dl) despite diet control, start metformin.		
Antiplatelet	Harm > benefit. Do not prescribe.	Harm = benefit. Do not prescribe.	Unclear benefit. Probably should not be given.	Give low-dose aspirin.
Drugs *not* recommended for reduction of CVD	Hormone replacement, vitamin B, vitamin C, vitamin E, folic acid.			

Source: adapted from World Health Organization (2007).
ACE, angiotensin-converting enzyme; LDL, low-density lipoprotein.

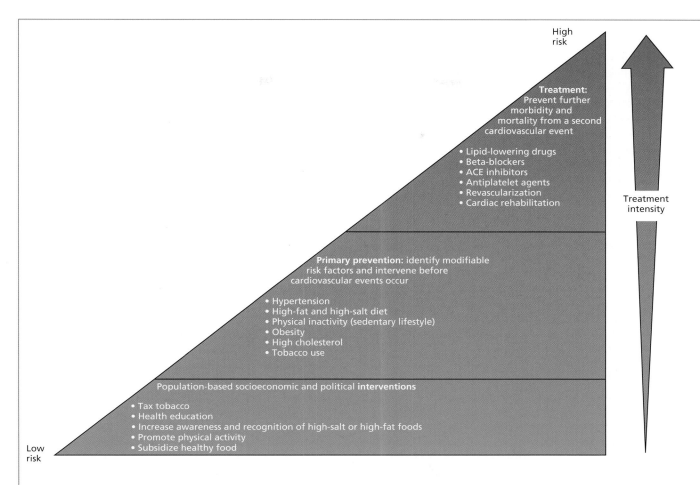

Figure 21.4 A graduated approach to interventions as cardiovascular risk increases. Adapted from Prevention of Cardiovascular Diseases, World Health Organization (2007) and Yusuf *et al.* (2001b).

and Noncommunicable Disease Control, Moscow, 28–29 April, 2011. http://www.who.int/nmh/events/moscow_ncds_2011/en/

- World Health Organization. Global Action Plan for the Prevention and Control of Non-communicable Diseases 2013–2020. Available at http://www.who.int/nmh/publications/ncd_action_plan/en/index.html
- World Health Organization. STEPwise approach to surveillance (STEPS) Questionnaire. WHO recommended tool for community surveillance of NCDs. Available at http://www.who.int/chp/steps/en/
- World Health Organization. Prevention of cardiovascular disease: pocket guidelines for assessment and management of cardiovascular risk. Available at http://www.who.int/cardiovascular_diseases/guidelines/Pocket_GL_information/en/

- For more information regarding international meetings and ongoing projects related to global cardiovascular medicine, see http://www.world-heart-federation.org
- For more information regarding international collaborations and guidelines for stroke care, see http://www.world-stroke.org
- For WHO data regarding NCDs in all regions of the world, see http://apps.who.int/gho/data/node.main.A858?lang=en
- Médecins Sans Frontières. *Clinical Guidelines: Diagnosis and Treatment Manual for Curative Programmes in Hospitals and Dispensaries Guidance for Prescribing*, 2013 edn. Available online at http://www.refbooks.msf.org/

REFERENCES

Avezum A, Braga J, Santos I, Guimarães HP, Marin-Neto JA, Piegas LS (2009) Cardiovascular disease in South America: current status and opportunities for prevention. *Heart* 95:1475–82.

Dalal S, Beunza JJ, Volmink J *et al*. (2011) Non-communicable diseases in sub-Saharan Africa: what we know now. *Int J Epidemiol* 40:885–901.

Harries AD, Zachariah R, Jahn A, Schouten EJ, Kamoto K (2009) Scaling up antiretroviral therapy in Malawi: implications for managing other chronic diseases in resource-limited countries. *J Acquir Immune Defic Syndr* 52(Suppl. 1):S14–16.

Ibrahim MM, Damasceno A (2012) Hypertension in developing countries. *Lancet* 380:611–19.

Kwan GF, Bukhman AK, Miller AC *et al*. (2013) A simplified echocardiographic strategy for heart failure diagnosis and management within an integrated noncommunicable disease clinic at district hospital level for sub-Saharan Africa. *JACC Heart Fail* 1:230–6.

Lim SS, Vos T, Flaxman AD *et al*. (2012) A comparative risk assessment of burden of disease and injury attributable to 67 risk factors and risk factor clusters in 21 regions, 1990–2010: a systematic analysis for the Global Burden of Disease Study 2010. *Lancet* 380:2224–60.

Mittal BV, Singh AK (2010) Hypertension in the developing world: challenges and opportunities. *Am J Kidney Dis* 55:590–8.

Ntsekhe M, Hakim J (2005) Impact of human immunodeficiency virus infection on cardiovascular disease in Africa. *Circulation* 112:3602–7.

Peck RN, Green E, Mtabaji J *et al*. (2013) Hypertension-related diseases as a common cause of hospital mortality in Tanzania: a 3-year prospective study. *J Hypertens* 31:1806–11.

Remenyi B, Carapetis J, Wyber R, Taubert K, Mayosi BM (2013) Position statement of the World Heart Federation on the prevention and control of rheumatic heart disease. *Nat Rev Cardiol* 10:284–92.

World Health Organization (2007) *Prevention of Cardiovascular Disease: Pocket Guidelines for Assessment and Management of Cardiovascular Risk*. Geneva: World Health Organization.

World Health Organization (2011a) The First Global Ministerial Conference on Healthy Lifestyles and Noncommunicable Disease Control, Moscow, 28–29 April, 2011. Moscow Declaration.

World Health Organization (2011b) Prevalence of elevated blood pressure. Available at http://gamapserver.who.int/mapLibrary/Files/Maps/Global_BloodPressurePrevalence_BothSexes_2008.png

World Health Organization (2013) A Global *Brief* on Hypertension: Silent Killer, Global Public Health Crisis. Geneva: World Health Organization.

Yusuf S, Reddy S, Ounpuu S, Anand S (2001a) Global burden of cardiovascular diseases. Part I. General considerations, the epidemiologic transition, risk factors, and impact of urbanization. *Circulation* 104:2746–53.

Yusuf S, Reddy S, Ounpuu S, Anand S (2001b) Global burden of cardiovascular diseases. Part II. Variations in cardiovascular disease by specific ethnic groups and geographic regions and prevention strategies. *Circulation* 104:2855–64.

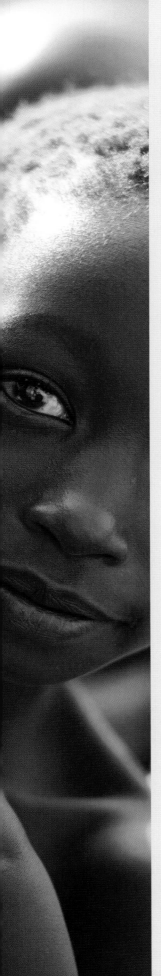

CHAPTER 22
Chronic Respiratory Disease

Peter P. Moschovis[1] and David C. Christiani[1,2]
[1]Massachusetts General Hospital, Boston, MA, USA
[2]Harvard School of Public Health, Boston, MA, USA

Key learning objectives

■ Review the epidemiology of chronic respiratory disease in low- and middle-income countries.

■ Understand the presentation of respiratory illnesses and how to distinguish from diseases with similar presentations.

■ Identify the optimal diagnostic tools for evaluating a patient with suspected respiratory disease in low-resource settings.

■ Understand diagnosis and management of the most common chronic respiratory diseases.

Abstract

Upwards of 1 billion people worldwide are estimated to suffer from chronic respiratory disease, including asthma, chronic obstructive pulmonary disease (COPD), occupational lung diseases, bronchiectasis, pulmonary interstitial diseases (including pneumoconioses), and pulmonary hypertension. This chapter reviews the risk factors, presentation, evaluation, diagnosis, and management of the major chronic respiratory diseases in low-resource settings.

Key words: chronic respiratory disease, chronic obstructive pulmonary disease, asthma, occupational lung disease, bronchiectasis, pneumoconioses, pulmonary hypertension, tobacco smoking, household air pollution, spirometry, radiography

Essential Clinical Global Health, First Edition. Edited by Brett D. Nelson.
© 2015 John Wiley & Sons, Ltd. Published 2015 by John Wiley & Sons, Ltd.
Companion website: www.essentialseries.com/globalhealth

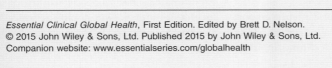

Introduction and epidemiology

As communicable disease mortality has decreased in many low- and middle-income countries (LMICs), chronic non-communicable disease has become a major cause of disability and death. Chronic respiratory disease now ranks third in global causes of death (Lozano *et al.*, 2012) and ninth in causes of disability (Murray *et al.*, 2012). Upwards of 1 billion people worldwide are estimated to suffer from chronic respiratory disease, including asthma, chronic obstructive pulmonary disease (COPD), occupational lung diseases, bronchiectasis, pulmonary interstitial diseases (including pneumoconioses), and pulmonary hypertension (Bousquet *et al.*, 2010).

As the burden of illness in chronic respiratory disease increases, the capacity for providing care has not kept pace. A combination of lack of diagnostic equipment, medicines, and expert pulmonary care makes diagnosis and treatment of chronic lung disease difficult in low-resource settings. A World Health Organization (WHO)-sponsored survey of 231 health facilities in 12 African countries found that only 44% of the facilities had access to an uninterrupted oxygen source, and only 35% had a consistent supply of electricity (Belle *et al.*, 2010).

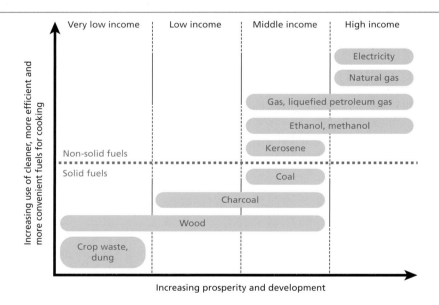

Figure 22.1 The "energy ladder": the relationship of wealth to type of household energy. *Source*: WHO (2006), figure 2, p. 9. Reproduced with permission of the World Health Organization.

Risk factors

The most successful efforts at prevention of chronic respiratory disease focus on reducing risk factors. Notably, many risk factors are associated with multiple respiratory diseases, including airways disease (asthma, COPD, and bronchiectasis), interstitial disease (e.g., pneumoconiosis), pulmonary vascular disease, lung cancer, and respiratory infections.

Tobacco smoking

Tobacco smoking is the leading global cause of preventable death, responsible for 6 million deaths annually (WHO, 2006; Lim *et al.*, 2012). Although smoking is declining in high-

income countries, a growing prevalence of tobacco smoking in LMICs will likely continue to drive the burden of chronic respiratory illness for several decades. In view of this epidemiologic transition, the WHO developed the Framework Convention on Tobacco Control, an international treaty designed to use policy measures (including taxation and regulation) to reduce tobacco smoking.

Household air pollution

An estimated 3 billion people worldwide cook with solid fuels, including biomass (wood, crop residues, dung, and charcoal) and coal (Figure 22.1) (Smith *et al.*, 2013). Through products of incomplete combustion, household air pollution is a major risk factor for COPD, asthma, lung cancer, interstitial lung disease, and pediatric acute respiratory infection, in addition to several non-respiratory diseases such as coronary artery disease, cerebrovascular disease, and cataracts (Lim *et al.*, 2012; Smith *et al.*, 2013). Household air pollution is estimated to be responsible for 18% of all disability-adjusted life years lost globally, and an even greater fraction in countries with a high prevalence of solid fuel use (Lim *et al.*, 2012).

While it is difficult to change a household's cooking fuel, many large-scale projects have attempted to reduce exposure to household air pollution. The most effective programs to date have focused on improving cookstove fuel efficiency, thereby reducing release of products of incomplete combustion. Other strategies include increasing access to cleaner fuels, improving ventilation, or changing location of cookstoves within a household (Schwela, 2000). The largest international effort is the Global Alliance for Clean Cookstoves, a public–private partnership whose goal is to enable the adoption of clean cookstoves and fuels in 100 million households by 2020.

Outdoor air pollution

Outdoor air pollution is rapidly becoming a major cause of respiratory morbidity in urban centers in LMICs. Several constituents of polluted outdoor air are known to cause harmful effects, including fine particulate matter, sulfur dioxide, nitrogen dioxide, carbon monoxide, and ozone (Lai *et al.*, 2013). Exposure to high levels of air pollution is associated with both acute and chronic declines in respiratory function, and many studies have found an increased risk of respiratory-related illnesses during periods of peak pollution (WHO, 2011).

Occupational risk factors

Many occupational exposures are associated with chronic respiratory disease, including agricultural exposures, asbestos, and mineral dusts (e.g., silica, coal, metals). Commonly exposed occupations include farmers, pest sprayers, miners, textile workers, and construction and craft workers. Despite bans on asbestos in 52 countries because of its known deleterious health effects, many industries in LMICs continue to manufacture and utilize asbestos (Collegium Ramazzini, 2010).

Infections

Respiratory infections, especially when untreated, can be associated with permanent airway injury and scarring, leading to bronchiectasis (irreversible dilation and scarring of the airway) and chronic airflow obstruction (Edmond *et al.*, 2012). A number of chronic systemic infections, including HIV and schistosomiasis, are associated with an increased risk of pulmonary arterial hypertension (Bloomfield *et al.*, 2012; Barnett & Hsue, 2013).

Presentation

Several chronic respiratory illnesses present with similar features, and few diseases have a single pathognomonic history or examination findings. Nonetheless, it is essential to obtain a detailed history and physical on patients in whom chronic respiratory disease is suspected. Many of these symptom histories vary across cultures and language, and it is important for the provider to remember that a patient's geographic location affects not only the local epidemiology of disease but also the way that symptoms are perceived and communicated.

History

- Dyspnea (shortness of breath): patients with respiratory disease often describe breathlessness, or a sensation of inability to get enough air. It is essential to determine the time course of a patient's dyspnea (acute/chronic), activities that elicit it (exertion, work/home, day/night), and any accompanying symptoms (e.g., chest tightness often suggests asthma).
- Cough can be a sign of airway inflammation or irritation. When patients report cough, one must elicit details of time course (acute/chronic, episodic), sputum production (presence, amount, color, hemoptysis), and accompanying symptoms (e.g., fever, chest pain, dyspnea).
- Chest pain: pleuritic chest pain is a useful sign of pleural inflammation or irritation, while other types (e.g., exertional, substernal, chest pressure) are less specific.
- Social history: a history of environmental or occupational exposures can be key in making a diagnosis as well as in formulating a treatment plan.

Physical examination

- Vital signs: respiratory rate and oxygen saturation via pulse oximetry.
- General appearance: work of breathing, use of accessory muscles, pursed-lip breathing, cyanosis.
- Neck: location/displacement of trachea, lymphadenopathy.
- Pulmonary examination: adventitious or "extra" breath sounds (e.g., crackles, wheezing, pleural rub), airflow, inspiratory-to-expiratory (I:E) ratio, percussion (dull/ hyperresonant).
- Cardiac examination: murmurs, gallops, loudness of P2, jugular venous pressure (JVP).
- Extremities: clubbing, edema (which can indicate volume overload or right heart failure).

Differential diagnosis

A variety of non-pulmonary diseases can present with similar symptoms, but several distinguishing features may be helpful.

Cardiac disease (see Chapter 21)

Congestive heart failure usually presents with dyspnea, but is often accompanied by signs of volume overload (e.g., edema, elevated JVP). It may be challenging to distinguish left ventricular failure from right ventricular failure, although crackles indicating pulmonary edema favor the former. Chest pain with typical anginal features points toward ischemic heart disease rather than pulmonary disease. In many cases, further testing may be required to distinguish cardiac from respiratory causes of dyspnea.

Anemia (see Chapter 24)

Severe anemia (e.g., from nutritional deficiencies or malaria) often presents with exertional dyspnea. Inspection for conjunctival pallor is a useful screening test for anemia.

Respiratory infections (see Chapters 8 and 19)

Acute respiratory infections (primarily caused by bacteria and viruses) can generally be distinguished by the acuity of presentation. Chronic respiratory infections (more often caused by

mycobacteria and fungi) are often accompanied by pleuritic pain and constitutional symptoms (e.g., fever, weight loss) and are much more prevalent among HIV-positive patients.

Evaluation of the patient with suspected chronic respiratory disease

After a careful history, physical examination, and consideration of the differential diagnosis, further testing may be helpful. Diagnostic equipment is often limited in low-resource settings, but in some cases a definitive diagnosis may not be possible without further testing.

Chest radiography

While generally not available in rural health facilities, most referral hospitals have basic radiographic capacity. Along with spirometry, a chest radiograph can help providers distinguish between most major chronic respiratory diseases (Figure 22.2).

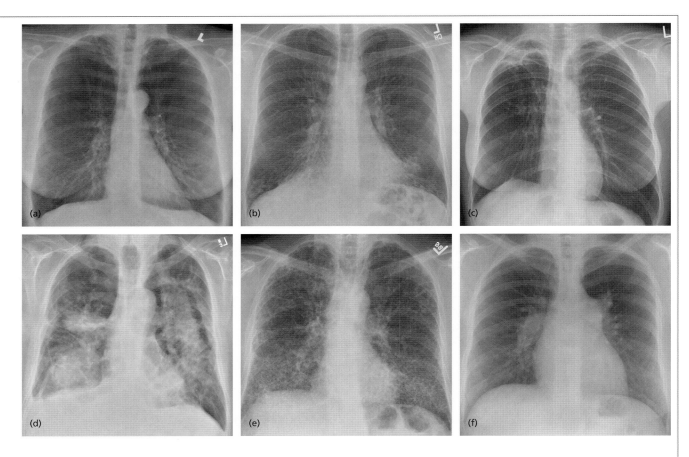

Figure 22.2 Chest radiography in major chronic respiratory diseases. (a) COPD: hyperinflation and decreased vascular markings. (b) Bronchiectasis: "tram-track" appearance of thickened airways, primarily in the right middle lobe and lingual. (c) Apical scarring related to prior tuberculosis infection. (d) Silicosis: extensive scarring from progressive massive fibrosis. (e) Interstitial fibrosis: extensive fibrosis which can be associated with workplace exposures or with idiopathic pulmonary fibrosis. (f) Pulmonary hypertension: enlarged pulmonary arteries. *Source*: Dr Matthew Gilman, Massachusetts General Hospital, MA, USA. Reproduced with permission.

Spirometry

Pulmonary function testing is critical for diagnosing many lung diseases, and while full testing (i.e., lung volume and diffusion capacity measurements) is rarely available in low-resource settings, inexpensive portable spirometry has become more accessible. Although spirometric testing requires some training and standardization, it allows a provider to distinguish between obstructive and restrictive diseases, as well as grading the severity of a ventilatory defect. The two primary measures of lung function are FVC (forced vital capacity, or the total amount of air that a patient can blow out after a maximal inspiration) and FEV_1 (forced expiratory volume in 1 s, or the amount of air that a patient can forcibly blow out in the first second of the FVC maneuver). Reductions in FEV_1 and FVC can be seen in both obstruction and restriction, and a reduced FEV_1/FVC ratio is diagnostic of obstruction (Figure 22.3). Definitive confirmation of restriction requires lung volume measurement (typically performed with body plethysmography or helium dilution); these tests are rarely available in low-resource settings.

Echocardiography

Cardiac ultrasound is a useful screening test for pulmonary hypertension, and can complement the pulmonary evaluation of dyspnea.

Diagnosis and treatment of major diseases

Asthma

Although asthma has traditionally been considered a disease of high-income countries, worldwide differences in prevalence have decreased, especially among children (Asher *et al.*, 2006). Asthma is usually diagnosed clinically based on a history of episodic dyspnea, wheezing, chest tightness, or cough. There is often seasonal variability to symptoms, with worse symptoms at night. Asthma often coexists with other allergic diseases, including rhinitis and eczema, and there is often a positive family history of atopy. Spirometry demonstrating airway obstruction that is reversible after

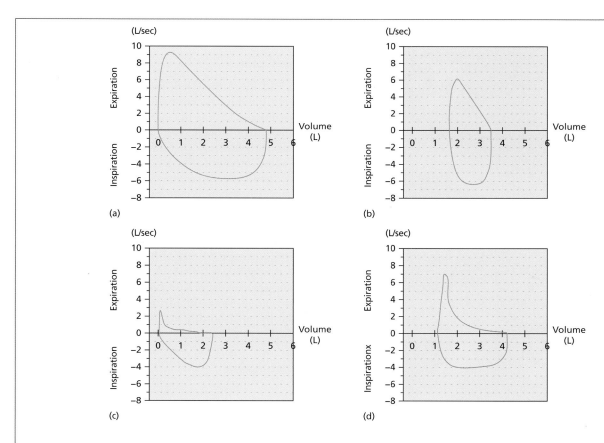

Figure 22.3 Spirometry findings in (a) normal, (b) restrictive, (c) obstructive, and (d) combined obstructive and restrictive ventilatory deficits.

administration of a bronchodilator can confirm the diagnosis of asthma.

Prevention of asthma by reducing indoor and outdoor air pollution and minimizing exposure to known triggers may be effective in reducing exacerbations. Medical treatment is based on severity and frequency of symptoms. For patients with mild and infrequent symptoms, short-acting beta-agonists (e.g., albuterol or salbutamol) are sufficient, but for patients with more severe or persistent symptoms addition of an inhaled corticosteroid (ICS) or an inhaled corticosteroid/long-acting beta-agonist (ICS/LABA) combination provides better control and decreases risk of exacerbations. Both low-dose ICS and low-dose ICS/LABA combinations are cost-effective interventions in low-resource settings (Aït-Khaled *et al.*, 2008; Stanciole *et al.*, 2012). Delivery of inhaled medications is substantially improved by the use of spacers, and in low-resource settings a home-made spacer can be easily constructed using a 500-mL plastic bottle (Figure 22.4) (Rodriguez *et al.*, 2008).

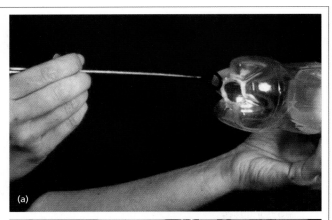
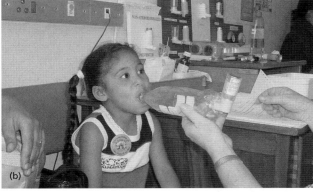

Figure 22.4 How to make an inhaler spacer from a plastic water bottle. *Source*: Zar *et al.* (2005), figures (a) and (b). Reproduced with permission of *South African Medical Journal* and H. Zar.

Chronic obstructive pulmonary disease

According to the Global Initiative for Chronic Obstructive Lung Disease (GOLD), COPD is "characterized by persistent airflow limitation that is usually progressive and associated with an enhanced chronic inflammatory response in the airways and the lung to noxious particles or gases" (Global Initiative for Chronic Obstructive Lung Disease, 2013). The disease is characterized by small airway inflammation that drives progressive airway damage and increased airways resistance, as well as parenchymal destruction that results in loss of elastic recoil and diffusion impairment. A diagnosis of COPD may be suspected when risk factors (smoking, household air pollution) and examination findings (wheezing) are present, and the diagnosis is confirmed by spirometry that demonstrates obstruction that is not fully reversible with a bronchodilator (post-bronchodilator FEV_1/FVC <70%, according to GOLD criteria).

For all patients who smoke, smoking cessation is key. Other supportive measures include vaccination against influenza and pneumococcus (if available), as well as encouragement to maintain physical activity. For hypoxemic patients, oxygen therapy has been demonstrated to reduce mortality (Kim *et al.*, 2008), although this may not be feasible in low-resource settings. Medications may be beneficial in both relieving symptoms and reducing exacerbations (Table 22.1).

Bronchiectasis

Bronchiectasis (from the Greek *bronchion*, meaning "airway" and *ektasis*, meaning "stretched") is irreversible dilation or scarring of the airways, leading to recurrent respiratory infections, chronic productive cough, airflow obstruction, and often hemoptysis. Early bacterial, viral, and mycobacterial (especially *M. tuberculosis*) infections are common causes of bronchiectasis worldwide, and once bronchiectasis is established a vicious cycle ensues, wherein infection begets airway inflammation that in turn makes clearing the infection more difficult (Jordan *et al.*, 2010).

Prompt identification and treatment of childhood respiratory infection reduces the risk of bronchiectasis. Once bronchiectasis is established, airway clearance mechanisms (chest physical therapy) are the mainstay of therapy. Judicious use of antibiotics during acute exacerbations of bronchiectasis will reduce the bacterial burden but risks selecting for resistant bacteria.

Pneumoconioses

Pneumoconioses, defined by the United Nation's International Labour Organization (ILO) as "the accumulation of dust in the lungs and the tissue reactions to its presence" (Stellman, 1998), encompass a variety of diseases in response to various exposures. The three most common forms are described below.

Table 22.1 Staging of COPD based on severity of obstruction (GOLD criteria) in patients with post-bronchodilator FEV_1/FVC <70%.

GOLD stage	Severity	Spirometric criteria	Treatment
GOLD 1	Mild	FEV_1 >80% of predicted	Short-acting bronchodilator as needed with or without long-acting bronchodilator (beta-agonist or anticholinergic) if moderate to severe symptoms
GOLD 2	Moderate	FEV_1 50–80% of predicted	Long-acting bronchodilator
GOLD 3	Severe	FEV_1 30–50% of predicted	Combination long-acting bronchodilator and inhaled corticosteroid
GOLD 4	Very severe	FEV_1 <30% of predicted	Combination long-acting bronchodilator and inhaled corticosteroid

Source: Global Initiative for Chronic Obstructive Lung Disease (2013).

Silicosis

Silicosis is found in individuals exposed to respirable crystalline silica dust (e.g., quartz, sand) and can manifest as chronic silicosis and airflow obstruction or progressive massive fibrosis (PMF), a severe destructive disease (Rees & Murray, 2007). Chest radiography typically demonstrates rounded nodular opacities, which are larger and can coalesce in PMF (see Figure 22.2d). "Eggshell" calcifications of hilar lymph nodes are strongly suggestive although not pathognomonic of silicosis. Silica exposure increases the risk of pulmonary tuberculosis, especially among those who also have HIV, and aggressive treatment of latent tuberculosis infection is indicated in these individuals (see Chapter 19). Silicosis also increases the risk of lung cancer.

Coal workers' pneumoconiosis

A result of exposure to coal dust, this condition most often presents as COPD (both emphysema and chronic bronchitis), but like silicosis it may also present as PMF. Chest radiography findings are similar to those in silicosis (rounded nodular opacities), and spirometry usually demonstrates obstruction (Wang & Christiani, 2000).

Asbestosis

Exposure to natural mineral silica fibers, as well as synthetic substitutes, can manifest as pulmonary parenchymal fibrosis (asbestosis), pleural plaques, or benign effusions. Asbestos exposure also increases the risk of mesothelioma and lung cancer and is synergistic with cigarette smoking for the latter. Asbestosis usually manifests as a restrictive deficit on spirometry, although some patients have mixed obstructive/restrictive deficits. Chest imaging demonstrates irregular linear markings in the lower lateral lung zones, and these often coexist with other markers of asbestos exposure (e.g., pleural plaques) (Collegium Ramazzini, 2010).

Treatment of Pneumoconioses

Unfortunately, there is no specific treatment for any of the pneumoconioses. Focus must instead be on primary preven-

> **Clinical experience**
>
> "During my elective in the Dominican Republic, I had the opportunity to work with an international NGO that delivers low-cost health services through mobile clinics. Many of the patients we served had chronic diseases like asthma, diabetes, and hypertension. In participating in this work and in talking with patients, it became evident that the community truly valued the organization's efforts to partner with local schools and churches in coordinating the mobile clinics. Key to the success of the program was continued support from local community leaders to disseminate information and share newly learned best practices for health and hygiene. As a result of this community partnership, the organization was able to provide a vital sustainable product, in this case chronic disease care and management through mobile clinics."
>
> Sam, medical student working in the Dominican Republic

tion through exposure reduction. The ILO recommends that employers institute several measures to reduce hazardous exposures, including engineering control (e.g., improving ventilation, water suppression of dusts), substitution of hazardous materials with non-hazardous replacements, work practices and administrative controls to minimize degree of exposure to workers, worker training in best practices, and provision of personal protective equipment (Alli, 2008).

Pulmonary hypertension

Despite a substantial burden of pulmonary hypertension among those infected with HIV and schistosomiasis, few pulmonary hypertension-specific medications (e.g., phosphodiesterase type 5 inhibitors, endothelin receptor agonists, and prostanoids) are currently available in low-resource settings. Thus, focus is generally on supportive care (e.g., diuretics, treating heart failure) and treatment of any underlying conditions (Bloomfield *et al.*, 2012; Barnett & Hsue, 2013).

Additional resources

- Global Initiative for Chronic Obstructive Lung Disease (GOLD). Global Strategy for the Diagnosis, Management and Prevention of COPD. Available at http://www.goldcopd.org/
- Global Initiative for Asthma (GINA). Pocket guide for asthma management and prevention. Available at http://www.ginasthma.org/
- Alli BO (2008) *Fundamental Principles of Occupational Health and Safety*. Geneva: International Labour Office. Available at http://www.ilo.org/publns
- World Health Organization. Fuel for life: household energy and health. Available at http://www.who.int/indoorair/publications/fuelforlife.pdf

REFERENCES

Aït-Khaled N, Enarson DA, Chiang C, Marks G, Bissell K (2008) *Management of Asthma: A Guide to the Essentials of Good Clinical Practice*, 3rd edn. Paris: International Union Against Tuberculosis and Lung Disease.

Alli BO (2008) *Fundamental Principles of Occupational Health and Safety*, 2nd edn. Geneva: International Labour Office.

Asher MI, Montefort S, Bjorksten B *et al.* (2006) ISAAC Phase Three Study Group. Worldwide time trends in the prevalence of symptoms of asthma, allergic rhinoconjunctivitis, and eczema in childhood: ISAAC Phases One and Three repeat multicountry cross-sectional surveys. *Lancet* 368:733–43.

Barnett CF, Hsue PY (2013) Human immunodeficiency virus-associated pulmonary arterial hypertension. *Clin Chest Med* 34:283–92.

Belle J, Cohen H, Shindo N *et al.* (2010) Influenza preparedness in low-resource settings: a look at oxygen delivery in 12 African countries. *J Infect Dev Ctries* 4:419–24.

Bloomfield GS, Lagat DK, Akwanalo OC *et al.* (2012) Waiting to inhale: an exploratory review of conditions that may predispose to pulmonary hypertension and right heart failure in persons exposed to household air pollution in low- and middle-income countries. *Glob Heart* 7:249–59.

Bousquet J, Kiley J, Bateman ED *et al.* (2010) Prioritised research agenda for prevention and control of chronic respiratory diseases. *Eur Respir J* 36:995–1001.

Collegium Ramazzini (2010) Asbestos is still with us: repeat call for a universal ban. *Arch Environ Occup Health* 65:121–6.

Edmond K, Scott S, Korczak V *et al.* (2012) Long term sequelae from childhood pneumonia: systematic review and meta-analysis. *PLoS ONE* 7(2):e31239.

Global Initiative for Chronic Obstructive Lung Disease (2013) Global strategy for the diagnosis, management and prevention of COPD. http://www.goldcopd.org/guidelines-global-strategy-for-diagnosis-management.html

Jordan TS, Spencer EM, Davies P (2010) Tuberculosis, bronchiectasis and chronic airflow obstruction. *Respirology* 15:623–8.

Kim V, Benditt JO, Wise RA, Sharafkhaneh A (2008) Oxygen therapy in chronic obstructive pulmonary disease. *Proc Am Thorac Soc* 5:513–18.

Lai HK, Tsang H, Wong CM (2013) Meta-analysis of adverse health effects due to air pollution in Chinese populations. *BMC Public Health* 13:360.

Lim SS, Vos T, Flaxman AD *et al.* (2012) A comparative risk assessment of burden of disease and injury attributable to 67 risk factors and risk factor clusters in 21 regions, 1990–2010: a systematic analysis for the Global Burden of Disease Study 2010. *Lancet* 380:2224–60.

Lozano R, Naghavi M, Foreman K *et al.* (2012) Global and regional mortality from 235 causes of death for 20 age groups in 1990 and 2010: a systematic analysis for the Global Burden of Disease Study 2010. *Lancet* 380:2095–128.

Murray CJ, Vos T, Lozano R *et al.* (2012) Disability-adjusted life years (DALYs) for 291 diseases and injuries in 21 regions, 1990–2010: a systematic analysis for the Global Burden of Disease Study 2010. *Lancet* 380:2197–223.

Rees D, Murray J (2007) Silica, silicosis and tuberculosis. *Int J Tuberc Lung Dis* 11:474–84.

Rodriguez C, Sossa M, Lozano JM (2008) Commercial versus home-made spacers in delivering bronchodilator therapy for acute therapy in children. *Cochrane Database Syst Rev* (2):CD005536.

Schwela D (2000) Air pollution and health in urban areas. *Rev Environ Health* 15:13–42.

Smith KR, Frumkin H, Balakrishnan K *et al.* (2013) Energy and human health. *Annu Rev Public Health* 34:159–88.

Stanciole AE, Ortegon M, Chisholm D, Lauer JA (2012) Cost effectiveness of strategies to combat chronic obstructive pulmonary disease and asthma in sub-Saharan Africa and South East Asia: mathematical modelling study. *BMJ* 344:e608.

Stellman JM (1998) *Encyclopaedia of Occupational Health and Safety*, 4th edn. Geneva: International Labour Office.

Wang XR, Christiani DC (2000) Respiratory symptoms and functional status in workers exposed to silica, asbestos, and coal mine dusts. *J Occup Environ Med* 42:1076–84.

WHO (2006) *Fuel for Life: Household Energy and Health.* Geneva: World Health Organization.

WHO (2011) *WHO Report on the Global Tobacco Epidemic, 2011*. Geneva: World Health Organization.

Zar HJ, Motala C, Weinberg EG (2005) Incorrect use of a homemade spacer for treatment of recurrent wheezing in children: a cause for concern. *S Afr Med J* 95:388–390.

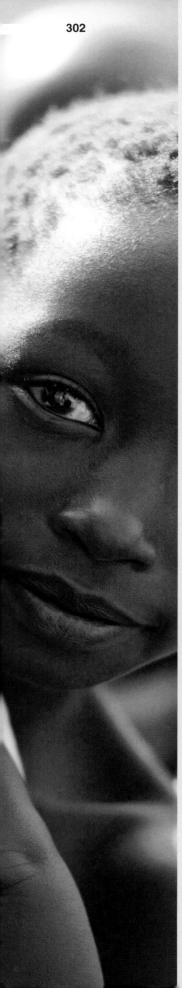

CHAPTER 23
Diabetes and Endocrinology

Julia E. von Oettingen[1], Diane Stafford[1], and Francine R. Kaufman[2]

[1]Boston Children's Hospital, and Harvard Medical School, Boston, MA, USA

[2]Medtronic Diabetes, The University of Southern California, and The Center for Diabetes, Endocrinology and Metabolism, Children's Hospital Los Angeles, Los Angeles, CA, USA

Key learning objectives

- Learn when to suspect and how to diagnose diabetes in children and adults.
- Recognize key features of type 1 and type 2 diabetes.
- Learn the principles of treating diabetic ketoacidosis and hyperglycemic hyperosmolar coma and understand the basics of chronic diabetes care.
- Understand the principles of diagnosis and treatment of common endocrine disorders in children and adults.

Abstract

Diabetes is an important non-communicable chronic disease with increasing prevalence globally. Type 1 diabetes is the predominant form in children, whereas type 2 diabetes is more common in adults. In certain populations, other forms including malnutrition-related and ketosis-prone diabetes need to be considered. Management strategies of diabetes should be adapted to the local setting. In resource-limited settings, basic equipment such as glucometer, urine ketone strips, and subcutaneous insulin are the principal tools to successfully manage diabetic emergencies and chronic care. Other endocrine conditions the global health clinician should be able to diagnose and manage include hypertension, thyroid disorders, and adrenal insufficiency. Vitamin D deficiency and rickets are more common in developing countries; early recognition and prompt treatment prevents long-term sequelae and morbidity.

Key words: endocrine, diabetes, type 1, type 2, thyroid, adrenal insufficiency, hypertension, Vitamin D, rickets

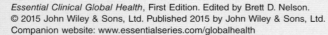

DIABETES

Introduction and epidemiology

More than 371 million people have diabetes worldwide, and the incidence of both type 1 diabetes (T1D) and type 2 diabetes (T2D) is rising (International Diabetes Federation, 2013). Other types of diabetes more common in sub-Saharan Africa, such as malnutrition-related diabetes, ketosis-prone atypical diabetes, and fibrocalculous pancreatitis leading to diabetes, have been well described (Hall *et al.*, 2011), but their exact incidence and prevalence rates are less well understood. Half of the population with diabetes remains undiagnosed, with this percentage approaching 80% in developing countries. Four out of five persons with diabetes live in low- or middle-income countries, with China and India being home to the greatest numbers of cases.

T2D accounts for the majority of diabetes (85–95%), while 5–10% of those diagnosed have T1D, including an estimated 490,000 children less than 14 years of age. As many as 4.8 million people die of diabetic complications and comorbidities every year (International Diabetes Federation, 2013). In the developing world, lack of access to healthcare and absence of simple diagnostic tools such as glucose meters lead to high rates of non-recognition, misdiagnosis, and death from acute or chronic complications. Insulin and other glucose-lowering medications are frequently not readily available, impairing proper treatment. In sub-Saharan Africa, 5-year mortality rates from diabetes are up to 57% and may be even higher in rural settings (Gill *et al.*, 2009).

Clinical experience: a 3-year-old boy with diabetes in Liberia

"I was called to see a 3-year-old boy in the emergency department. The boy had come to the hospital the previous night because of rapid breathing, abdominal pain, and fevers. The malaria smear was "2+," and he was treated with quinine. Because this medication can cause hypoglycemia, he was also given a D50% glucose bolus. His mental status deteriorated overnight; he was increasingly sleepy and less responsive. When I assessed him the next morning, the child looked critically ill and dehydrated, was minimally responsive, and showed labored breathing but had clear lungs. I ordered a blood sugar, thinking the child may have hypoglycemia. The reading was "HI" on the meter (i.e. >600 mg/dL [>33.3 mmol/L]) and we repeated the test to be sure it was correct, especially since the mother denied the child had had any symptoms of increased thirst or urination. We weren't able to confirm the blood sugar in the lab, but we were able to find a urine glucose strip that showed glucose above 1000 mg/dL (>55.6 mmol/L). We began treatment according to a setting-appropriate DKA protocol, and the child gradually improved. The next morning he was sitting up, smiling, and asking to eat. It was a new and incredible experience to the staff, most of whom had never diagnosed or treated diabetes in a child. I had learned the important lesson that DKA can look like any other critical illness, particularly in settings where children present late to care. We all agreed: any child with impaired mental status needs a blood sugar check, even in settings where US$1 per glucometer test strip seems unaffordable."

Julia, physician working in Liberia

Diagnosis

A diagnosis of diabetes should be suspected in a patient who presents with classic symptoms, including increased thirst (polydipsia), increased urination (polyuria), and weight loss. Children frequently present with bedwetting (enuresis), while adolescents and adults often wake up several times at night to urinate (nocturia). A fruity breath may have been noticed by family members. Other symptoms of diabetes may be less specific, such as headaches, fatigue, mood changes, and abdominal pain. Vomiting, abnormally deep and rapid breathing (Kussmaul respirations), a decreased level of consciousness, and coma appear late and may indicate diabetic ketoacidosis (DKA), with or without its major complication of cerebral edema. Diabetic symptoms may go unrecognized for weeks or months, and T2D patients may be asymptomatic for years or present with complications at diagnosis. DKA is a fairly common presentation for all types of diabetes. Moderate to severe DKA may resemble any other critical illness, such as gastroenteritis with severe dehydration, pneumonia, sepsis, or cerebral malaria. A bedside blood or urine glucose test is the first step in making the appropriate diagnosis.

It may often be difficult to distinguish T1D from T2D, or these from other types of diabetes. Typical clinical features can help to make a presumptive diagnosis. The presence of obesity, acanthosis, and high blood pressure suggest T2D, while normal weight, other autoimmune disorders, and insulin dependence suggest T1D (Table 23.1). Screening and diagnostic criteria for diabetes are presented in Tables 23.2 and 23.3.

Table 23.1 Difference between type 1 and type 2 diabetes.

	Type 1 diabetes	Type 2 diabetes	Comment
Pathophysiology	Absolute insulin deficiency. Autoimmune process leads to pancreatic β-cell destruction.	Relative insulin deficiency. Fat and muscle cells are less responsive to insulin, leading to increased insulin secretion.	Diabetes autoantibodies (GAD, IA-2, insulin and zinc transporter 8) are positive in >85% of T1D. These are not usually available in resource-poor settings.
Age	Younger	Older	T1D is thought to have a decade later onset in sub-Saharan Africa. Increasing rates of obesity have led to a significant increase in T2D diagnoses in the young.
Body habitus	Thin	Overweight/obese; central fat distribution	With rates of obesity increasing worldwide, even patients with T1D can be very overweight at presentation.
Race	More prevalent in Caucasians	Blacks, Hispanics, Asians seem to be at greater risk	
Polyuria, polydipsia	+++	−/++	T2D can often be asymptomatic.
Weight loss	+++	+	Weight loss >10–20% of body weight is not uncommon in T1D. Weight loss in T2D is variable but can be significant if diagnosis is delayed for a long time.
Acanthosis nigricans	−	++	Darkened and rough skin around the neck, axillae, elbows.
Glycosuria	+++	+++	
Ketones	+++	−/+	Ketones are almost always present in T1D unless diagnosis is made very early. Ketones in T2D are less common.
Diabetic ketoacidosis (DKA)	++	−/+	In resource-poor settings, DKA is a very common presentation of T1D. Occasionally, DKA or ketosis can be seen in T2D, particularly in black people.
Hyperglycemic hyperosmolar state (HHS)	−	+	Much more common in T2D.
Diabetes complications	−/+	++	Complications can include retinopathy (poor vision), nephropathy (impaired renal function), and neuropathy (foot ulcer, neuropathic pain).
Response to oral hyperglycemics	−	++	T2D responds initially, most patients eventually become insulin dependent.
Insulin level	Low	High	Often unavailable
C-peptide	Low	Low-normal-high	Often unavailable

Table 23.2 Screening criteria for diabetes.

Type 1 diabetes

No screening

Type 2 diabetes

Adults

Age 45 years and above; if normal, repeat every 3 years

At a younger age or more frequently if BMI >25 kg/m² or if additional risk factors:
- physical inactivity
- first-degree relative with diabetes
- high-risk ethnic population (African descent, Latino, Native American, Asian descent, Pacific Islander)
- GDM or history of delivering a baby >4 kg
- hypertension (>140/90 mmHg)
- hyperlipidemia
- polycystic ovary syndrome (PCOS)
- history of impaired glucose tolerance or impaired fasting glucose
- acanthosis nigricans
- history of vascular disease

Children

BMI or weight >85th percentile *or* weight >120% of ideal for height *plus* two of the following risk factors:
- history of T2D in first- or second-degree relative
- race/ethnicity (as above in adult criteria)
- acanthosis nigricans, hypertension, dyslipidemia, or PCOS

Start screening at age 10 years or at onset of puberty, whichever is earlier, then screen every 3 years

Fasting blood glucose is preferred method

Gestational diabetes (GDM)

High-risk pregnancy: first antepartum visit *and* 24–28 weeks

Average pregnancy: 24–28 weeks

Low-risk pregnancyᵃ: No screening

Screen women with GDM for persistent diabetes 6–12 weeks postpartum and every 3 years for development of diabetes

ᵃAge <25 years, normal pre-pregnancy weight, low ethnic prevalence, no history of poor obstetric outcome, no history of abnormal glucose tolerance, no first-degree relatives with diabetes.
Source: adapted from Anon. (2012).

Diabetic ketoacidosis and hyperglycemic hyperosmolar state

DKA and hyperglycemic hyperosmolar state (HHS) are the two major hyperglycemic emergencies. They are thought to be two different manifestations of the same underlying pathologic

state of insulin deficiency (Figure 23.1). DKA is more common than HHS, especially in T1D. The distinguishing features are presence of ketosis and acidosis in DKA and more pronounced hyperglycemia, hyperosmolarity, and profound dehydration without acidosis in HHS. Clinically, the conditions are often difficult to differentiate, and therefore, in the absence of a thorough laboratory evaluation and diagnosis, they are treated similarly by correcting dehydration and restoring adequate insulinization.

Formal criteria for DKA include hyperglycemia (glucose >300 mg/dL, 16.6 mmol/L), pH below 7.3, and bicarbonate below 15 mmol/L, while criteria for HHS include hyperglycemia (glucose >600 mg/dL, 33.3 mmol/L), osmolarity above 320 mmol/L, pH above 7.3, and bicarbonate above 15 mmol/L. Standard laboratory evaluation for a hyperglycemic crisis usually includes plasma glucose, electrolytes, venous blood gas (VBG), complete blood count with differential, urinalysis, and hemoglobin (Hb)A1c. When limited diagnostic testing is available, diagnosis is made based on clinical symptoms, elevated blood sugar and, if available, presence of urine ketones.

Principles of DKA treatment include hydration, insulin (Figure 23.2), and eventual glucose administration, all of which are crucial in correcting the patient's hyperglycemia *and* acidosis. Figure 23.3 outlines the general treatment of DKA in children and adults. Detailed guidelines with flowcharts for well-equipped settings are available from the American Diabetes Association (2004). In HHS, acidosis is classically absent, and although treatment is very similar to DKA, emphasis should be placed on sufficient initial fluid resuscitation. During treatment of a hyperglycemic crisis, the most important tool is monitoring the patient's vital signs and clinical status (Figure 23.4). If possible, electrolytes and acid–base status should be assessed every 2–4 hours. However, if these are not available, hourly to 2-hourly blood sugars and, if possible, urinary ketone measurements combined with careful clinical monitoring is indicated. In particular, development of cerebral edema must be detected and treated promptly (Table 23.4).

DKA has resolved once the acid–base status is normalized (as defined by pH >7.3), bicarbonate is above 18 mmol/L, and there is a normal anion gap. When these parameters are not available, careful assessment of clinical status, glycemia, and ketonuria (if possible) are useful. Resolution of DKA is suggested by a well-appearing patient who is hungry and feels ready to eat, has blood sugars below 250 mg/dL, and decreasing levels of ketones in the urine.

Chronic medical management

Insulin therapy

Patients in whom a diagnosis of T1D or an atypical form of diabetes is suspected are treated with insulin. Patients with T2D who present with significant symptoms of hyperglycemia also require insulin when they are first diagnosed, although usually in higher quantities than in T1D due to

Table 23.3 Diagnostic criteria and alternative diagnostic tools for diabetes.

	Diabetes mellitus	Pre-diabetes	Gestational diabetes
Diagnostic tools			
Fasting blood glucose	>126 mg/dL (>7.0 mmol/L)	100–125 mg/dL (5.6–6.9 mmol/L)	>126 mg/dL (>7.0 mmol/L)
Random blood sugar	>200 mg/dL (>11.1 mmol/L)[a]	140–199 mg/dL (7.8–11.0 mmol/L)	>200 mg/dL (>11.1 mmol/L)
Oral glucose tolerance test after at least 8 hours of fasting 75 g glucose (adults) 3 g/kg glucose (children)	>200 mg/dL (>11.1 mmol/L) at 2 hours[b]	140–199 mg/dL (7.8–11.0 mmol/L) at 2 hours	>92 mg/dL (>5.1 mmol/L) fasting >180 mg/dL (>10.0 mmol/L) at 1 hour >155 mg/dL (>8.6 mmol/L) at 2 hours
Hemoglobin A1c	>6.5%	5.7–6.4%	
Alternative diagnostic tools			
Urine glucose strip	+++	−/+	−/+
Urine ketones strip	T1D: usually + T2D: +/−	−	−
Ant attraction test	If no other diagnostic tools are available, one could consider the ancient test of pouring the patient's urine on an outside spot and observing whether the urine attracts ants. If so, the urine is likely to contain glucose.		

[a] Plus classic symptoms of diabetes of hyperglycemic crisis.
[b] Must be confirmed on a subsequent day by any of the other criteria for a diagnosis of diabetes mellitus.

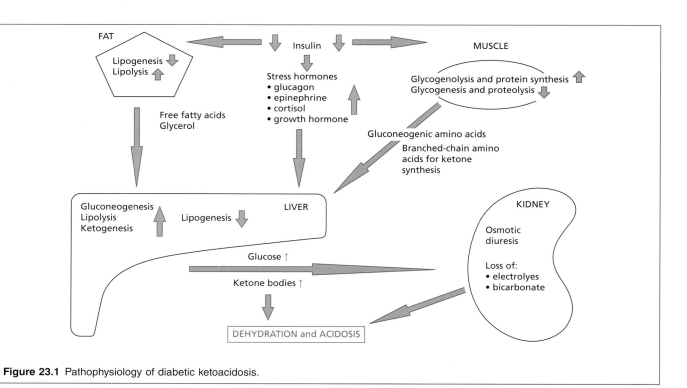

Figure 23.1 Pathophysiology of diabetic ketoacidosis.

insulin resistance. Typical insulin starting doses for a type 1 patient who fully depends on insulin are as follows.

- Less than 5 years old: 0.25–0.5 units/kg daily.
- Prepubertal child (5–11 years): 0.5 units/kg daily.
- Pubertal child (11–16 years): 0.8–1 units/kg daily.
- Postpubertal adolescent and adult (>16 years): 0.7–0.8 units/kg daily.

Many patients with T1D undergo a so-called "honeymoon" or remission phase, during which their pancreatic insulin production temporarily improves, allowing for a decrease in exogenous insulin dosages. This phase can last for weeks or months, rarely up to 1–2 years. During this period, insulin requirements can be as low as a few units per day, although it is not suggested that insulin be discontinued. The clinical course in ketosis-prone atypical diabetes is characterized by intermittent unpredictable episodes of DKA with high insulin requirements for a few weeks, followed by remission with close to normal insulin production of varying duration.

Types of insulin are depicted in Figure 23.5. In most resource-poor settings, Regular, NPH and a premixed insulin containing 70% NPH and 30% Regular are available. Typical regimens are 70/30 premixed insulin given twice daily, or NPH twice daily with Regular twice daily (Figure 23.6). In these regimens, NPH functions as a "basal" insulin for maintenance requirements and Regular as a "bolus" insulin for food.

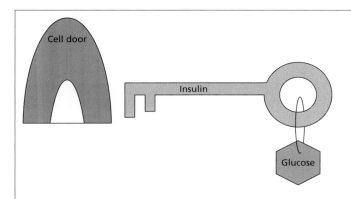

Figure 23.2 Insulin serves as a key to glucose entry into the cell.

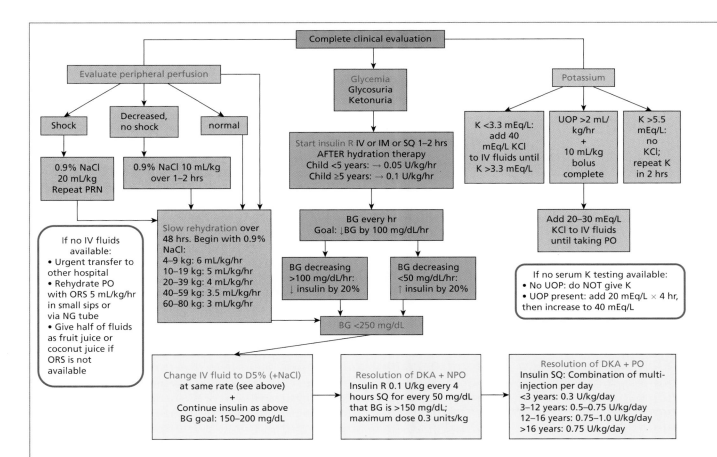

Figure 23.3 Algorithm for the treatment of DKA in adults and children. BG, blood glucose; ORS, oral rehydration solution; SQ, subcutaneous; UOP, urine output. Adapted from International Diabetes Federation (2011).

Name: Age: Weight:				Hospital ID: Date:					
Time	GCS	HR	RR	Glucose	Ketones	Urine output	K+	IV fluid type and rate	Insulin
1AM									
2AM									
....									

Figure 23.4 An example of a form that can be used for monitoring a patient in DKA.

Table 23.4 Cerebral edema treatment.

Mannitol: 0.25–1 g/kg per dose infused over 20–30 min, repeat every 6–8 hours as needed

3% saline: 5–10 mL/kg over 30 min

Other measures: reduce rate of fluid administration, 30° elevation of head of bed, consider intubation and mechanical ventilation

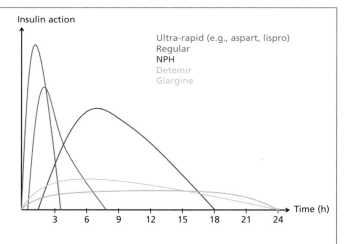

Figure 23.5 Types of insulin.

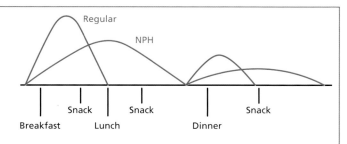

Figure 23.6 Twice-daily insulin regimen.

Both have in common that they peak at a relatively predictable time. Thus, once given, the patient has to consume a certain amount of food to match the peaks of the administered insulin. This feeding helps avoid hypoglycemia at the time of insulin peak. Ideally, patients eat three scheduled meals and two to three snacks to coincide with the insulin peaks.

Oral hyperglycemic medications

T2D frequently responds to oral glucose-lowering medications in the early stages of the disease. T2D patients started on insulin at diagnosis can often be tapered off with introduction of oral agents. Because of the progressive nature of T2D, one oral medication may not control glycemia for more than a few months to years, after which additional oral agents or other injectables, and eventually insulin, are required. Depending on which medications and combinations are used, the cost may be high and the addition of insulin and weaning from other medications may reduce the cost of treatment.

Metformin is the preferred initial oral hyperglycemic medication (Inzucchi *et al.*, 2012). Patients suspected to have T2D who were started on insulin should simultaneously receive metformin, and a subsequent insulin wean should be attempted. If metformin monotherapy at maximal tolerated dose does not achieve or maintain goal blood sugars (or, if available, goal HbA1c), a second oral agent such as a sulfonylurea (e.g., glibenclamide), meglitinide (e.g., repaglinide), thiazolidinedione (e.g., pioglitazone), newer oral agents such as inhibitors of dipeptidyl peptidase 4 (e.g., gliptins) and glucagon-like peptide 1 antagonists (e.g., exenatide), or insulin should be added. Additional resources are available for more detailed use of oral hyperglycemic medications (Inzucchi *et al.*, 2012).

Blood sugar testing

Diabetes management in resource-poor settings is largely limited by the availability of glucose meters and strips. Glucose strips, in particular, are expensive and can be as much as US$1 each. Many patients are therefore only able to check their blood sugar a maximum (at best) of one to two times daily. For patients on insulin, priority glucose measurements should be before the first insulin dose in the morning (the fasting glucose level) and before the second insulin dose in the evening.

One to two times per week, a bedtime and/or lunchtime blood sugar measurement should be obtained. Ideally, four blood sugars (pre-meal and at bedtime) are measured each day.

Insulin adjustments

Goal blood sugars are 100–200 mg/dL in adolescents and adults and up to 250 mg/dL in children under 5 years of age, and insulin doses should be titrated to avoid hypoglycemia. As a principle, the morning blood sugar reflects the evening dose, and the evening blood sugar reflects the morning dose. In general, doses are adjusted by about 5–10% at a time, and adjustments are made after 2–3 days of a consistent pattern and insulin dose.

Nutrition, exercise, and lifestyle

Food insecurity is a common problem in resource-limited settings. Many patients may not have stable access to food and may not be accustomed to consuming more than one or two meals per day. Quantity and timing of meals tends to be unpredictable. A key feature of diabetes education in these settings is the above outlined insulin regimen and meal plan. Patients can be taught to divide their daily meal portion into four to six small meals in order to adhere to the meal plan as best as possible.

Besides insulin and glucose-lowering agents, healthy nutrition, exercise, and lifestyle modifications are the mainstay of diabetes treatment. Patients should receive education about the components of a healthy diet with a balanced intake of protein, fat, and carbohydrates. In many cultures, the latter is a principal source of energy, and an effort should be made to uncover alternative, affordable, and palatable food choices from the local diet. Simple sugars should be avoided. Exercise is strongly encouraged, and patients should receive education on the positive effect of exercise on glucose metabolism and their overall health.

Hypoglycemia

Hypoglycemia in a patient with diabetes is defined as a blood glucose below 70 mg/dL. Symptoms of hypoglycemia include neuroglycopenic symptoms (irritability, confusion, mental status changes, coma, seizures) and symptoms related to sympathetic activation (heart racing, shakiness, extreme hunger). However, hypoglycemia unawareness is a common phenomenon, especially in patients with recurrent hypoglycemic episodes. Patient education regarding recognition and treatment of hypoglycemia is thus crucial. In the conscious patient, any blood sugar level below 70 mg/dL should prompt the following treatment:

1. 15 g of rapid-acting sugar (e.g., three to four glucose tablets, half glass of juice, or three to four hard candies);
2. recheck blood sugar 15 min later;
3. if >70 mg/dL, provide small snack;
4. if still <70 mg/dL, repeat treatment in steps 1–3.

> ### Clinical experience: a diabetic waistpack
>
> "When we realized that our pediatric patients didn't have a place to put their glucose meter and diabetes supplies when they were going outside or traveling from their home to the clinic, and that they were neither carrying snacks nor would they have an immediate ability to buy one if they were hypoglycemic, we came up with the idea of a diabetic waistpack. Not only did they look fun and fashionable to the kids, but the packs had just enough room for a glucometer, log book, glucose tabs, and a small snack. Our patients soon adopted the packs as their constant companions."
>
> Julia, physician working in Haiti

If the patient is unconscious or having seizure activity, treatment with glucagon 1 mg i.m. for adults and 0.015 mg/kg i.m. for children is preferred and most effective, although frequently unavailable. The oral route should not be used in these situations due to a high risk of aspiration. Patients may need to be transferred to the nearest hospital for intravenous dextrose administration. Alternatively, a nasogastric tube can be placed for enteral glucose administration, or glucose gels or solutions can be rubbed into the gums.

Complications of diabetes

Table 23.5 summarizes many of the complications seen in individuals with diabetes and includes recommendations for the prevention and management of these complications.

Psychosocial and cultural implications

Patients with diabetes are often stigmatized, and there are myths and misconceptions about diabetes worldwide. Health beliefs are often hard to correct, and medical and psychosocial consequences can be significant. The notion of diabetes being the patient's fault due to a lazy lifestyle or unhealthy food consumption is common in wealthier countries, whereas the concept of diabetes being contagious, a curse, a poison, or the result of witchcraft may be more common in different cultures. While providers should listen to and understand the health beliefs of patients, families, and communities, it is important to provide education in order to foster understanding and integration of patients back into their families and communities. Finding local resources and support groups may motivate patients and provide essential support. National diabetes associations frequently provide such services, and contacts can be found through the International Diabetes Federation's website (www.idf.org).

Table 23.5 Complications of diabetes.

Complication	Monitoring	Frequency	Treatment
Hypertension	Check blood pressure (BP)	Every visit	*Goal*: systolic <120 mmHg and diastolic <80 mmHg BP >120/80: recommend lifestyle changes[a] BP >140/80: add pharmacologic therapy (ACE inhibitor)
Dyslipidemia	Fasting lipid profile (total cholesterol, LDL, HDL, triglycerides)	Every 1–2 years	*Goal*: LDL <100 mg/dL (<2.6 mmol/L), HDL >50 mg/dL (>1.3 mmol/L), triglycerides >150 mg/dL (>1.7 mmol/L) *Lifestyle modifications*: reduce saturated fat, *trans* fats, and cholesterol intake; increase omega-3 fatty acids, viscous fiber, and plant stanols/sterols; weight loss; physical activity. If unsuccessful, consider statin therapy
Nephropathy	Urine microalbumin Serum creatinine (adults only)	Yearly	Initiate ACE inhibitor (or angiotensin-receptor blocker) if micro- or macro-albuminuria. Treat ensuing chronic kidney disease; consult with nephrologist if possible
Retinopathy	Dilated and comprehensive eye examination by an ophthalmologist or optometrist	At diagnosis, then yearly	Refer to ophthalmologist experienced in treating diabetic retinopathy for possible laser photocoagulation and/or other necessary treatments
Distal peripheral neuropathy	Pinprick sensation, vibration perception, 10-g monofilament, pressure sensation (on distal plantar aspect of great toes and metatarsal joints), ankle reflexes	At diagnosis, then yearly	Optimize glycemic management. Provide symptomatic relief for specific symptoms
Autonomic neuropathy	History: resting tachycardia, exercise intolerance, orthostatic hypotension, constipation gastroparesis, erectile dysfunction, sweating dysfunction, impaired neurovascular function	At diagnosis, then yearly	Optimize glycemic control, supportive treatment (pain management, dietary changes in gastroparesis, sildenafil for erectile dysfunction)
Foot ulcers	Comprehensive foot examination	Yearly	Patient self-foot care education (daily self-examination, daily moisturizer, proper footwear, no barefoot walking), early detection of ulcers, symptomatic care for ulcers, referral for amputation in refractory cases

[a]Weight loss, avoid alcohol, increase activity level, reduce sodium intake to <1500 mg/day.
ACE, angiotensin-converting enzyme; LDL, low-density lipoprotein; HDL, high-density lipoprotein. Source: American Diabetes Association (2012).

ENDOCRINE DISORDERS

Thyroid disorders

Common disorders of thyroid function include iodine deficiency, leading to goiter and eventually hypothyroidism, and autoimmune thyroid disease, resulting in hypothyroidism (Hashimoto thyroiditis) or hyperthyroidism (Graves disease). It is important not to delay the diagnosis of congenital hypothyroidism, which is part of newborn screening programs in high-income countries. Thyroid cancer, although rare, should be part of the differential in the evaluation of a neck mass. Table 23.6 outlines the general diagnoses of thyroid function tests and the types of conditions they can indicate.

Hypothyroidism

Common signs and symptoms are cold intolerance, constipation, dry skin, dry and coarse hair, low heart rate, depression and, in severe cases, myxedema. In the growing child,

Table 23.6 Interpretation of thyroid function tests.

TSH	T4/free T4	Interpretation	Example
↑	↓	Primary hypothyroidism	Hashimoto's, iodine deficiency
↑	Normal	Subclinical hypothyroidism	Early stages of Hashimoto's
↓	↑	Hyperthyroidism	Graves disease, thyroid adenoma
↓	Normal	Subclinical hyperthyroidism	Early Graves disease, acute thyroiditis
↓/normal	↓	Central hypothyroidism	Pituitary hormone deficiency, sick euthyroid

linear growth failure in the setting of weight gain is the hallmark of hypothyroidism. In infants and toddlers less than 3 years of age, developmental delay can suggest congenital hypothyroidism.

Congenital hypothyroidism

Where newborn screening is available, infants should be treated with levothyroxine 15 μg/kg as soon as the diagnosis of hypothyroidism is made. Doses should be titrated to maintain thyroxine (T4) in the upper normal range and thyroid-stimulating hormone (TSH) at 1–2 μIU/mL. In the absence of newborn screening, any child with developmental delay of unexplained etiology, poor growth with sustained weight gain, or other typical features of congenital hypothyroidism (umbilical hernia, thick tongue, open fontanels) should be evaluated and treated promptly as needed.

Iodine deficiency

Suspicion should be high in persons with goiter who live in endemic areas of iodine deficiency. Diagnosis can be made based on the presence of an often nodular goiter, although clinically it may be difficult to differentiate from autoimmune thyroiditis (see next section). While treatment needs to focus on the hypothyroid individual, in areas of iodine deficiency there also needs to be a population-based preventive approach utilizing iodized salt. Pregnant and breastfeeding women should all take a multivitamin containing at least 150 μg iodine per day.

Autoimmune hypothyroidism (Hashimoto thyroiditis)

A diagnosis of autoimmune hypothyroidism should be suspected in patients with symptoms of hypothyroidism and goiter, although in rare instances the autoimmune process causes thyroid atrophy and a goiter is not present. The thyroid gland feels firm and more granular but is usually without nodularity. Diagnosis can be confirmed by an elevated TSH and low T4 or free T4, and if available by positive thyroid peroxidase and/or thyroglobulin antibodies. Treatment is with levothyroxine, titrated to normalize thyroid function tests. A

typical target dose for adults is 1.7 μg/kg and for children 2–5 μg/kg. In long-standing hypothyroidism, the dose should be titrated upward slowly (e.g., every 2–4 weeks) to avoid atrial fibrillation, congestive heart failure, or idiopathic intracranial hypertension.

Hyperthyroidism

Classic symptoms of hyperthyroidism include heat intolerance, nervousness and anxiety, oily skin and hair, frequent (rarely liquid) bowel movements, tachycardia, hypertension with widened pulse pressure, weight loss, fatigue, proximal muscle weakness, often inability to fall asleep at night, and exophthalmus.

Graves disease

In addition to hyperthyroidism, patients with Graves disease often present with exophthalmus and a large goiter. TSH is typically suppressed, T4 and free T4 are elevated, and triiodothyronine (T3) is characteristically very elevated. Thyroid-binding inhibitory immunoglobulin is positive. Ultrasound can help to distinguish Graves from multinodular goiter or an autonomous ("hot") nodule. A beta-blocker (e.g., atenolol) is frequently used for symptomatic relief. Treatment is either medical (methimazole or propylthiouracil, titrate dose to effect), radioactive iodine ablation (often not available), or surgical resection.

Thyroid storm

Thyroid storm is a clinical diagnosis that should be suspected in any patient with severe signs of hyperthyroidism, fever, and mental status changes. If possible, it should be managed in a critical care unit. Treatment is as follow.

- High-dose propylthiouracil (PTU; unlabeled use): typically 200–300 mg every 4–6 hours.
- Iodide or iodine (at least 1–2 hours after PTU):
  ○ Lugol's solution 20 drops/mL (8 mg iodine/drop): take 10 drops three times daily; children 4–8 drops every 6–8 hours; or

○ Potassium iodide (SSKI) 20 drops/mL (38 mg iodide/drop): take 5 drops four times daily; children 5 drops two to four times daily.
- Glucocorticoids: 100 mg i.v. every 8 hours; children 50 mg/m^2 per dose every 8 hours.
- Beta-blocker and antipyretics for symptomatic relief.

Adrenal disorders

Congenital adrenal hyperplasia

Congenital adrenal hyperplasia (CAH) results from an enzyme defect in the cortisol synthesis pathway, the most common etiology being 21-hydroxylase deficiency. The defect results in insufficient cortisol production and build-up of precursor steroid hormones, including androgens. In its classic salt-wasting form, both glucocorticoids and mineralocorticoids are deficient. Female infants frequently present with virilized or ambiguous genitalia. Male infants are typically normal appearing. Salt wasting with subsequent electrolyte imbalances (hyperkalemia and hyponatremia) due to mineralocorticoid deficiency ensues at around 1 week of age and is life-threatening if left untreated. Investigations include electrolytes, and 17-hydroxyprogesterone, if available. Treatment should be initiated promptly with hydrocortisone at doses of 10–12 mg/m^2 daily in three divided doses. The goal is to suppress the adrenal axis in an attempt to suppress further androgen excess. Patients with salt-wasting CAH require fludrocortisone, usually given at 0.05–0.1 mg per day. All patients require stress-dose steroids for periods of illness (see section below).

CAH also exists as a late-onset, non-classic form that presents outside of the neonatal period and does not include salt wasting. Typical clinical features are very early adrenarche, clitoromegaly, growth acceleration with an advanced bone age, early virilization in boys, and hirsutism in girls. Young women may present with hirsutism, irregular menses, or amenorrhea. Treatment is similar to that for classic CAH. Optimal suppression of the adrenal axis must be carefully weighed against overtreatment with steroids to ensure normal growth and prevent compromised adult stature.

Adrenal insufficiency

Adrenal insufficiency is a rare but potentially life-threatening condition. Dysfunctional adrenal glands lead to primary adrenal insufficiency; more rarely, a lack of central adrenocorticotropin (ACTH) stimulus leads to secondary adrenal insufficiency. Causes for primary adrenal insufficiency prevalent in developing countries include infectious diseases (HIV, meningococcemia, tuberculosis, malaria) and, more rarely, autoimmune disease (Addison's). Classic symptoms are hypotension, hyperpigmentation, salt craving, abdominal pain, and nausea, and diagnostic laboratory findings are hyperkalemia and hyponatremia due to mineralocorticoid deficiency. If possible, diagnosis should be confirmed with cortisol and ACTH levels; the gold standard is an ACTH stimulation test. Treatment must be prompt to avoid adrenal crisis and consists of hydrocortisone replacement (6–8 mg/m^2 daily every 8 hours), with stress-dose steroids (hydrocortisone 50 mg/m^2 daily divided every 6 hours) given for critical illness, fever above 38.5°C, vomiting, or surgical procedures.

Vitamin D deficiency/rickets

Vitamin D deficiency is prevalent worldwide. Risk factors include dark skin, limited sun exposure, full or partial veiling, and diet low in Vitamin D. Infants and children with Vitamin D deficiency are at risk for rickets, which should be suspected in any child with hypocalcemia, tetany, and/or skeletal findings such as bowed legs, rachitic rosary (prominent bumps at the costochondral joints), craniotabes (thinning or softening of skull), and bony tenderness. If possible, calcium, phosphorus, alkaline phosphatase, and 25-hydroxyvitamin D levels should be obtained. Knee and/or wrist radiography confirm the diagnosis. Vitamin D repletion therapy should be instituted promptly with 1000 IU (infants <12 months) and 2000 IU (children >12 months) daily for 2–3 months. During Vitamin D treatment, prophylactic calcium supplementation to avoid hungry bone syndrome should be given with **elemental calcium** 30–75 mg/kg divided three times daily (e.g., calcium carbonate 75–180 mg/kg divided three times daily), although higher doses may be required. Following acute therapy, maintenance replacement therapy with 400–800 IU Vitamin D is recommended if feasible. A change in diet to increase daily calcium and Vitamin D is recommended to avoid recurrence.

Hypertension

The definition of hypertension is systolic/diastolic blood pressure above 139/89 mmHg (pre-hypertension, 120–139/80–89; stage I, 140–159/90–99; stage II, >160/100 mmHg) and in children, blood pressure above the 99th percentile for age, gender, and height (pre-hypertension, >95th percentile; stage I, 95–99th percentile + 5 mmHg; stage II, >99th percentile + 5 mmHg) (Brady, 2012). Measurements should be confirmed manually on three separate occasions. About 95% of hypertensive adults have essential (primary) hypertension, whereas up to 70–85% of hypertensive children have secondary hypertension due to an underlying cause (Brady, 2012). The younger the patient, the more carefully underlying pathology should be excluded, including pathology of the cardiovascular system (coarctation of the aorta), endocrine system (hyperthyroidism, pheochromocytoma, Cushing syndrome, hyperaldosteronism, diabetes mellitus, and CAH), neurological system (increased intracranial pressure), renal system (parenchymal, glomerulonephritis, pyelonephritis, polycystic kidneys, reflux nephropathy), and systemic conditions such as lupus erythematosus.

Treatment for primary hypertension consists of weight loss, exercise, salt restriction, healthy diet, and smoking cessation. Medical therapy with an angiotensin-converting enzyme (ACE) inhibitor, furosemide, beta-blocker, or calcium-channel blocker is indicated if hypertension persists after 6 months of lifestyle changes, if there is presence of stage II hypertension, or for symptomatic treatment of secondary hypertension. See Chapter 21 for additional management of hypertension.

Additional resources

- Brink SJ, Rhen W, Lee W, Pillay K, Kleinebreil L (2010) *Diabetes in Children and Adolescents: Basic Training Manual for Healthcare Providers in Developing Countries.*

Novo Nordisk with International Society for Pediatric and Adolescent Diabetes. Available at http://www.changingdiabetesaccess.com/pdfs/training_manuals_and_presentations/CDiC_Manual_UK_Jan_2011_001_LOW.pdf
- International Diabetes Federation: www.idf.org
- Life for a Child: www.idf.org/lifeforachild, including video on type 1 diabetes at http://www.youtube.com/watch?v=A8iFbduZF14
- American Diabetes Association: www.diabetes.org
- Thyroid Manager, for online thyroid resources: http://www.thyroidmanager.org/
- EndoText, for online endocrine resources: http://www.endotext.org/

REFERENCES

American Diabetes Association (2004) Hyperglycemia crises in diabetes. *Diabetes Care* 27(Suppl. 1):S94–102.

American Diabetes Association. (2012) Standards of medical care in diabetes, 2012. Position statement. *Diabetes Care* 35(Suppl. 1):11–63.

Brady TM (2012) Hypertension. *Pediatr Rev* 33:541–52.

Gill GV, Mbanya JC, Ramaiya KL, Tesfaye S (2009) A sub-Saharan African perspective of diabetes. *Diabetologia* 52:8–16.

Hall V, Thomsen RW, Henriksen O, Lohse N (2011) Diabetes in sub-Saharan Africa 1999–2011: epidemiology and public health implications, a systematic review. *BMC Public Health* 11:564.

International Diabetes Federation (2011) Global IDF/ISPAD guideline for diabetes in childhood and adolescence. Available at http://www.idf.org/global-idfispad-guideline-diabetes-childhood-and-adolescence

International Diabetes Federation (2013) *IDF Diabetes Atlas*, 6th edn. Brussels, Belgium: International Diabetes Federation. Available at http://www.idf.org/diabetesatlas

Inzucchi SE, Bergenstal RM, Buse JB *et al.* (2012) Management of hyperglycemia in type 2 diabetes: a patient-centered approach: position statement of the American Diabetes Association (ADA) and the European Association for the Study of Diabetes (EASD). *Diabetes Care* 35(6):1364–79.

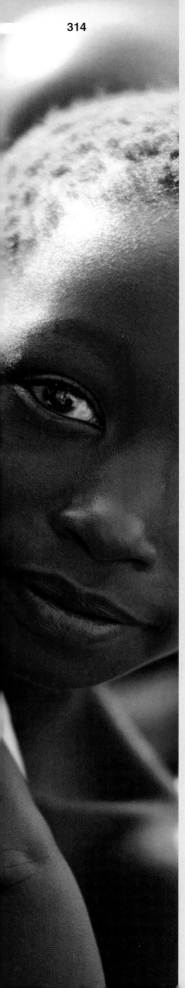

CHAPTER 24

Cancer and Blood Disorders

Natasha M. Archer and Carlos Rodriguez-Galindo

Dana-Farber/Boston Children's Cancer and Blood Disorders Center, and Harvard Medical School, Boston, MA, USA

Key learning objectives

- Review the epidemiology of cancer and blood disorders in low- and middle-income countries.
- Learn how to elicit a history from, and perform a thorough physical examination on, a patient with a suspected cancer or blood disorder.
- Understand the basic evaluation of a person with a suspected cancer or blood disorder.
- Understand the diagnosis and management of the most common cancer and blood disorders in adults and children.

Abstract

More than 80% of patients with cancer and blood disorders live in low- and middle-income countries. Despite the large need for hematology and oncology programs in these settings, very few exist. Therefore, it is imperative that the general practitioner has a healthy suspicion for these disorders as well as basic knowledge regarding the screening, presentation, evaluation, diagnosis, and management of cancer and blood disorders. This chapter reviews these general principles and provides a more detailed description of the most common cancer and blood disorders encountered in both adults and children worldwide.

Key words: hematology, oncology, blood, cancer, anemia, iron-deficiency anemia, sickle cell anemia, breast cancer, prostate cancer, acute lymphoblastic leukemia

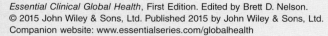

Introduction and epidemiology

Cancer and blood disorders are a significant cause of morbidity and mortality worldwide (Boyle & Levin, 2008; Bray *et al.*, 2012). While advances in the two fields have led to a significant decrease in the incidence, morbidity, and mortality in high-income countries, the burden of disease is particularly significant in low- and middle-income countries (LMICs), where greater than 80% of people with blood disorders and 80% of children and adults diagnosed with cancer every year live (Farmer *et al.*, 2010; Stonebraker *et al.*, 2010; Weatherall, 2011; Pasricha *et al.*, 2013; Rodriguez-Galindo *et al.*, 2013). Even more concerning is the disproportionate number of deaths that are a direct result of these diseases. LMICs face challenges of inaccurate disease epidemiology due to the paucity of cancer and blood disorder registries, late presentation of disease, lack of infrastructure to diagnose and treat even the most basic conditions, and high prevalence of abandonment when treatment is attempted. While these challenges can be discouraging, they should never be used as an excuse for lack of care.

Screening

Focused efforts on the screening and early diagnosis of cancer and blood disorders in high-income countries have significantly decreased the morbidity and mortality associated with these diseases. Classically, a good screening test is inexpensive and has a high sensitivity. It also yields major reductions in morbidity and mortality worldwide. Ideally, management of the disease being screened would also be made available not only because it is ethically appropriate but also because it will encourage individuals to come for screening. Table 24.1 lists screening and early diagnosis procedures for common cancer and blood disorders.

Presentation

Many people with cancer and blood disorders can present with non-specific symptoms like fatigue, fever, night sweats, or weight loss, while others present with pathognomonic signs such as a large breast mass. It is not only essential that clinicians maintain a high suspicion of disease but that they also create an environment that allows people to be open about their health and not fear being turned away.

Although the histories of patients with cancer and blood disorders may be vague and complicated, it is important to attempt to obtain as detailed a history as possible and complete a thorough physical examination, which although difficult is necessary even in a setting with non-private rooms. Remember that late presentation is common not only secondary to denial and fear of stigma on the part of the patient, but also possibly misdiagnosis by practitioners.

History

Fatigue
Patients in LMICs often present with fatigue. It is important to investigate the time course of the fatigue (when it started, does it come and go) and whether any changes in the patient's ability to accomplish activities of daily living have occurred. For example, is the patient still able to walk up the mountain to the clinic or complete daily chores like the laundry and field work?

Fever
Fever can often be mistaken for a sensation of feeling hot, which is not uncommon in tropical environments. Most patients will not have access to a thermometer to effectively measure their temperature. Therefore, it is important to ask about associated symptoms such as rigors and chills, which may be more instructive.

Night sweats
Night sweats in a tropical environment may also be difficult to ascertain. Asking whether the patient actually woke in the night and changed their night clothes may be more helpful than sweating at night.

Weight loss
Most people will not have access to a scale and may not know if they have actually lost weight. It is therefore important for the practitioner to use creative ways to ask this question, including whether the individual has noticed a change in dress or pant size, whether they are using a different hole to fasten their belt, or whether other people have noticed that they are smaller in size. Weight loss is also complicated by the lack of food security, so common in LMICs. It is important to get a diet history to ensure that the weight loss experienced is not a function of poverty.

Mass
A mass should always be assumed malignant; it is too risky to suggest that it is probably benign and ask the patient to return if it changes. Most will not return because they heard "benign" and not "probably benign"; they may assume they will be sent home again, and thus they seek help elsewhere. Alternatively, they may be in denial and do not want to hear what they fear

Table 24.1 List of recommended risk-reduction strategies, screening, and early diagnostic procedures for cancer and blood disorders, specifically in LMICs.

	Condition	Risk-reduction strategies	Screening and early diagnosis	
			Low-income countries	**Middle-income countries**
Adult cancers	Breast	Maintain healthy body weight, increase physical activity, minimize alcohol intake	Clinical breast examination	Mammography
	Cervical	Human papillomavirus (HPV) vaccination program	Visual inspection of cervix with acetic acid (VIA)	Papanicolaou (pap) smear
	Colorectal	Decrease smoking, consumption of red meat, and excessive alcohol; increase physical activity	One-time flexible sigmoidoscopy	Colonoscopy
	Esophageal and gastric	Treatment of *Helicobacter pylori*; decrease tobacco, alcohol, and betel liquid exposure; increase physical activity	No screening recommended	No screening recommended
	Lung	Tobacco control interventions including raising price of cigarettes, banning smoking in public places, treating tobacco dependence; provide safe cooking stoves for families to replace unventilated coal-fuel stoves	No screening recommended	No screening recommended
	Prostate	No preventable risk factors	No screening recommended	No screening recommended
	Hepatocellular	Hepatitis B virus (HBV) vaccine program; screen blood for hepatitis C virus (HCV), needle exchange for injection drug users, crop substitution, improve grain storage practices that reduce contamination with aflatoxin B1	Newborn HBV vaccine programs	Newborn HBV vaccine programs
	Skin	Limit sun exposure	Clinical skin examination	Clinical skin examination
Pediatric cancers	Retinoblastoma	No preventable risk factors; however, should educate mothers about leukocoria	Red reflex examination	Red reflex examination, followed as needed by examination under anesthesia
	Testicular	No preventable risk factors; however, boys and young men should be educated about the presentation of testicular cancer	No screening recommended	No screening recommended
Blood disorders	Iron-deficiency anemia	Breastfeeding up to 6 months; at 6 months, provide iron or iron-fortified formula; provide pregnant women with iron supplementation	Hemoglobin (infants and women of childbearing age)	Hemoglobin and iron studies if hemoglobin low
	Infectious causes of anemia	Malaria treatment, helminthic treatment	Malaria smear especially in already anemic population; stool ova and parasites	Malaria smear, especially in already anemic population; stool ova and parasites
	Sickle cell disease	Parental genetic counseling	Isoelectric focusing (IEF)	High-performance liquid chromatography (HPLC)

you will tell them. All masses should be evaluated with imaging, which should be reviewed by both a radiologist and an oncologist. Remember that revealing a mass to a patient may result in some rejection from family and friends as well as loss of work. This can be a very vulnerable time for many patients. They do not need to be reminded that they should have come earlier. They need to be supported and assured that you will do everything in your power to address their condition, you will keep them comfortable, and they will live their lives in dignity.

Social history
Knowing the patient's social situation and exposures is extremely important in helping to confirm or exclude cancer, blood disorders, as well as other conditions in your differential diagnosis.

Physical examination

Vital signs
In the evaluation of cancer and blood disorders, all vital signs are important, including temperature, heart rate, blood pressure, respiratory rate, oxygen saturation, weight, and height. Temperature, heart rate, and blood pressure can be very informative regarding potential septicemia in a sick patient with cancer or a blood disorder, especially if their suspected diagnosis involves the lack or dysfunction of white blood cells, a key line of defense against serious bacterial infections. Respiratory rate and oxygen saturation can be a clue that there is involvement of the heart, lungs, or abdomen (in children a full abdomen can compress the lungs, making it hard to breath). Weight and height can objectively measure weight loss and are needed to determine weight-based chemotherapy.

General appearance
Assessment of cachexia, which often reflects a debilitating chronic disease, should be performed.

Head, eyes, ears, nose and throat
Tongue pallor was found to be the most sensitive of the pallor sites (conjunctiva, palmar, nail beds) in a recent study from India in patients with hemoglobin below 7 g/dL (Kalantri *et al.*, 2010). Loss of papillation of the tongue can be seen in iron-deficiency anemia. The head (and neck) are commonly affected in pediatric cancers. For example, retinoblastoma, the most common intraocular malignancy of childhood, can present with leukocoria, an abnormal white pupil. When it is detected at this stage, when still intraocular, enucleation is curative in greater than 90% of patients. Nasal obstruction and proptosis of the eye can be signs of rhabdomyosarcoma. A wait-and-see approach to such a tumor can lead to inoperable disease and greatly decreased chance of cure.

Neck
Lymphadenopathy is a common finding in blood and solid tumor cancers.

Pulmonary examination
Breath sounds, percussion, and tactile fremitus can help determine whether there is pulmonary involvement.

Cardiac examination
Elevated jugular venous pressure (JVP) and a cardiac rub can suggest a pericardial effusion.

Abdominal examination
Hepatosplenomegaly and the presence of abdominal masses should always be assessed.

Skin
Petechiae, rashes, and jaundice are common skin findings that can support a particular diagnosis or organ involvement.

Extremities
Lower extremity edema can suggest cardiac involvement. In the case of soft tissue or bone cancers, masses can occur in the extremities. Mid-upper arm circumference (MUAC) is a useful assessment of nutritional status in children (see Chapter 12).

Differential diagnosis

When a patient presents with a mass, the differential diagnosis should include a variety of neoplastic conditions, depending on the site of the mass, as well as two common non-neoplastic conditions, human immunodeficiency virus (HIV) and tuberculosis, both of which can present with cytopenias, masses, and a weakened immune system. Other infectious diseases such as dengue can present with signs associated with leukemia.

HIV (see Chapter 18)
HIV can cause cytopenias, including thrombocytopenia and anemia, as well as lymphadenopathy concerning for lymphoma or a neck mass. In addition, patients with AIDS also present with diseases only seen in people with a weakened immune system such as *Pneumocystis jiroveci* pneumonia. Lastly, Kaposi sarcoma, a vascular tumor associated with human herpesvirus (HHV)-8, is an AIDS-associated condition. It is characterized by cutaneous, linear, non-painful lesions on the lower extremities, face, or genitalia. These can be mistaken for hematomas or purpura (red or purple discoloration >3 mm in size that do not blanch under pressure and are caused by bleeding underneath the skin).

Tuberculosis (see Chapter 19)
Tuberculosis is a very common respiratory infection in resource-limited settings. It can present with non-specific symptoms very similar to those of people with a suspected cancer or blood disorder, including fatigue, fever, weight loss, and night sweats. Lymphadenopathy is very common and can be confused for lymphoma. Chest X-ray obtained in the setting of respiratory symptoms can reveal large opacities, which can be concerning for lung metastases or a primary lung cancer. Given how

similar tuberculosis can appear to so many different cancer and blood disorders, a detailed history (noting exposures), physical examination, and laboratory data are imperative in distinguishing this disease.

Dengue (see Chapter 20)

Dengue is a virus transmitted by the *Aedes aegypti* mosquito. It typically presents with fever, headache, myalgia, joint pain, and rash. In a small number of cases it can develop into dengue hemorrhagic fever, characterized by thrombocytopenia, subsequent bleeding, and significant capillary leakage. As fever, myalgia, and thrombocytopenia are often presenting symptoms of acute leukemia, it is important to look at a peripheral blood smear of those with suspected dengue in order to not delay or, worse, miss the diagnosis of acute leukemia.

Evaluation

Evaluation of the patient with a blood disorder

Informed by findings from a detailed history and a thorough physical examination, laboratory data are often required to make the definitive diagnosis of a blood disorder.

Complete blood count

Laboratory evaluation should always begin with a complete blood count (CBC), including red blood cell indices such as red cell distribution width (RDW), mean corpuscular volume (MCV), mean corpuscular hemoglobin (MCH), mean corpuscular hemoglobin concentration (MCHC) and a differential (which can be done manually by the clinician or a laboratory technologist). The MCV represents the size of the red blood cells, and the MCH and MCHC represent the average hemoglobin content of red blood cells. RDW and MCV are particularly useful in classifying anemias, while the MCH and MCHC, when elevated, can suggest the presence of spherocytes, smaller and denser red blood cells that resemble a sphere as opposed to a discoid shape and are commonly found in hemolytic anemia conditions. If the CBC is abnormal, preparation and examination of a peripheral blood smear (PBS) should follow (Box 24.1). A PBS can be especially helpful in distinguishing the many forms of anemia, disorders that lead to abnormal bleeding and clotting, as well as malignant disorders such as leukemia (Figure 24.2). Because of limited resources, a PBS is usually only performed in the setting of an abnormal CBC or clinical features, such as petechiae, easy bruising, or jaundice. The review of a PBS

Box 24.1 How to prepare a peripheral blood smear for blood disorder evaluation

Materials
Two glass slides, dropper, blood sample, staining kit, microscope, gloves

Technique (Figure 24.1)
The steps for preparing a thick and thin peripheral blood smear are also discussed in Chapter 31. However, for the evaluation of blood disorders, a thin smear is sufficient.

1. Place a drop of blood on the bottom slide approximately one-third of the way from one end of the slide.
2. Position the other top slide at a 45° angle in front of the drop of blood. Pull back toward the blood until you touch the blood and it spreads along the edge of the top slide.
3. Without lifting the slide, spread the drop of blood over the slide with one fluid movement in the opposite direction.
4. Allow the slide to dry for 2–3 min.
5. Stain the slide. There are several staining kits available. Most kits use a version of the Wright and Giemsa stains, but the specific staining instructions differ based on solutions used. Follow the instructions that come with your stain for the optimal results.
6. Once you have successfully stained your slide, view it under a light microscope.

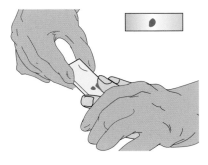
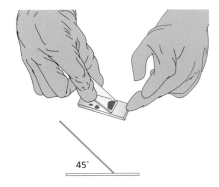

Figure 24.1 Preparation of thin peripheral blood smears.

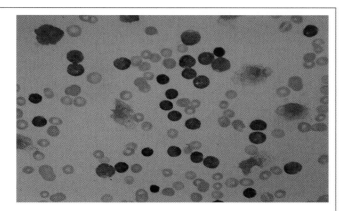

Figure 24.2 Peripheral blood smear of a 2-year-old boy with acute lymphoblastic leukemia (ALL) and a high presenting white blood cell count at risk for tumor lysis syndrome. Note the large number of lymphoblasts. They are larger than the red blood cells and have very little cytoplasm.

requires a consistent systematic approach, for example reviewing the size, shape, content, and number of red blood cells, white blood cells, and platelets every time a PBS is examined.

Bone marrow aspirate and biopsy

When two or more cell lines are decreased and confirmed on review of the PBS, a bone marrow aspirate and biopsy may need to be performed. The bone marrow is the factory where blood cells are made. A bone marrow aspirate and biopsy can distinguish between a hypocellular marrow as seen in aplastic anemia, a hypercellular marrow as seen in leukemia, and a marrow replaced by solid tumors or fibrosis. Bone marrow aspirates and biopsies are understandably difficult to examine for non-specialists. However, we recommend investing resources in the ability to perform bone marrow aspirates and aspirate smears. Then, with the use of telemedicine, bone marrow aspirate images using a simple camera phone can be shared with hematopathologist colleagues widely.

Other laboratory investigations

Based on results of the CBC, PBS, and bone marrow aspirate and biopsy, together with the clinical context, further studies may be needed. Some particularly useful laboratory tests, if available, include testing for iron-deficiency anemia (iron, ferritin, total iron binding capacity), hemoglobinopathies (isoelectric focusing or hemoglobin electrophoresis), factor VIII and IX deficiency or coagulations studies (prothrombin time or partial thromboplastin time), and cross-matching to facilitate any necessary transfusions.

Evaluation of a patient with a suspected non-solid tumor

The initial evaluation of hematologic malignancies (leukemia and lymphoma) is similar to that of benign blood disorders.

Laboratory assessment

After a detailed history and physical examination, standard laboratory assessment includes a CBC with differential, coagulation studies, and a type and cross for the blood bank.

Bone marrow aspirate and biopsy

Bone marrow aspirate and biopsy should be performed if abnormalities in two or more cell lines exist or if the presence of blasts is noted on the PBS.

Lumbar puncture

A lumbar puncture for evaluation of cerebrospinal fluid (CSF) cytology is performed for therapeutic and staging purposes in leukemia and some types of lymphoma. In the setting of a diagnosis of leukemia, intrathecal chemotherapy is administered at the time of the diagnostic procedure for both the treatment of the central nervous system (CNS) and to avoid contamination of the CSF by leukemic cells.

Lymph node biopsy

An excisional biopsy is preferred over a needle biopsy since it is important to evaluate the entire architecture of the lymph node for a proper diagnosis.

Tumor lysis

Tumor lysis is an oncologic emergency (Tables 24.2 and 24.3). Unlike with patients with suspected benign blood disorders, those suspected of a blood cancer can be at risk for tumor lysis syndrome, the sudden lysis of cancer cells that leads to life-threatening electrolyte abnormalities. Laboratory results consistent with tumor lysis include increased potassium, phosphate, uric acid, creatinine, and lactate dehydrogenase (LDH) and decreased calcium. These should be checked regularly (approximately every 8–12 hours and at least daily), especially in patients with rapidly dividing cancers, such as Burkitt lymphoma, or in patients with a high presenting white blood cell count. In settings where laboratory data are not easily obtained, one should focus on checking potassium, uric acid, creatinine, and calcium. These are the tumor lysis labs that will most affect your management.

Infectious work-up

Patients with hematologic malignancies often present with a degree of immunosuppression. When infection is suspected, a thorough infectious work-up should be performed that includes blood culture in the presence of fever, chest X-ray and sputum Gram stain and culture if respiratory symptoms exist, and urinalysis and urine culture if urinary symptoms are present.

Table 24.2 Common adult oncologic emergencies.

Emergency	Associated cancer	Signs and symptoms	Evaluation	Treatment
Febrile neutropenia	All cancers	Fever	↓ANC	Antipseudomonal antibiotics, fungal coverage
Tumor lysis syndrome	Burkitt lymphoma and leukemias (ALL, AML, CML)	Renal failure	↑K, ↑uric acid, ↑phosphate, ↓Ca; ECG if K high	Intravenous hydration, allopurinol
Hypercalcemia	Multiple myeloma, breast, and lung	Lethargy, confusion, constipation, anorexia, nausea, muscle weakness, polyuria, polydipsia, acute kidney injury	↑Ca, ↑creatinine	Hydration, bisphosphonates, dialysis
Hyperleukocytosis	Multiple myeloma, AML, and CML	Oronasal bleeding, blurred vision, neurologic symptoms, confusion, heart failure	↑WBC, clinical	Plasmapheresis
Superior vena cava syndrome	Small cell lung, lymphoma, and metastatic lesions to supraclavicular area	Dyspnea, facial fullness, venous engorgement of the neck and chest wall	Chest X-ray, CT	Elevation of head, chemotherapy or radiation therapy
Pericardial tamponade	Lung, breast, lymphoma, leukemia, and melanoma	Chest pain, dyspnea, anxiety	Pulsus paradoxus, ECG	Periocardiocentesis
Pulmonary embolus	All cancers	Dyspnea, pleuritic chest pain	CT pulmonary angiography, *V/Q* scan	Anticoagulation
Biliary obstruction	Pancreatic, bile duct carcinoma, lymphoma, and metastatic breast, colon, lung, and ovarian	Jaundice, pain	Endoscopic retrograde cholangiopancreatography (ERCP)	ERCP with stent or percutaneous transhepatic drain placement
Bowel obstruction	Gastric, colonic, and metastatic lung, breast, and melanoma	Nausea, vomiting, obstipation	Abdominal X-ray and CT	Nil by mouth, nasogastric tube, exploratory laparotomy
Spinal cord compression	Multiple myeloma and metastatic lesions from lung, breast, and prostate	Back pain, weakness, autonomic dysfunction (urinary retention, decreased anal sphincter tone)	Full spine MRI	Dexamethasone, surgical decompression, radiation therapy

ALL, acute lymphoblastic leukemia; ANC, absolute neutrophil count; AML, acute myeloid leukemia; CML, chronic myeloid leukemia.

Evaluation of a patient with a suspected solid tumor

As mentioned earlier, any mass in a patient should be thoroughly and promptly evaluated.

Laboratory assessment

While arranging for imaging of the mass, which can admittedly be challenging in resource-limited settings, standard laboratory studies should be assessed, such as a CBC with differential, chemistry panel (including tumor lysis data), type and cross, and clotting times.

Imaging

Cancers involving the bone should be examined with radiography that always includes the joint above and below the suspected lesion. Additionally, as available, computed tomography (CT) or magnetic resonance imaging (MRI) will clarify

Table 24.3 Common pediatric oncologic emergencies.

Emergency	Associated cancer	Symptoms	Evaluation	Treatment
Febrile neutropenia	All cancers	Fever	↓ANC	Antipseudomonal antibiotics, fungal coverage
Tumor lysis syndrome	Burkitt lymphoma, leukemias (ALL, AML, CML), hepatoblastoma, and 4S neuroblastoma	Renal failure	↑K, ↑uric acid, ↑phosphate, ↓Ca; ECG if K high	Intravenous hydration, allopurinol
Hyperleukocytosis	Leukemia	Respiratory distress, lethargy, confusion	↑WBC, clinical	Hydration, leukopheresis
Hypercoagulability	All cancers	Pulmonary embolism (dyspnea, pleuritic chest pain), DVT (extremity swelling and pain)	CT pulmonary angiography, V/Q scan, ultrasound	Anticoagulation
Bleeding	Leukemia, and Wilms tumor	Mucosal bleeding, increased bruising, hematuria, cerebrovascular accident	↓platelets, ↑PT, PTT, ↓fibrinogen, vWF	Platelet transfusion, Vitamin K, fresh frozen plasma, DDAVP
Superior vena cava syndrome	Non-Hodgkin lymphoma, T-cell leukemia, teratoma, thyroid cancer, Hodgkin lymphoma, sarcoma, and neuroblastoma	Shortness of breath, facial swelling, syncope, tracheal compression symptoms including cough, dyspnea, air hunger, wheezing, occlusion of central venous catheter	Chest X-ray, CT showing mass	Chemotherapy, radiation therapy
Mediastinal mass	Non-Hodgkin lymphoma, T-cell leukemia, teratoma, thyroid cancer, Hodgkin lymphoma, sarcoma, and neuroblastoma	Tracheal compression symptoms including cough, dyspnea, air hunger, wheezing, occlusion of central venous catheter	Chest X-ray, CT showing anterior mediastinal mass	Chemotherapy, radiation therapy
Massive hepatomegaly	4S neuroblastoma	Respiratory distress, emesis, decreased urine output, DIC	Abdominal CT	Chemotherapy
Increased intracranial pressure (ICP) with brain herniation	Brain tumors (most often astrocytomas, primitive neuroectodermal tumors including medulloblastoma)	Vomiting, lethargy, seizures, increased head circumference, headache, focal neurologic deficits, Cushing's triad (bradycardia, widened pulse pressure, irregular breathing)	Brain CT, brain MRI	Dexamethasone, antiseizure prophylaxis, maintain platelets >50,000 cells/μL
Spinal cord compression	Brain tumors, neuroblastoma, osteosarcoma, rhabdomyosarcoma, Ewing sarcoma, non-Hodgkin lymphoma, and Hodgkin lymphoma	Back pain, paralysis, sensory loss, anal sphincter incompetence	Neurologic examination, MRI	Dexamethasone, laminectomy, radiation therapy, chemotherapy

ALL, acute lymphoblastic leukemia; AML, acute myeloid leukemia; ANC, absolute neutrophil count; CML, chronic myeloid leukemia; DDAVP, desmopressin; DIC, disseminated intravascular coagulation; DVT, deep venous thrombosis; PT, prothrombin time; PTT, partial thromboplastin time; vWF, vonWillebrand factor; WBC, white blood cell count.

the disease extent and any compromise of vital structures. Soft tissue masses in the neck and abdomen can be first assessed using ultrasound. CT and MRI often prove most helpful especially if surgical resection is being considered. Cancer in the chest is often discovered on chest X-ray, and a CT should follow to further define the disease.

Pathology

While imaging may be helpful, in order to make a definitive diagnosis, a biopsy is required. This should be performed as soon as it is safe, and the biopsied tissue should be reviewed by a pathologist who understands cancer is in your differential diagnosis.

Diagnosis and treatment of common cancer and blood disorders

Cancer and blood disorders encompass a vast array of diseases. This chapter, therefore, is by no means a comprehensive over-view of either hematology or oncology, and it is recommended that clinicians seek advice from hematologists and oncologists while managing individual patients. The sections that follow highlight the most common cancer and blood disorders in adults and children. Tables 24.4, 24.5 and 24.6 also provide some basic information about less common, but equally important, conditions found in both adults and children that one may encounter while working in LMICs. It is important to remember that no patients with cancer or a blood disorder should ever be turned away; if treatment and cure are not possible, palliation can and should be offered to all patients who suffer from symptoms related to their disease, regardless of prognosis. Palliation is not meant to hasten or postpone death, but to offer support in living as actively and comfortably as possible.

Breast cancer

Breast cancer typically presents with a hard, irregular, fixed, and non-tender mass. As with all solid tumors, it is

Table 24.4 Common oncologic diseases in adults.

Cancer type	Presenting symptoms	Diagnosis	Treatment
Nasopharyngeal	Nasal obstruction, epistaxis, cervical lymphadenopathy, sore throat, recurrent otitis media, tinnitus	Fiberoptic endoscopic examination with biopsy, CT, EBV titers	Surgery, radiation, chemotherapy
Breast	Breast mass	Mammography, ultrasound, breast biopsy	Surgery, radiation, chemotherapy
Lung	Respiratory symptoms, chest pain, hemoptysis, lymphadenopathy	Lung biopsy, CT chest	Surgery, radiation, chemotherapy
Esophageal and gastric	Dysphagia, weight loss, regurgitation, odynophagia, cough	Esophagogastroduodenoscopy (EGD), endoscopic ultrasound with biopsy, CT chest and abdomen	Surgery, radiation, chemotherapy
Renal cell carcinoma	Hematuria, abdominal mass, flank pain	CT abdomen, biopsy, partial/total nephrectomy	Surgery, radiation, chemotherapy
Hepatocellular carcinoma	Abdominal pain, jaundice, bleeding or bruising	α-Fetoprotein, abdominal ultrasound, CT or MRI, liver biopsy	Liver transplant, liver tumor resection if localized, systemic and intra-arterial chemotherapy, ablation, chemoembolization
Colorectal	Change in bowel habits, rectal bleeding, weakness, fatigue	Colonoscopy, biopsy, CT, MRI	Surgery, radiation, chemotherapy
Bladder	Hematuria	Urine cytology, cystoscopy and biopsy, CT or MRI	TURBT (transurethral resection of bladder tumor), radial cystectomy, washes with BCG and immunotherapy agents
Cervical	Irregular and heavy bleeding	Cervical cytology and biopsy	Surgery, radiation, chemotherapy
Prostate	Urinary frequency, urgency, nocturia, hesitancy	Prostate examination, biopsy using transrectal ultrasound	Surgery, chemotherapy, radiation

Table 24.4 Common oncologic diseases in adults. (*Continued*)

Cancer type	Presenting symptoms	Diagnosis	Treatment
Kaposi sarcoma	Purplish reddish-blue macules, nodules, or plaques in patient with HIV	Clinical and biopsy	Surgery, radiation, chemotherapy
Chronic myeloid leukemia	Fatigue, abnormal blood counts, weight loss, abdominal fullness	Peripheral blood smear and bone marrow aspirate, FISH for *BCR/ABL1*	Hydroxyurea to reduce WBC count, tyrosine kinase inhibitors, stem cell transplant
Acute myeloid leukemia	Fever, fatigue, bone pain	Blood smear, bone marrow aspirate and biopsy with flow cytometry	Chemotherapy, stem cell transplant
Hodgkin lymphoma	Fever, weight loss, lymphadenopathy, masses	Excisional lymph node biopsy	Chemotherapy, radiation, stem cell transplant
Non-Hodgkin lymphoma	Fever, weight loss, lymphadenopathy, masses	Bone marrow aspirate and biopsy, excisional lymph node biopsy	Chemotherapy, radiation, stem cell transplant

EBV, Epstein–Barr virus; FISH, fluorescence *in situ* hybridization; WBC, white blood cell count.

Table 24.5 Common oncologic diseases in children.

Cancer type	Presenting symptoms	Diagnosis	Treatment
Brain tumors	Headache, vomiting, ataxia	CT, MRI	Surgery, radiation, chemotherapy
Retinoblastoma	Leukocoria, buphthalmos, orbital mass	Retinal examination under anesthesia	Enucleation, chemotherapy, radiation
Neuroblastoma	Abdominal mass, bone pain	CT of area of mass and abdomen, urine VMA, HVA	Surgery, chemotherapy, radiation, autologous stem cell transplant
Wilms tumor	Abdominal mass	Ultrasound and CT abdomen	Surgery, radiation, chemotherapy
Osteosarcoma	Pain, mass, pathologic fracture	X-ray including joint above and below lesion, CT of lesion and of chest	Surgery and neoadjuvant/adjuvant multiagent chemotherapy
Ewing sarcoma	Pain, mass in midshaft of long bones	X-ray including joint above and below lesion, CT of lesion and of chest	Surgery and neoadjuvant/adjuvant multiagent chemotherapy
Testicular	Testicular mass	Testicular ultrasound	Orchiectomy, chemotherapy
Acute lymphoblastic leukemia	Fever, fatigue, bone pain	Blood smear, bone marrow aspirate and biopsy with flow cytometry	Chemotherapy, radiation, stem cell transplant
Acute myeloid leukemia	Fever, fatigue, bone pain	Blood smear, bone marrow aspirate and biopsy with flow cytometry	Chemotherapy, stem cell transplant
Chronic myeloid leukemia	Fever, fatigue, bone pain, abdominal pain	Blood smear, bone marrow aspirate and biopsy with flow cytometry	Chemotherapy, stem cell transplant
Hodgkin lymphoma	Fever, weight loss, lymphadenopathy, masses	Bone marrow aspirate and biopsy, excisional lymph node biopsy	Chemotherapy, radiation, stem cell transplant
Non-Hodgkin lymphoma	Fever, weight loss, lymphadenopathy, masses	Bone marrow aspirate and biopsy, excisional lymph node biopsy	Chemotherapy, radiation, stem cell transplant

HVA, homovanillic acid; VMA, vanillylmandelic acid.

Table 24.6 Common hematologic diseases in adults and children.

	Presenting symptoms	Diagnosis	Treatment
Red blood cell disorders			
Iron-deficiency anemia	Fatigue, palpitations, pre-syncope	↓hemoglobin, ↓iron	Iron replacement
Hemolytic anemia	Fatigue, palpitations, pre-syncope, jaundice	↑bilirubin, ↑LDH, ↑reticulocyte count	Steroids
Red blood cell aplasia	Fatigue, palpitations, pre-syncope	↓hemoglobin	Red blood cell transfusion if severe
Sickle cell anemia	Infection, splenic sequestration, pain	Isoelectric focusing, hemoglobin electrophoresis	Penicillin prophylaxis, if ≤5 years of age immunizations, patient education, stem cell transplant
Thalassemia	Symptoms of anemia, slowed growth, jaundice	↓MCV, +/− hemoglobin electrophoresis	Transfusions with attention to iron overload, stem cell transplant
Neutrophil disorders			
Neutropenia	None or signs of infection	↓WBC	Observation, G-CSF
Leukocytosis	None or oronasal bleeding, blurred vision, neurologic symptoms, confusion, heart failure	↑WBC	Leukopheresis
Platelet disorders			
Immune thrombocytopenia	Petechiae, easy bruising, mucosal bleeding	↓platelets	Observation, steroids
Thrombotic thrombocytopenic purpura	Acute kidney injury, mental status changes, fever	↓platelets, ↑schistocytes, ↓ADAMTS13	Plasmapheresis, immunosuppressive therapy
Hemolytic–uremic syndrome	Diarrhea, acute kidney injury	↓platelets, ↑schistocytes	Supportive care
Heparin-induced thrombocytopenia	Bleeding and/or clotting	↓platelets, ↓platelet factor 4	Stop heparin
Bleeding and clotting			
Hemophilia	Spontaneous bleeding, hemarthrosis	Factor level	Factor replacement
Venous thrombus/ pulmonary embolus	Pain and swelling in extremity, respiratory distress with pulmonary embolism	Ultrasound, *V/Q* scan, CT scan	Heparin
Von Willebrand disease	Mucocutaneous bleeding (epistaxis, menorrhagia), easy bruising, prolonged post-dental bleeding	vWD assays (vWF:RCo, vWF:Ag, FVIII:Co)	DDAVP, human plasma-derived VWF
Disseminated and localized intravascular coagulopathy	Bleeding and/or clotting	PT, PTT, ↓platelets	
Vitamin K deficiency	Bleeding, purpura, intracranial bleeding in newborn	↓Vitamin K, ↓Factors II, VII, IX, X	Vitamin K
Bone marrow failure			
Acquired	Fatigue, pallor, infections, bleeding	Bone marrow aspirate and biopsy	Immunosuppressive agents, stem cell transplant
Fanconi	Short stature, hypopigmented spots and café-au-lait spots, abnormality of thumbs, microcephaly, hydrocephaly, hypogonadism developmental delay	Increased chromosomal breakage in lymphocytes	Stem cell transplant
Myelodysplasia	Fatigue, pallor, infections, bleeding	Bone marrow aspirate and biopsy	Stem cell transplant

DDAVP, desmopressin; LDH, lactate dehydrogenase; PT, prothrombin time; PTT, partial thromboplastin time; vWD, vonWillebrand disease; WBC, white blood cell count.

Table 24.7 Simplified staging system for breast cancer.

Stage	Characteristic
0	Carcinoma *in situ* and Paget disease
IA	Tumor ≤2 cm without other disease
IA	Tumor ≤2 cm with lymph node involvement
IIA	Tumor >2 cm or mobile axillary nodes
IIB	Tumor 2–5 cm with lymph node involvement or tumor >5 cm
IIIA	Any tumor size with internal mammary or fixed axillary nodes
IIIB	Any tumor size with direct extension to chest wall or skin
IIIC	Any tumor size with infraclavicular or supraclavicular nodes
IV	Any tumor size with distant masses

Source: What you need to know about breast cancer. Available at http://www.cancer.gov/cancertopics/wyntk/breast/page6

Table 24.8 Staging of prostate cancer use the TNM staging system, which evaluates tumor size (T), involvement of lymph nodes (N), and any metastasis (M).

Stage	Tumor	Nodes and metastasis
I	T1a: non-palpable, not visible on imaging	N0, M0, Gleason[a] <6
II	T1/T2: within prostate	N0, M0
III	T3: extends through capsule	N0, M0
IV	T4: invades adjacent structures	N0, M0
	Any T	N1, M0
	Any T	Any N, M1

[a]The Gleason grade is the sum of the cancer's differentiation score (1 = best, 5 = worst) of the two most prevalent patterns in the biopsy. Low grade is a sum <6.
Source: National Cancer Institute (2014).

important to perform a thorough physical examination, including the contralateral breast and bilateral axillary lymph nodes. It is also essential to image the lesion and determine the stage of the disease. Imaging is usually accomplished using mammogram and ultrasound. The presence of metastatic disease can be assessed using chest radiography or chest CT and ultrasound of the abdomen or abdominal CT, as available or by referral.

Breast cancer can be staged using a simplified staging system for breast cancer (Table 24.7). All forms of treatment include some form of local control – either surgery or radiation to treat existing disease and prevent local recurrence – as well as systemic therapy, including chemotherapy, biologics, and/or hormonal inhibitors.

Prostate cancer

Prostate cancer is the most common cancer in adult men. It typically presents with urinary obstructive symptoms (hesitancy, decreased stream, or retention) or irritative symptoms (dysuria or increased frequency). On digital rectal examination, the clinician can often palpate a large, irregularly shaped prostate. Transrectal ultrasound and guided biopsy that includes 6–12 core specimens is ideally performed for diagnosis, while metastatic disease can be assessed using bone scan or abdominal/pelvic CT, as available or by referral. TNM staging is used to stage prostate cancer (Table 24.8). Treatment ranges from active surveillance to radical prostatectomy. In addition, chemotherapy, androgen deprivation, and radiation therapy are commonly used therapies.

Anemia

Anemia, a group of acquired and hereditary blood disorders characterized by low hemoglobin, is the most common blood disorder in both adults and children: 1.6 billion people worldwide are anemic (Pasricha *et al.*, 2013). Two of the most common forms of anemia are iron-deficiency anemia and sickle cell anemia.

Iron-deficiency anemia

Iron-deficiency anemia is a microcytic anemia, with generally a low MCV (80 fL – age [in years]) or, on PBS, a red blood cell smaller than a non-activated lymphocyte. Other aspects of the blood smear that suggest iron-deficiency anemia are hypochromia (red blood cells with a central pallor greater than one-third of the cell), pencil cells (red blood cells shaped like an unsharpened pencil), and thrombocytosis (Figure 24.3). Common causes include occult blood loss and/or poor iron intake or absorption. Therefore, treatment should involve decreasing blood loss and increasing iron intake or absorption. Iron deficiency is most often treated with oral iron supplementation in the form of ferrous sulfate. Oral iron should not be taken with calcium-containing drinks or foods (e.g., milk, dairy, dark leafy greens, fortified grains), which block iron absorption. Instead, iron is best absorbed in the presence of Vitamin C-containing beverages like (non-calcium-fortified) orange juice. Intravenous iron supplementation is reserved for those who cannot absorb oral supplementation. In this case, injectable iron dextran is regularly used in high-income countries. A test dose must first be administered to assess for side effects, including anaphylaxis. If the setting is not equipped to manage anaphylaxis, iron dextran should not be used, and

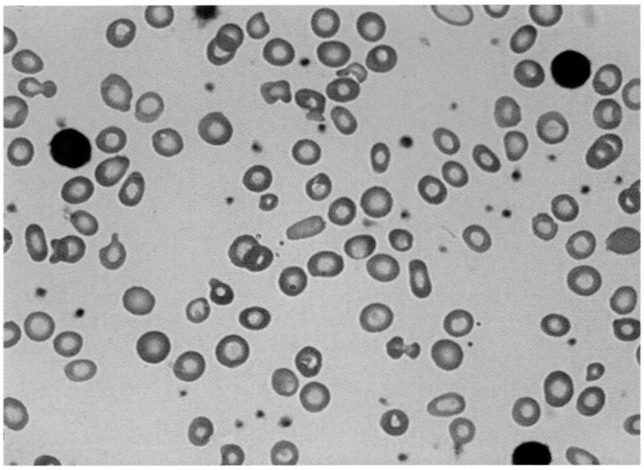

Figure 24.3 Peripheral blood smear of a 2 year old with iron-deficiency anemia. Note the large central pallor of the erythrocytes, small size compared with neighboring lymphocyte, and pencil cells, often seen in iron-deficiency anemia. *Source*: Oski *et al.* (in press). Reproduced with permission of Elsevier and C. Brugnara.

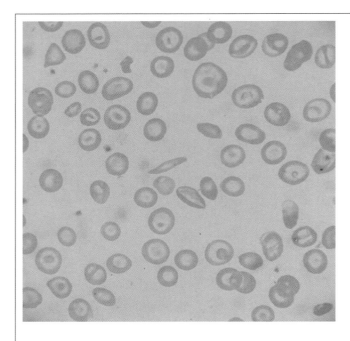

Figure 24.4 Peripheral blood smear of child with HbS β^0-thalassemia, a type of sickle cell anemia. Note the sickle-shaped cell located in the center of the blood smear and surrounded by target cells, which are characteristic in HbS β^0-thalassemia and HbSC disease.

injectable ferric gluconate is an alternative. Both of these preparations are costly, however. In communities with a high helminth infection burden, consider deworming as it has been shown to increase hemoglobin and reduce the prevalence of anemia (Gulani *et al.*, 2007).

Sickle cell anemia

Sickle cell anemia is the most common hemoglobinopathy worldwide. It is an inherited blood disease characterized by a point mutation in the β-globin chain of hemoglobin that causes a hydrophilic glutamic acid to be replaced by a hydrophobic valine at the sixth position. This single-point mutation results in sickle hemoglobin (HbS). HbS is passed from parents to children through the genes. When a person has sickle cell trait, there is one gene for normal hemoglobin (HbA) and one gene for HbS, and because there is still one gene for HbA, the individual does not have the disease. On the other hand, an individual who inherits two genes for HbS (one from each parent) will have sickle cell disease.

In sickle cell disease, due to polymerization of deoxygenated HbS, the red blood cells often irreversibly adopt a sickle shape (Figure 24.4) in the presence of an infection, low oxygen, or dehydration. These hard and sickle-shaped cells cause the complications associated with sickle cell anemia. The sickle blood cells are less flexible and break down during circulation. This hemolysis leads to a chronically low blood count, or anemia. The sickle cells can also become trapped within blood vessels in the body, thus interfering with normal blood flow.

The resulting obstruction can lead to ischemia, which causes sudden pain anywhere in the body, and to damage to the body tissues and organs over time. Because HbA and HbF (fetal hemoglobin) inhibit polymerization, there are less sickle cells in the presence of these hemoglobins. As a result, people with sickle cell trait (HbAS) and newborns (HbFS) often do not have any sickle cell symptoms.

Individuals with sickle cell anemia must be treated as if functionally asplenic in the first 5 years of life. They require penicillin prophylaxis as well as pneumococcal, *Haemophilus influenza*e, and meningococcal immunization. They should also be evaluated by physical examination and blood culture, and treated empirically with antibiotics every time they have a temperature above 38.5°C (101.3°F). Pain should be treated aggressively with heat packs, ibuprofen, and opioids, when necessary. Hydroxyurea is often used for moderate to severe sickle cell anemia; it increases HbF, thereby reducing the occurrence of sickling-related complications (Ware, 2010).

Leukemia

Leukemia is a type of blood cancer characterized by an abnormal increase in the percentage of immature white blood cells or blasts in the bone marrow. For the diagnosis of leukemia, greater than 20% of cells in the bone marrow should be blasts.

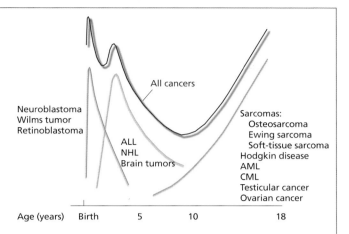

Age (years)   Birth   5   10   18

Figure 24.5 While childhood cancers can occur at any age, they tend to occur within certain age groups. This helps narrow the differential diagnosis; however, the final diagnosis must be confirmed via biopsy in almost all cases. ALL, acute lymphoblastic leukemia; AML, acute myeloid leukemia; CML, chronic myeloid leukemia; NHL, non-Hodgkin lymphoma.

Where available, flow cytometry, cytogenetic studies, and molecular studies of blood or bone marrow aspirate help determine the type of leukemia.

Acute lymphoblastic leukemia (ALL) is the most common cancer in children (Figures 24.2 and 24.5). There is no staging system for ALL, but risk groups (based on factors such as age at diagnosis, presenting white blood cell count, cytogenetics/ploidy, and CNS involvement) are being established to determine the optimal approach to treatment.

Chemotherapy is the standard therapy for hematologic malignancies. ALL in children requires 2 years of therapy, which involves an induction phase (during which the illness is brought into remission), followed by consolidation, and finally maintenance. While chemotherapy regimens differ, they almost always include treatment with corticosteroids, methotrexate, vincristine, mercaptopurine, asparaginase, and an anthracycline such as doxorubicin. Given the cardiotoxicity associated with doxorubicin, all patients should have an echocardiogram prior to the start of treatment to assess for baseline cardiac function.

Additional resources

- Blood disorder guidelines: www.nhlbi.nih.gov/guidelines/current.htm
- Physician's Data Query by National Cancer Institute: www.cancer.gov/cancertopics/pdq
- International Network for Cancer Treatment and Research (INCTR) palliative care handbook. Available at www.inctr-palliative-care-handbook.wikidot.com/
- Palliative care toolkit by the Worldwide Palliative Care Alliance and Help the Hospices. Available at http://www.thewpca.org/resources/

REFERENCES

Boyle P, Levin B (2008) *World Cancer Report 2008*. Lyon: International Agency for Research on Cancer.

Bray F, Jemal A, Grey N, Ferlay J, Forman D (2012) Global cancer transitions according to the Human Development Index (2008–2030): a population-based study. *Lancet Oncol* 13:790–801.

Farmer P, Frenk J, Knaul FM *et al.* (2010) Expansion of cancer care and control in countries of low and middle income: a call to action. *Lancet* 376:1186–93.

Gulani A, Nagpal J, Osmond C, Sachdev HP (2007) Effect of administration of intestinal antihelminthic drugs on haemoglobin: systematic review of randomised controlled trials. *BMJ* 334:1095–100.

Kalantri A, Karambelkar M, Joshi R, Kalantri S, Jajoo U (2010) Accuracy and reliability of pallor for detecting anaemia: a hospital-based diagnostic accuracy study. *PLoS ONE* 5(1):e8545.

National Cancer Institute (2014) Stage information for prostate cancer. Available at http://www.cancer.gov/cancertopics/pdq/treatment/prostate/healthprofessional/page2. Last modified April 11, 2014.

Oski FA, Brugnara C, Nathan DG (in press) A diagnostic approach to the anemic patient. In: Orkin SH, Nathan DG, Ginsburg D, Look TA, Fisher DE, Lux SE (eds) *Hematology of Infancy and Childhood*, 8th edn. Philadelphia: Saunders Elsevier.

Pasricha SR, Drakesmith H, Black J, Hipgrave D, Biggs BA (2013) Control of iron-deficiency anemia in low- and middle-income countries. *Blood* 121:2607–17.

Rodriguez-Galindo C, Friedrich P, Morrissey L, Frazier L (2013) Global challenges in pediatric oncology. *Curr Opin Pediatr* 25:3–15.

Stonebraker JS, Brooker M, Amand RE, Farrugia A, Srivastava A (2010) A study of reported factor VIII use around the world. *Haemophilia* 16:33–46.

Ware R (2010) How I use hydroxyurea to treat young patients with sickle cell anemia. *Blood* 115:5300–11.

Weatherall DJ (2011) The challenge of haemoglobinopathies in resource-poor countries. *Br J Haematol* 154:736–44.

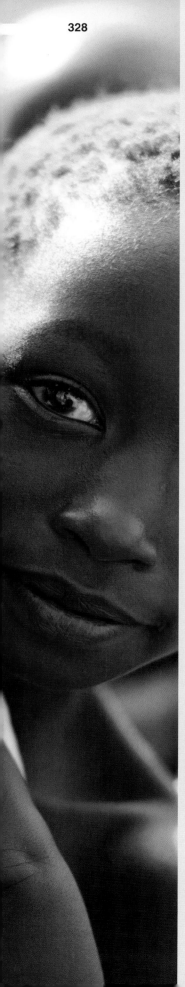

CHAPTER 25
Trauma and Emergency Care

Susan C. Lipsett[1], Michelle L. Niescierenko[1,2], and Lois K. Lee[1,2]

[1]Boston Children's Hospital, Boston, MA, USA
[2]Harvard Medical School, Boston, MA, USA

Key learning objectives

■ Identify the need for organized trauma and emergency care in the developing world.

■ Cultivate a systematic approach to the initial trauma evaluation.

■ Develop the skills to diagnose and manage life-threatening injuries immediately.

■ Highlight the importance of the physical examination and conservative management in a resource-limited setting.

■ Recognize key differences in the management of pediatric emergencies.

Abstract

Developing countries face unique challenges related to trauma and emergency care as they have substantial rates of serious injuries but a relative dearth of systematic trauma care. However, organized care has been shown to improve survival and be cost-effective. The aim of this chapter is to give a practical introduction to the management of trauma and other emergencies in the resource-limited setting. The principles of Advanced Trauma Life Support® (ATLS) are introduced. Recommendations are made for essential equipment to be available for the emergent resuscitation of a patient. Given the resource constraints in developing countries, the chapter focuses on use of physical examination and basic diagnostic studies, as well as simple life-saving procedures.

Key words: abdominal injury, head injury, neck injury, primary survey, secondary survey, spine injury, thoracic injury, trauma, emergency

Essential Clinical Global Health, First Edition. Edited by Brett D. Nelson.
© 2015 John Wiley & Sons, Ltd. Published 2015 by John Wiley & Sons, Ltd.
Companion website: www.essentialseries.com/globalhealth

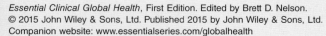

Introduction

The burden of traumatic injury in the developing world is high and has been largely ignored compared with infectious diseases and nutritional deficiencies (Gosselin *et al.*, 2009). The lack of systematic care affects immediate survival and may result in lifelong disability for trauma patients. Organized trauma care has been shown to improve survival and be cost-effective (American College of Surgeons Committee on Trauma, 2012; Gosselin *et al.*, 2009). The aim of this chapter is to give a practical introduction to the management of trauma and other emergencies in the resource-limited setting by focusing on the physical examination, basic diagnostic studies, and simple life-saving procedures.

Initial trauma evaluation

Preparation

The availability of essential equipment (Table 25.1) and resources should be assessed in advance of receiving trauma patients. Useful imaging modalities most frequently available include X-ray and ultrasound. The availability of, and the time needed to obtain, safe blood products should also be understood. In addition, there is wide regional variation in the availability of critical care or advanced resources; therefore, an understanding of regional transport and referral capabilities is essential.

Primary survey

The primary survey is performed as the initial assessment of the trauma patient to evaluate the vital functions and to immediately treat any life-threatening injuries as they are identified. The steps in the trauma patient's evaluation are Airway, Breathing, Circulation, Disability (neurologic examination), and Exposure (ABCDE). These steps are followed in the same order every time to ensure that no critical injuries are overlooked. Any abnormality must be addressed before moving on to the next step in the assessment. For example, if a trauma patient has abnormal breathing, this should be addressed with appropriate maneuvers (e.g., supplemental oxygen, bag-valve mask ventilation) before proceeding to assessment of the circulatory status. The goal of the primary survey is to keep the patient alive until definitive management is feasible (American College of Surgeons Committee on Trauma, 2012).

Spinal immobilization

While the primary survey is being conducted, one provider should initiate and then maintain cervical spine (C-spine) stabilization at all times during the evaluation. C-spine stabilization can be accomplished in a number of ways (Figure 25.1). The C-spine should remain immobilized until it is evaluated and cleared for concern of spine or spinal cord injury.

Airway

First, assess the patient's airway for patency and security. A patient without a secure airway will not be able to ventilate or oxygenate adequately. If the patient is talking or moaning, the airway is patent and being maintained. Noisy breathing (snoring, stridor, or gurgling) is a sign of an unsecured airway at risk for obstruction. If the patient is not vocalizing, the provider must assess for signs of breathing by looking for chest rise and listening for breath sounds as evidence of a patent airway.

Red flag

If the airway is not patent and secure, stop and attempt the following maneuvers.

- Lift the angles of the lower jaw with each hand, displacing the mandible anteriorly with the thumbs. This will open up the pharynx and relieve obstruction from the epiglottis and tongue (Figure 25.2).
- Place a nasopharyngeal airway in the awake patient or an oropharyngeal airway in the minimally conscious or unconscious patient to relieve obstruction caused by the tongue (Figure 25.3).
- If unable to maintain a patent airway, consider securing the airway with endotracheal intubation where available. Endotracheal intubation is rarely useful where ventilators are not readily available.

Breathing

Next in the primary survey is an evaluation of the patient's breathing for oxygenation and ventilation. First inspect the chest wall for symmetric chest rise, flail segments, or penetrating trauma. Palpate for crepitus or subcutaneous air, as these may indicate a pneumothorax. Determine the tracheal position by inspection and palpation; a deviated trachea is highly concerning for tension pneumothorax. Auscultate for breath

Table 25.1 Essential equipment for trauma care.

Basic supplies

Scissors/shears
Scalpel
Clamps
Sterile gauze
Syringes
Needles (including large-bore)
Blankets
Penlight or flashlight
Skin tape

Airway

Oral/nasal airways
Bag-valve mask
Suction device
Suction tubing
Oral (Yankauer) suction catheter

Breathing

Pulse oximeter
Stethoscope
Oxygen (cylinder or concentrator)
Oxygen tubing
Nasal prongs
Facemask
Chest tube set-up
Three-way dressing
Large-bore needles

Circulation

Clock with second hand
Blood pressure cuff
Intravenous supplies and tubing
Intraosseous needles or spinal needles
Normal saline or Lactated Ringer's solution
Blood, if available
Urinary catheter with collection bag
Nasogastric tube

Source: Mock *et al.* (2004).

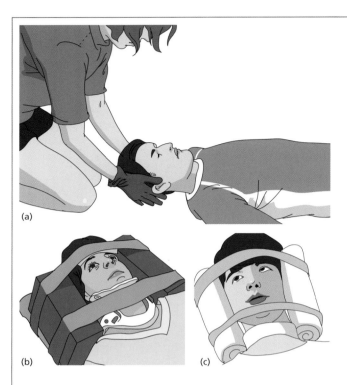

Figure 25.1 Cervical spine stabilization. (a) Manual cervical spine stabilization should be maintained immediately, followed by application of a cervical collar and backboard. (b) Full spinal immobilization. (c) Spinal immobilization can be improvised if the standard cervical collar, backboard and head blocks are not available. Sandbags, rolled towels, or T-shirts may be used.

sounds bilaterally. Assess for hypoxia using pulse oximetry. Supplemental oxygen should be provided to all trauma patients during the initial evaluation.

Red flag

Assess for the following conditions: tension pneumothorax, open pneumothorax, massive hemothorax, or flail chest.

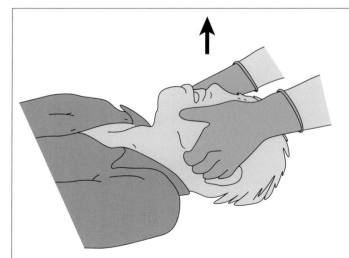

Figure 25.2 Jaw thrust. Use the index and middle fingers to push the posterior aspect of the jaw anteriorly, preventing the tongue from occluding the airway. The jaw thrust is the preferred method of opening the airway in patients with potential C-spine injury.

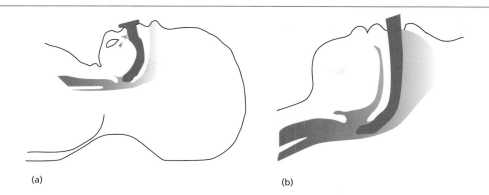

Figure 25.3 Oropharyngeal and nasopharyngeal airways. The oropharyngeal airway (a) should be inserted in the anatomic position, using a tongue depressor to keep the tongue out of the way. The nasopharyngeal airway (b) should be lubricated and inserted into the more patent nare.

Tension pneumothorax is a potentially life-threatening pneumothorax. This is a clinical diagnosis made by the identification of chest pain, tachypnea, tachycardia, decreased breath sounds with hyperresonance to percussion, tracheal deviation, respiratory distress, and sometimes hypotension. Immediate needle decompression on the side of the pneumothorax should be performed by inserting a large-bore intravenous catheter immediately above the second rib in the mid-clavicular line to relieve the tension caused by air (Figure 25.4). The intravenous catheter is left in place with a closed three-way stopcock until tube thoracostomy placement can be completed.

Open pneumothorax, or "sucking chest wound," occurs with a penetrating injury and is treated by immediately placing an occlusive dressing taped on three sides, allowing air to escape out the fourth side. This prevents additional air from entering the chest cavity on inspiration but allows air to escape the chest cavity on expiration (Figure 25.5).

Massive hemothorax is the presence of a large amount of blood in the pleural space. Assume this is present if there are decreased breath sounds and dullness to percussion in the setting of major blunt torso trauma or penetrating trauma. Tachycardia and/or hypotension suggest significant internal blood loss. Immediate tube thoracostomy, or chest tube (Box 25.1), is essential to prevent respiratory and circulatory compromise (Figure 25.6).

A flail segment is created by two or more contiguous rib fractures and is a significant threat to effective respiration. Examination is notable for paradoxical motion of the flail segment during inspiration. Initial management of a flail segment involves positioning the patient with the injured side down and providing pain control (Fleisher & Ludwig, 2010).

Circulation

The third step in the primary survey is the evaluation of the patient's circulatory status. The trauma patient is at risk for

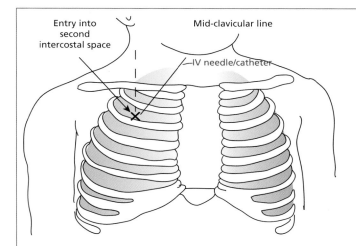

Figure 25.4 Needle decompression. A large-bore intravenous catheter is inserted into the second intercostal space in the mid-clavicular line until a rush of air is heard. The needle should be removed and the catheter left in place until a chest tube can be placed.

life-threatening internal and external hemorrhage. It is critical to identify the hemodynamically unstable patient in shock and provide immediate fluid resuscitation. First assess the skin for color and warmth, capillary refill, and pulses. Early hypovolemic shock, so-called warm shock, is manifested by tachycardia, tachypnea, and a widened pulse pressure. As shock progresses, the patient will have a declining mental status, narrow pulse pressure, and hypotension. The skin will become cool (so-called cold shock) and pale with less palpable pulses. In the absence of a blood pressure cuff, a palpable radial pulse indicates a systolic blood pressure of at least 80 mmHg, and a palpable carotid pulse indicates a systolic blood pressure of

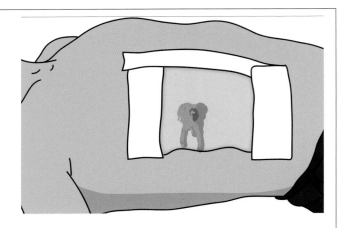

Figure 25.5 Three-way taped occlusive dressing. Apply petroleum-soaked gauze or a foil wrapper to the chest wound and tape on three sides.

at least 50 mmHg (Fleisher & Ludwig, 2010). Be aware that the signs of shock may be more subtle in children, who have a relatively fixed cardiac contractility and become heart rate-dependent in the hypovolemic state. They may present initially only with tachycardia, with hypotension being a late sign of hypovolemic shock (Pokota & Saladino, 2005). The major sites of blood loss are from visible wounds or internal wounds of the chest, abdomen, retroperitoneum, and pelvis.

Red flag

Assess for massive external hemorrhage or cardiac tamponade.

Box 25.1 Tube thoracostomy placement (Thomsen *et al.*, 2006)

Materials
Sterile gloves, sterile drapes, betadine or chlorhexidine, lidocaine and needles for local anesthesia, syringe for aspirating fluid, scalpel, hemostats or Kelly clamp, chest tube, drainage system, suture, scissors.

Procedure
- Abduct ipsilateral arm to expose mid-clavicular to axillary area of the chest.
- Locate fourth intercostal space in anterior axillary line (level of nipple).
- Don sterile gloves.
- Clean the area with betadine or chlorhexidine and drape with sterile drapes.
- Anesthetize the skin overlying the sixth rib with the needle at a shallow angle to create a subcutaneous wheal of lidocaine. Aspirate before injecting to assess for possible venous penetration of the needle. Next, readjust the needle to track over the rib and then into the area just superior to the rib to anesthetize the deeper spaces.
- Make a 2-cm skin incision in the anesthetized skin wheal parallel to the sixth rib.
- Enter the incision using hemostats or a Kelly clamp, and then bluntly dissect the subcutaneous tissue. Tunnel superiorly to the fifth rib, using the top of the rib to provide balance as you dissect the intercostal muscles.

- Aiming for the area just superior to the rib avoids the neurovascular bundle, which runs along the rib's inferior aspect.
- Use your finger or the closed Kelly clamp to bluntly enter the parietal pleura; use controlled pressure, and stop as soon as you feel the release of pressure, indicating that you are inside the pleural cavity. This makes a track through the subcutaneous tissue and muscle for the thoracostomy tube.
- Open the clamp widely to dilate this track through the intercostal muscle, then withdraw the clamp and ensure with your finger that the lung has fallen away from the parietal pleura by inserting it into the track and moving it around 360° in the pleural space.
- Pass the thoracostomy (chest) tube through the incision, aiming posterior–inferior for hemothorax and posterior–superior for pneumothorax.
- Secure the tube in place with sutures and cover with occlusive dressing.
- Attach the tube to a vacuum container.
- Confirm placement with chest radiography.

Potential complications
Bleeding, infection, pneumothorax, hemothorax, perforation of vascular or visceral structures.

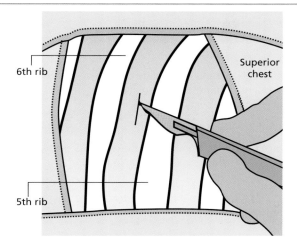

Figure 25.6 Insertion of a thoracostomy tube, as described in Box 25.1.

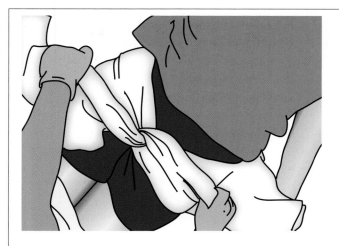

Figure 25.7 Pelvic binding sheet. In suspected pelvic injuries, prevent exsanguination by wrapping a folded bedsheet circumferentially around the patient's pelvis, pulling the ends to apply adequate compression.

Massive external hemorrhage should be visible; however, assess the patient's back for bleeding that might otherwise go undetected. Control significant hemorrhage immediately with direct pressure. A tourniquet should be applied for any limb-threatening extremity wound. Traction should be applied to displaced femur fractures. Open pelvic fractures should be stabilized with a binding sheet (Figure 25.7).

Cardiac tamponade is a hemodynamic emergency caused by blood accumulating in the pericardium. Warning signs of cardiac tamponade include muffled heart sounds, neck vein distension, tachycardia, and a narrowed pulse pressure. Hypotension is a late sign. Pericardiocentesis should be performed immediately in the unstable trauma patient with suspected cardiac tamponade. Blind pericardiocentesis, although potentially life-saving, comes with significant risk of damage to vital structures. Ultrasound should be used, if available, to confirm location.

Disability

The fourth step in the primary survey is the evaluation of the trauma patient's gross neurological status by assessing the patient's level of consciousness (mental status) and spontaneous movement. The Glasgow Coma Scale (GCS) quantifies mental status and is a prognostic indicator of neurological outcome (Table 25.2). This scale has been validated for adults, children, and infants.

Exposure

Finally, remove all clothing, with shears as needed, so as to completely expose the patient and allow a thorough assessment of injuries. Once the primary survey is complete, the patient and the resuscitation environment should be kept warm to prevent hypothermia. Children are even more sensitive to hypothermia and should be warmed as soon as it is feasible.

Initial fluid resuscitation

Obtaining intravenous access and initiating fluid resuscitation should be achieved as soon as possible. Two large-bore (16–20 gauge) intravenous lines should be obtained (American College of Surgeons Committee on Trauma, 2012). If intravenous access is unsuccessful after two attempts or within 90 seconds, intraosseous access should be obtained. All medications and fluids can be infused through an intraosseous line safely and reliably. It is essential to send blood samples to the laboratory for measurement of serum hemoglobin/hematocrit, blood type, and serum glucose.

The trauma patient showing any signs of hypovolemia should be rapidly volume-resuscitated. Initial resuscitation typically includes 1–2 L (or 20 mL/kg for pediatric patients) of an isotonic fluid such as normal saline or Lactated Ringer's solution, which may be repeated (but see Clinical pearl box for an important caveat to aggressive fluid resuscitation among children presenting with shock in Africa). If there is no response after a second fluid bolus and safe blood is accessible, the patient should be given 1–2 units (or 10 mL/kg for pediatric patients) of packed red blood cells or whole blood (American College of Surgeons Committee on Trauma, 2012). If no blood is available for transfusion, fluid resuscitation should be continued to optimize circulatory status. A lack of response to timely fluid resuscitation is an indicator of internal injury with ongoing hemorrhage, and the patient requires an emergent laparotomy.

Table 25.2 Glasgow Coma Scale in adults, children, and infants. Whenever different, the corresponding response of pre-verbal children/infants is noted in parentheses.

Points	Eye opening	Verbal	Motor
6			Obeys commands (*Infant*: moves spontaneously and purposefully)
5		Oriented (*Infant*: smiles, babbles or coos)	Localizes pain
4	Spontaneous	Confused (*Infant*: cries but consolable)	Withdraws in response to pain
3	To speech	Inappropriate words (*Infant*: persistent inappropriate crying or screaming)	Abnormal flexion – decorticate posturing
2	To pain	Incomprehensible sounds (*Infant*: moans or grunts)	Abnormal extension – decerebrate posturing
1	None	No response	No response

Source: Teasdale & Jennett (1974) and Holmes *et al.* (2005).

Clinical pearl: special considerations in pediatric shock

A notable exception to aggressive fluid resuscitation for children is that bolus resuscitation may actually increase mortality among febrile children presenting with shock in an African setting with a high prevalence of malnutrition and anemia. This is based on the results of a large multi-country trial in sub-Saharan Africa (Maitland *et al.*, 2011). At least under these circumstances, fluid resuscitation in children should be done much more judiciously, with current evidence supporting giving febrile children in shock maintenance intravenous fluids rather than boluses. However, this study did not include children with hemorrhagic shock from trauma, where fluid resuscitation with boluses is recommended to replace ongoing blood loss.

Secondary survey

The secondary survey is a detailed examination of the entire body performed after the primary survey and initial stabilization are complete. The head should be examined for scalp hematomas, skull depression, hemotympanum (blood in the inner ear, behind the tympanic membrane), ecchymoses, pupillary response, and movements of the eyes. The neck and chest should be palpated for crepitus. The abdomen should be examined for distension, bowel sounds, bruising, or tenderness. The extremities should be assessed for fractures, and the pubis and anterior iliac spines should be gently com-

pressed and depressed for any signs of pelvic instability. The patient should be log-rolled and the spine palpated for step-offs or focal tenderness. If any of these are present, radiography of the thoracic, lumbar, and sacral spine should be considered to assess for fracture, which can lead to the immediate complication of neurogenic (spinal) shock or long-term disabling injuries like paralysis. A rectal examination can assess for rectal tone and presence of blood in the rectal vault (suggesting intestinal injury). Urethral examination should inspect for lacerations or blood. The neurological examination should assess the pupils and strength and sensation of the extremities.

If bedside ultrasound is available, the focused assessment with sonography for trauma (FAST) should be performed to evaluate for fluid in the pericardium and peritoneum, which indicates hemorrhage. A urinary catheter allows close monitoring of urine output, but it should not be placed if there is concern for pelvic fracture or urethral injury. Placement of a nasogastric tube should be considered in trauma with any altered mental status or obvious intra-abdominal injury, but this should not be placed if there is any evidence of significant facial injury (American College of Surgeons Committee on Trauma, 2012). Open wounds should be cleaned and irrigated, and tetanus prophylaxis should be considered (Table 25.3) (Hospenthal *et al.*, 2011).

Head trauma

The fixed space of the skull poses a challenge in head trauma, as intracranial hemorrhage or brain edema can result in brain herniation and death (Fleisher & Ludwig, 2010). The lack of

Table 25.3 Tetanus vaccination and tetanus immune globulin (TIG).

No. of prior doses	Clean minor wounds		All other wounds	
	Tetanus vaccine[a]	TIG	Tetanus vaccine[b]	TIG
<3 or unknown	Yes	No	Yes	Yes
3 or more	If last vaccine >10 years ago	No	If last vaccine >5 years ago	No

[a]Combined vaccines sometimes available; consult local guidelines and use either combined or tetanus alone.
[b]Infants <6 weeks should receive TIG without vaccine for dirty wounds.
Source: Centers for Disease Control and Prevention (2012).

Box 25.2 Severe mechanisms for head injury (Kuppermann *et al.*, 2009)

- Motor vehicle crash with rollover, patient ejection, or death of another passenger
- Pedestrian or bicyclist without helmet struck by motor vehicle
- Falls >1.5 m for patients 2 years and older
- Falls >1 m for patients younger than 2 years
- Head struck by high-impact object

Box 25.3 Criteria for discharge of the patient with minor head trauma (Haydel *et al.*, 2000; Stiell *et al.*, 2001; Sun *et al.*, 2007; Kuppermann *et al.*, 2009)

- No loss of consciousness or amnesia
- GCS 15
- No alcohol or drug intoxication
- Normal vital signs
- Normal neurologic examination
- No signs of skull fracture or basilar skull fracture
- No evidence of trauma above the clavicles
- No seizures
- No headache or vomiting
- Tolerating oral intake
- Ambulating normally
- Low-risk mechanism

---

advanced neuroimaging in resource-limited settings forces reliance on history and physical examination for evaluation. The skull should be inspected and palpated for evidence of trauma. Signs of a basilar skull fracture include hemotympanum and mastoid or periorbital ecchymosis. It should be noted that plain radiography of the skull is not reliable in diagnosing intracranial hemorrhage or skull fracture and should not be included in the evaluation of head trauma (Hofman *et al.*, 2000). A detailed neurologic examination, including a repeat mental status and pupillary examination, should be performed in order to identify lateralizing signs of intracranial or spinal cord injuries. A dilated non-reactive pupil in an unconscious patient is indicative of cerebral herniation.

As intracranial pressure (ICP) increases from intracranial hemorrhage or cerebral edema, a patient may develop bradycardia, hypertension, and irregular respirations. These are referred to as Cushing's triad and are a sign of impending herniation. In this situation, mannitol and/or hypertonic saline should be administered emergently to decrease ICP (Fleisher & Ludwig, 2010). Patients with signs of increased ICP require emergent neurosurgical intervention or stabilization and referral, if available. Non-surgical management of increased ICP includes elevating the head of the patient 30° and treating hypoxia and hypotension. The beneficial effects of hyperventilation are short-lived, as the body equilibrates within minutes, making this technique less useful. Corticosteroids are not recommended for the management of increased ICP or head injury.

Traumatic seizures should be managed with benzodiazepines as a rescue therapy. Ongoing seizures may be controlled with antiepileptic drugs including phenytoin, fosphenytoin, or phenobarbital (Fleisher & Ludwig, 2010). The benefit of seizure prophylaxis with antiepileptic drugs is variable depending on the diagnosis and is not routinely recommended.

All patients with a severe mechanism for head injury (Box 25.2) should be observed for at least 6 hours following the injury, regardless of examination findings. Frequent vital sign measurements and neurologic examinations should be performed. In pediatric patients with a severe mechanism of injury *and* other signs or symptoms of head injury, 24-hour observation should be considered. Patients with minor head trauma should be observed for 6 hours after the injury, if space and staffing allow. In limited-resource settings, adult patients meeting discharge criteria (Box 25.3) may be discharged home without observation. All pediatric patients should be observed for 4–6 hours, and then if they meet criteria may be discharged. If any of the discharge criteria are not met, the patient requires continued hospital observation for signs of progressing injury.

Neck trauma

With any significant trauma there is risk for C-spine injury (Rathore, 2013). An unstable C-spine fracture can easily lead to spinal cord injury if the patient is not properly immobilized after trauma. After the primary survey, the neck should be examined for signs of injury by removing the stabilization or collar and holding the neck in alignment by a clinical provider for the examination. The C-spine can be cleared in adults by

Box 25.4 NEXUS criteria
(Hoffman *et al.*, 2000)

- Normal level of alertness
- No posterior midline cervical tenderness
- No focal neurologic deficit
- No evidence of intoxication
- No clinically apparent distracting painful injury

clinical examination using the NEXUS criteria (Box 25.4). If any of the criteria are present, C-spine radiographs should be obtained (Hoffman *et al.*, 2000). These consist of a lateral, anteroposterior, and open-mouth odontoid view. It is important to visualize from the odontoid all the way to the C7–T1 junction. If radiography is negative and there is low suspicion of C-spine injury, the examiner should ask the patient to move the neck in flexion, extension, and lateral rotation, and ask the patient to stop any movement if they experience pain. The examiner should not manipulate the patient's neck. If there is no pain with these movements, stabilization is no longer required (Fleisher & Ludwig, 2010). If radiography is negative but there is a high suspicion of injury, the patient should remain immobilized. Hospital admission should be considered in order to reassess with serial physical examinations and repeat radiography.

C-spine injuries are much less common in children under 8 years of age. When they occur in this age group, they are usually at the level of C3 and higher, which carries a significant risk of mortality (Khanna & El-Khoury, 2007). The pediatric spine is more flexible than the adult's, so force significant enough to stretch and injure the spinal cord may not result in spinal fractures; therefore, spinal cord injury without radiographic abnormality (SCIWORA) may be present. Children under 8 years old should have C-spine radiography performed after significant head, neck, or torso trauma. As with adults, if radiography is negative and there is a low suspicion of C-spine injury, the C-spine may be cleared clinically. A high suspicion of injury, regardless of radiography, warrants continued immobilization and inpatient admission for serial examinations.

Thoracic trauma

After initial stabilization, a more thorough examination of the thorax should be performed. The tracheal position should be reevaluated for signs of tension pneumothorax. Inspection should be done for bruising, lacerations, or penetrating wounds. Auscultation should be performed for subtly decreased aeration, concerning for apical pneumothorax, or crackles, concerning for pulmonary contusion. The chest wall should be palpated for crepitus or focal tenderness. Percussion may differentiate between potential pneumothorax and hemothorax. Response to any supplemental oxygen applied should be assessed with pulse oximetry. With signs of thoracic trauma,

or in any major trauma, chest radiography should be obtained. Electrocardiogram (ECG) may show characteristic changes in some cases of traumatic cardiac injury. Table 25.4 details the diagnosis and initial management of the most important traumatic thoracic injuries.

Clinical pearl: special considerations in pediatric thoracic trauma

Thoracic injuries in children are rare but often serious. The child's ribcage is more flexible than the adult's, so a child may have a pulmonary contusion even with no rib fractures. The most common traumatic thoracic injuries in children are pulmonary contusion, pneumothorax, and hemothorax (Pitetti & Walker, 2005; Thomsen *et al.*, 2006).

Indications for operative management of thoracic injuries include large-volume chest tube output in massive hemothorax or the need for a pericardial window in the definitive management of cardiac tamponade. There are very few situations in which emergent resuscitative thoracotomy is useful; thus, it is not recommended in resource-limited settings (Fleisher & Ludwig, 2010).

"Pulmonary toilet" (e.g., deep breaths, ambulation, coughing) is essential in thoracic injuries, especially in pulmonary contusion and flail chest, to prevent atelectasis and subsequent pneumonia. Opioids should be used for pain control to allow patients to actively participate in these activities. Intercostal nerve blocks offer additional analgesia in rib fractures (Mock *et al.*, 2004). Children can be motivated to breathe deeply by activities like blowing on a piece of paper or tissue.

Abdominal trauma

Abdominal injuries in trauma are common and include splenic, hepatic, or renal injury; intestinal injury including hematoma, perforation, or bowel ischemia; and pancreatic injury. Children are at risk for multiple organ injuries at the same time due to the lack of protection from ribs and subcutaneous tissue and the close proximity of intra-abdominal organs. Specific intra-abdominal injuries are difficult to diagnose without CT, which makes the history and physical examination crucial for management decisions in resource-limited settings.

The details of the traumatic event should be determined. Key details include use of seatbelts/restraints/helmet, presence of abdominal pain, time since the injury, and any history of vomiting. It is important to determine if there are signs of peritonitis, such as rebound tenderness or involuntary contraction of the abdominal muscles. Splenic injury may present with left upper quadrant tenderness, a contusion over the left upper

Table 25.4 Common thoracic injuries and management.

Condition	Presentation	Diagnostic studies	Management
Immediately life-threatening conditions already identified in primary survey			
Tension pneumothorax	Tracheal deviation, hypotension, shortness of breath, hypoxia, tachypnea, pleuritic chest pain, diminished breath sounds on ipsilateral side, hyperresonance to percussion on ipsilateral side	None (clinical diagnosis)	Needle decompression followed by tube thoracostomy
Open pneumothorax	Same as simple pneumothorax in presence of penetrating injury	None (clinical diagnosis)	Three-sided occlusive dressing
Massive hemothorax	Shortness of breath, hypoxia, tachypnea, diminished breath sounds on ipsilateral side, hyporesonance to percussion on ipsilateral side, tachycardia, hypotension	Chest X-ray (hypolucency)	Tube thoracostomy if any respiratory or circulatory compromise. Bring to OR if >1500 mL blood returned from chest tube
Flail chest	Unequal excursion, paradoxical chest movement, contiguous ribs with more than two fractures	Chest X-ray (rib fractures)	Position injured side down, splinting, pain control
Cardiac tamponade	Tachycardia (hypotension is late sign), narrowed pulse pressure, muffled heart sounds, distended neck veins	Chest X-ray (enlarged heart), ECG (low voltages; but low sensitivity), ultrasound (fluid in pericardium)	Maintain preload through intravenous fluid administration, pericardiocentesis
Additional thoracic injuries to identify after initial stabilization			
Simple pneumothorax	Same as tension pneumothorax without tracheal deviation or hypotension	Chest X-ray (hyperlucency)	Tube thoracostomy
Pulmonary contusion	Shortness of breath, hypoxia, tachypnea. Auscultation may reveal focal crackles or may be normal	Chest X-ray (non-anatomic regions of hypolucency; may be normal early on)	Oxygen, pulmonary toilet, fluid restriction
Cardiac contusion	Chest pain, hypotension, dysrhythmia	ECG (ST changes, tachycardia, premature beats, atrial arrhythmia), troponin (elevated)	Supportive, monitoring

Source: American College of Surgeons Committee on Trauma (2008); Pitetti & Walker (2005); Thomsen *et al.* (2006).

quadrant or left lower chest, left-sided rib fractures, referred left shoulder pain, or a medially displaced gastric bubble on radiography (Pokota & Saladino, 2005; Thomsen *et al.*, 2006; Wegner *et al.*, 2006). Hepatic injury may show similar findings on the right side (Pokota & Saladino, 2005; Wegner *et al.*, 2006). Renal injury is suggested by flank pain and tenderness, contusion over the flank, or hematuria. Multiple rib fractures should raise suspicion for associated hepatic, splenic, or renal injuries (Pitetti & Walker, 2005).

Laboratory testing is of some use in the assessment of abdominal trauma. Serum hemoglobin/hematocrit should be trended for evidence of ongoing blood loss. If available, increased liver transaminases in the setting of abdominal trauma are suggestive of hepatic injury, and increased pancre-

atic enzymes (e.g., amylase, lipase) are concerning for pancreatic injury (Schonfeld & Lee, 2012; Holmes *et al.*, 2013). Isolated hematuria (>5–20 red blood cells per high-power field) may be an indicator of renal injury (Fleisher & Ludwig, 2010).

Abdominal radiography should be performed in all cases of suspected abdominal trauma to assess for pneumoperitoneum (free air), which would indicate hollow viscous injury and require laparotomy. The FAST ultrasound examination has been shown to be sensitive for free fluid in adults, indicating intra-abdominal hemorrhage. It is not sensitive for hollow viscous injury, so it cannot reliably exclude all intra-abdominal injuries. Use of the FAST examination in pediatrics is increasing, although studies have shown variable sensitivity and specificity for detecting intra-abdominal injuries (Schonfeld & Lee, 2012).

The initial management of blunt abdominal trauma involves fluid resuscitation and pain control (Fleisher & Ludwig, 2010). Most blunt abdominal injuries will heal with supportive care. The only indications for surgical intervention (laparotomy) in this setting are persistent hemodynamic instability, pneumoperitoneum, or peritonitis (Pokota & Saladino, 2005; Wegner *et al.*, 2006). Box 25.5 outlines principles of non-operative management of suspected intra-abdominal injury.

Clinical pearl: seatbelt sign

While seatbelts unequivocally save lives, there is a risk of intra-abdominal injury from seatbelts in a high-speed motor vehicle collision. The "seatbelt sign" (Sokolove *et al.*, 2005; Schonfeld & Lee, 2012) is a pattern of ecchymoses or abrasions in the distribution of a seatbelt found over the patient's abdomen and/or chest after a motor vehicle collision. A seatbelt sign along with abdominal tenderness is highly concerning for intra-abdominal injury, especially intestinal injury, and may also be associated with a lumbar spine fracture. Any patient with a positive seatbelt sign and abdominal tenderness should be admitted for overnight observation and bowel rest.

Box 25.5 Non-operative management of suspected intra-abdominal injury (Pokota & Saladino, 2005; Kuzma & Atua, 2008; Parks *et al.*, 2011)

- Bed rest
- Nothing by mouth for the first 24 hours, in case surgical intervention needed
- Serial abdominal examinations
- Serial hemoglobin measurements
- Blood transfusion, as indicated
- Pain control
- Careful management of fluid status
- Hospitalization until tolerating solid diet, ambulating, normal vital signs, stable hematocrit
- Work/activity restriction for 1–4 weeks depending on severity of injury; should be reexamined prior to return to work
- Patients with suspected splenic injury should be vaccinated against encapsulated organisms (*Streptococcus pneumoniae*, *Haemophilus* spp., *Neisseria meningitidis*)

Risk stratification to determine which patients are safe for discharge home is essential in the resource-limited environment where CT is not available. A patient with any of the following factors is considered at risk for intra-abdominal injury: abdominal pain, abdominal tenderness, evidence of abdominal wall trauma/ecchymosis from a seatbelt, evidence of thoracic wall trauma, decreased breath sounds, hematuria (>5–20 red blood cells per high-power field), and GCS under 14 (Holmes *et al.*, 2009, 2013). Patients with none of these factors, and who are able to reliably verbalize symptoms, may be discharged home. Both pre-verbal children and adults with any significant mechanism of injury merit consideration for 24- to 48-hour hospital admission, regardless of symptoms, to assess for any evolving intra-abdominal injury (Wegner *et al.*, 2006). In settings where inpatient monitoring is not available, patients should have daily outpatient follow-up, explicit counseling about signs of worsening injury, and instructions for complete rest.

Penetrating abdominal trauma has a high rate of intra-abdominal injury. The colon and small bowel are the most frequently injured organs, due to their anterior location in the abdomen, followed by the liver, spleen, and major vessels (Fleisher & Ludwig, 2010). The examination should assess for hypovolemia based on vital signs, indicating blood loss, and peritonitis from leakage of enteric contents. General management includes fluid resuscitation, broad-spectrum antibiotics, and definitive surgical intervention. Gunshot wounds, due to their highly destructive nature, require immediate laparotomy. Stab wounds, especially anterior stab wounds, have a high risk of major vessel injury. Posterior stab wounds are less critical, as the paraspinal musculature is protective and the bleeding often self-tamponades. However, all stab wounds, even the most minor, require local exploration to rule out injury to deeper structures.

Conclusion

Trauma accounts for a significant burden of disease in the developing world. Advance preparation and a systematic algorithmic approach to trauma and other emergencies should be adapted. While advanced diagnostics are often not available in these settings, careful history and physical examination can guide life-saving treatment.

Additional resources

- American College of Surgeons Committee on Trauma (2012) *Advanced Trauma Life Support for Doctors: Student Course Manual*, 9th edn. Chicago, IL: American College of Surgeons.
- World Health Organization. WHO Guidelines for essential trauma care. Available at http://www.who.int/violence_injury_prevention/publications/services/guidelines_traumacare/en/

REFERENCES

American College of Surgeons Committee on Trauma (2012) *Advanced Trauma Life Support for Doctors: Student Course Manual*, 9th edn. Chicago, IL: American College of Surgeons.

Centers for Disease Control and Prevention (2012) *CDC Health Information for International Travel 2012*. New York: Oxford University Press.

Fleisher G, Ludwig S (eds) (2010) *Textbook of Pediatric Emergency Medicine*, 6th edn. Philadelphia: Lippincott Williams & Wilkins.

Gosselin RA, Spiegel DA, Coughlin R, Zirkle LG (2009) Injuries: the neglected burden in developing countries. *Bull WHO* 87:246.

Haydel MJ, Preston CA, Mills TJ, Luber S, Blaudeau E, DeBlieux PMC (2000) Indications for computed tomography in patients with minor head injury. *N Engl J Med* 343:100–5.

Hoffman JR, Mower WR, Wolfson AB, Todd KH, Zucker MI (2000) Validity of a set of clinical criteria to rule out injury to the cervical spine in patients with blunt trauma. National Emergency X-Radiography Utilization Study Group. *N Engl J Med* 343:94–9. Erratum in *N Engl J Med* 2001;344:464.

Hofman PA, Nelemans P, Kemerink GJ, Wilmink JT (2000) Value of radiological diagnosis of skull fracture in the management of mild head injury: meta-analysis. *J Neurol Neurosurg Psychiatry* 68:416–22.

Holmes JF, Palchak MJ, MacFarlane T, Kuppermann N (2005) Performance of the pediatric Glasgow Coma Scale in children with blunt head trauma. *Acad Emerg Med* 12:814–19.

Holmes JF, Wisner DH, McGahan JP, Mower WR, Kuppermann N (2009) Clinical prediction rules for identifying adults at very low risk for intra-abdominal injuries after blunt trauma. *Ann Emerg Med* 54: 575–84.

Holmes JF, Lillis K, Monroe D *et al.* (2013) Identifying children at very low risk of clinically important blunt abdominal injuries. *Ann Emerg Med* 62:107–16.e2

Hospenthal DR, Murray CK, Andersen RC *et al.* (2011) Guidelines for the prevention of infections associated with combat-related injuries: 2011 update. *J Trauma* 71(2 Suppl. 2):S210–34.

Khanna G, El-Khoury GY (2007) Imaging of cervical spine injuries of childhood. *Skeletal Radiol* 36: 477–94.

Kuppermann N, Holmes JF, Dayan PS *et al.* (2009) Identification of children at very low risk of clinically-important brain injuries after head trauma: a prospective cohort study. *Lancet* 374:1160–70.

Kuzma J, Atua V (2008) Conservative management of splenic injury in the tropics. *Trop Doct* 38:210–13.

Maitland K, Kiguli S, Opoka RO *et al.* (2011) Mortality after fluid bolus in African children with severe infections. *N Engl J Med* 364:2483–95.

Mock C, Lormand JD, Goosen J, Joshipura M, Peden M (2004) *Guidelines for Essential Trauma Care*. Geneva: World Health Organization.

Parks NA, David JW, Forman D, Lemaster D (2011) Observation for nonoperative management of blunt liver injuries: how long is long enough? *J Trauma* 70:626–9.

Pitetti RD, Walker S (2005) Life-threatening chest injures in children. *Clin Pediatr Emerg Med* 6:16–22.

Pokota DA, Saladino RA (2005) Blunt abdominal trauma in the pediatric patient. *Clin Pediatr Emerg Med* 6:23–31.

Rathore FA (2013) Spinal cord injuries in the developing world. In: Stone JH, Blouin M (eds) *International Encyclopedia of Rehabilitation*. Center for International Rehabilitation Research Information and Exchange. Available at http://cirrie.buffalo.edu/encyclopedia/en/article/141/

Schonfeld D, Lee LK (2012) Blunt abdominal trauma in children. *Curr Opin Pediatr* 24:314–18.

Sokolove PE, Kuppermann N, Holmes JF (2005) Association between the "seat belt sign" and intra-abdominal injury in children with blunt torso trauma. *Acad Emerg Med* 12:808–13.

Stiell IG, Wells GA, Vandemheen K *et al.* (2001) The Canadian CT Head Rule for patients with minor head injury. *Lancet* 357:1391–6.

Sun BC, Hoffman JR, Mower WR (2007) Evaluation of a modified prediction instrument to identify significant pediatric intracranial injury after blunt head trauma. *Ann Emerg Med* 49:325–32.

Teasdale G, Jennett B (1974) Assessment of coma and impaired consciousness: a practical scale. *Lancet* ii:81–4.

Thomsen TW, DeLaPena J, Setnik G (2006) Thoracentesis. *N Engl J Med* 355:e16.

Wegner S, Colletti J, Van Wie D (2006) Pediatric blunt abdominal trauma. *Pediatr Clin North Am* 53:243–56.

CHAPTER 26
Critical Care

Asya Agulnik[1] and Traci A. Wolbrink[1,2]
[1]Boston Children's Hospital, Boston, MA, USA
[2]Harvard Medical School, Boston, MA, USA

Key learning objectives

- Describe the essential components of an intensive care unit (ICU).
- Understand which patients may benefit from ICU care in the low-resource setting.
- Identify the monitoring and intervention strategies that lead to improved patient outcomes in the ICU.
- Understand management strategies and priorities for common diseases encountered in the ICU.
- Describe possible iatrogenic complications and how they may be prevented.

Abstract

An intensive care unit (ICU) represents the concentration of critical care expertise, medication, and equipment. In a low-resource setting, patients presenting to the hospital are frequently in the late stages of their illness and regularly require intensive care. These patients can often be successfully managed with simple, timely interventions. The goal of this chapter is to describe the components of an ICU in a low-resource setting. Recommendations are made for patient selection, patient monitoring, and avoidance of iatrogenic complications. Common ICU diagnoses and their management strategies are discussed.

Key words: intensive care, critical care, oxygen, respiratory distress, sepsis, altered mental status, seizures, nosocomial infections

Essential Clinical Global Health, First Edition. Edited by Brett D. Nelson.
© 2015 John Wiley & Sons, Ltd. Published 2015 by John Wiley & Sons, Ltd.
Companion website: www.essentialseries.com/globalhealth

Introduction

Critical care is an integral part of hospital-based care. According to the World Health Organization (WHO), every hospital where surgery and anesthesia is performed should have an ICU (World Health Organization, 2003). In the resource-limited environment, patients frequently present to the hospital late in the course of their illness and often in critical condition, making the inclusion of an ICU even more imperative. Many of these illnesses, such as infections, trauma, and surgical emergencies, are acute problems readily curable with simple interventions. Unlike in the developed world, most severely ill patients are young, without comorbidities, and are more likely to respond to appropriate and timely interventions with few complications (Baker, 2009; Firth & Ttendo, 2012).

When physicians from high-resource settings conceptualize an ICU, images of ventilators, infusion pumps, and other technologic interventions come to mind. In its basic form, however, an ICU or a high-dependency unit (HDU) is not necessarily technology reliant. It represents the concentration of critical care expertise, medications, and equipment in one physical space to improve the management of severely ill patients (Riviello *et al.*, 2011). This organization allows the appropriate monitoring and intervention for these patients.

By providing appropriate care for the sickest patients, hospitals can build community confidence in the quality of their services. Also, providing treatment options for these patients trains physicians to identify signs of critical illness and manage patients' changing clinical status, regardless of the environment in which they practice (Baker, 2009).

Box 26.1 Sample admission criteria for an ICU

Patients requiring monitoring and management of the following:

- Respiratory distress/failure
- Hemodynamic instability
- Acute change in mental status
- Seizures
- Post-surgical care

Intensive care units

Triage and admission criteria

Early recognition and appropriate triage of critically ill patients at all levels of medical care (outpatient clinic, emergency/casualty department, general wards) is integral to improving patient outcomes. Critically ill patients who present to the emergency department should be transferred directly to the ICU after stabilization, with minimal interruption of care and without first going to the general ward. Patients admitted to the general wards may deteriorate during the course of their illness; hospitals should be encouraged to have protocols in place for prompt identification and transfer of these patients to the ICU (Baker & Rylance, 2012). Delays in patient transfer may result in slower interventions with worse outcomes.

Every ICU should have criteria for which patients can be admitted to the unit (Box 26.1). These should be determined based on the hospital's patient population and resources. Emphasis should be placed on patients with acute illness modifiable with available interventions and who have a good likelihood of successful recovery (Nichols, 2008).

Layout and equipment

An ideal ICU has individual patient rooms to protect patient confidentiality and aid in infection control. In low-resource hospitals, however, physical space is often limited. Individual patient rooms require more space and increase the number of staff necessary for adequate monitoring. ICUs in low-resource settings are typically organized as a large room with individual beds. For infection control reasons, beds should be spaced out as much as possible (Basnet *et al.*, 2011).

Locations should specifically be set aside for emergency equipment, medications, monitors, and medical records (Table 26.1). Protocols commonly used in the unit should be posted in easily visible areas. All staff should be familiar with the location of the available equipment and resuscitation supplies for times when these are emergently needed.

Staffing and training

A major characteristic of an ICU is a higher staff-to-patient ratio. This distinction is particularly important in low-resource hospital settings, where nursing and physician staffing are strained. The goal should be a higher staffing ratio than the general wards to provide adequate monitoring and care for patients whose clinical status is expected to change rapidly. When caring for a critically ill patient, an ideal nurse to patient

Table 26.1 ICU resources. It is important to have the following equipment and medications immediately available on-site.

Equipment

Oxygen with delivery device
Pulse oximeter
Suction
Nebulization machine
Blood pressure measurement tool (manual or automatic)
Manual ventilation bag with masks of various sizes
Nasal and oral airways of various sizes
Intravenous/intraosseus supplies with tubing
Hand hygiene equipment
Dressings, gauze, disinfectant solution

Medications

Intravenous fluids: normal saline (NS) or lactated Ringer's, D5NS, higher dextrose concentrations
Antibiotics
Antiepileptics
Pain medications
Reversal agents (naloxone, flumazenil, neostigmine)
Antiemetics
Steroids
Nebulization medications (salbutamol, racemic epinephrine)
Vasopressors (dopamine, epinephrine)
Antihypertensives

Box 26.2 AVPU scale for monitoring a patient's mental status

Alert
Responsive to **V**oice
Responsive to **P**ain
Unresponsive

Source: Limmer & Monosky (2002).

ratio is 1:1 or 1:2; however, a ratio of 1:3 or 1:4 may be more realistic in a low-resource setting. Careful attention must be made to distribute the sickest patients amongst the ICU nursing staff to ensure that each patient receives appropriate attention.

All ICU staff members should be trained to appropriately recognize and manage common ICU emergencies in a timely manner. The nurses and physicians working in the ICU should have undergone specialized training in advanced care, such as advanced cardiac life support (ACLS) (Baker & Rylance, 2012).

Teamwork and simulation

ICUs are environments where patients have life-threatening illnesses and are at risk for rapid deterioration. To appropriately care for patients in these high-stress scenarios, clinicians should be comfortable and effective working as a team. Regular simulation of common scenarios can teach hands-on skills and communication strategies integral to successful patient care (Nichols, 2008).

Monitoring

One of the benefits of ICU care is the ability to closely monitor the progression of illness in critical patients (Baker & Rylance,

2012). Changes in patient status are often reflected in their vital signs before other signs and symptoms are present. Recognizing these changes allows clinicians to intervene early, before a disease process becomes irreversible.

Critically ill patients should have heart rate, blood pressure, respiratory rate, oxygen saturation, and consciousness level monitored every 1–2 hours, and more frequently if unstable (World Health Organization, 2003). Level of consciousness can be recorded simply using the AVPU scale (Box 26.2). Basic monitoring data can be collected by trained personnel using physical examination, blood pressure cuff, and pulse oximeter. When choosing equipment, it is important to select devices that are easily serviced and replaced locally.

Active monitoring of patients should also include intake (intravenously, by mouth, nasogastric tube) of fluid and nutrition, output (stool, gastric, urine, blood loss), and overall fluid balance (World Health Organization, 2003). Special attention should be paid to monitoring urine output. In children, urine output can be monitored by weighing or counting diapers. When exact measurement of urine output is critical, a urinary catheter can be placed. Adequate urine output can be defined as at least 0.5–1 mL/kg per hour (Nichols, 2008). Urine output below this is concerning for volume depletion, renal failure, and/or the syndrome of inappropriate secretion of antidiuretic hormone (SIADH).

Vital signs, fluid balance, and other data should be recorded in a flowchart to facilitate trending the patient's progress (Figure 26.1) (World Health Organization, 2011). For the ICU to be effective, monitoring must be in place at all hours of the day and night (World Health Organization, 2003). There should be a mechanism in place to help staff alert the physician if significant changes are noted (e.g., tachycardia, hypotension, desaturation, decreased urine output, mental status changes). All staff should have training on normal vital sign ranges for patients of different ages (Table 26.2), and it is helpful to have these clearly posted in the unit.

Transfers and handoffs

Each ICU should have defined criteria for when a stabilized patient is ready for transfer to the general wards. Usually, this occurs when a patient has sufficiently improved that they no

Severe illness monitoring form (first 6 hours)

Name: ___   Patient No.: ___   Birth date: _/_/_   Age: ___   Sex: M / F   Admission date: ___   Admission time: ___

Diagnosis:

Circle if test sent and record result: Electrolytes ___ AFB ___ Blood culture ___ Urine dipstick ___ Malaria ___ Gram stain ___ CXR ___ Other ___

Allergies:

Pregnant Yes/No   EDD:

		0	30	60 (1 hr)	90	120 (2 hrs)	150	180 (3 hrs)	210	240 (4 hrs)	270	300 (5 hrs)	330	360 (6 hrs)	390
	Time of day														
	Monitoring interval (minutes) from arrival or start														
Q30–60 min (until normal)	SpO₂														
	Heart rate														
	Systolic BP														
	Respiratory rate														
	Conscious level (AVPU)														
Q1–6 hours, repeat if abnormal	Temperature (°C)														
	Glucose														
	Urine output*														
	Hemoglobin														
Exam															
Assess															
Response	Fluids (type, rate)														
	Oxygen (method/flow)														
	Salbutamol														
	Vasopressor (type/rate)														
	Glucose														
	Antibiotics														
	Antimalarial														
	Antiviral														
	Furosemide														
	Blood														
	Other														
Clinician (initials)															

Figure 26.1 Sample patient monitoring chart for the ICU. *Source:* World Health Organization (2011), p. 209. Reproduced with permission of the World Health Organization.

Table 26.2 Normal vital sign ranges by age.

Age (years)	Heart rate (beats/min)	Respiratory rate (breaths/min)	Systolic blood pressure (mmHg)
<1	120–160	30–40	70–90
1–5	100–120	25–30	80–90
5–12	80–100	20–25	90–110
>12	60–100	15–20	100–120

Source: Nichols (2008).

Box 26.3 Common causes of respiratory distress

- Pneumonia
- Asthma/bronchiolitis
- Congenital heart disease (child)
- Chronic obstructive pulmonary disease (adult)
- Congestive heart failure
- Chest wall trauma
- Pleural effusion
- Metabolic acidosis (e.g., diabetic ketoacidosis, dehydration)

longer need intensive monitoring and their risk of requiring acute resuscitation is low.

Handoff should occur directly between the physicians and nurses caring for the patient to the receiving care team at every point of patient transfer. Information presented in the handoff should include the patient identifiers, medical history, allergies, details of their illness and hospital course, current medications, and ongoing management plan.

Disease processes and interventions

Respiratory distress

The purpose of respiration is to facilitate oxygen absorption in the alveolar capillaries, or oxygenation, and CO_2 elimination, or ventilation. Impairment of either of these processes can cause respiratory distress; frequently, both are affected in lung disease. Oxygenation failure can be identified by low oxygen saturation; ventilation failure can be measured as an elevated serum CO_2 in a blood gas analysis. Where CO_2 measurement is not possible, ventilation failure should be suspected in a patient with respiratory symptoms and physical examination findings of hypercarbia, such as tachycardia and altered mental status.

Respiratory distress, especially due to pneumonia, is one of the most common disease processes necessitating critical care (Box 26.3). Unrecognized and untreated pneumonia can rapidly progress to respiratory failure and death, particularly in children. Early identification and management of respiratory disease improves survival in low-resource settings (Duke *et al.*, 2009; Riviello *et al.*, 2011).

Management strategies

All patients admitted to the ICU should have close monitoring of respiratory rate and oxygen saturation. Oxygen should be the first intervention for patients with respiratory distress, hypoxia ($Spo_2 < 90\%$), or clinical symptoms of hypoxemia (Duke *et al.*, 2009; Duke, 2011). Lower saturation standards should be used for special populations, such as patients with suspected chronic obstructive pulmonary disease (COPD) or congenital heart disease. After initial stabilization, oxygen support can be slowly weaned to room air with frequent oxygen saturation checks. If the saturation remains above 90% on room air, the patient can be monitored off oxygen (Duke, 2011).

In low-resource hospitals, oxygen is typically supplied through oxygen cylinders or oxygen concentrators (Panel 26.1). Oxygen cylinders must be replaced at appropriate intervals to provide a steady source of oxygen. If oxygen concentrators are used, oxygen cylinders must be available for back-up during power outages and patient transport. It is also important to periodically test the function of oxygen concentrators using oxygen analyzers (World Health Organization, 2003; Duke *et al.*, 2009).

Oxygen can be delivered via a nasal cannula, face-mask, or nasal tube (Panel 26.1). Some hospitals may offer face tents to deliver oxygen to infants; however, the Fio_2 delivered by these devices are highly variable. It is impossible to deliver 100% Fio_2 to a patient without using a non-rebreather mask with a reservoir. If a patient remains hypoxic on low-flow nasal cannula, an effort should be made to deliver higher Fio_2.

For patients with severe respiratory disease, low-flow oxygen may be insufficient to maintain adequate oxygenation. High-flow oxygen may be delivered through a simple mask, non-rebreather mask, or humidified high-flow nasal cannula (flow rates $>4\,L/min$). In most low-resource settings, equipment and oxygen capacity is insufficient for these techniques. However, bubble continuous positive airway pressure (CPAP) providing positive end-expiratory pressure (PEEP) can be established using supplies commonly available in most hospitals (Figure 26.2). It is important to note that patients on bubble CPAP are dependent on a steady flow of oxygen; cessation of oxygen flow can quickly lead to suffocation. Therefore, bubble CPAP should only be used in settings where there is close and preferably continuous monitoring of patients and where there is staff trained in using the device.

The above interventions are helpful in supporting patients with impaired oxygenation but are insufficient to treat impaired ventilation secondary to lung disease or hypoventilation.

Panel 26.1 Common oxygen sources and oxygen delivery devices

Common oxygen sources

Oxygen cylinder

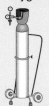

Pressurized oxygen source
Limited oxygen capacity depending on size
Lifespan influenced by the oxygen flow rate

Oxygen concentrator

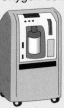

Create >90% oxygen by separating oxygen from room air using electricity
Designed to provide around 4 L/min of oxygen to a single patient; if one concentrator is used for multiple patients, the flow rate will be split between them (Duke *et al*., 2009)

Oxygen delivery devices

Nasal cannula

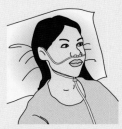

1 L/min flow increases FiO_2 delivered by roughly 4% above room air (21%) (e.g., a patient on 2 L/min by nasal cannula is receiving 29% FiO_2) (Nichols, 2008)

Face mask

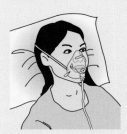

100% oxygen provides 35–60% FiO_2 (Nichols, 2008)

Non-rebreather mask

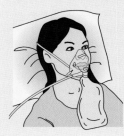

If tight-fitting mask with good seal, 100% FiO_2 may be administered (Nichols, 2008)

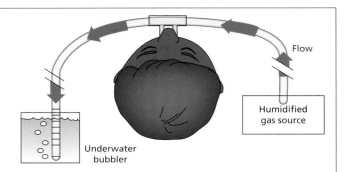

Figure 26.2 Simple bubble CPAP can be made from common hospital supplies (adapted from AdaptAir.org). The PEEP delivered with bubble CPAP can be adjusted by changing the depth the tubing is immersed in water.

Table 26.3 Common causes of shock.
Hypovolemic
Hemorrhage
Gastrointestinal losses (diarrhea, vomiting)
Burns
Inadequate intake (dehydration)
Cardiogenic
Heart failure
Arrhythmia
Myocarditis
Distributive
Sepsis
Anaphylaxis
Neurogenic
Obstructive
Pneumothorax
Cardiac tamponade
Pulmonary embolism

Invasive or non-invasive methods, such as bilevel positive airway pressure or mechanical ventilation, may be needed to deliver positive pressure inhalations to patients with impaired ventilation. The equipment necessary for these interventions is generally not available in low-resource settings and therefore will not be discussed in this chapter.

Patients with respiratory disease, particularly children, often have difficulty handling excessive secretions. Frequent and aggressive respiratory toilet, including suctioning and chest physical therapy, can reduce a patient's respiratory distress by removing mucus from the nares and oropharynx and assist in expectorating mucus from the patient's lower airway, especially when the patient's own respiratory muscles are weakened (Nichols, 2008).

Various pathologies causing respiratory distress, such as asthma or COPD, present with wheezing. Wheezing should be treated with inhaled beta-agonists, frequently salbutamol in low-resource settings. Salbutamol nebulization can be administered every 10–20 min until patient improvement, or continuously. For patients with suspected reactive airway disease, steroids such as prednisone should also be given to reduce airway inflammation. In life-threatening wheezing, magnesium sulfate can be given intravenously, preceded by a fluid bolus to avoid hypotension (World Health Organization, 2003, 2011, 2013).

> ### 🔍 Clinical pearl
>
> Metabolic acidosis – caused by, for example, diabetic ketoacidosis, sepsis with lactic acidosis, or poisoning – produces a compensatory respiratory alkalosis. If a patient has tachypnea without history or physical examination elements suggestive of respiratory pathology, consider another cause for the elevated respiratory rate.

Shock

Shock is a state of acute circulatory dysfunction resulting in failure to adequately deliver oxygen to end organs and tissues. Shock can occur as a result of infection, hypovolemia, anaphylaxis, and cardiac or neurologic dysfunction (Table 26.3). In low-resource settings, shock is frequently the result of the late presentation of hemorrhage, gastrointestinal fluid losses, or overwhelming infection.

Management strategies

Sepsis is a systemic host response to infection leading to organ dysfunction and hypotension (Table 26.4). Outcomes of patients with sepsis depend on rapid administration of appropriate therapy. For this reason, early identification of sepsis-like physiology in critically ill patients is the key to improving survival. In a patient with a suspected infection, early signs of sepsis include fever or hypothermia, tachycardia (or bradycardia in infants), tachypnea, and poor distal perfusion. Basic laboratory changes include hyperglycemia (or hypoglycemia in infants) and leukocytosis or leukopenia. Hypotension is a late finding of severe disease and should never be used as a threshold to initiate therapy. Patients with sepsis should have close monitoring for signs of end-organ dysfunction, including altered mental status and decreased urine output. If laboratory investigations are available, concerning results include thrombocytopenia, coagulopathy, rising creatinine, elevated transaminases, and hyperbilirubinemia (Dellinger et al., 2013).

Table 26.4 Definitions of sepsis syndromes.

Systemic inflammatory response syndrome (SIRS)

Two of the following (and at least one of those marked *)
 *Hyperthermia or hypothermia
 Tachycardia, or bradycardia in children <1 year old
 Tachypnea
 *Leukocytosis or leukopenia

Sepsis

SIRS in the presence of suspected or proven infection

Severe sepsis

Sepsis with organ dysfunction or acute respiratory distress syndrome

Septic shock

Sepsis plus hypotension not reversed by fluid administration

Source: Dellinger et al. (2013).

Box 26.5 Calculating maintenance intravenous fluids using drip factor

Calculating hourly maintenance intravenous fluid rate for children (4:2:1 rule)

$$\text{First 10 kg} = \text{weight} \times 4\,\text{mL/h}$$

$$+10\text{–}20\,\text{kg} = \text{additional weight} \times 2\,\text{mL/h}$$

$$+ >20\,\text{kg} = \text{additional weight} \times 1\,\text{mL/h}$$

Calculating the drip rate

$$\frac{\text{Fluid rate (mL/h)} \times \text{Drip factor (drops/mL)}}{60\,\text{min/h}}$$
$$= \text{Desired drip rate (drops/min)}$$

Example
Maintenance fluids for 25-kg child, intravenous (IV) bag with drip rate of 15 drops/mL:

$$\text{Desired IV fluid rate} = (10 \times 4\,\text{mL/h})$$
$$+ (10 \times 2\,\text{mL/h})$$
$$+ (5 \times 1\,\text{mL/h}) = 65\,\text{mL/h}$$

$$\text{Desired drip rate}$$
$$= \frac{65\,\text{mL/h} \times 15\,\text{drops/mL}}{60\,\text{min/h}}$$
$$= \sim 16\,\text{drops/min}$$

Box 26.4 Sepsis management
(Dellinger et al., 2013)

- Rapid fluid resuscitation using isotonic fluid[a]
- Early and appropriate antibiotic delivery
- Place patient on 100% oxygen even in the absence of hypoxia
- Optimize hemoglobin through transfusion to improve oxygen-carrying capacity
- Prevent and monitor for hypoglycemia
- Consider need for stress-dose hydrocortisone (50 mg/m^2 daily) (especially in patients with possible adrenal insufficiency, chronic steroid use, young children)

[a] May increase mortality in in low-resource settings with high prevalence of malnutrition or anemia (Maitland et al., 2011)

Early goal-directed therapy with rapid volume repletion, appropriate antibiotic administration within the first hour, and utilization of vasopressors has been shown to reduce shock-related mortality (Box 26.4) (Dellinger et al., 2013), even when adapted to the low-resource setting (Dunser et al., 2012; Mahavanakul et al., 2012). However, a recent study demonstrated increased mortality with aggressive fluid resuscitation in febrile African children, questioning the role of aggressive fluid resuscitation in low-resource settings with a high prevalence of malnutrition and anemia (Maitland et al., 2011). It remains unclear whether these findings are generalizable to all low-resource settings and adult patients.

After initial resuscitation, it is important to maintain optimum fluid balance in all ICU patients. Ongoing losses from diarrhea, vomiting, or hemorrhage should be replaced with isotonic fluid or blood. Many low-resource settings do not have infusion pumps to deliver hourly maintenance fluids. Hanging intravenous bags without attention to maintenance requirements can easily result in fluid overload, particularly in small children. In the absence of intravenous pumps, flow rates can be adjusted to approximate maintenance fluids by counting the drops per minute (Box 26.5) in the intravenous tubing drip chamber. Each intravenous set-up has a "drip factor" specified on the packaging describing the number of drops per milliliter delivered.

According to the Surviving Sepsis guidelines, vasopressors should be initiated after 1 hour of interventions if the patient continues to have hypotension despite adequate volume resuscitation (Dellinger et al., 2013). Vasopressors, however, are rarely available in low-resource settings. If vasopressors are available but infusion pumps are not, infusion rates can be calculated and adjusted using the drip-rate technique. Vasopressors should be given through central venous access if possible; if not, vasopressors should be delivered through the largest vein available due to risk of skin necrosis from extravasation.

Patients with sepsis need to be closely monitored for clinical changes, and interventions should be continued until normal physiology has been restored. Specific therapeutic endpoints include normal heart rate, capillary refill less than 2 s, normal peripheral pulses, warm extremities, normal mental status, and urine output more than 1 mL/kg per hour. Normalization of blood pressure is not a reliable endpoint for resuscitation, especially in children and young adults who often have normal blood pressures in the setting of sepsis. In low-resource settings, resuscitation efforts may be limited by availability of interventions, so therapy should be optimized utilizing available resources.

> ### Clinical pearl
>
> Be vigilant for clinical deterioration after rapid fluid administration in a patient with suspected septic shock. Patients with cardiogenic shock from myocarditis, myocardial ischemia, severe anemia, or malnutrition may acutely worsen after fluid resuscitation due to fluid overload, demonstrating tachypnea from pulmonary edema, hepatomegaly from liver congestion, and/or worsening perfusion. If cardiogenic shock is suspected, give a smaller initial fluid bolus (10 mL/kg) and monitor effects.

Table 26.5 Common causes of altered mental status.

Neurologic
Trauma (hemorrhage, diffuse axonal injury)
Stroke
Seizures
Space-occupying lesion (mass)
Endocrine
Hypoglycemia
Electrolyte abnormality (hyponatremia, etc.)
Acid–base abnormality
Thyroid disease
Adrenal insufficiency
Diabetic ketoacidosis
Infectious
Sepsis
Meningitis/encephalitis
Cerebral malaria
Severe pneumonia (respiratory failure)
Renal
Uremia
Gastrointestinal
Liver failure
Toxic ingestion

Altered mental status

Patients may be admitted to the ICU for close neurological monitoring or intervention secondary to acute changes in mental status that occur as the result of derangements of the brain's metabolic activity, through insufficient nutrient delivery or toxic effects (Table 26.5). The Glasgow Coma Scale may be used to evaluate the patient's mental status (see Chapter 25). In low-resource settings, ongoing monitoring of patient mental status can be performed using the AVPU scale (see Box 26.2).

Management strategies

Seizures

Convulsive or non-convulsive status epilepticus is a neurologic emergency and prompt intervention must be taken to prevent patient deterioration. As in all critical scenarios, initial attention must be paid to assessing and protecting the patient's airway, breathing, and circulation. The patient should be placed in a recovery position to prevent aspiration (Figure 26.3). Intravenous or intraosseus access should be obtained. If possible, dextrose levels should be emergently checked, as hypoglycemia is a common and reversible cause of seizures in critically ill patients (Nichols, 2008). If glucometers are not available, dextrose can be given empirically.

The initial intervention for seizures is administration of a benzodiazepine; diazepam is generally available in low-resource settings. If intravenous access is not established, the intravenous formulation of diazepam can be administered rectally. If seizures continue beyond 10 min, a repeat dose can be given. For ongoing seizures, a second antiepileptic, commonly phenobarbital in children and phenytoin in adults, should be administered with a loading dose, then a maintenance dose. With repeated administration of antiepileptic medications, special attention should be paid to the patient's airway and respiration. If hypopnea or apnea develop, temporary bag-valve mask ventilation or intubation and mechanical ventilation may be necessary until the patient recovers their respiratory drive (World Health Organization, 2011, 2013).

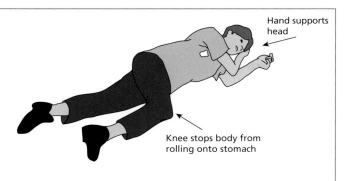

Hand supports head

Knee stops body from rolling onto stomach

Figure 26.3 Seizure recovery position.

🔍 Clinical pearl

Any deterioration in mental status in a previously stable patient is an ominous sign of new or unrecognized pathology. A previously tachypneic child who becomes sleepy, for example, is concerning for worsening hypercarbia and impending respiratory failure. An awake trauma victim who suddenly loses consciousness may have a new cerebral hemorrhage. Any new changes in a patient's mental status should prompt nursing staff to alert physicians for a full reevaluation of the underlying cause.

Pain management

Pain is a frequent complication of severe illness. Beyond its psychological effects on the patient, untreated pain can also significantly interfere with treatment and prevent improvement. The stress of experiencing pain increases the metabolic demands on the body when the ability to meet those demands is already stressed. Shallow rapid breathing from pain can prevent optimum oxygenation and ventilation in patients, making them more susceptible to respiratory complications. Patients experiencing severe pain may be unable to cooperate with necessary interventions (Nichols, 2008). In low-resource settings, the treatment of pain is sometimes seen as a low-priority intervention; however, appropriate pain management is a crucial component of ICU care. When available, opioids and non-opioid drugs should be administered via intravenous or enteral routes. Doses should be carefully titrated to provide adequate analgesia while limiting complications such as hypoventilation. Anxiety can be treated with benzodiazepines. In children, distraction and the presence of a parent can significantly reduce discomfort and aid with patient care.

Patient safety and quality

Infection prevention and control

Hospital-acquired infections are a challenge in any intensive care setting due to high illness severity and number of invasive interventions performed (Rosenthal *et al.*, 2012a). While nosocomial infections lead to high morbidity and mortality in these patients, simple low-cost infection control measures can lead to significant reduction in their occurrence. Infection control guidelines and practice bundles can help reduce hospital-acquired infections in low-resource settings (Rosenthal *et al.*, 2012b,c,d).

General concepts of hospital infection control include hand hygiene, personal protective equipment, isolation, and adherence to sterile practice (World Health Organization, 2011). All hospital staff should be expected to perform hand hygiene before and after any patient contact. Alcohol-based rubs are highly effective in preventing spread of infection (Nichols, 2008). Soap and water should be used when hands are visibly soiled or when alcohol-based rubs are not available. Protective gloves should be used during any contact with body fluids, such as dressing changes, blood draws, or accessing intravenous lines. If available, gowns, eye protection, and masks should be used when caring for patients with suspected communicable disease. If possible, these patients should be separated from others in separate rooms, via curtains, or physical space. When performing any invasive procedure, efforts to establish and maintain sterility should be emphasized.

Skin breakdown

Critically ill patients often have impaired ability to communicate discomfort and decreased mobility, putting them at risk for complications such as skin breakdown or intravenous infiltrates. Special attention should be paid by nursing staff to actively monitor for these conditions. Immobile patients should be regularly repositioned in bed and their skin inspected for any signs of pressure ulcer development. Intravenous cannulas should be checked frequently for signs of inflammation, swelling, or infection, and the site changed if any problem is identified (World Health Organization, 2011).

Ethical considerations

Family/patient involvement

Families of critically ill patients are affected beyond the emotional stress of the illness itself. Hospitals are often located far from patients' communities, isolating the family from their natural support system. By staying in the hospital, family members frequently miss work, adding to the significant financial burden of the hospitalization and illness itself.

The patient's wishes should always guide the care provided. Critically ill patients are often not able to advocate for their own care. For this reason, it is vital to involve the family in treatment decisions and frequently update them on the progress of the patient. For pediatric patients, the presence of the parents at the bedside can significantly aid in the therapy of the child by reducing anxiety and discomfort.

In low-resource settings, family members can be trained to carry out simple tasks of monitoring and caring for the patient. Examples include feeding and washing the patient, rotating the patient to prevent ulcers, notifying staff if there is a change in clinical status or when intravenous fluid bags are empty, or, in special situations, short-term manual ventilation (World Health Organization, 2011).

End of life

Despite receiving all available care, many patients with critical illness will die. The role of healthcare providers in these cases is to maintain the patient's comfort and dignity and offer support to the family in this difficult period. The decision to redirect care to provide only comfort measures is a complex decision and is based on the likelihood for recovery from illness and the patient's and family's wishes. Pain and other symptoms, such as dyspnea, should be treated. Patient and family preferences around end-of-life care should be supported if at all possible (Nichols, 2008; World Health Organization, 2011).

Additional resources

- World Health Organization (2003) *Surgical Care at the District Hospital: the WHO Manual*. Available at http://www.who.int/surgery/publications/scdh_manual/en/
- World Health Organization (2011) *IMAI District Clinician Manual: Hospital Care for Adolescents and Adults*, Vols 1 and 2. Available at http://www.who.int/hiv/pub/imai/imai2011/en/
- World Health Organization (2013) *Pocket Book of Hospital Care for Children*, 2nd edn. Available at http://www.who.int/maternal_child_adolescent/documents/child_hospital_care/en/index.html
- Duke T (ed.) (2011) The clinical use of oxygen in hospitals with limited resources. Available at http://video.rch.org.au/cich/The_Clinical_Use_of_Oxygen_November_2011.pdf

REFERENCES

Baker T (2009) Critical care in low-income countries. *Trop Med Int Health* 14:143–8.

Baker T, Rylance J (2012) Critical care where there is no ICU: basic management of critically ill patients in a low income country. *Update in Anaesthesia* 28:27–30. Available at http://www.google.com/url?url=http://www.wfsahq.org/archive-update-in-anaesthesia/update-in-anaesthesia/update-028/download&rct=j&frm=1&q=&esrc=s&sa=U&ei=TfSfU8HpJY2SyASE5YDQDw&ved=0CBkQFjAB&usg=AFQjCNGsr5GmWUru3z_RtaNzyzy8JqjL3A

Basnet S, Adhikari N, Koirala J (2011) Challenges in setting up pediatric and neonatal intensive care units in a resource-limited country. *Pediatrics* 128:e986–92.

Dellinger RP, Levy MM, Rhodes A *et al.* (2013) Surviving sepsis campaign: international guidelines for management of severe sepsis and septic shock, 2012. *Intensive Care Med* 39:165–228.

Duke T (ed.) (2011) The clinical use of oxygen in hospitals with limited resources. World Health Organization. Available at http://video.rch.org.au/cich/The_Clinical_Use_of_Oxygen_November_2011.pdf

Duke T, Subhi R, Peel D, Frey B (2009) Pulse oximetry: technology to reduce child mortality in developing countries. *Ann Trop Paediatr* 29:165–75.

Dunser MW, Festic E, Dondorp A *et al.* (2012) Recommendations for sepsis management in resource-limited settings. *Intensive Care Med* 38:557–74.

Firth P, Ttendo S (2012) Intensive care in low-income countries: a critical need. *N Engl J Med* 367:1974–6.

Limmer D, Monosky K (2002) Assessment of the altered mental status patient. *Emerg Med Serv* 1(3):54–8, 81.

Mahavanakul W, Nickerson EK, Srisomang P *et al.* (2012) Feasibility of modified Surviving Sepsis campaign guidelines in a resource-restricted setting based on cohort study of severe *S. aureus* sepsis. *PLoS ONE* 7(2):e29858.

Maitland K, Kiguli S, Opoka RO *et al.* (2011) Mortality after fluid bolus in African children with severe infections. *N Engl J Med* 364:2483–95.

Nichols DG (ed.) (2008) *Roger's Textbook of Pediatric Intensive Care*, 4th edn. Philadelphia: Lippincott Williams &Wilkins.

Riviello ED, Letchford S, Achieng L, Newton MW (2011) Critical care in resource poor settings: lessons learned and future directions. *Crit Care Med* 39:860–7.

Rosenthal VD, Bijie H, Maki DG *et al.* (2012a) International Nosocomial Infection Control Consortium (INICC) report, data summary of 36 countries, for 2004–2009. *Am J Infect Control* 40:396–407.

Rosenthal VD, Rodrigues C, Alvarez-Moreno C *et al.* (2012b) Effectiveness of a multidimensional approach for prevention of ventilator-associated pneumonia in adult intensive care units from 14 developing countries of four continents: findings of the International

Nosocomial Infection Control Consortium. *Crit Care Med* 40:3121–8.

Rosenthal VD, Ramachandran B, Dueñas L *et al.* (2012c) Findings of the International Nosocomial Infection Control Consortium (INICC), Part I: Effectiveness of a multidimensional infection control approach on catheter-associated urinary tract infection rates in pediatric intensive care units of 6 developing countries. *Infect Control Hosp Epidemiol* 33:696–703.

Rosenthal VD, Todi SK, Alvarez-Moreno C *et al.* (2012d) Impact of a multidimensional infection control strategy on catheter-associated urinary tract infection rates in the adult intensive care units of 15 developing countries:

findings of the International Nosocomial Infection Control Consortium (INICC). *Infection* 40:517–26.

World Health Organization (2003) *Surgical Care at the District Hospital.* Available at http://www.who.int/surgery/publications/scdh_manual/en/

World Health Organization (2011) *IMAI District Clinician Manual: Hospital Care for Adolescents and Adults*, Vols 1 and 2. Available at http://www.who.int/hiv/pub/imai/imai2011/en/

World Health Organization (2013) *Pocket Book of Hospital Care for Children*, 2nd edn. Available at http://www.who.int/maternal_child_adolescent/documents/child_hospital_care/en/index.html

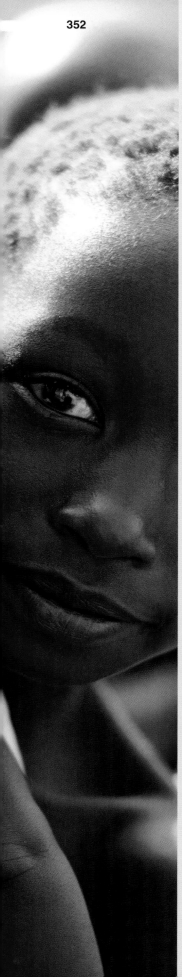

CHAPTER 27

Mental Health and Neurological Disorders

Mark Tomlinson[1,2], Amelia van der Merwe[1,2], and Peter S. Azzopardi[3,4]

[1]Alan J. Flisher Centre for Public Mental Health, Stellenbosch, South Africa
[2]Stellenbosch University, Stellenbosch, South Africa
[3]Centre for Adolescent Health, Royal Children's Hospital, Murdoch Childrens Research Institute, Department of Paediatrics, University of Melbourne, Melbourne, Australia
[4]Wardliparingga Aboriginal Research Unit, South Australian Health and Medical Research Institute, Adelaide, Australia

Key learning objectives

- Understand that mental, neurological, and substance use disorders are among the foremost contributors to the global burden of disease.

- Review the significant mental health treatment gap between high-income countries (HICs) and low- and middle-income countries (LMICs), due in part to inadequate resources, trained personnel, and stigma.

- Discuss the principles of good mental health care, including addressing stigma and ensuring sensitive and confidential care.

- Discuss the Mental Health Global Action Program (mhGAP) as an excellent set of intervention guidelines to help clinicians address mental, neurological, and substance use disorders in non-specialized health settings.

Abstract

Mental disorders are among the foremost contributors to the global burden of disease, deeply affecting the health and well-being of individuals, families, and communities. There is a significant mental health treatment gap between HICs and LMICs. Significant challenges to reducing the treatment gap and decreasing the burden of mental disorders include insufficient resources, stigma and discrimination, cultural and contextual factors, and the continued compartmentalization and separation of mental health systems from general health services. However, significant advances have been made in recent years in promoting recognition and response to mental health globally. These include the World Health Organization's Mental Health Global Action Program intervention guidelines, the Grand Challenges in Global Mental Health, and the Movement for Global Mental Health. This chapter outlines key principles in providing mental health care in resource-limited settings. It outlines common symptoms and presentations of the common mental disorders – depression, self-harm, alcohol use disorders, psychosis, dementia, and seizure disorder – and discusses principles of assessment and management.

Key words: mental health, depression, alcohol use disorders, psychosis, self-harm, dementia, common mental disorders, mhGAP, treatment gap, mental health systems

Introduction

Positive mental health is a value in its own right; it contributes to the individual's well-being and quality of life; and also contributes to society and the economy by increasing social functioning and social capital. Positive mental health refers to human qualities and life skills such as cognitive functioning, positive self-esteem, social and problem-solving skills, the ability to manage major changes and stresses in life, and to influence the social environment, the ability to work productively and fruitfully and to make contributions to the community, and a state of emotional, spiritual, and mental well-being

(Jané-Llopis *et al.*, 2005, p. 9).

Mental disorders are among the leading contributors to the burden of disease for children, adolescents, and adults globally (Vos *et al.*, 2012). The burden of mental disorders is projected to grow significantly over the coming two decades as a result of demographic transitions (including rapid urbanization) and epidemiological transitions (Mathers & Loncar, 2006) and is estimated to result in the loss of US$16.1 trillion over this period (Bloom *et al.*, 2011). Globally, suicide remains a significant cause of preventable early death, with 86% of suicides occurring in LMICs, the majority of cases between the ages of 15 and 44 years. Mental disorders are associated with socioeconomic disadvantage; poverty increases the risk of mental illness due to increased stress, poor nutrition, and violence. Furthermore, mental health problems can result in poverty due to loss of earning potential and disengagement from the community due to stigma (Patel & Thornicroft, 2009; Lund *et al.*, 2011).

There is a significant "treatment gap" for mental disorders; 80% of the world's population live in LMICs yet these areas receive less than 20% of the available mental health resources. In sub-Saharan Africa, for example, over 90% of people living with schizophrenia and other psychoses remain untreated (Patel *et al.*, 2011). This treatment gap is a function of not only limited resources but also poor detection of common mental disorders. For example, more than 75% of those reporting significant anxiety, mood, impulse control, or substance use disorders in the World Mental Health Surveys in LMICs did not receive any preventive care or treatment. In many settings, mental health services are compartmentalized and not integrated with the broader health system, despite the fact that many mental disorders co-occur with other acute and chronic health conditions and can worsen associated health outcomes (Moussavi *et al.*, 2007). An additional contributing factor to the treatment gap is the extent to which mental disorders are stigmatized, leading to significant barriers to accessing care and social exclusion once a diagnosis is made (Thornicroft *et al.*, 2009; Tsai & Tomlinson, 2012). In India, for example, stigma is such a significant barrier that only 10% of people with mental disorder receive any form of evidence-based treatment (Shidhaye & Kermode, 2013).

Global initiatives focused on closing the treatment gap between HICs and LMICs

Addressing the treatment gap for mental disorders in LMICs involves increasing the awareness and demand for services; enhancing the capacity of healthcare teams; addressing stigma; reducing the cost of treatments (particularly pharmacological treatments); integrating care with the management of other related health and social problems; and using an evidence-based, practice-based, and community-based approach to treatment (de Jesus *et al.*, 2009; Patel & Thornicroft, 2009; Prince *et al.*, 2009; Flisher *et al.*, 2010).

A number of global initiatives have been developed in the past several years which focus on the treatment gap between HICs and LMICs in terms of mental health disorders, including the World Health Organization (WHO)'s Mental Health Global Action Program (mhGAP) intervention guidelines, the Grand Challenges in Global Mental Health, the *Lancet* series on global mental health, and the Movement for Global Mental Health (Patel *et al.*, 2011).

In particular, the mhGAP intervention guidelines provide simple algorithms to guide clinicians in the recognition, assess-

ment, and management of common mental, neurological, and substance use disorders in non-specialized health settings (see Additional resources section). In this chapter we do not intend to replicate these excellent guidelines but rather help orientate readers to these resources and introduce key concepts and principles. We reproduce the mhGAP diagnostic and treatment algorithms for depression (the most prevalent mental disorder) and suicide/self-harm (a clinical emergency). We also include some key points around diagnosis and management of alcohol use disorders, dementia, psychosis, and seizures. While seizures are not strictly mental disorders, they are often included as part of mental, neurological, and substance-use (MNS) disorders; chronicity, stigma, impact on quality of life, insufficient investment, and a treatment gap are common to these conditions (WHO, 2008). The mhGAP guidelines include guidelines on the common MNS disorders, including seizures.

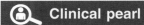 **Clinical pearl**

"There can be no health without mental health" (WHO, 2005 cited in Prince *et al.*, 2007, p. 859).

Providing mental health care in resource-limited settings: task-shifting

A critical issue in responding to the treatment gap for mental disorder in resource-limited settings is the shortage of specialist mental health staff. A substantial body of research currently suggests that cost-effective, affordable, and efficacious interventions can be developed and implemented by assembling members of the community and by restructuring tasks among healthcare teams. This process is known as "task-shifting" and is an increasingly important approach for many interventions in global health (MacArthur, 2008). Task-shifting involves the handover of particular tasks from specialist health workers to health workers who have received less training and have fewer qualifications, for the more economic use of the limited available resources for promoting mental health in LMICs. In scaling up community-based interventions such as these, the role of highly qualified health workers consequently changes to facilitate a context-specific and necessary reform of mental health services in LMICs. Specialists' new roles include providing training and supervision of community health workers and less time spent in one-to-one clinical activities. Task-shifting directly addresses the shortage of trained psychiatrists, and scientific evidence shows that this approach is likely to have a significant effect on reducing the treatment gap between HICs and LMICs (MacArthur, 2008). The mhGAP strategy uses task-shifting as a basis to the WHO guidelines (Patel & Prince, 2010; Bass *et al.*, 2012).

In addition to task-shifting, effective interventions to close the treatment gap involve patient empowerment, capacity building, community outreach, health systems strengthening, research, and sound program management, including monitoring and evaluation (Raja *et al.*, 2012). A supportive policy framework (including government partnerships that prioritize mental health) are also key to addressing the mental health treatment gap.

Providing mental health care in resource-limited settings

It should be emphasized that providing mental health services can be challenging (even for specialized teams in resource-rich settings). If possible, assemble and work as part of a team, allowing for case discussion, reflection, and the sharing of tasks and responsibilities. It is also useful to identify what resources are available in the local community, including human resources (counselors, key support people such as community leaders and traditional healers), social resources (housing, finances), and treatment resources (medications).

Key principles of providing mental health care

Principles of providing good mental health care echo those of providing good clinical care (see Chapter 1). However, given the stigma and barriers to accessing healthcare for mental disorder, there are some principles worth highlighting.

Mental health should be explored and addressed at each clinical encounter using communication that is clear, respectful, and non-judgmental. This is not only part of providing comprehensive healthcare, but it also helps address the mental health treatment gap (Patel *et al.*, 2013). Going beyond the presenting complaint is especially important for adolescents (see Chapter 14) as many mental disorders have their onset during adolescence, and young people may face significant barriers in accessing health services including poor health literacy (especially where health services are fragmented) and concerns around confidentiality.

Conversely, the physical health and well-being of people with mental disorders should also be addressed. Many of the determinants of mental disorders are common to physical illness. People living with mental disorder are more likely to be socioeconomically disadvantaged, and they may experience additional barriers to preventive and essential healthcare. Regularly perform physical health checks and provide education around healthy behaviors (nutrition, smoking, substance use, contraception, and safe sex).

Confidentiality should be assured and maintained, recognizing when confidentiality should be breached for the safety of the individual (risk of suicide) or community (risk of harm to others). An example of a confidentiality statement is provided in Chapter 14.

A challenge to confidentiality in the assessment of mental illness is the value of third-party history, for example from a partner or parent. Explain early in the consultation that you may talk to other people (e.g., family members, community members, members of the treatment team) in order to better understand and address the patient's health needs. Involve the patient as much as possible in these decisions. Reassure them that any discussion you have is to help them.

While people with mental illness may not be competent to provide consent for treatment or withholding of treatment, they may be able to provide assent or agreement. Involve them as much as possible in the management plan.

Disclosure of distressing information (such as self-harm or sexual assault) should be responded to sensitively.

Given the challenges of identifying mental disorder in cross-cultural settings, visiting clinicians should work closely with local healthcare workers to assist identification and interpretation of symptoms. This may involve seeing patients together. Local healthcare workers are likely to have an understanding of the social context and supports available to the patient. In small communities, healthcare workers may be related to patients; empower local professionals while reinforcing confidentiality.

Other considerations
- Evidence-based information should be provided to patients in terms they can understand.

- Patients and their families should be engaged as much as possible in the decision-making process. Ask and respond to patient fears and concerns around diagnosis and treatment.
- Facilitate linkage of patients with community supports. Ask the patient to help identify suitable support people and support for basic services (e.g., food, shelter, safety).
- Actively follow-up with patients. Individuals with mental disorders are among those at the highest risk of poor clinical follow-up. Use family and community resources to contact individuals who have not returned for follow-up. Patients who have missed follow-up appointments should never be punished or scolded.

Symptoms and presentation of common mental disorders

Table 27.1 shows the typical presenting symptoms of the more common mental disorders and may serve as a guide in screening for mental health conditions. If individuals present with features of more than one condition, all relevant conditions should be assessed. However, mental health presentations are often non-specific or are only seen when other circumstances bring the individual into contact with the healthcare system, especially in settings with significant social stigma. For example, a person with an alcohol use disorder may only present to a health facility in the setting of an injury. Therefore,

Table 27.1 Common presentations of mental health disorders.

Mental health disorder	Presentation
Depression	Low energy; fatigue; sleep or appetite problems Persistent sad or anxious mood; irritability Low interest or pleasure in activities that used to be interesting or enjoyable Difficulties in carrying out usual work, school, domestic, or social activities Multiple symptoms with no clear physical cause (e.g., aches and pains, palpitations, numbness)
Self-harm/suicide	Current thoughts, plan, or act of self-harm or suicide History of thoughts, plan, or act of self-harm or suicide
Alcohol use disorder	Appearing to be under the influence of alcohol (e.g., smell of alcohol, looks intoxicated, hangover) Presenting with an injury Somatic symptoms associated with alcohol use (e.g., insomnia, fatigue, anorexia, nausea, vomiting, indigestion, diarrhea, headaches) Difficulties in carrying out usual work, school, domestic, or social activities
Psychosis	Abnormal or disorganized behavior (e.g., incoherent or irrelevant speech, unusual appearance, self-neglect, unkempt appearance) Delusions (a false firmly held belief or suspicion) Hallucinations (hearing voices or seeing things that are not there) Neglecting usual responsibilities related to work, school, domestic, or social activities Manic symptoms (several days of being abnormally happy, too energetic, too talkative, very irritable, not sleeping, reckless behavior)
Dementia	Decline or problems with memory (severe forgetfulness) and orientation (awareness of time, place, and person) Mood or behavioral problems such as apathy (appearing uninterested) or irritability Loss of emotional control: easily upset, irritable, or tearful Difficulties in carrying out usual work, domestic, or social activities
Seizure disorder	Convulsive movement or fits/seizures During the convulsion: loss of consciousness or impaired consciousness, stiffness, rigidity, tongue bite, injury, incontinence of urine or feces After the convulsion: fatigue, drowsiness, sleepiness, confusion, abnormal behavior, headache, muscle aches, or weakness on one side of the body

Source: adapted from WHO (2010).

mental health conditions should be considered at all patient encounters. Chapter 14 (Figure 14.3 and Table 14.4) illustrates a framework for assessing the broader health and well-being of adolescents and may provide an example of broader health assessments of all patients.

Assessment and management

If a mental health disorder is suspected based on symptoms shown in Table 27.1, clinicians should systematically assess the patient to see if the condition is present and if a diagnosis should be made. As part of the systematic assessment, organic or physical illness should also be considered. For example, anemia or hypothyroidism can both present with low energy or fatigue as seen in depression.

 Clinical pearl

Medical illness (organic disease) can present with symptoms similar to those of mental health disorders. Specific conditions are included in the mhGAP guidelines. All patients presenting with symptoms of mental disorder should have a medical history and examination.

In this chapter we have reproduced the diagnostic algorithm for depression, which is the most common mental health disorder, and suicide or self-harm, which is a clinical emergency. For all other mental health disorders, we refer the reader to the full mhGAP guidelines.

Depression

Figure 27.1 outlines the assessment and management of moderate to severe depression. Core diagnostic criteria include at least 2 weeks of at least two of the following: depressed mood, loss of interest or pleasure in normally pleasurable activities and/or decreased energy or easily fatigued. Recent meta-analysis showed that psychosocial interventions implemented in outpatient and primary care contexts enhance social functioning in individuals with depression and should be integrated into efforts to scale up services (De Silva *et al.*, 2013). Psychoeducation is an important component of management and involves explaining to the patient, and to their family as appropriate, that depression is common and effective treatment is possible. Psychoeducation includes promoting positive behaviors (good nutrition, sleep, physical activity, social activity), education around harmful behaviors (such as substance use or social withdrawal), and a safety plan of where to seek help if the person has feelings of self-harm or suicide. Exploring and addressing current psychosocial stressors is important in managing depression. This may involve talking through issues in the clinic or helping the person identify people with whom they can talk. Managing depression may also involve specific psychological interventions, such as interpersonal therapy, or

antidepressant medication, outlined in detail in the mhGAP guidelines. Antidepressant therapy should not be used as first-line treatment in adolescents or in people who have experienced recent bereavement or loss, and they should be used with caution in pregnant women. All people living with depression should be offered regular follow-up.

Self-harm and suicide

Discussing self-harm and suicide does not provoke acts of self-harm, but rather often helps alleviate the fear and anxiety with which these individuals are living (WHO, 2008). Figure 27.2 outlines the assessment and diagnostic algorithm for self-harm and suicide. Self-harm and suicide are deeply personal issues and are best discussed in the context of rapport and trust. Clinicians should use a sensitive non-judgmental line of questioning. A notification of intent to self-harm usually requires the clinician to breach confidentiality to guarantee the safety of the patient. Explain why you are breaching confidentiality, and involve the patient as much as possible. Key principles of management include guaranteeing the immediate safety of the individual; treat any injury or poisoning, remove means of self-harm, and care for the patient in a secure, supervised, and supportive environment while they are being assessed or at imminent risk (i.e., do not leave them alone). Consult specialist advice, if available, and activate psychosocial supports. This may include mobilizing family, friends, and community supports. Comorbidities such as depression, psychosis, or chronic pain should also be managed. When the person is safe to return home, provide a safety plan of whom to contact during crisis and maintain regular contact and follow-up.

Alcohol use disorders

Key diagnostic criteria for alcohol use disorders (AUDs) are shown in Boxes 27.1 and 27.2. AUDs are a significant cause for concern as they cause a great deal of harm for individuals, families, and communities. However, they often go unnoticed and untreated for long periods. This is despite the fact that brief, easily delivered interventions have been shown to be

Clinical experience

"I volunteered as a nursing student on a reservation in rural North Dakota, and at times I would see patients who struggled with issues of mental health. One of the things that struck me was the need that existed to support not only the individual patients, but also the family and friends who accompanied them. The burden of illness often reaches beyond the person seeking help. It is important to involve caretakers and loved ones in the treatment plan, and to also consider if the need for treatment and support extends throughout this network."

Elizabeth, registered nurse working
in the rural United States

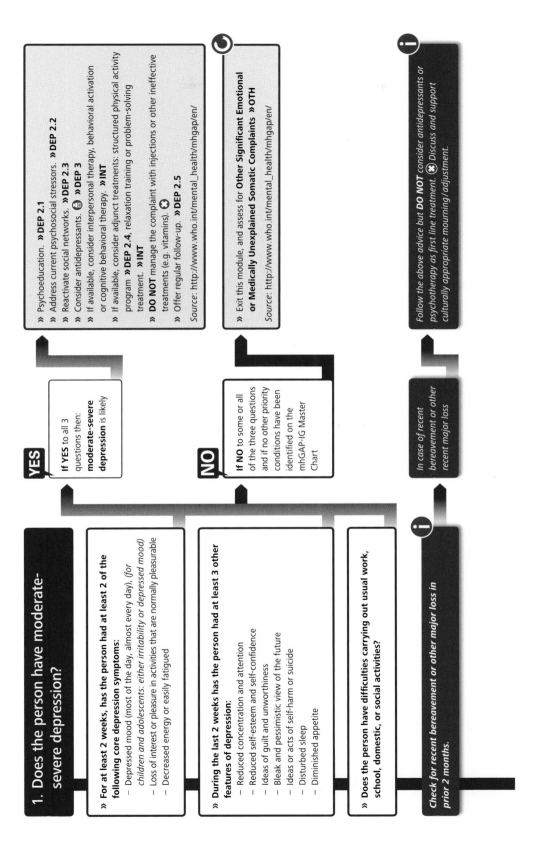

1. Does the person have moderate-severe depression?

» **For at least 2 weeks, has the person had at least 2 of the following core depression symptoms:**
  – Depressed mood (most of the day, almost every day), *(for children and adolescents: either irritability or depressed mood)*
  – Loss of interest or pleasure in activities that are normally pleasurable
  – Decreased energy or easily fatigued

» **During the last 2 weeks has the person had at least 3 other features of depression:**
  – Reduced concentration and attention
  – Reduced self-esteem and self-confidence
  – Ideas of guilt and unworthiness
  – Bleak and pessimistic view of the future
  – Ideas or acts of self-harm or suicide
  – Disturbed sleep
  – Diminished appetite

» **Does the person have difficulties carrying out usual work, school, domestic, or social activities?**

YES

If **YES** to all 3 questions then: **moderate-severe depression** is likely

» Psychoeducation. **»DEP 2.1**
» Address current psychosocial stressors. **»DEP 2.2**
» Reactivate social networks. **»DEP 2.3**
» Consider antidepressants. **»DEP 3**
» If available, consider interpersonal therapy, behavioral activation or cognitive behavioral therapy. **»INT**
» If available, consider adjunct treatments: structured physical activity program **»DEP 2.4**, relaxation training or problem-solving treatment. **»INT**
» **DO NOT** manage the complaint with injections or other ineffective treatments (e.g. vitamins).
» Offer regular follow-up. **»DEP 2.5**

Source: http://www.who.int/mental_health/mhgap/en/

NO

If **NO** to some or all of the three questions and if no other priority conditions have been identified on the mhGAP-IG Master Chart

» Exit this module, and assess for **Other Significant Emotional or Medically Unexplained Somatic Complaints »OTH**

Source: http://www.who.int/mental_health/mhgap/en/

ⓘ **Check for recent bereavement or other major loss in prior 2 months.**

In case of recent bereavement or other recent major loss

ⓘ *Follow the above advice but DO NOT consider antidepressants or psychotherapy as first line treatment. ⊗ Discuss and support culturally appropriate mourning/adjustment.*

Figure 27.1 Assessment and management guide for depression. *Source:* WHO (2010), pp. 10–12. Reproduced with permission of the World Health Organization.

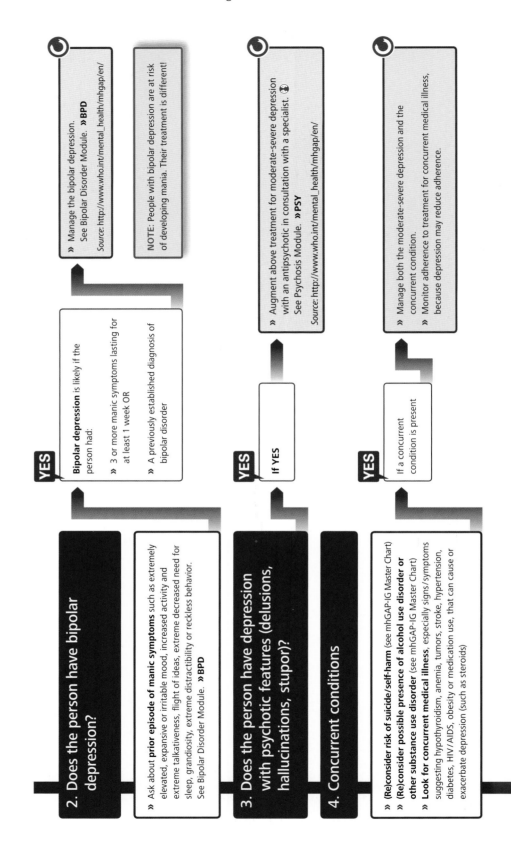

Figure 27.1 *(Continued)*

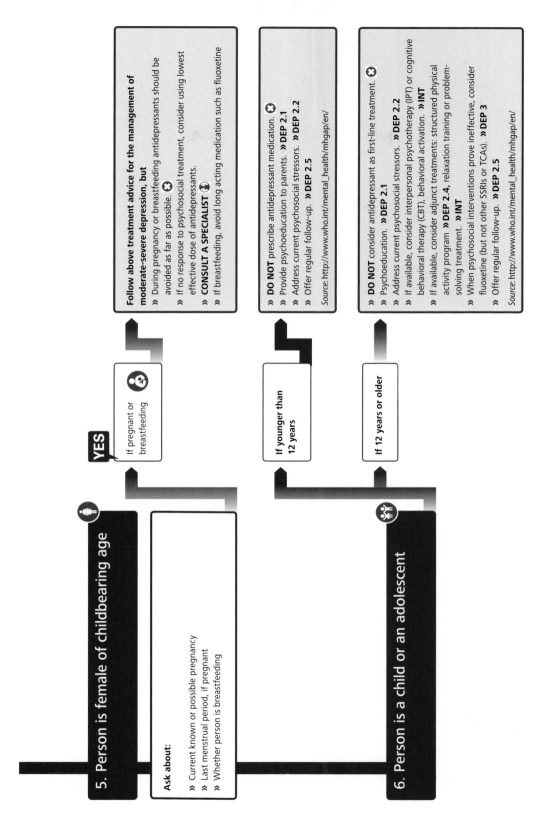

Figure 27.1 (*Continued*)

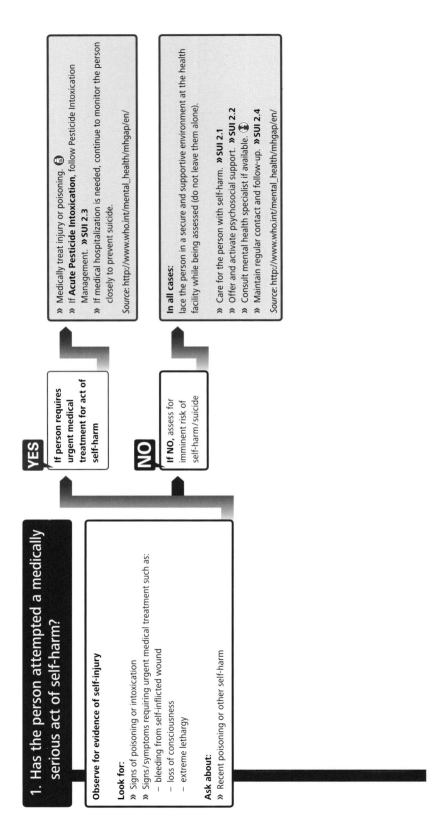

1. Has the person attempted a medically serious act of self-harm?

Observe for evidence of self-injury

Look for:
» Signs of poisoning or intoxication
» Signs/symptoms requiring urgent medical treatment such as:
  – bleeding from self-inflicted wound
  – loss of consciousness
  – extreme lethargy

Ask about:
» Recent poisoning or other self-harm

YES

If person requires urgent medical treatment for act of self-harm

» Medically treat injury or poisoning. 🔵
» If **Acute Pesticide Intoxication**, follow Pesticide Intoxication Management. **» SUI 2.3**
» If medical hospitalization is needed, continue to monitor the person closely to prevent suicide.

Source: http://www.who.int/mental_health/mhgap/en/

NO

If NO, assess for imminent risk of self-harm/suicide

In all cases:
lace the person in a secure and supportive environment at the health facility while being assessed (do not leave them alone).

» Care for the person with self-harm. **» SUI 2.1**
» Offer and activate psychosocial support. **» SUI 2.2**
» Consult mental health specialist if available. 🔵
» Maintain regular contact and follow-up. **» SUI 2.4**

Source: http://www.who.int/mental_health/mhgap/en/

Figure 27.2 Assessment and management guideline for self-harm or suicide. *Source:* WHO (2010), pp. 74–76. Reproduced with permission of the World Health Organization.

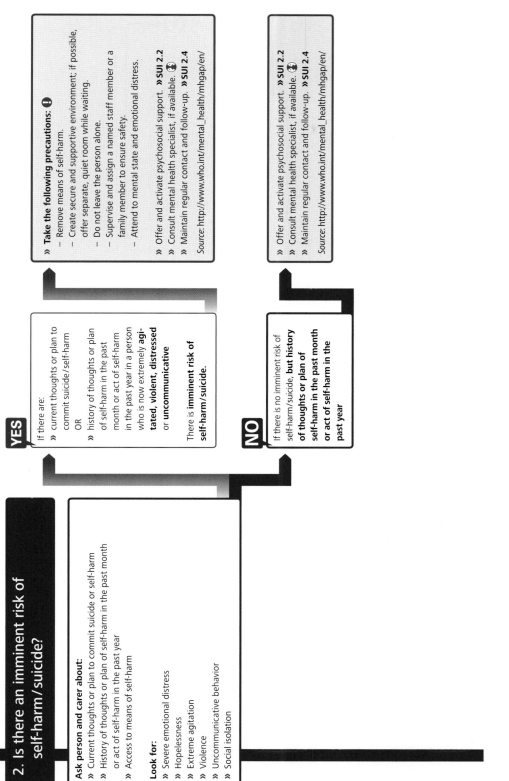

Figure 27.2 (*Continued*)

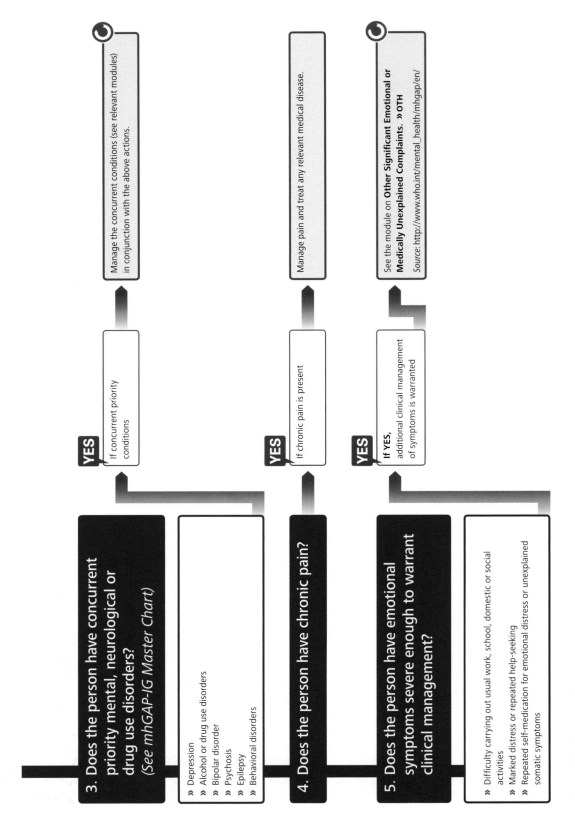

Figure 27.2 (*Continued*)

Box 27.1 Diagnosis of alcohol or drug dependence (Patel, 2002)

The person must have at least two of the following symptoms for at least 1 month:

- Drinking (or drug use) that has led to personal problems such as losing job or health problems such as accidents or jaundice.
- Difficulty in controlling the use of alcohol (or the drug) even though there are problems being caused by its use.
- Alcohol (or the drug) is used throughout the day.
- Feeling sick or unwell unless drinking alcohol (or taking the drug).
- Using gradually increasing amounts of alcohol (or the drug).

Box 27.2 Definitions of alcohol use disorders (WHO, 1992; Saunders et al., 1993; Benegal et al., 2009)

Hazardous use (ICD 10; Z72.1)
A pattern of alcohol consumption that carries with it a risk of harmful consequences to the drinker. These consequences may be damaging to mental or physical health, or social consequences to the drinker or others. Other potential consequences include worsening of existing medical conditions or psychiatric illnesses, injuries caused to self or others due to impaired judgment after drinking, high risk sexual behaviors while intoxicated, and worsening of personal or social interactions.

Hazardous use is often operationalized as an average consumption of 21 drinks or more per week for men and 14 drinks or more per week for women. It is recognized by the WHO as a disorder distinct from other AUDs (Saunders et al., 1993).

Harmful use (ICD 10; F10.1)
A pattern of drinking that is already causing damage to health. The damage may be either physical (e.g., liver damage from chronic drinking) or mental (e.g., depressive episodes secondary to drinking). Harmful patterns of use are often criticized by others and are sometimes associated with adverse social consequences of various kinds. However, the fact that a family or culture disapproves of drinking is not by itself sufficient to justify a diagnosis of harmful use (WHO, 1992; Saunders et al., 1993).

Alcohol dependence (ICD10; F10.2)
A cluster of behavioral, cognitive and physiological phenomena that develop after repeated alcohol use and that typically include a strong desire to take alcohol, difficulties in controlling its use, persisting in its use despite harmful consequences, a higher priority given to alcohol use that to other activities and obligations, increased tolerance, and sometimes a physical withdrawal state (WHO, 1992).

effective (Benegal et al., 2009). Management of AUD involves a stepped-care approach. The first stage involves early detection and brief intervention: exploring reasons for alcohol use, avoiding going to places where alcohol is served, removing alcohol sources from the home. The next level of intervention involves psychosocial approaches to preventing relapse, including structured interventions and self-help groups. The third level of intervention includes pharmacotherapy for detoxification and relapse prevention, which requires specialized input and is the most costly option (Benegal et al., 2009). An important consideration is supporting families and other loved ones of individuals with AUD and exploring social networks and finances (which may either be the cause or be caused by AUD). Additional, more detailed guidance for the management of AUD is provided in mhGAP.

Psychosis

Psychosis is characterized by delusions, such as believing things to be true which are not (e.g., being controlled by outside forces), and/or by hallucinations (e.g., seeing or hearing things that others cannot) (Box 27.3). People with psychosis often have withdrawn disorganized behavior and find it difficult to work, participate in education, or engage with society. Psychotic symptoms are usually terrifying. Management of psychotic illness can be challenging in resource-limited settings. Management includes psychoeducation for individuals, and their families as appropriate, and antipsychotic medication. Key messages of psychoeducation include the ability to recover, importance of maintaining social interaction as much as possible, and that medication taken regularly can alleviate symptoms. Combined interventions that include low doses of conventional antipsychotics in addition to brief and simple psychoeducational interventions have been identified as an important and cost-effective means of closing the treatment

gap for schizophrenia between HICs and LMICs (de Jesus et al., 2009). In some settings, people with psychotic illness are thought to be "possessed." Protecting the human rights of individuals with a psychotic illness may involve educating community leaders around this disease and the potential for treatment. If possible, involve people with psychosis, their families, and community leaders in the design, implementation, and evaluation of interventions (WHO, 2008).

Box 27.3 Psychotic symptoms (WHO, 2010)

- Incoherent or irrelevant speech
- Delusions
- Hallucinations
- Withdrawal, agitation, disorganized behavior
- Beliefs that thoughts are being inserted or broadcast from one's mind
- Social withdrawal and neglect of usual responsibilities related to work, school, domestic or social activities

If multiple symptoms are present, psychosis is likely. The presence of these symptoms for more than 3 months suggests chronic psychosis is likely.

Dementia

Dementia usually occurs in older adults (>60 years) and is characterized by cognitive impairment (orientation, language) and/or memory problems that have been present for at least 6 months, are progressive in nature, and which are associated with impairment in social function (Box 27.4) (WHO, 2008). An assessment of dementia usually involves an interview with a third party or key informant. The primary goals for management of dementia are enhancing physical health, cognition, activity levels, and general well-being; observing and responding to behavioral and psychological symptoms of dementia; and providing appropriate information and long-term support to caregivers. There are a number of interventions available to individuals living with dementia, including psychological, sensory therapy, caregiver-focused interventions, and pharmacological interventions. However, most of the evidence that exists is for the effectiveness of caregiver-focused interventions and pharmacological interventions. The most effective caregiver-focused interventions include psychoeducational interventions, cognitive behavioral therapy counseling, caregiver support, and respite care (Prince *et al.*, 2009). Indications for pharmacological treatment include cognitive impairment, behavioral symptoms (agitation and aggression), and psychological symptoms (depression, anxiety, and psychosis). In these cases, there is a strong evidence base for the efficacy of donepezil, rivastigmine, and galantamine. Haloperidol and atypical antipsychotic drugs are more effective for the treatment of aggression than for the treatment of agitation or behavioral and psychological symptoms of dementia (Prince *et al.*, 2009). Atypical antipsychotic drugs have also been routinely prescribed for psychosis in dementia, but a meta-analysis of their treatment effects indicated that only aripiprazole had a statistically and clinically significant effect. The data on the effectiveness of antidepressants are inconclusive. Finally, rigorous research on anticonvulsants to treat behavioral and psychological symptoms of dementia demonstrate that sodium

---

Box 27.4 Diagnostic criteria for dementia (Prince *et al.*, 2009)

Persons with **mild dementia** have noticed a deterioration in memory for recent events. For example, they may forget that their daughter had visited the previous day. They also find it difficult to concentrate, think flexibly, plan, and take decisions. They are likely to feel bewildered, anxious and sad. They may become angry and defensive when others point out errors.

Persons with **moderate dementia** have severe memory problems. Only early memories are retained. Recent events are not remembered, or rapidly forgotten. They may not know the day, date or time of day. They often do not know where they are. They cannot communicate clearly, having problems finding the right word and using the wrong words. They may hear voices or see things that are not there, and can develop false beliefs, for example that children are entering their house and stealing things. They are likely to be anxious, sad, bewildered, and can become agitated or aggressive.

Persons with **severe dementia** have complete memory loss. They may no longer recognize their close family. They have severe speech difficulties or are unable to communicate. They may be apathetic and totally inactive, but at times can be agitated and verbally and physically aggressive. They cannot coordinate their physical movements, may have lost the ability to walk and feed themselves, and have difficulty swallowing. They are likely to be incontinent.

---

valproate is ineffective and carbamazepine may be more effective.

Complete care should include a number of components, such as information about the diagnosis, routine needs assessments, physical health checks, and caregiver support. If necessary, caregiver training, respite care, and the assessment and treatment of behavioral and psychological symptoms of dementia should be included in the care package. In addition to mhGAP, see Prince *et al.* (2009) for a description of packages of care for those living with dementia in HICs and LMICs.

Seizure disorders

Acute seizure is a medical emergency due to the risk of airway compromise (see Chapter 26 for the acute management of seizures). Chronic seizure disorder, or epilepsy, is a heterogeneous group of chronic conditions resulting in abnormal electrical discharges in the brain. Causes of chronic seizure disorder include genetic, birth trauma, brain injury (infection, tumor, head injury), metabolic, or idiopathic. Not all seizures result in convulsions (uncontrolled movement of the muscles), but convulsive epilepsy is associated with the greatest morbidity, mortality, and stigma (WHO, 2008). Convulsions may be either focal (uncontrolled movement of one body part) or generalized, may include incontinence, and are usually followed by a period of drowsiness. Management principles include education (especially given the social stigma), provision of an acute management plan, and consideration of antiepileptic medication. An acute management plan should provide family members with information on what to do if a seizure occurs: remove the person from danger, place them on their side, do not place anything in their mouth, and call for help. For people with more than two seizures on two different days in the past year, consideration should be given to an anticonvulsant medication. Guidance around antiepileptic medication choice (and their side effects) is provided in mhGAP.

Additional resources

- World Health Organization. Mental Health Gap Action Programme (mhGAP). Available at http://www.who.int/mental_health/mhgap/en/
- Programme for Improving Mental Health Care (PRIME). Available at http://www.prime.uct.ac.za/
- Centre for Public Mental Health. Available at http://www.cpmh.org.za/
- *The Lancet* series on global mental health (2007 and 2011). Available at http://www.thelancet.com/journals/lancet/article/PIIS0140-6736(11)60891-X/fulltext
- Department of Mental Health, World Health Organization. Available at http://www.who.int/mental_health/en/
- Movement for Global Mental Health. Available at http://www.globalmentalhealth.org/
- Grand Challenges Canada Global Mental Health programme. Available at http://www.grandchallenges.ca/grand-challenges/global-mental-health/
- National Institute of Mental Health. Available at http://www.nimh.nih.gov/index.shtml
- Centre for International Mental Health, University of Melbourne. Available at http://cimh.unimelb.edu.au/
- University of Lisbon, Department of Mental Health Masters Programme in Mental Health Policy and Services. Available at http://www.fcm.unl.pt/main/index.php?option=com_content&view=article&id=673&catid=21

REFERENCES

Bass JK, Bornemann TH, Burkey M *et al.* (2012) A United Nations General Assembly Special Session for mental, neurological, and substance use disorders: the time has come. *PLoS Med* 9(1):e1001159.

Benegal V, Chand PK, Obot IS (2009) Packages of care for alcohol use disorders in low- and middle-income countries. *PLoS Med* 6(10):e1000170.

Bloom DE, Cafiero ET, Jané-Llopis E *et al.* (2011) *The global economic burden of non-communicable diseases.* Geneva: World Economic Forum.

de Jesus MJ, Razzouk D, Thara R, Eaton J, Thornicroft G (2009) Packages of care for schizophrenia in low- and middle-income countries. *PLoS Med* 6(10):e1000165.

De Silva MJ, Cooper S, Li HL, Lund C, Patel V (2013) Effect of psychosocial interventions on social functioning in depression and schizophrenia: meta-analysis. *Br J Psychiatry* 202:253–60.

Flisher AJ, Sorsdahl K, Hatherill S, Chehil S (2010) Packages of care for attention-deficit hyperactivity disorder in low- and middle-income countries. *PLoS Med* 7(2):e1000235.

Jané-Llopis E, Barry M, Hosman C, Patel V (2005) Mental health promotion works: a review. *Promot Educ* 12:9–25.

Lund C, De Silva M, Plagerson S *et al.* (2011) Poverty and mental disorders: breaking the cycle in low-income and middle-income countries. *Lancet* 378:1502–14.

MacArthur G (2008) Challenges and priorities for global mental health research in low- and middle-income countries: Symposium report. London: Academy of Medical Sciences. Available at www.acmedsci.ac.uk

Mathers CD, Loncar D (2006) Projections of global mortality and burden of disease from 2002 to 2030. *PLoS Med* 3:e442.

Moussavi S, Chatterji S, Verdes E, Tandon A, Patel V, Ustun B (2007) Depression, chronic diseases, and decrements in health: results from the World Health Surveys. *Lancet* 370:851–8.

Patel V (2002) *Where There is No Psychiatrist: A Mental Health Care Manual.* London: Royal College of Psychiatrists.

Patel V, Prince M (2010) Global mental health: a new global health field comes of age. *JAMA* 303:1976–7.

Patel V, Thornicroft G (2009) Packages of care for mental, neurological, and substance use disorders in low- and middle-income countries. *PLoS Med* 6(10):e1000160.

Patel V, Boyce N, Collins PY, Saxena S, Horton R (2011) A renewed agenda for global mental health. *Lancet* 378:1441–2.

Patel V, Belkin GS, Chockalingam A *et al.* (2013) Grand Challenges: integrating mental health services into priority health care platforms. *PLoS Med* 10(5):e1001448.

Prince M, Patel V, Saxena S *et al.* (2007) Global mental health: no health without mental health. *Lancet* 370:859–77.

Prince MJ, Acosta D, Castro-Costa E, Jackson J, Shaji KS (2009) Packages of care for dementia in low- and middle-income countries. *PLoS Med* 6(11):e1000176.

Raja S, Underhill C, Shrestha P *et al.* (2012) Integrating mental health and development: a case study of the basic needs model in Nepal. *PLoS Med* 9(7): e1001261.

Saunders J, Aasland O, Babor T, de la Fuente J, Grant M (1993) Development of the Alcohol Use Disorders Identification Test (AUDIT): WHO collaborative project on early detection of persons with harmful alcohol consumption: II. *Addiction* 88:791–804.

Shidhaye R, Kermode M (2013) Stigma and discrimination as a barrier to mental health service utilization in India. *Int Health* 5:6–8.

Thornicroft G, Brohan E, Rose D, Sartorius N, Leese M (2009) Global pattern of experienced and anticipated discrimination against people with schizophrenia: a cross-sectional survey. *Lancet* 373:408–15.

Tsai AC, Tomlinson M (2012) Mental health spillovers and the Millennium Development Goals: the case of perinatal depression in Khayelitsha, South Africa. *J Glob Health* 2(1):10302.

Vos T, Flaxman AD, Naghavi M *et al.* (2012) Years lived with disability (YLDs) for 1160 sequelae of 289 diseases and injuries 1990–2010: a systematic analysis for the Global Burden of Disease Study 2010. *Lancet* 380:2163–96.

WHO (1992) *The ICD-10 Classification of Mental and Behavioural Disorders: Clinical Descriptions and Diagnostic Guidelines*. Geneva: World Health Organization.

WHO (2008) mhGAP: Mental Health Gap Action Programme: Scaling up care for mental, neurological and substance use disorders. Available at http://www.who.int/mental_health/mhgap_final_english.pdf

WHO (2010) mhGAP Intervention guide for mental, neurological and substance use disorders in non-specialized health settings. Available at http://www.who.int/mental_health/publications/mhGAP_intervention_guide/en/

CHAPTER 28
Dermatology

Sara Ritchie[1], Brett D. Nelson[2], and Francisco Vega-Lopez[1,3]

[1]University College London Hospitals, London, UK
[2]Harvard Medical School and Massachusetts General Hospital, Boston, MA, USA
[3]National Medical Center, Universidad Nacional Autónoma de México, Mexico City, Mexico

Key learning objectives

- Understand the geographical distribution of infectious agents affecting the skin.
- Be aware of topographical diagnosis in dermatology according to body site affected.
- Learn the descriptive morphological terms of skin lesions.
- Learn the important infectious skin conditions to which the traveller may be at risk.

Abstract

Knowledge of dermatology is important in the practice of global health. Skin problems sometimes affect mortality, but more frequently cause significant morbidity, disfigurement, or disability, which along with stigmatization can disproportionately affect people living in poor or rural areas of the world. Skin problems may be non-infective in nature, or can be infective due to a potentially very wide range of etiological agents, including bacteria, fungi, viruses, rickettsiae, parasites, and ectoparasites. The history is of vital importance, and skills in pattern recognition and lesion recognition are crucial in order to determine the correct diagnosis. Knowledge of global prevalence patterns of disease are also key, as is knowledge of the appropriate investigations to arrange, when available. While treatment options can sometimes be more limited in resource-poor settings, knowledge of appropriate common topical or oral treatments in dermatology is also important.

Key words: dermatology, skin conditions, pyogenic, mycobacterial, fungal, leishmaniasis, schistosomiasis, strongyloides, onchocerciasis, *Loa loa*

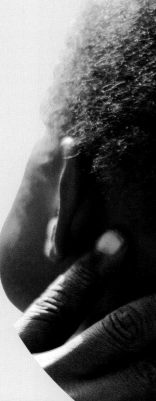

Introduction

Skin disease may represent a primary condition, or be a secondary manifestation of systemic illness, and the history and examination should be directed toward both. Both infective and non-infective etiological conditions need to be considered. In-depth epidemiological knowledge of the global geographical pathology is required in the practice of tropical dermatology. Knowledge of common body sites affected and morphological descriptive terms in dermatology is also important (Figure 28.1).

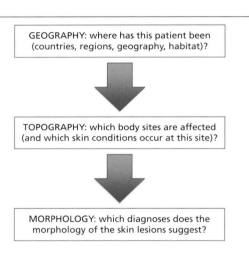

Figure 28.1 Algorithm for developing a dermatological differential diagnosis.

History

Dermatological diagnoses are frequently made from the history and physical examination alone. Laboratory investigations may have less of a role, particularly in resource-limited settings. A thorough history is therefore critical in order to develop an accurate differential diagnosis.

In the history, always consider asking about the following information:

- previous skin disease;
- precipitating factors;
- duration of signs and symptoms;
- evolution of clinical signs;
- medications;
- contact with wild or domestic animals (e.g., in caves);
- contact with fresh or salt water;
- contact with soil (e.g., tree planting);
- symptoms in relatives or household contacts;
- an assessment of the patient's immune status;
- countries and regions of residence or travel;
- occupation and hobbies.

Examination and morphology of skin lesions

A general physical examination is often required, including checks for extracutaneous signs such as fever, enlarged lymph nodes, and hepatosplenomegaly. Examination of hair, nails, buccal (cheek) mucosa, and the skin of the genital area may also be required. An ability to accurately describe skin lesions is an essential step which may often help lead to a diagnosis. The number, type, and distribution of all skin lesions should be observed. Some morphological types of skin lesions, together with common general and tropical examples, are shown in Table 28.1.

Distribution and characteristic patterns of skin lesions

Certain skin diseases have a predilection for manifestation on specific sites on the human body. Knowledge of common body sites affected and characteristic patterns may assist in determining a diagnosis. Figure 28.2 outlines topographical, or regional, diagnoses in dermatology, with examples of both general and tropical skin conditions common at each body site.

Skin problems can be due to bacteria, fungi, parasites, or viruses, and the suspected cause will determine which investigations to take and to which laboratories you will need to send each sample. Knowledge of the possible types of infecting organisms is therefore important. An introductory guide to some of the infectious causes of skin conditions in low- or middle-income countries is outlined in the following sections; however, for a more comprehensive list a textbook of tropical dermatology should be consulted.

Bacterial infections

Pyogenic infections

Pyogenic infections are purulent bacterial infections, or bacterial infections that produce pus. Most pyogenic skin infections are painful and the diagnosis is often clinical. The appearance of pyogenic infections ranges through impetigo with typical golden crust, folliculitis with pustules centered around hair follicles, and furunculosis or boils. At the more

Table 28.1 Nomenclature for description of skin lesions.

Morphology	Definition	Common examples
Macule	Flat blanching spot <1 cm which can be of any color	Infections Drug rashes
Papule	Small raised lump <1 cm in size	Papular urticaria Scabies Lichen planus
Pustule	A papule containing pus	Folliculitis Tinea Pustular psoriasis
Furuncle (abscess)	A boil >1 cm containing pus	Pyogenic Myiasis Trypanosomal chancre
Petechiae	Flat spots <1 cm which do not blanch with pressure and are purplish in color	Idiopathic thrombocytopenic purpura Vasculitis (e.g., Henoch–Schönlein purpura) Rickettsial infection Dengue
Patch	Flat lesions >1 cm which can be of any color	Eczema Tinea
Plaque	Flat-topped raised area >1 cm in size	Psoriasis (silvery scale) Lichen planus Sarcoidosis
Nodule	Solid lump >1 cm in size	Nodular prurigo Sarcoidosis Secondary syphilis Deep fungal infection Cutaneous tuberculosis Cutaneous leishmaniasis Malignancy
Eschar	Nodule with necrotic center	Tick typhus Lyme disease
Wheal (hives)	Raised areas of dermal edema which are transitory, resolving within 24 hours	Urticaria Strongyloidiasis *Loa loa* Gnathostomiasis
Erosion	Superficial area of partial loss of epidermis <1 cm	Pemphigus Porphyria cutanea tarda
Ulcer	Deeper area of broken skin with full loss of epidermis and some dermis >1 cm	Pyogenic Vasculitic Autoimmune Leishmaniasis Pyoderma gangrenosum Malignancy
Vesicle	Blister <1 cm containing clear fluid	Herpes simplex virus Pompholyx
Bulla	Blister >1 cm containing clear fluid	Bullous impetigo Bullous pemphigoid

(Continued)

Table 28.1 Nomenclature for description of skin lesions. (*Continued*)

Morphology	Definition	Common examples
Linear lesion	Lesion usually >1 cm which has appearance of a straight line	Lichen striatus Phytophotodermatitis Dermatitis artefacta
Serpiginous track	Wiggly, wavy, creeping line	Cutaneous larva migrans
Annular lesion	Ring-shaped lesion	Tinea Granuloma annulare Sarcoid Leprosy Syphilis Annular erythema
Circinate lesion	Arc-shaped lesion	Tinea Jessner lymphocytic infiltrate Erythema elevatum diutinum
Targetoid	Target-shaped lesions	Erythema multiforme
Lichenoid	A descriptive term to indicate a thickened or raised lesion with a shiny or rough appearance	Lichen planus Eczema
Lupoid	A specific descriptive term to indicate a shiny area	Lupoid leishmaniasis Lupoid tuberculosis Sarcoidosis
Hypopigmentation	Partial loss of pigment	Pityriasis versicolor Pityriasis alba Sarcoidosis Leprosy

severe end of the spectrum, pyogenic infections can cause cellulitis with well-demarcated sheets of erythema or necrotic ulceration of the skin. Bacteriological swabs with antibiotic sensitivity profile should be requested, if available. Mild infections are successfully treated with bathing or soaking the affected skin in potassium permanganate solution (1:10,000 dilution in water). Mild superficial infections respond well to antiseptic creams and ointments containing cetrimide, chlorhexidine, fusidic acid, or mupirocin. More severe infections require systemic β-lactam or macrolide antibiotics, such as a flucloxacillin, erythromycin, or clarithromycin. Recurrent infections may require an antimicrobial soap substitute and screening and eradication of methicillin-resistant *Staphylococcus aureus* (MRSA). Panton–Valentine leukocidin (PVL) is a particularly virulent toxin produced by some species of *Staphylococcus aureus*. Testing for this, if available, should be requested in severe, poorly responsive, or recurrent skin infections. PVL-MRSA may require dual therapy including rifampicin. Necrotizing soft tissue infections can have a high mortality and pose one of the few dermatological emergencies, with early diagnosis being crucial (Demos *et al.*, 2012).

Treponemal infections

Treponemes are a genus of bacterial spirochete infections that include venereal syphilis, non-venereal endemic syphilis, yaws, and pinta. Primary syphilis presents up to 3 months after infection and typically manifests with a single painless chancre around the genitals, mouth, rectum, or other skin. Secondary syphilis can present up to 6 months after infection with a generalized erythematous maculopapular rash. These lesions may evolve into nodules or plaques. Annular or circinate lesions may be seen. The mucous membranes are often involved, and there is frequently palmoplantar involvement (Figure 28.3). HIV seroconversion should also be considered in the differential diagnosis of secondary syphilis. Tertiary, or late, syphilis can occur 3–15 years after initial infection and can produce noduloulcerative lesions and gummas, or soft rubbery granulomas, which can be mistaken for cutaneous tuberculosis, leishmaniasis, deep fungal infection, or psoriasis. Primary syphilis can be diagnosed by darkfield microscopy of a chancre (specimen or fluid). Secondary or late syphilis is confirmed by serology. All the treponemal infections cause positive serology, which may be indistinguishable from syphilis. The treatment

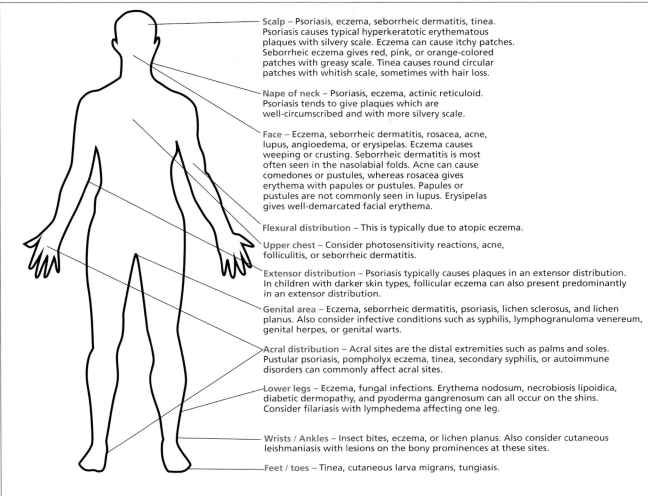

Scalp – Psoriasis, eczema, seborrheic dermatitis, tinea. Psoriasis causes typical hyperkeratotic erythematous plaques with silvery scale. Eczema can cause itchy patches. Seborrheic eczema gives red, pink, or orange-colored patches with greasy scale. Tinea causes round circular patches with whitish scale, sometimes with hair loss.

Nape of neck – Psoriasis, eczema, actinic reticuloid. Psoriasis tends to give plaques which are well-circumscribed and with more silvery scale.

Face – Eczema, seborrheic dermatitis, rosacea, acne, lupus, angioedema, or erysipelas. Eczema causes weeping or crusting. Seborrheic dermatitis is most often seen in the nasolabial folds. Acne can cause comedones or pustules, whereas rosacea gives erythema with papules or pustules. Papules or pustules are not commonly seen in lupus. Erysipelas gives well-demarcated facial erythema.

Flexural distribution – This is typically due to atopic eczema.

Upper chest – Consider photosensitivity reactions, acne, folliculitis, or seborrheic dermatitis.

Extensor distribution – Psoriasis typically causes plaques in an extensor distribution. In children with darker skin types, follicular eczema can also present predominantly in an extensor distribution.

Genital area – Eczema, seborrheic dermatitis, psoriasis, lichen sclerosus, and lichen planus. Also consider infective conditions such as syphilis, lymphogranuloma venereum, genital herpes, or genital warts.

Acral distribution – Acral sites are the distal extremities such as palms and soles. Pustular psoriasis, pompholyx eczema, tinea, secondary syphilis, or autoimmune disorders can commonly affect acral sites.

Lower legs – Eczema, fungal infections. Erythema nodosum, necrobiosis lipoidica, diabetic dermopathy, and pyoderma gangrenosum can all occur on the shins. Consider filariasis with lymphedema affecting one leg.

Wrists / Ankles – Insect bites, eczema, or lichen planus. Also consider cutaneous leishmaniasis with lesions on the bony prominences at these sites.

Feet / toes – Tinea, cutaneous larva migrans, tungiasis.

Figure 28.2 Typical locations of various dermatologic conditions.

of choice is penicillin, and allergic individuals respond to tetracyclines or erythromycin.

Mycobacterial infections

Cutaneous tuberculosis should be considered in patients from endemic areas. The clinical appearance of the skin lesions depends on the route of entry of the organism and the immune status of the patient. In lupus vulgaris, there is direct extension of underlying tuberculous foci causing crusted or scaly plaques or ulcers, often on the face, nose, or ears. Sarcoidosis or discoid lupus erythematosus may need to be considered in the differential of lupus vulgaris. Scrofuloderma is breakdown of the skin directly overlying tuberculosis-infected lymph nodes (Figure 28.4). Atypical mycobacterial skin infection should be considered in ecthyma (crusted pyogenic ulcers) that is suppurating or ulcerative and is unresponsive to penicillins or second-generation macrolides. Mycobacterial infection should

also be considered with a history of keeping tropical fish or after injury or abrasion of the skin from coral.

If mycobacterial infection is suspected, skin biopsies should be taken for histology and microbiology. Histology may show caseating granulomas. Culture is the gold-standard investigation, but can take a number of weeks to become positive and has low sensitivity in paucibacillary cases. Polymerase chain reaction (PCR) may be more sensitive, although PCR, microscopy, and culture can each be negative (Abdalla *et al.*, 2009). In the context of strong clinical suspicion, a trial of antituberculous therapy may be considered. All forms of skin tuberculosis respond to standard WHO antituberculosis regimens with four drugs for 2 months, followed by dual therapy for 4 months. Atypical mycobacteria should be treated with at least two antituberculous drugs.

Leprosy should be considered in individuals with a history of living for several years in endemic areas. Leprosy can affect the skin and peripheral nerves. Clinical features on the skin are

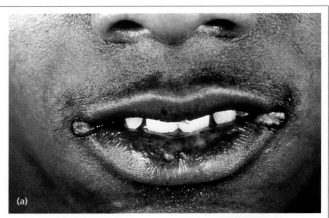

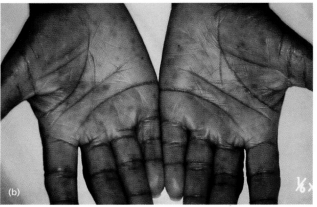

Figure 28.3 Secondary sphyilitic lesions. Secondary syphilis can present as mucous membrane lesions, like those located at the labial commissures (a), or as a maculopapular rash with frequent palmoplantar distribution (b). *Source*: (a) CDC Public Health Image Library/R. Sumpter; (b) CDC Public Health Image Library/M.F. Rein.

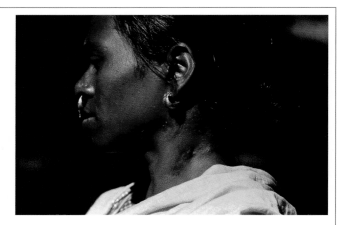

Figure 28.4 A young woman in Pakistan with a scrofulodermal scar resulting from the breakdown of skin directly overlying tuberculosis-infected lymph nodes. *Source*: CDC Public Health Image Library.

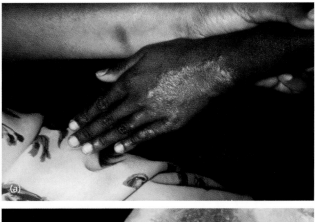

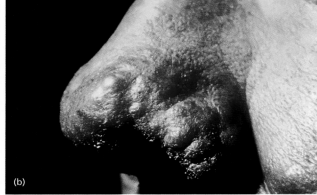

Figure 28.5 Examples of paucibacillary (a) and multibacillary (b) forms of leprosy. *Source*: (a) CDC Public Health Image Library/ A.J. Lebrun; (b) CDC Public Health Image Library/A.E. Kaye.

determined by the host immune response. In paucibacillary leprosy (those with a low bacterial burden), up to four skin lesions may be apparent clinically, which are usually flat, dyschromic, and anesthetic or insensitive to touch (Figure 28.5a). Bacilli may not be seen on slit-skin smear in paucibacillary leprosy. However, in multibacillary leprosy (those with a high bacillary burden), skin lesions may be diffuse, quite pronounced, or even nodular (Figure 28.5b), and nerve damage occurs late, giving lesions that may be only slightly anesthetic but which may eventually cause a glove-and-stocking anesthesia. In the case of multibacillary leprosy, bacilli are usually seen on microscopy. The patient should also be examined for signs of nerve damage and for signs of reversal reactions (immunologically mediated episodes of acute or subacute inflammation). The patient may be in reversal at diagnosis, which would be suggested by erythema or edema in the skin lesions, or by nerve tenderness. The investigation of choice is slit-skin smear to look for acid-fast bacilli. Biopsy may show granulomas. PCR is very sensitive. The World Health Organization (WHO) recommends a two-drug regimen for paucibacillary leprosy, and a three-drug regimen for multibacillary leprosy. If the patient is in reaction, they are at risk of rapid loss of nerve function and require urgent oral steroids. In HIV co-infection, relapse rates of leprosy appear unchanged; however, leprosy may begin as part of immune reconstitution, and these patients appear to be at increased risk of reactions (Ustianowski *et al.*, 2006).

Fungal infections

Superficial fungal infection

Superficial fungal infection can be caused by dermatophytes or *Malassezia*. Dermatophyte infections, or ringworm, may manifest as single or multiple coalescing circinate or annular plaques with erythema and variable degrees of scaling. Scalp infections in children can manifest with the kerion clinical form with patches of non-scarring alopecia and boggy inflammation of the skin. The symbiotic yeast *Malassezia* can cause a superficial infection called pityriasis versicolor, which is characterized by small coalescing patches or plaques showing hyperpigmentation or hypopigmentation. These diagnoses are usually clinical. Granuloma annulare or discoid eczema should be considered in the differential. Dermatophytes respond to triazole compounds, such as fluconazole, and allylamines, such as terbinafine or griseofulvin. Localized infections require topical therapy for 3–8 weeks. Oral antifungals are indicated in severe or disseminated skin infections, tinea capitis, and onychomycosis (fungal nail infection). Tinea capitis in children requires oral terbinafine (or griseofulvin) 15–20 mg/kg for 6–8 weeks. Pityriasis versicolor responds to topical selenium sulfur shampoo or the azole antifungals.

Subcutaneous fungal infection

Sporotrichosis is a worldwide fungal infection that can occur after exposure to abrasions from thorns or splinters. It classically disseminates into proximal satellite lesions via the lymphatic system, called sporotrichoid spread. The differential diagnosis of this pattern includes atypical mycobacteria or cutaneous leishmaniasis, and skin biopsies should be taken for each appropriate laboratory. Definitive diagnosis of sporotrichosis is based on identification in culture. Microscopy, histopathology, or serology, if available, may enable an earlier presumptive diagnosis (Bastos de Lima Barros *et al.*, 2011).

Mycetoma, or madura foot, comprises a clinical triad of a subcutaneous mass, sinus tract formation, and granular discharge affecting particularly one foot (Figure 28.6). It includes both fungal eumycetoma and bacterial actinomycetoma and can occur within the "mycetoma belt" (15° S to 30° N of the equator). The infection is acquired by direct inoculation, and local agricultural workers are at highest risk. Correct species identification is important for management, using deep-tissue biopsy, cultures, serology, or PCR. Radiography, ultrasound, CT, or MRI may detect underlying bone involvement. Antimicrobial or surgical therapy is usually protracted (Ameen & Arenas, 2008a,b).

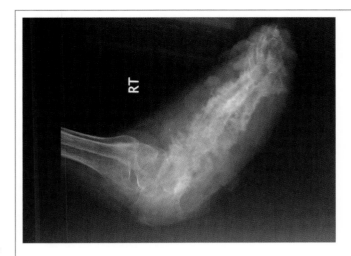

Figure 28.6 A radiograph image showing extensive subcutaneous fungal infection in madura foot. *Source*: Wikimedia © Haitham Alfalah. Reproduced under the Creative Commons license.

Deep fungal infection

A number of fungi can cause deep infection of the skin, including coccidioidomycosis, paracoccidioidomycosis, and histoplasmosis. These infections pose a particularly high risk in the context of immunosuppression. Coccidioidomycosis is acquired through inhalation of infective spores in subtropical desert regions of the world, most commonly in urban areas of the Americas. The skin becomes involved in a small proportion of cases, and lesions manifest as erythematous, verrucous (wart-like), scarring, or scaling nodules. Paracoccidioidomycosis occurs only on the American continent, particularly in Mexico and Central and South America. It predominantly affects male agricultural workers in rural rainforest areas. Infection is via inhalation or direct inoculation into the skin. It may present many years after an individual has left an endemic region, with painful nodular, hemorrhagic, ulcerated, or verrucous lesions. The skin is affected in the majority of cases, although it is also a systemic disease that can affect the pulmonary, endocrine, or neurological system. In addition to skin biopsies, a chest radiograph and lumbar puncture are necessary in all cases. A history of tree planting should be sought in tropical regions. Exposure to bat or bird droppings may pose a risk of histoplasmosis in caves or abandoned mines. Treatment requires specialist doctors in dermatology or infectious diseases if available.

Parasitic and ectoparasitic infections

Cutaneous larva migrans, tungiasis, myiasis, and scabies

Cutaneous larva migrans results from the accidental penetration of the human skin by hookworm larvae. It is a common worldwide infection that can occur after barefoot contact with infected sand or soil. It causes a creeping, erythematous, serpiginous larval track that moves at the rate of 1–2 cm/day, and the diagnosis is clinical (see Chapter 36, Figure 36.3). Treatment is with albendazole 400–800 mg (according to body weight) daily for 3 days or ivermectin 200 μg/kg one-time dose. Tungiasis, or skin infection by the sandflea, commonly affects one foot and is caused by the burrowing flea *Tunga penetrans*. The fleas usually penetrate the soft skin of the toe-web spaces. A cratered single nodule develops with a central hemorrhagic punctum. Cryotherapy, curettage, surgical excision, or application of petroleum jelly and then careful removal of the flea and eggs with a sterile needle are curative. Several worldwide fly larvae are also capable of colonizing the human skin, causing myiasis that can manifest as boils. The treatment of choice for myiasis is the mechanical removal or surgical excision of the larvae. Lesions can be covered by petroleum jelly to suffocate the larvae, which can subsequently be extracted via a cruciform incision. Scabies should be considered in any individual with an intensely itchy papular eruption. The itch is usually worse at night, and typically causes papules in the skin folds, including the fingerwebs, wrists, axillae, umbilicus, and buttocks. The diagnosis is usually clinical, with skin scrapings having low sensitivity, although dermoscopy may be a useful confirmatory tool. Treatment for scabies is with 5% topical permethrin or oral ivermectin.

Ticks

Infections transmitted by ticks include spotted fever, tick typhus, relapsing fever, and Lyme disease, among others. Ticks should be removed carefully with very fine forceps held as close to the skin as possible. Delay in removal increases the risk of transmission of infectious agents. The bite characteristically produces an eschar, or the expanding targetoid erythema migrans rash of Lyme disease. It is also important to consider rickettsial infection in any person returning from an African game park who has a febrile illness with a petechial or maculopapular rash. Empirical antibiotic therapy should be started early before awaiting confirmation of diagnosis if rickettsial infection is suspected or on diagnosing erythema migrans. The drugs of choice for treatment of rickettsial infection are doxycycline (100 mg twice daily by mouth) or tetracycline (500 mg four times daily by mouth). The duration of antibiotic therapy for Lyme disease is 2 weeks and for rickettsiae is related to clinical response, being continued for at least 3 days after the patient becomes afebrile to prevent recrudescence (Parola *et al.*, 2005).

Cutaneous leishmaniasis

Cutaneous leishmaniasis should be considered in anyone who has been to a country of endemicity who presents with slowly progressive skin lesions unresponsive to antibiotics. The protozoa are transmitted by sandflies and the disease is endemic in 88 countries, including all those bordering the Mediterranean.

The incubation period can be as short as 15 days but is more commonly 4–8 weeks. Clinical manifestations include nodules covered with crust or ulceration with a raised border (see Chapter 20, Figure 20.5a). The differential diagnosis of infections with lymphocutaneous sporotrichoid spread includes atypical mycobacterial infection or subcutaneous fungal infection. Classification of cutaneous leishmaniasis in geographical terms as "Old World" (eastern hemisphere) or "New World" (western hemisphere) is important to guide diagnosis and treatment. The infecting species must be determined in order to guide choice of treatment. Where available, investigation includes skin biopsies for histology to look for granulomas, direct microscopy with Giemsa stain to reveal intracellular amastigotes, culture in Novy–MacNeal–Nicolle (NNN) medium, and genetic analysis by PCR techniques (Goto & Lindoso, 2010). Antimonials, such as sodium stibogluconate and meglumine antimoniate, are the first-line treatment and can be injected intralesionally at weekly intervals for many Old World infections. Severe, mucosal, or New World infections may need parenteral treatment. In HIV co-infection, leishmaniasis can present atypically, be more severe, or may present as immune reconstitution. Immune response to treatment in HIV-positive patients depends on an adequate CD4 count, and amphotericin B may be more efficacious than antimonials or pentamidine, which both depend on T-cell response (Ameen, 2010).

Schistosomiasis

Consider swimmer's itch (or cercarial dermatitis) in any person who develops even a mild itchy papular rash (Figure 28.7) soon after swimming in a freshwater lake in endemic countries. Cercarial dermatitis is caused by penetration of the skin by the free-living larval stages of the helminth *Schistosoma*, which lives part of its life cycle in freshwater snails. The dermatitis occurs within hours of infection, resolves within 10 days, and is a

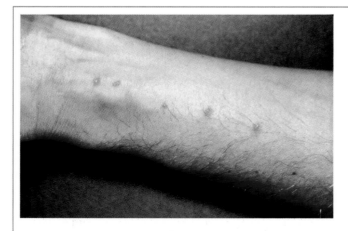

Figure 28.7 Cercarial dermatitis, or "swimmer's itch," as a result of acute schistosomiasis infection. *Source*: CDC Public Health Image Library.

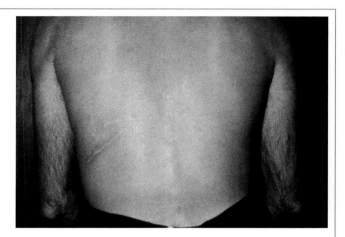

Figure 28.8 Larva currens rash in strongyloidiasis. *Source*: CDC Public Health Image Library.

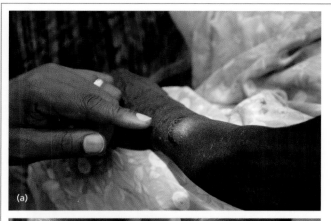

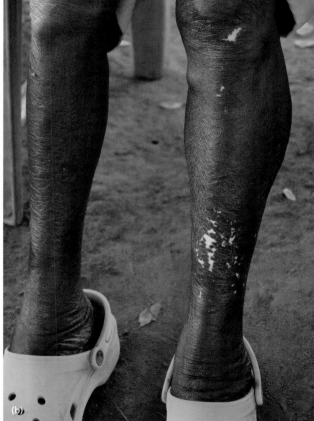

Figure 28.9 Dermatological findings among individuals in South Sudan with onchocerciasis. These lesions include fibrotic nodules called onchocercomata (a) and skin lichenification and "leopard skin"-like dyschromia (b). *Source*: D. Harris, Baltimore, 2012. Reproduced with permission of D. Harris.

clinical diagnosis. Schistosomiasis occurs in sub-Saharan Africa, Southeast Asia, and also parts of Brazil and Venezuela. At this stage serology may be negative, and in addition urine and stool may also be negative in the first 8 weeks after infection. Screening serology can take up to 3 months to become positive. Treatment with praziquantel, because it is effective against adult worms but not larvae, should be given 3 months after the last exposure.

Other parasitic infections

Strongyloidiasis is a common worldwide helminth infection transmitted via skin contact with infected soil or sand. It can present with the typically fast-moving rash of larva currens (Figure 28.8), which travels at several centimeters per hour, or as recurrent urticaria. It is diagnosed serologically and can be treated with the anthelminthic ivermectin as a single dose of 200 μg/kg body weight (or multiple doses in the context of immunosuppression). Ivermectin should be avoided during pregnancy.

Onchocerciasis is a filarial helminth endemic across equatorial Africa, Yemen, and Central and South America, although it may currently be approaching elimination in Latin America. Known as river blindness, it can also have chronic dermatological manifestations. Following an incubation period of approximately 1 year, the adult worms live freely in the skin or within fibrotic nodules called onchocercomata (Figure 28.9a). Skin lesions can also present with lichenification and dyschromia (hyper- and hypo-pigmentation) (Figure 28.9b). Most patients develop peripheral eosinophilia. Diagnosis by microscopy for microfilariae from skin snips taken from the back, hips, and thighs is less useful for early infections and has lower sensitivity than newer biochemical methods such as skin-snip PCR, serology, and antigen dipstick tests (Stingl, 2009).

Loa loa is a filarial helminth transmitted by the *Chrysops* fly, which is only found in West Africa. Symptoms may not appear until several years after the patient has left an area of endemicity. As the larvae mature, they migrate away from the bite site around the body in the subcutaneous tissues or deep fascial layers and periodically produce transient, itchy, nontender, edematous lumps called Calabar swellings (Figure 28.10a). These swellings can last between a few hours to a few

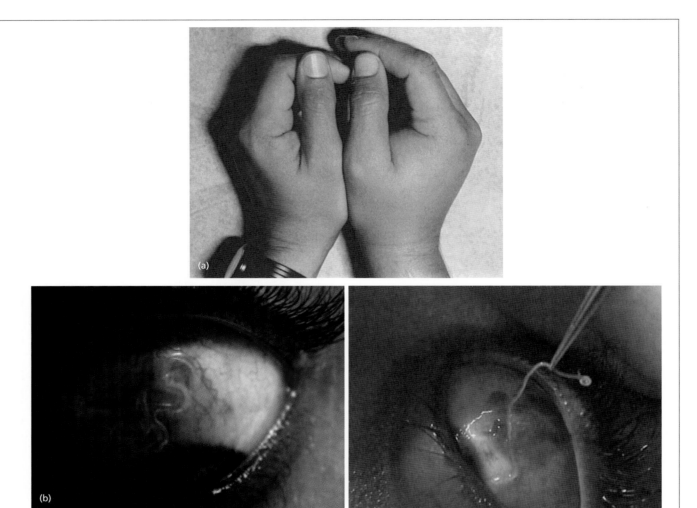

Figure 28.10 *Loa loa* can present as transient Calabar swelling (a, on right hand) as well as visible migration of the worm across the conjunctiva (b). *Source*: (a) Guerrant *et al.* (1999), reproduced with permission of Elsevier; (b) reprinted from *Eye* 25, 389–391 by permission from Macmillan Publishers Ltd, copyright 2011, figures 1 and 2, p. 390.

days. Visible migration of the worms across the conjunctiva is pathognomonic (Figure 28.10b). The eosinophil count may be normal initially. Diagnosis can be made by microscopy for microfilariae on a blood smear collected around midday or by PCR (Boussinesq, 2006).

Viral skin infections

Viral infections that are prevalent globally include molluscum contagiosum in children, the wart virus, and herpesviruses. In an infected individual, herpes simplex virus (HSV) can cause grouped vesicles at any site of skin injury, which can subsequently intermittently recur at this same site. Varicella zoster virus should be considered with blisters in a dermatomal distribution. Patients with HIV infection commonly suffer from a variety of skin conditions. With the advent of highly active

antiretroviral therapy, there has been a change in the common skin conditions seen from infective to inflammatory. These HIV-related skin conditions include pruritus, xerosis (dry skin), eczema, seborrheic dermatitis, folliculitis, pruritic papular eruption, recalcitrant viral warts, psoriasis, pityriasis rubra pilaris, granuloma annulare, erythema elevatum diutinum, alopecia, photosensitivity, and non-melanoma skin cancer. The frequency and number of infectious skin disorders increase with progressing AIDS-established illness to include cytomegalovirus, severe dermatophyte infections, cutaneous cryptococcosis, and Kaposi sarcoma.

Conclusion

Skin conditions are often neglected in resource-limited settings, but are common and can cause significant morbidity, which can cause disability, stigmatization, and can affect livelihood. Skin conditions can be due to non-infective causes, infective causes, or can be a manifestation of systemic disease.

Additional resources

- Tyring SK, Lupi O, Hengge UR (2005) *Tropical Dermatology*. Oxford: Churchill Livingstone.

REFERENCES

Abdalla CMZ, Prado de Oliveira ZN, Sotto MN, Leite KRM, Canavez FC, Muraro de Carvalho C (2009) Polymerase chain reaction compared to other laboratory findings and to clinical evaluation in the diagnosis of cutaneous tuberculosis and atypical mycobacteria skin infection. *Int J Dermatol* 48:27–35.

Ameen M (2010) Cutaneous and mucocutaneous leishmaniasis: emerging therapies and progress in disease management. *Expert Opin Pharmacother* 11:557–69.

Ameen M, Arenas R (2008a) Emerging therapeutic regimes for the management of mycetomas. *Expert Opin Pharmacother* 9:2077–85.

Ameen M, Arenas R (2008b) Developments in the management of mycetomas. *Clin Exp Dermatol* 34:1–7.

Bastos de Lima Barros M, de Almeida Paes R, Schubach AO (2011) *Sporothrix schenckii* and sporotrichosis. *Clin Microbiol Rev* 24:633–54.

Boussinesq M (2006) Loiasis. *Ann Trop Med Parasitol* 100:715–31.

Demos M, McLeod MP, Nouri K (2012) Recurrent furunculosis: a review of the literature. *Br J Dermatol* 167:725–32.

Goto H, Lindoso JAL (2010) Current diagnosis and treatment of cutaneous and mucocutaneous leishmaniasis. *Expert Rev Anti Infect Ther* 8:419–33.

Guerrant RL, Walker DH, Weller PF (eds) (1999) *Tropical Infectious Diseases*. Philadelphia: Churchill Livingstone.

Parola P, Paddock CD, Raoult D (2005) Tick-borne rickettsioses around the world: emerging diseases challenging old concepts. *Clin Microbiol Rev* 18:719–56.

Stingl P (2009) Onchocerciasis: developments in diagnosis, treatment and control. *Int J Dermatol* 48:393–6.

Ustianowski A, Lawn SD, Lockwood DN (2006) Interactions between leprosy and HIV: a paradox. *Lancet Infect Dis* 6:350–60.

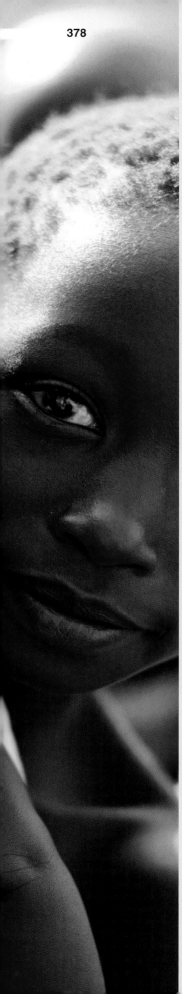

CHAPTER 29
Oral Health

Brittany A. Seymour[1,2] and Lisa E. Simon[1,3]
[1]Harvard School of Dental Medicine, Boston, MA, USA
[2]Harvard Global Health Institute, Boston, MA, USA
[3]Cambridge Health Alliance, Boston, MA, USA

Key learning objectives

- Recognize normal oral landmarks and anatomy and distinguish from abnormal.
- Learn how to assist patients in proper oral hygiene, nutrition, and prevention of common oral conditions.
- Learn how to identify, screen for, triage, and treat common oral conditions, particularly in resource-limited settings.
- Learn how to recognize early oral manifestations of common systemic conditions in low-income regions of the world.

Abstract

Oral diseases are the most common chronic diseases worldwide, inhibiting adequate nutritional intake and growth in children and negatively impacting the general well-being of most populations worldwide. This chapter assists healthcare practitioners in how to recognize and distinguish normal oral landmarks and anatomy from abnormal. Readers will learn how to assist patients in proper oral hygiene, nutrition, and prevention of common oral conditions. Additionally, the chapter addresses how to identify, screen for, triage, and treat common oral conditions, particularly in resource-limited settings. Finally, readers will learn how to recognize associations and early oral manifestations of common systemic conditions in low-income regions of the world.

Key words: global oral health, dental caries, periodontal disease, oral hygiene, oral disease prevention, common oral conditions, oral manifestations, oral systemic connection

Essential Clinical Global Health, First Edition. Edited by Brett D. Nelson.
© 2015 John Wiley & Sons, Ltd. Published 2015 by John Wiley & Sons, Ltd.
Companion website: www.essentialseries.com/globalhealth

Introduction

Oral diseases are the most common chronic diseases worldwide, inhibiting adequate nutritional intake and growth in children and negatively impacting the general well-being of most populations worldwide. Many known links exist between oral and other systemic diseases, including shared common risk factors such as poor diet, stress, lack of clean water, poor sanitation, tobacco, and alcohol abuse (Petersen, 2003; Petersen *et al.*, 2005a,b; Sheiham, 2005; Watt, 2005). Following the United Nations Summit on Non-Communicable Diseases, oral diseases were formally recognized by a UN Resolution as a public health problem that poses a major health burden on many countries (Benzian *et al.*, 2012). The Global Burden of Diseases, Injuries, and Risk Factors Study 2010, recognized as the most comprehensive effort since the last global survey in 1990, highlighted oral diseases among the top 50 most prevalent non-fatal but disabling conditions in the world (Vos *et al.*, 2012). Growing awareness is important in understanding these neglected yet highly prominent health challenges that are inhibiting school performance and attendance, improved health, and economic development in many low- and middle-income countries around the world. By recognizing normal oral landmarks and anatomy and distinguishing normal from abnormal, health practitioners can assist in early detection and even avoidance of these highly preventable conditions.

Pediatric and adult tooth numbers and normal oral anatomy

Children have 20 primary teeth, also known as deciduous teeth but often called "baby teeth." Each of these teeth is identified by a letter of the alphabet (A–T). Adults typically have 32 permanent teeth, and each adult tooth is numbered 1–32 (Figure 29.1). Teeth consist of three layers: (i) the enamel on the crown or cementum on the roots, (ii) the dentin, and (iii) the pulp where the nerve and blood supply are housed (Figure 29.2). The periodontal ligament attaches each tooth to either the mandible or the maxillary bone. The last row of molars in adult dentition are the third molars, often referred to as "wisdom teeth;" it is not uncommon for a person to experience impaction, partial eruption, or to be completely missing one or more third molars. Mixed dentition occurs during childhood and adolescence, when the primary teeth are exfoliated and the permanent teeth erupt. Table 29.1 illustrates normal exfoliation and eruption patterns of the primary and adult dentition. It should be noted that normal oral anatomy includes not only the teeth but also the maxilla and mandible (upper and lower jaw bones), muscles of mastication (chewing), hard and soft palate, uvula, tonsils, and the lining of the throat.

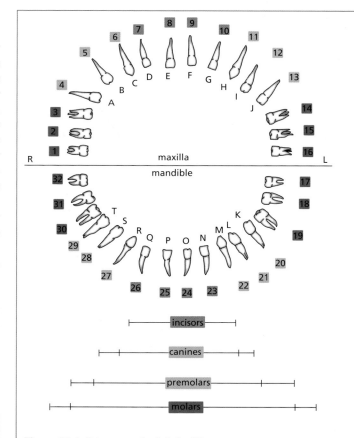

Figure 29.1 Primary and adult dentition.

🔍 Clinical pearl

Healthy primary teeth affect the long-term health of the permanent teeth and are essential to guiding the eruption process of normal permanent dentition.

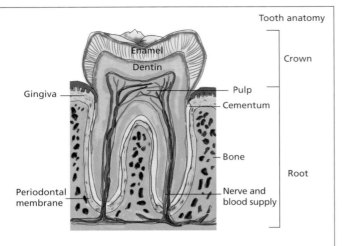

Figure 29.2 Normal anatomical characteristics of a tooth and supporting periodontal structures.

Table 29.1 Tooth eruption chart (primary, mixed, permanent dentition).

Age	Dentition stage	Description	Notes
0–6 months	Primary	No teeth	N/A
6–25 months	Primary	By 25–33 months all primary teeth have erupted	Mandibular central incisor first tooth to erupt
6 years	Mixed	Exfoliation of primary teeth; eruption of secondary teeth	Mandibular incisors first primary teeth to exfoliate; Mandibular incisors first permanent teeth to erupt
12 years	Mixed	Primary teeth completely exfoliated	Permanent molars and premolars may still be erupting
18–21 years	Permanent	All permanent teeth have now erupted	

Basic oral hygiene and risk factors for oral disease

The most common oral diseases – dental caries (also known as cavities or tooth decay) and periodontal disease (gum disease) – can be prevented by addressing relatively simple modifiable risk factors.

Red flag

Plaque control is one of the most important measures a person can take to improve his or her oral health or that of children.

Plaque is an adhesive bacterial biofilm that is formed on teeth and just below the gingiva. It contains upwards of 300 species of bacteria, many of which are indigenous microbiota that inhabit the oral cavity as early as just after birth or within the first months of life. Certain species of bacteria, the most predominant being *Streptococcus mutans*, cause caries by producing acid waste resulting from the metabolism of sugars in foods. Caries occur when bacterial plaque accumulates on tooth surfaces without adequate removal over time. Periodontal disease is more complex, caused by a wider variety of bacteria that is associated with disease severity, but it still begins with the accumulation of plaque around and between the teeth and gingiva.

Factors involved in producing dental caries are sugar substrate, bacteria living in plaque, a host tooth, and enough time for these factors to develop a cavity (Figure 29.3). Elimination of any of these factors can reduce or prevent caries altogether.

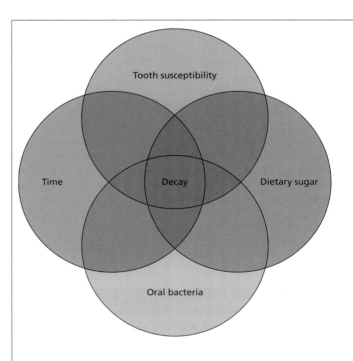

Figure 29.3 A Venn diagram of the causes of dental caries.

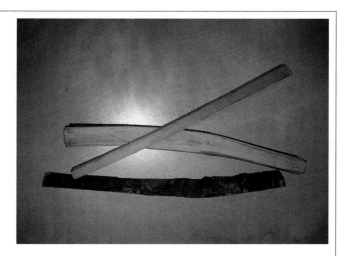

Figure 29.4 Examples of chewing sticks. *Source*: R. Khandelwal, Harvard School of Dental Medicine, Boston, USA. Reproduced with permission of R. Khandelwal.

Mechanical removal of plaque can be achieved using a toothbrush or chewing sticks (Figure 29.4) when toothbrushes are not available. Chewing sticks can be as effective as toothbrushes when properly used (Al-Otaibi *et al.*, 2003). In addition, a fluoride source should be used. Fluoride inhibits bacterial enolase and replaces the hydroxide ion in enamel, leading to stronger teeth and a reduced oral bacterial load. The World Health Organization (WHO) recommends consuming up to 1.5 mg fluoride per liter of drinking water, but in areas where clean and fluoridated drinking water is not available alternatives should be used. The use of fluoride toothpaste or fluoridated milk or salts should be encouraged, even for young children (Petersen & Lennon, 2004). Depending on the level of fluoride in the water, these can be used as supplements to fluoridated water as well. Finally, removal of plaque between the teeth to prevent caries and periodontal disease can be achieved using dental floss or some type of similar fibrous material, such as thread or plant fibers. Any materials used for plaque removal should be cleaned well after each use and replaced after they become uncleanable.

Adequate nutrition is another leading method of oral disease prevention. The risk of dental caries increases with both frequency and quantity of exposure to cariogenic (decay-causing) foods, such as sugary foods and fermentable carbohydrates, sugar-sweetened beverages, and sticky processed foods that stay in the grooves of teeth longer. Someone consuming cariogenic foods should remove any plaque and remaining food particles soon after consumption. For infants and young children without teeth, parents or caretakers should wipe the child's gingiva with a soft cloth to reduce caries-producing bacterial counts following breastfeeding or bottle use. Nighttime bottle use, a leading risk factor for early childhood caries, should be discouraged since salivary flow is at its lowest during

sleep. Between meals, and as often as possible for both oral and general health, patients should be encouraged to drink water frequently and eat low-sugar snacks consisting of whole fruits and vegetables whenever possible. Finally, caretakers should avoid sharing utensils or any other devices with their children, as this is the leading way that highly cariogenic bacteria are passed on to children.

🔍 Clinical pearl

Each time a sugary substrate is eaten, the pH of the oral cavity drops, increasing the risk for caries. Limiting the frequency of sugar intake each day reduces the number of times the oral pH drops, which in turn reduces caries risk. Additionally, saliva is a natural defense against caries; limiting sugar intake to meal times when salivary flow is highest also reduces the risk of dental caries.

Identification, diagnosis, and treatment of common oral conditions in developing settings

Most dental diseases can be diagnosed and treated before they cause symptoms such as discomfort and pain for the patient. Dental screenings are a very important tool for identifying individuals who can benefit from treatment. Anyone of any age, including infants and older people who are edentulous (without teeth), should be screened for oral diseases and conditions. In addition to identifying individuals who will benefit from treatment, all patients should be asked about their diet and oral hygiene habits, encouraged to brush and floss regularly, and urged to avoid consumption of sugar-sweetened beverages and sugary foods. Box 29.1 lists the equipment necessary for dental screenings and triage in developing settings.

Gingivitis and periodontal disease

Periodontal disease is an inflammatory condition leading to loss of attachment between the teeth and the mandible or maxilla, along with swelling, friability, and sensitivity of the gingival tissues. Periodontal disease has a multifactorial etiology, including host factors such as immune system response and bacterial colonization with certain anaerobic bacteria.

Red flag

People with certain systemic conditions, such as diabetes mellitus and malnutrition, as well as alcoholics and smokers, are at increased risk for periodontal disease.

Box 29.1 Equipment and supplies for dental screenings and triage in developing settings

- Examination gloves (non-latex preferable due to risk for allergic reaction)
- Mask
- Protective eyewear
- Flashlight
- Tongue depressor
- Metal dental explorer
- Metal periodontal probe
- Dental mirror

- Temporary restoration material such as Cavit, IRM, or Fuji II.

As dental care often involves intimate contact with bodily fluids, universal precautions should always be taken. Reusable instruments (Figure 29.5) should be sterilized or cleaned between use via autoclave, boiling, or chemical means.

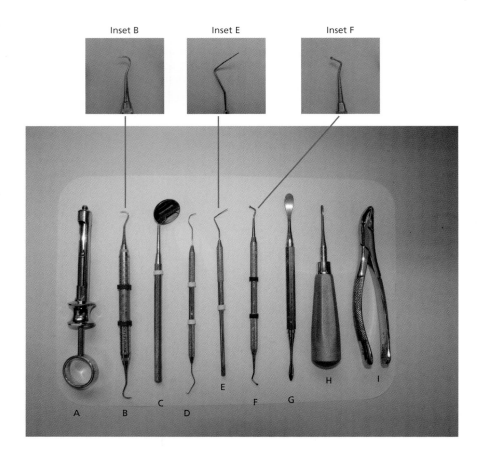

Inset B   Inset E   Inset F

A B C D E F G H I

Figure 29.5 Dental instruments discussed in this chapter. (a) Anesthetic syringe; (b) hand scaler (close-up in inset); (c) mirror; (d) explorer; (e) periodontal probe (close-up in inset); (f) spoon excavator (close-up in inset); (g) periodontal elevator; (h) periosteal elevator; (i) forceps.

Prevalence of periodontal disease also tends to be higher in individuals of lower socioeconomic status. While these are known risk factors, anyone can get periodontal disease, which affects up to 20% of the adult population globally (Petersen & Ogawa, 2005). Prevalence of periodontal disease also increases with age.

Periodontal disease can affect only a few teeth (localized periodontal disease) or most teeth (generalized periodontal disease). The gingiva around periodontally involved teeth will be erythematous, swollen, and "boggy" in appearance, and patients may report increased sensitivity and tendency to bleed in these areas. The gingiva may recede from the teeth, resulting

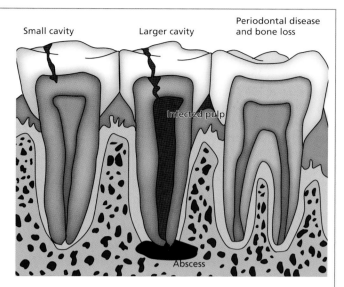

Figure 29.6 Examples of dental caries, infected pulp, abscess, gingival inflammation (gingivitis), and periodontal disease.

in teeth that appear "longer." At more advanced stages of periodontal disease, the teeth may become mobile. Gingivitis is a milder form of periodontal disease, in which the gingival tissue may become inflamed but the bony attachment of the teeth is not affected (Figure 29.6).

During a periodontal screening, the gingiva should be assessed for all these signs and symptoms. Using a gloved finger, gently palpate the gingiva above each tooth for tenderness. A metal periodontal probe should be gently inserted into the sulcus of each tooth on the buccal (cheek) and lingual (tongue) side close to where it touches the adjacent tooth (or where the adjacent tooth should be). In a healthy individual, the epithelial attachments of the tooth to the gingiva should be at a depth of 2–3 mm; probing depths greater than this likely indicate disease. Diseased tissue will also be more friable and inflamed; one may note bleeding from the sulcus, or the patient may report pain during probing, but pain is not always present. Following probing, check each tooth for mobility using the blunt end of a probe and a gloved finger.

The ideal treatment for periodontal disease is the removal of plaque and other irritants such as calculus (tartar) both supragingivally and subgingivally. Remind individuals to floss and brush twice a day, angling the bristles of the toothbrush into the sulcus between the gums and teeth. Cleansing of the deep pockets of diseased teeth can be accomplished using a specialized instrument called a scaler, if available. Highly symptomatic individuals can benefit from systemic antibiotics effective against anaerobic bacteria, such as amoxicillin or metronidazole (Mombelli, 2012). Teeth that are very mobile (especially those that can be depressed into the socket), have

multiple pockets deeper than 8 mm, or are suppurating or painful should be extracted (Box 29.2).

Dental caries

Dental caries is the most common bacterial infection in the world, affecting almost 100% of adults by the age of 35.

Red flag

Although rates of decay are highest in more developed countries, they are on the rise in developing countries, particularly low- and middle-income countries that have adopted the high-sugar "Western" diet (Petersen *et al.*, 2005b).

Enamel has the highest mineral content and takes the longest to become demineralized when in prolonged contact with plaque; demineralization is the beginning of the caries process. Once demineralization extends beneath the enamel into the dentin, the caries process can progress much more rapidly. Decay that has reached the pulp of the tooth will likely cause pain and can lead to localized or even systemic infection (Figure 29.6). Pulpal decay can only be alleviated through pulpectomy, known as endodontic therapy ("root canal" treatment), or by extracting the tooth (Box 29.2).

Signs and symptoms of dental caries will vary depending on how advanced the decay. Decay that has not yet penetrated the enamel can be considered "incipient" and may not require treatment. Different levels of decay can be identified and treated as described in Table 29.2. Dental decay can also occur around the edges of older restorations, know as recurrent caries. The margins of these restorations should be examined with a dental explorer for softness during screening, indicating marginal leakage and failure.

Clinical pearl: atraumatic restorative treatment

Atraumatic restorative treatment (ART) is a technique for eliminating decay and restoring teeth in resource-poor settings where electricity may not be available. Following excavation of a decayed tooth with a metal spoon excavator, a substance called glass ionomer (GI) is used to fill the cavity. GI does not require light to set to hardness (it is autocurable) and can be transported as separate liquid and powder components to be mixed when needed. GI also releases fluoride for up to a year after placement, preventing further decay. GI is more brittle than conventional restoration materials but still has a 65% 10-year survival rate. People with anxiety surrounding dental care or limited dental exposure may also find the experience of restoration with ART more pleasant because it is less invasive and less technology-dependent (Frencken *et al.*, 2012).

Box 29.2 How to extract a tooth (Langdon et al., 2010)

Equipment
- Gloves (nitrile or latex)
- Face mask
- Protective eyewear
- Flashlight
- Periodontal elevator
- Periosteal elevator
- Forceps

Inspect
Assess the patient's general health and anxiety level. Confirm which tooth you plan to extract, and examine adjacent teeth. When removing mandibular teeth, the plane of occlusion (chewing surfaces of the teeth) should be parallel with the floor. When removing maxillary teeth, the plane of occlusion should be roughly 60°.

Anesthetize
Administer a local anesthetic, such as 2% lidocaine with 1 in 100,000 epinephrine, in the soft tissue area around the root of the tooth. Anesthesia should take a few minutes to take effect, and more than one carpule (1.7 mL) of anesthesia may be necessary. A complete inferior alveolar nerve block is often necessary for extraction of mandibular molars or premolars.

Loosen periodontal and periosteal ligaments
Insert a sterile periodontal elevator into the periodontal ligament space (the space between the gingiva and the tooth) to loosen the periodontal fibers with a gentle rotational movement. Start on the side of the tooth closest to the front of the mouth and work backward, avoiding the lingual side of the tooth. When the gingiva feels loosened, complete the same movements with the periosteal elevator until the tooth feels freely mobile within the socket. Use care not to loosen the ligaments of the neighboring teeth.

Extract
Place a sterile gauze or clean cloth in the back of the patient's mouth to prevent aspiration of the tooth. Insert forceps as apically (toward the tip of the tooth) as possible and luxate (push with the forceps, instead of pulling, while applying apical pressure toward the root of the tooth) gently toward the buccal to expand the alveolar bone and allow the tooth to be removed. If you are not sure whether the tooth has more than one root, don't rotate it. Extract the tooth towards the buccal, as the lingual alveolar plate is thicker. Confirm that the entire tooth and root has been removed by curetting the bony socket. This will also help to remove granulation tissue. In maxillary teeth, curette the apex of the socket gently to see if the extraction socket communicates with the sinus. If you are uncertain if a sinus communication has been exposed, have the patient close his or her nose and gently blow; small air bubbles can be seen in the extraction socket if a communication is present.

Postoperative instructions
Ensure adequate hemostasis and have the patient bite on a sterile gauze or clean cloth for at least half an hour following extraction. Ice packs or cold compresses can reduce swelling. Non-steroidal anti-inflammatory drugs or narcotics can be prescribed for pain management. If a maxillary tooth was extracted, discourage the patient from drinking through a straw or blowing their nose for 1 week to prevent opening of a sinus communication. Warn the patient of the risk of alveolar osteitis ("dry socket"), which occurs when the blood clot is dislodged, resulting in painful exposed bone. The risk increases greatly with the use of tobacco products or alcohol. See the patient for a follow-up appointment within 1 week of extraction.

Table 29.2 Triage and treatment of dental caries.

Type of decay	Signs	Symptoms	Treatment
Incipient	"White spot" most visible on dry teeth, which might feel "sticky" if probed with a sharp metal object	None	Monitor for growth in size or occurrence of symptoms and counsel patient on oral hygiene and diet (avoiding sugary foods and beverages). Apply fluoride if available.
Primary	Larger areas of softness or pitting, or dark "shadow" visible on tooth	None, or some cold sensitivity may occur	Conventional restoration (composite or amalgam filling) or ART (see Clinical pearl: atraumatic restorative treatment).
Urgent	Grossly visible decay with 50% or greater loss of tooth structure. Draining sinus tracts may be present on palate or buccal plate and can be traced to affected tooth using sterile probe	Spontaneous pain, especially at night, or prolonged sensitivity (30 s or longer) or pain caused by consuming cold, hot, or sweet foods	Pain will not resolve unless the pulp is removed (endodontic therapy/"root canal") or the tooth is extracted (see Box 29.2).

Dental trauma

Injury to the teeth and oral tissues is most prevalent in toddlers and school-aged children but is growing with the increasing incidence and morbidity of injuries worldwide. Approximately 15% of children worldwide will experience some form of traumatic injury to their teeth. The most commonly affected teeth are the two maxillary central incisors. Diagnosis and treatment of dental trauma depends on whether the teeth have been broken, moved, or removed by the accident. Furthermore, treatment varies based on whether the tooth is a permanent tooth or deciduous tooth. Diagnoses and treatments are described below in Table 29.3. Before treating a dental injury, first assess the neurological status of the patient and ensure that he or she is hemodynamically stable.

Oral cancer

Red flag

Oral cancer is the eighth most common type of cancer worldwide, and the third most prevalent in certain parts of the world (Beaglehole et al., 2009).

Of oral cancers, 90% are squamous cell carcinomas (van der Waal et al., 2011). Consumers of alcohol, tobacco, and betel quid (a carcinogenic mixture of tobacco, areca nut, lime, and betel leaf common in Southeast Asia) are all at increased risk of oral cancer, as are people with oral forms of human papillomavirus (HPV)-16. The HPV vaccine is effective against oral cancer. Alcohol and tobacco use increase the risk of oral cancer, and multiplicatively increase oral squamous cell carcinoma risk by 300 times (Pelucchi et al., 2006). However, oral cancer can arise in any individual, and everyone should be screened for signs of the disease.

Presentation of oral cancer and its rate of growth can vary considerably. On screening, cancerous or precancerous lesions may appear as irregular asymmetrical plaques of white (leukoplakia), red (erythroplakia), or red and white (erythroleukoplakia), or as ulcerations that have not healed in longer than 2 weeks. Patients may also report spontaneous loosening of teeth or changes in the fit of their dentures if they wear any. Symptoms such as pain or parasthesia can also be present.

When screening for oral cancer, it is important to be thorough and methodical so that no surfaces are skipped. Complete an examination in the same systematic way each time. Inspect the labial and buccal mucosa, the gingiva, the top, sides, and bottom of the tongue, the floor of the mouth, the palate, and

Table 29.3 Diagnosis and treatment of dental trauma in permanent and deciduous teeth.

Trauma type	Signs and symptoms	Treatment for primary teeth	Treatment for permanent teeth
Subluxation	Tooth is slightly mobile with sulcular bleeding	Observe; changes in color or pain mean the tooth is necrotic and should be extracted.	Observe; changes in color or pain mean the tooth is necrotic and should be extracted.
Lateral luxation	Crown is pushed backward toward the hard palate (upper tooth) or tongue (lower tooth)	Apply local anesthetic and position tooth back into socket by gently pushing forward and upward into socket. Then observe and manage like subluxation.	Apply local anesthetic and position tooth into socket. If tooth is mobile, splint with a "figure 8" suture.
Intrusive luxation	Tooth is pushed into the socket	Extract	Extract; in 8–10 year old children, tooth may retrude naturally in a few days. If this does not happen, extract.
Avulsion	Tooth is knocked completely out of the mouth	None; permanent tooth will erupt to replace lost tooth, although eruption may be delayed due to trauma.	Re-implant as quickly as possible, then splint: <60 min is ideal. Gently rinse socket only if there is a blood clot present. If the tooth cannot be placed immediately back in the socket, place in Hank's balanced salt solution (if available), milk, or saliva.
Crown fracture	Part of the tooth crown has broken off	Extract	If painful or a red "blushing" spot is visible, place calcium hydroxide paste (if available) and cover with restoration material (IRM or Cavit if available; soft wax or tape if not).

oropharynx for signs of asymmetry or lesions. Gently bimanu-ally palpate the floor of the mouth to feel for enlarged lymph nodes. Then palpate the lymph nodes of the cervical chain and the submandibular nodes. Firm, fixed, and tender nodes should be noted. Be sure to rule out dental infection as a cause of lymphadenopathy.

While some oral cancers may be curable simply through surgical excision, many oral cancers must be treated by combination chemotherapy and radiation therapy. Individuals with suspected oral cancer or lesions that appear abnormal, no matter how small, should be referred to tertiary care for biopsy and further assessment.

Noma

Noma is a necrotizing gingival infection that can rapidly spread to adjacent soft tissues, causing rampant tissue necrosis (Challacombe *et al.*, 2011). Noma is an opportunistic infection of normal oral flora that occurs in immunocompromised individuals and children living in extreme poverty. Noma is correlated with a combination of risk factors that include poverty, malnutrition, poor sanitation, and poor oral hygiene. Of the estimated 140,000 annual cases globally, approximately 100,000 occur in sub-Saharan Africa in young children between the ages of 1 and 7 years. Children who survive noma are often left permanently disfigured due to the extent of tissue destruction (Beaglehole *et al.*, 2009).

> **Red flag**
>
> Without treatment, 70–90% of children with noma will die (Petersen *et al.*, 2005b).

Noma may initially have signs and symptoms of gingival inflammation or periodontal disease, but systemic symptoms such as pain, fever, and lymphadenopathy will soon develop. Tissue death in the oral cavity gives the patient's breath a distinctive odor (fetor oris). Many children first develop noma following a period of acute illness.

Any signs of periodontal infection in a young child or immunocompromised individual should be closely monitored. If available, penicillin and metronidazole can be administered as first-line therapies. However, noma is a medical emergency, and referral to tertiary care should occur as quickly as possible.

Early oral manifestations of common systemic conditions in low-income regions

HIV/AIDS

Oral manifestations of common systemic conditions in low-income regions can increase early detection of these conditions.

Table 29.4 Common oral manifestations of HIV/AIDS.

Manifestation	Signs and symptoms
Candidiasis	Angular cheilitis (painful cracks at the corners of lips)
	Pseudomembranous membrane (white cottage cheese-like)
	Erythematous/atrophic regions
Kaposi sarcoma	Reddish-purple proliferations on gingiva or palate
Oral ulcers	Small or large painful macules on mucosal surfaces. Can be erythematous or covered with a white-yellow keratin membrane

The oral manifestations of HIV/AIDS decrease the ability for adequate nutritional intake, and poor nutrition compounds impaired immune status (Coogen *et al.*, 2005; Moynihan, 2005). Table 29.4 describes common oral manifestations of HIV/AIDS.

With all HIV/AIDS oral manifestations, improvement of CD4 counts is of course the main objective. In addition, antifungals can be administered for oral candidiasis. Oral ulcers are often viral and due to reactivation in immunocompromised patients. The depth and size of oral ulcers will be larger in immunocompromised people, so health practitioners should monitor pain levels and observe for the possibility of dysphagia, malnutrition, and dehydration. Topical anesthetics, such as benzocaine or lidocaine, can be applied for palliative care. Most oral ulcers should resolve within 2 weeks but can take longer depending on the immune status of the patient.

> **Red flag**
>
> Oral lesions are often early clinical manifestations of the progression of HIV to AIDS, appearing in 80% of those with AIDS (Coogen *et al.*, 2005).

Malnutrition

As with HIV/AIDS, early signs of malnutrition, such as micronutrient deficiencies, can be seen in the oral cavity (Moynihan, 2005). Table 29.5 describes these oral signs of malnutrition. Improved nutrition and appropriate micronutrient supplements can eliminate most of these oral conditions.

Table 29.5 Oral manifestations of malnutrition.

Disorder	Signs and symptoms
Sialadenosis	Non-inflammatory enlargement of salivary glands
Hypoplastic spots	Brown spots on teeth due to childhood malnutrition during enamel formation
Pellagra (B$_6$ deficiency)	Glossitis and stomatitis (raw, red, smooth tongue)
Pyridoxine (B$_{12}$) deficiency	Glossitis and stomatitis (raw, red, smooth tongue). Distinguish from pellagra due to neurological deficits
Iron-deficiency anemia	Angular cheilitis and atrophic glossitis. Patient may complain of burning sensation in oral cavity
Necrotizing ulcerative periodontitis	Loss of bone and soft tissue attachment around teeth, with suppuration

Non-communicable diseases

Clinical pearl

Non-communicable diseases (NCDs) are gaining more attention than ever as their global burden, particularly in developing regions, becomes better understood (Fineberg, 2010). Oral health is directly associated with NCDs. Because of the high numbers of individuals suffering from both non-communicable and oral diseases, patients and providers must be informed of their interconnectivity and how to manage them.

Patients suffering from cardiovascular disease (CVD) may have an increased risk for complications due to periodontal disease (Gaetti-Jardim et al., 2009; Hokamura & Umemura, 2010; Mahendra et al., 2010). Therefore, to prevent escalating disease or initial CVD, patients at risk for or who currently have CVD should have oral examinations and cleanings on a regular basis. Diabetes and periodontal disease are also closely associated. Patients with diabetes are much more susceptible to infection, are less able to manage infection once it is present, and often have delayed healing (Little & Falace, 2002). Therefore, those with diabetes are at greater risk for periodontal infection and disease (Griffin et al., 2009; Acharya et al., 2010; Bandyopadhyay et al., 2010). Conversely, patients with periodontal disease may have more difficulty controlling their blood glucose levels (Demmer et al., 2010; Montoyta-Carralero et al., 2010). Thus, patients with diabetes must be extremely disciplined and practice good oral hygiene habits daily. Control of oral health can enhance a patient's ability to control his or her diabetes and reduce the risk of long-term tooth loss and oral disease.

Conclusions

It is important to create a mutual understanding that oral health is directly associated with general health. Providing routine oral screenings and addressing the common risk factors for oral diseases and other systemic and non-communicable diseases will provide a deeper understanding of this relationship. All healthcare providers, including community health workers, physicians, dentists, and specialists, must collaborate in the treatment of their patients. The result can lead to improved health outcomes for all patients worldwide.

Additional resources

- Beaglehole R, Benzian H, Crail J, Mackay J (2009) *The Oral Health Atlas: Mapping a Neglected Global Health Issue.* Cointrin, Switzerland: FDI World Dental Education and Myriad Editions.
- World Health Organization Oral Health Programme. Available at http://www.who.int/oral_health/en/
- Dickson M (2010) *Where There is no Dentist.* Berkeley, CA: Hesperian Foundation.
- Langlais RP, Miller CS (1998) *Color Atlas of Common Oral Diseases,* 2nd edn. Philadelphia: Williams & Wilkins.
- Frencken JE, Holmgren C, van Palenstein Helderman WH (2002) Basic Package of Oral Care. World Health Organization Collaborating Center for Oral Health Care Planning and Future Scenarios and College of Dental Science, University of Nijmegen. Available at http://www.chdentalinstitute.org/images/BPOC.pdf
- World Health Organization (1997) *Oral Health Surveys: Basic Methods,* 4th edn. Geneva: World Health Organization. Available at: http://www2.paho.org/hq/dmdocuments/2009/OH_st_Esurv.pdf

REFERENCES

Acharya AB, Satyanarayan A, Thakur SL (2010) Status of association studies linking diabetes mellitus and periodontal disease in India. *Int J Diabetes Dev Ctries* 30:69–74.

Al-Otaibi M, Al-Harthy M, Söder B, Gustafsson A, Angmar-Månsson B (2003) Comparative effect of chewing sticks and toothbrushing on plaque removal and gingival health. *Oral Health Prev Dent* 1:301–7.

Bandyopadhyay D, Marlow NM, Fernandes JK, Leite RS (2010) Periodontal disease progression and glycaemic control among Gullah African Americans with type E diabetes. *J Clin Periodontol* 37:501–9.

Beaglehole R, Benzian H, Crail J, Mackay J (2009) *The Oral Health Atlas: Mapping a Neglected Global Health Issue.* Cointrin, Switzerland: FDI World Dental Education and Myriad Editions.

Benzian H, Bergman M, Cohen LK, Hobdell M, Mackay J (2012). The UN high-level meeting on prevention and control of non-communicable diseases and its significance for oral health worldwide. *J Public Health Dent* 72:91–3.

Challacombe S, Chidzonga M, Glick M *et al.* (2011) Global oral health inequalities: oral infections. Challenges and approaches. *Adv Dent Res* 23:227–36.

Coogen MM, Greenspan J, Challacombe SJ (2005) Oral lesions in infection with human immunodeficiency virus. *Bull WHO* 83:700–6.

Demmer RT, Desvarieux M, Holtfreter B *et al.* (2010) Periodontal status and A1C change: longitudinal results from the study of health in Pomerania (SHIP). *Diabetes Care* 33:1037–43.

Fineberg H (2010) The under-appreciated burden: chronic illness in the developing world. Harvard School of Public Health lecture series, November 8, 2010.

Frencken JE, Leal SC, Navarro MF (2012) Twenty-five-year atraumatic restorative treatment (ART) approach: a comprehensive overview. *Clin Oral Investig* 16:1337–46.

Gaetti-Jardim E Jr, Marcelino SL, Feitosa AC, Romito GA, Avila-Campos MJ (2009) Quantitative detection of periodontopathic bacteria in atherosclerotic plaques from coronary arteries. *J Med Microbiol* 58:1568–75.

Griffin SO, Barker LK, Griffin PM, Cleveland JL, Kohn W (2009) Oral health needs among adults in the United States with chronic disease. *J Am Dent Assoc* 140:1266–74.

Hokamura K, Umemura K (2010) Roles of oral bacteria in cardiovascular diseases. From molecular to clinical cases: *Porphyromonas gingivalis* is the important role of intimal hyperplasia in the aorta. *J Pharmacol Sci* 113:110–14.

Langdon J, Patel M, Ord R, Brennan P (eds) (2010) *Operative Oral and Maxillofacial Surgery*, 2nd edn. London: Hodder Arnold.

Little JW, Falace D (2002) *Dental Management of the Medically Compromised Patient*, 6th edn. St Louis, MO: Mosby, p. 53.

Mahendra J, Mahendra L, Kurian VM, Jaishankar K, Mythili R (2010) 16S rRNA-based detection of oral pathogens in coronary atherosclerotic plaque. *Indian J Dent Res* 21:248–52.

Mombelli A (2012) Antimicrobial advances in treating periodontal diseases. *Front Oral Biol* 15:133–48.

Montoyta-Carralero JM, Saura-Perez M, Canteras-Jordana M, Morata-Murcia IM (2010) Reduction of HbA1c levels following nonsurgical treatment of periodontal disease in type 2 diabetes. *Med Oral Patol Oral Cir Bucal* 15:808–12.

Moynihan PJ (2005) The role of diet and nutrition in the etiology and prevention of oral disease. *Bull WHO* 83:694–9.

Pelucchi C, Gallus S, Garavello W, Bosetti C, La Vecchia C (2006) Cancer risk associated with alcohol and tobacco use: focus on upper aero-digestive tract and liver. *Alcohol Res Health* 29:193–8.

Petersen PE (2003) The World Oral Health Report 2003. Continuous improvement of oral health in the 21st century: approaches of the WHO Global Oral Health Programme. Available at http://www.who.int/oral_health/media/en/orh_report03_en.pdf

Petersen PE, Lennon MA (2004) Effective use of fluorides for the prevention of dental caries in the 21st century: the WHO approach. *Community Dent Oral Epidemiol* 32:319–21.

Petersen PE, Ogawa H (2005) Strengthening the prevention of periodontal disease: the WHO approach. *J Periodontol* 76:2187–93.

Petersen PE, Estupinan-Day S, Ndiaye C (2005a) WHO's action for continuous improvement in oral health. *Bull WHO* 83:642.

Petersen PE, Bourgeois D, Ogawa H, Estupinan-Day S, Ndiaye C (2005b) The global burden of oral diseases and risks to oral health. *Bull WHO* 83:661–9.

Sheiham A (2005) Oral health, general health and quality of life. *Bull WHO* 83:644.

van der Waal I, de Bree R, Brakenhoff R, Coebergh JW (2011) Early diagnosis in primary oral cancer: is it possible? *Med Oral Patol Oral Cir Bucal* 16:e300–5.

Vos T, Flaxman AD, Naghavi M *et al.* (2012) Years lived with disability (YDLs) for 1,160 sequelae of 289 diseases and injuries, 1990–2010: a systematic analysis for the Global Burden of Disease Study 2010. *Lancet* 380:2163–96.

Watt RG (2005) Strategies and approaches in oral disease prevention and health promotion. *Bull WHO* 83:711–18.

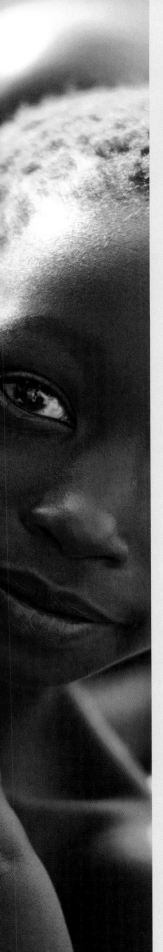

CHAPTER 30
Blindness and Visual Impairment

Michael G. Morley[1,2], Katharine E. Morley[2,3], Thuss Sanguansak[4], and Suwat Kusakul[5]

[1]Ophthalmic Consultants of Boston, Boston, MA, USA
[2]Harvard Medical School, Boston, MA, USA
[3]Massachusetts General Hospital, Boston, MA, USA
[4]Khon Kaen University, Khon Kaen, Thailand
[5]Nakhon Phanom Hospital, Nakhon Phanom, Thailand

Key learning objectives

- Understand the epidemiology of blindness and impaired vision.
- Understand the overwhelming importance of cataracts in global blindness and how they are curable with highly effective, low-cost surgical interventions.
- Learn about other common causes of global blindness including glaucoma, macular degeneration, corneal diseases, and diabetic retinopathy.
- Understand how some causes of global blindness are diminishing due to effective public health interventions while others are increasing due to an aging population and obesity.
- Learn about innovative transformative interventions that have measurably affected rates of global blindness.

Abstract

Progress is being made in the fight against global blindness. The prevalence of trachoma, onchocerciasis, and Vitamin A deficiency is decreasing due to groundbreaking partnerships between pharmaceutical companies, non-governmental organizations, and government blindness programs. In addition, innovative eye care institutions such as Aravind Eye Care System and Tilganga Institute of Ophthalmology have developed innovative and effective methods to address the problem of blindness in developing countries. However, there are large challenges remaining in the quest to eliminate avoidable blindness. Cataract, glaucoma, and macular degeneration continue to grow as the population ages, and diabetic retinopathy is rapidly emerging as a major global cause of blindness.

Key words: global blindness, cataract, glaucoma, trachoma, onchocerciasis, Vitamin A deficiency, diabetic retinopathy

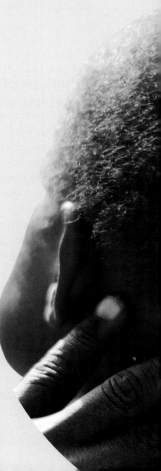

Essential Clinical Global Health, First Edition. Edited by Brett D. Nelson.
© 2015 John Wiley & Sons, Ltd. Published 2015 by John Wiley & Sons, Ltd.
Companion website: www.essentialseries.com/globalhealth

Introduction

Being blind in the developing world is more than a personal tragedy for the affected individual. The ramifications extend far beyond the loss of vision. The economic sequelae impact the well-being of affected individuals, their immediate family, and their community. Poverty is more common in households with blind non-working individuals, and mortality rates are significantly higher for blind individuals living in the developing world.

Table 30.1 WHO definitions of blindness and visual impairment.

Classification	Visual acuity in better eye (feet)	Visual acuity in better eye (meters)
Normal vision	20/20 to 20/60	6/6 to 6/18
Visual impairment	20/60 to 20/200	6/18 to 6/60
Blindness	20/400 to light perception	6/120 to light perception
Complete blindness	No light perception	No light perception

Blindness includes patients who have vision equal to or worse than 20/400. In worsening order of severity, blindness may be further characterized by the patient's ability to "count fingers at x feet or meters" (CF), see "hand motions" (HM), see light perception (LP), and no light perception (NLP).
Source: World Health Organization (2013c).

Box 30.1 How to measure visual acuity

Visual acuity is the "vital sign" of the eye. It is easy to do and critically important for diagnosis and monitoring of eye diseases. If there is an ophthalmic complaint, visual acuity should be checked, in both eyes separately.

Supplies
A well-lit Snellen chart, an illiterate "E" chart, a child's chart, or a small near-vision reading card.

Procedure
For all vision tests, always measure only one eye at a time and watch to ensure the patient does not "peek" with second eye.

1. Patients should wear their distance or reading glasses, depending on whether the eye chart is for distance or near vision.
2. Measure the right eye first by occluding the left eye with a hand, tissue, or occluder (fingers are easy to "peek" through).
3. Ask the patient to read the letters of the eye chart, starting at the top.
4. Record the lowest line on the chart at which patients are able to correctly read at least half of the letters/numbers. Repeat process for left eye.

For illiterate patients and young children
A "tumbling E" chart may be used in which the letter E is oriented with the three bars pointing to the right, left, up, or down. Ask patients to indicate the direction of the letter E by pointing with their fingers in the direction corresponding to the three bars on the E.

Definition of blindness and visual impairment

The World Health Organization's (WHO) definitions of blindness and visual impairment are listed in Table 30.1. Loss of vision in only one eye does not meet the definition of blindness. As a reference point, an unrestricted driver's license in the United States, for example, typically requires best corrected visual acuity of 20/40 or better in at least one eye; 20/40 visual acuity means that the individual being tested can see at 20 feet what a person with "normal" vision can see at 40 feet. Another way to understand visual acuity measurements is that a patient with 20/40 visual acuity requires an object to be twice as large (or half as close) to be seen clearly when compared to a patient who has 20/20 visual acuity. Box 30.1 describes how visual acuity is measured.

Outside the United States, vision is often expressed in a similar ratio, but meters are used instead of feet, e.g., 6/12 (in meters) in place of 20/40 (in feet). Note that the definition of blindness does not require "no light perception"; rather it reflects a profound inability to see clearly.

Epidemiology of blindness and refractive error

Approximately 40 million people worldwide are blind according to World Health Organization (2013a). The prevalence of blindness varies throughout the world with lower-income

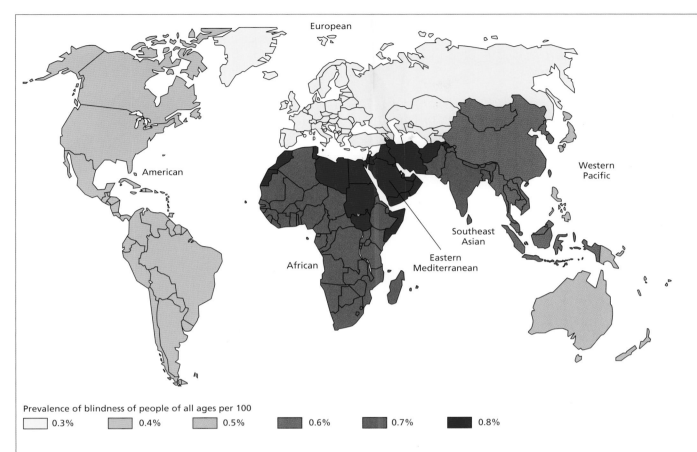

Figure 30.1 Prevalence of global blindness. *Source*: adapted from World Health Organization (2010) with permission.

countries generally having higher rates (Figure 30.1). In fact, 90% of blind people live in developing countries. The highest rates of blindness are seen in individuals older than 50, the poor, and in women. Africa has the highest rates of blindness on a per-capita basis. Fully 80% of global blindness is preventable or treatable.

Cataracts cause 50% of all global blindness, by far the largest cause. This is important because cataracts are easily cured with proven cost-effective interventions. Following cataracts, in descending order of frequency, glaucoma, macular degeneration, corneal diseases, and trachoma are the top causes of global blindness (Figure 30.2).

Several effective public health programs, some of which are discussed in this chapter, have measurably reduced the rates of blindness due to trachoma, onchocerciasis, and Vitamin A deficiency. In contrast, cataracts, glaucoma, macular degeneration, and diabetic retinopathy are increasing in prevalence due to an aging population and increasing obesity.

Uncorrected refractive error – myopia (near-sightedness), hyperopia (far-sightedness), astigmatism (non-spherical curvature of the cornea), and presbyopia (loss of ability with age to focus up close) – is the largest cause of visual impairment worldwide, impacting 285 million people. Uncorrected refrac-

tive error is nearly completely curable with glasses, contact lenses, or refractive surgery.

Common causes of global blindness

Cataract

The term "cataract" comes from the Latin word for waterfall due to the white appearance of a mature cataract in the pupil. Some 20 million people worldwide are blind from cataracts. Cataracts occur most commonly in people aged 50 and older. Cataract blindness is more common in females than in males with a ratio of about 1.6 : 1 (Abou-Gareeb *et al.*, 2001), in part due to the increased longevity of women compared with men and because of social, financial, and societal factors that reduce opportunities for surgical intervention (Lewallen & Courtright, 2002). Not surprisingly, the poor are affected more than the rich.

Cataracts typically present with painless progressive loss of vision. Patients may complain of blurred vision at either near or far, and they may also complain of glare, i.e., diminished acuity in bright lights due to scattered defocused light. The diagnosis of cataract is quite simple in most cases; a penlight

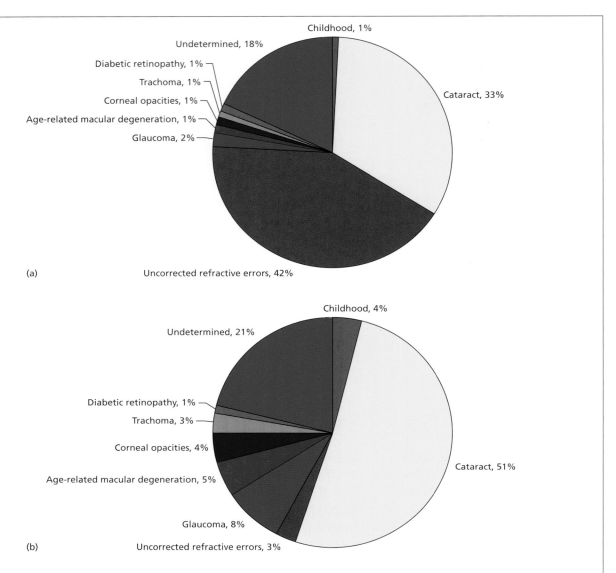

(a)

(b)

Figure 30.2 Causes of global visual impairment (a) and blindness (b) (Pascolini & Mariotti, 2012). (a) The common causes of visual impairment (visual acuity 20/60 to 20/200). Refractive error and cataract account for more than three-quarters of the cases. (b) The common causes of blindness (visual acuity 20/400 or less). Cataract accounts for half of the cases. Glaucoma, macular degeneration, and corneal diseases also cause significant numbers of cases. *Source*: reproduced from *Br J Ophthalmol*, Pascolini and Mariotti, 96(5):614–18, 2012, with permission from BMJ Publishing Group Ltd.

or slit-lamp examination demonstrates a cloudy lens that may be white or brownish-yellow in color (Figure 30.3). Treatment of cataract consists of surgical extraction of the cataractous lens followed by implantation of an artificial, clear lens. Surgical outcomes are generally excellent with most patients recovering 20/40 or better vision. In general, the cost of cataract surgery around the world approximates 1 month's salary. Data from the WHO show that cataract surgery is a cost-effective intervention throughout the world (Lansingh *et al.*, 2007).

An example of a successful cataract surgical program is the partnership between the Himalayan Cataract Project and Tilganga Institute of Ophthalmology in Kathmandu, Nepal. They have made significant contributions to the fight against blindness in the developing world through innovative developments in surgical technique, conducting "cataract camps" in remote locations, training of providers, and raising the awareness of eye diseases in impoverished populations.

Despite the excellent outcomes and high cost-effectiveness, cataract prevalence is rising. There are significant barriers to the eradication of blindness due to cataract: a growing number of aged people, patients' unawareness of diagnosis or treatment, inadequate surgical manpower, lack of access to

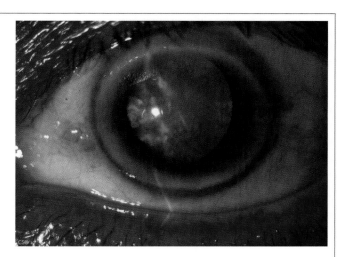

Figure 30.3 Clinical photograph of cataract. The whitish-gray-brown color in the pupil is the cataract. This cataract has reduced visual acuity to a level of count fingers at 3 feet (legal blindness). The white ring around the edge of the cornea is called arcus senilis, a common finding in elderly patients.

treatment for geographic reasons, cultural beliefs, patients' fear, economic constraints, lack of family support, and acceptance of blindness as a normal part of old age. There is no known prevention of cataract.

Glaucoma

Glaucoma is a heterogeneous collection of conditions that cause optic nerve damage and result in irreversible vision loss. Nearly all have in common a triad of features: (i) elevated eye pressure, (ii) optic nerve damage ("cupping"), and (iii) progressive loss of visual field. Total blindness may occur in the end stage in any of the forms.

Glaucoma represents about 12% of global blindness. It is more common in older individuals, those with a family history, and those with African ancestry. There are two main subtypes of glaucoma, open angle and narrow angle, which refers to the anatomy of the "angle" formed by the cornea and iris through which aqueous fluid egresses from the eye. Open-angle glaucoma is the most common subtype in the Americas, Europe, and Africa, but in East Asia narrow-angle glaucoma is the most common subtype due to anatomical variations in angle structure (Glaucoma Research Foundation, 2011).

Open-angle glaucoma is known as the "silent thief" due to the stealthy, slow, and relentless way that vision is lost. Slow progressive peripheral visual field loss is usually asymptomatic until advanced field loss occurs, which is irreversible even with treatment. Angle closure, in contrast, can present with dramatic pain, redness, haloes around light, and a markedly narrow or occluded angle. Sometimes angle closure is subacute and chronic with the same end result.

The diagnosis of glaucoma requires specialized ophthalmic instruments to measure intraocular pressure (tonometry), examine the angle (gonioscopy), and assess the optic nerve. Therefore, referral to a high-level facility is usually required. The treatment of glaucoma depends on the subtype. Open-angle glaucoma is generally treated with topical eyedrops (e.g., timolol, pilocarpine, brimonidine, latanoprost) to lower pressure in milder cases. Laser and/or surgical procedures can also be performed to lower pressure in more difficult cases. By lowering pressure, loss of vision is slowed, but vision is not improved. Narrow-angle glaucoma is generally treated with laser iridotomy (a small hole in the iris) that is curative in many cases. There is no known prevention for glaucoma, but treatment to reduce intraocular pressure slows the progression of loss of visual field.

Glaucoma has several characteristics that make it particularly challenging to manage on a global scale. The diagnosis is frequently made only after there has already been advanced irreversible vision loss. In most cases, treatment is chronic, expensive, inconvenient and, most importantly from a patient acceptance standpoint, not improving (i.e., treatment stabilizes the disease but does not restore lost visual acuity or improve vision). Earlier detection of glaucoma through improved patient awareness and better screening may help to reduce blindness from glaucoma.

Trachoma

Trachoma, caused by the organism *Chlamydia trachomatis*, is the most common cause of preventable global blindness. Trachoma typically presents initially as a chronic conjunctivitis with redness and discharge from the eyes. Repeated infections cause scarring of the tarsal (inner) aspect of the eyelids (Figure 30.4 and see Box 30.2 for how to examine the lids for scarring), which ultimately results in trichiasis, or inward rotation of the eyelashes. Chronic rubbing of the eyelashes on the cornea results in painful abrasions and scarring of the cornea, and ultimately blindness results. Some 21 million people are infected with trachoma; 8 million have trichiasis, and 1.2 million are blind as a result of trachoma (Burton & Mabey, 2009; World Health Organization, 2013b).

Trachoma is a disease of the poor. Chronic persistent reservoirs of infection, often involving communally raised children or even whole communities, are typically found in low-income settings with suboptimal hygiene, lack of access to clean water, and insufficient access to healthcare. Repeated infections typically involve transmission of infected eye discharge into the eyes from fingers, clothes, towels, or flies seeking liquid from tears. Women, who tend to do more of the child rearing and have more exposure to infected children, have a higher prevalence of trachoma. Treatment of trachoma is based on the WHO's SAFE campaign (Box 30.3). Whole communities are treated if trachoma is endemic, i.e., the prevalence of infection is 10% or more in children under 10 years

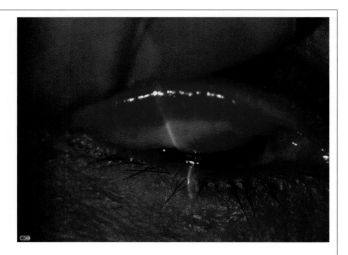

Figure 30.4 Clinical photograph of eyelid scarring from chronic infection with *Chlamydia trachomatis*. The horizontal white fibrotic scar (Arlt line) causes contraction of the inner (conjunctival) surface of the upper lid and inward rotation of the eyelashes. Corneal scarring and blindness occur after prolonged and painful scratching of the cornea by the inturned lashes.

old or if trichiasis is present in more than 1% of the population older than 15 years.

Trachoma is an important, in-progress, success story in public health. The prevalence of blindness due to trachoma is decreasing due to a variety of factors, especially the WHO's Global Eradication of Trachoma (GET) project (Mathew *et al.*, 2009). One of the most noteworthy aspects of the GET program is the novel collaborations between the WHO, pharmaceutical companies, eye care non-governmental organizations (NGOs), and government health ministries. In particular, 225 million doses of azithromycin (valued at US$5 billion) have been donated by the pharmaceutical industry to the GET project, thereby providing an important example of using profits from a commercially successful drug (azithromycin) to support healthcare in developing countries afflicted by trachoma. In addition, the GET program uses a population-based approach to treat community reservoirs, while also treating individuals with active disease. Oral azithromycin is much more effective than topical tetracycline ointment (the previous standard treatment) due to its ease of use and longer duration of action. The prevalence of trachoma has begun to drop due to the effective interventions in infected communities, especially in countries like Morocco that have diligently applied the GET recommendations (Center for Global Development, 2007).

Onchocerciasis (river blindness)

Onchocerciasis is a parasitic disease caused by the organism *Onchocerca volvulus*, which is transmitted through the bites of the blackfly *Simulium damnosum*. The disease is also called

river blindness because the blackfly vectors breed in the fast flowing waters of rivers in West and Central Africa and Latin America. The great majority (99%) of blindness from onchocerciasis is found in sub-Saharan Africa, with only 1% found in South America and Yemen.

Like trachoma, onchocerciasis is an important public health success story in global health and ophthalmology. The prevalence of blindness due to onchocerciasis has dropped by an estimated 77% in the past two decades due to the Onchocerciasis Control Program (Coffeng *et al.*, 2013; TDR for Research on Diseases of Poverty, 2013). This program has several important elements: a robust collaboration between the WHO, NGOs such as the International Agency for the Prevention of Blindness and the Lions Clubs International Foundation, pharmaceutical company Merck, government ministries of health, and use of community health workers to control and deliver the drug, ivermectin, to their communities. Merck has agreed to donate ivermectin to NGOs who are then responsible, in conjunction with ministries of health, for delivery of the drug to affected populations. Ivermectin lends itself well to this project because it is stable, safe (wide therapeutic window), does not require refrigeration, and can be delivered orally. A single dose on a yearly basis can keep the disease under control. Vector control (i.e., aerial spraying of areas infected with blackflies) has been an important element of the program, and there is great interest in assessing the efficacy and environmental impact of this element of the public health intervention. However, full eradication of onchocerciasis is difficult due to the reservoir of flies and certain disease characteristics, including a 14-year lifespan of the parasite.

Other important ophthalmic conditions

Table 30.2 lists some other common and important causes of global blindness.

Innovations in the delivery of eye care in the developing world

Several innovative approaches have been established to reduce global blindness. Aravind Eye Care System (AES) is perhaps the prototypical model for self-sustaining eye care in the developing world (Bill and Melinda Gates Foundation, 1999–2013; Rosenberg, 2013). Started by Dr Govindappa Venkataswamy in Madurai, India in 1976, AES is the largest provider of eye care in the world. AES uses a tiered pricing model in which well-to-do patients pay a premium for superior service (less waiting, private rooms, premium intraocular lenses, private nurses, etc.) and profits from that activity subsidize high-quality but basic services (ward rooms, shared nurses, monofocal lenses, etc.) for the poor. The same surgeons perform surgery on both rich and poor. Aravind has also been very progressive and entrepreneurial, unafraid to think "outside the box" with innovative enterprises that help support the core mission to "eliminate needless blindness, providing

Box 30.2 How to flip an eyelid and remove a foreign body

Foreign bodies may become lodged under the eyelid and cause painful abrasions and corneal scars. By everting the lid, foreign bodies can be removed with a cotton-tipped swab (Figure 30.5).

Supplies
Topical anesthetic drops (proparacaine, tetracaine or lidocaine), sterile cotton-tipped swab.

Procedure
1. Wash your hands.
2. Explain to the patient what you plan to do.
3. Grasp the eyelashes of the upper lid and gently pull down and away from the globe.
4. Place a finger or the handle of a cotton-tipped swab about 1 cm from the lid margin.
5. Pull the lashes up and push gently down on the finger or cotton-tipped swab, resulting in eversion of the lid.
6. Hold the lash firmly against the superior orbital bone to prevent it from reverting to its normal position.
7. Use a cotton-tipped swab to sweep the foreign body from the inner lid surface.

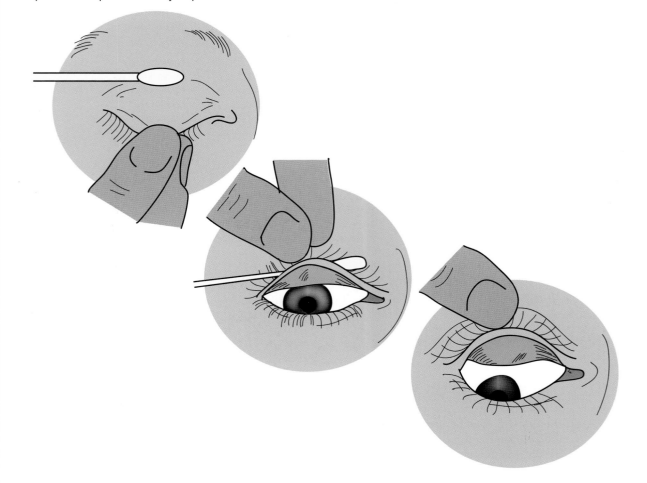

Figure 30.5 Lid eversion.

Box 30.3 The World Health Organization's SAFE campaign for the elimination of trachoma

Surgical repair of entropion (inward rotation of the lid and lashes)
Antibiotics to individuals and communities infected with trachoma
Facial cleanliness
Environmental improvements (closed latrines, clean water, etc.)

Table 30.2 Other important causes of global blindness.[a]

Condition	Etiology	Presentation	Diagnosis	Treatment	Epidemiology	Comments
Macular degeneration	Aging changes, genetic and environmental factors	Blurred, distorted vision	Fundus examination	Intraocular injections of anti-VEGF medicines	Most common in the elderly, smokers, lightly pigmented skin/eyes	Leading cause of blindness in developed countries
Corneal scarring	Multiple causes including trachoma, trauma, degenerations, pterygium	Trauma, degenerative diseases resulting in a white scar	Slit-lamp examination	Corneal transplantation	4% of global blindness; causes include trauma, infections, degenerations, Vitamin A deficiency	Corneal transplants require close postoperative monitoring
Diabetic retinopathy	Elevated blood sugar levels cause retinal damage, edema, and bleeding	Most common: blurred vision from macular edema, floaters from bleeding due to proliferative diabetic retinopathy (PDR)	Fundus examination	Glycemic control, intravitreal injection of anti-VEGF medicines, laser treatment	Dramatically rising rates in developing countries, especially China and India	Cataracts commonly also present
Vitamin A deficiency	Diet low in Vitamin A	Night blindness, Bitot spots (corneal keratinization, corneal scarring)	Serum Vitamin A levels, clinical diagnosis	Vitamin A supplementation, orally or in fortified foods	Increased mortality from infections (e.g., measles, pneumonia, diarrhea) in Vitamin A deficiency	Considerable progress in past decade, one of the most cost-effective interventions in medicine

[a]These causes of global blindness are important because of their public health impact due to their prevalence (macular degeneration), growing impact (diabetes), or successful control (Vitamin A deficiency).
VEGF, vascular endothelial growth factor.

compassionate and high quality eye care to all." The AES model includes partnering with local businesses to support eye camps; reducing costs by manufacturing and selling their own intraocular lenses and pharmaceuticals; enhancing revenue and human resources by developing an institute for ophthalmic facility management; and training physicians and ancillary personnel including ophthalmic assistants, equipment engineers, and surgical techs. They have used modern management and business techniques to maximize their success while at the same time keeping a clear focus on their core humanitarian goal of eradicating blindness for all.

Other innovative approaches to blindness in the developing world include ORBIS International, which has implemented a "flying eye hospital" and teaching facility located on a jet that travels to developing countries and provides training and surgical procedures.

Tilganga Institute of Ophthalmology (TIO) has also been a leader in promoting eye care for the poor around the world. TIO is a tertiary-care eye hospital in Kathmandu, Nepal with resident and fellow training programs, an intraocular laboratory, efficient cataract surgical outreach programs, and an ophthalmic research program. Their high-volume cataract surgical camps are an efficient mechanism for addressing cataract blindness in some of the most rural and impoverished areas of the world.

Finally, some of the most important and effective developments in the delivery of eye care have occurred because of partnerships between organizations that merge their strengths and resources to tackle what was once seen as formidable unsolvable problems. For example, the partnership between the WHO and the International Agency for the Prevention of Blindness (IAPB) to create the Vision 2020 program has measurably

Clinical experience

"While a second-year medical student, I had the amazing opportunity to join a postoperative cataract clinic in northern Thailand. The surgeons had been there a month earlier for cataract extraction, and then I went back with the team to check visual acuity and refractive error, dispense glasses, and survey patients on their overall satisfaction. I was so glad that I could help promote eye health and be part of the care structure for an international mission. The patients were deeply grateful for our care, thanking me multiple times just for checking their vision with a pinhole occluder and Snellen chart. Many patients had not learned to read letters but could read numbers or the tumbling E, and they were as willing and eager to read the chart as I was for them to do it! They were so happy once they were given their glasses and could see."

Jesse, medical student working in Thailand

affected rates of blindness in the world (World Health Organisation, 2007). As noted above, partnerships between pharmaceutical companies and NGOs and the Vision 2020 program have also significantly impacted millions of people.

Additional resources

Books

• Ruit S, Tabin G, Wykoff C (2006) *Fighting Global Blindness: Improving World Vision Through Cataract Elimination.* Washingto, DC: American Public Health Association.
• Gerstenblith AT, Rabinowitz MP (eds) (2012) *Wills Eye Manual: Office and Emergency Room Diagnosis of Eye Disease,* 6th edn. Philadelphia: Lippincott, Wilkins & Wilkins.

• Friedman NJ, Kaiser PK, Pineda R (2009) *Massachusetts Eye and Ear Infirmary Illustrated Manual of Ophthalmology,* 3rd edn. Philadelphia: Saunders Elsevier.

Apps

• Eye Handbook: Ophthalmology for Your Smartphone. Available at http://www.eyehandbook.com/index.php

Websites

• American Academy of Ophthalmology. Available at http://www.aao.org/
• World Health Organization. Prevention of Blindness and Visual Impairment. Available at http://www.who.int/blindness/en/
• International Agency for the Prevention of Blindness (IAPB) Vision 2020. Available at http://www.iapb.org/vision-2020

Institutes of ophthalmology

• Tilganga Institute of Ophthalmology. Available at http://www.tilganga.org
• Aravind Eye Care System. Available at http://www.aravind.org/

Non-government organizations

• Himalayan Cataract Project. Available at http://www.cureblindness.org/
• Lions Clubs International. Available at http://www.lionsclubs.org/EN/index.php
• Fred Hollows Foundation. Available at http://www.hollows.org.au
• Seva Foundation. Available at http://www.seva.org/
• Sightsavers. Available at http://www.sightsavers.org
• Eye Care Foundation. Available at http://www.eyecarefoundation.nl/english/
• Orbis. Available at http://www.orbis.org

REFERENCES

Abou-Gareeb I, Lewallen S, Bassett K, Courtright P (2001) Gender and blindness: a meta analysis of population-based prevalence surveys. *Ophthalmic Epidemiol* 8:39–56.

Bill and Melinda Gates Foundation (1999–2013) Pioneering eye surgery network receives 2008 Gates Award for Global Health. Available at http://www.gatesfoundation.org/Media-Center/Press-Releases/2008/05/Pioneering-Eye-Surgery-Network-Receives-2008-Gates-Award-for-Global-Health

Burton MJ, Mabey DC (2009) The global burden of trachoma: a review. *PLoS Negl Trop Dis* 3(10): e460.

Center for Global Development (2007) Millions Saved: Case 10: Controlling Trachoma in Morocco. Available at http://www.cgdev.org/page/case-10-controlling-trachoma-morocco

Coffeng LE, Stolk WA, Zouré HG *et al.* (2013) African Programme For Onchocerciasis Control 1995–2015: model-estimated health impact and cost. *PLoS Negl Trop Dis* 7(1):e2032.

Glaucoma Research Foundation (2011) Glaucoma in Asian populations. Available at http://www.glaucoma.org/gleams/glaucoma-in-asian-populations.php

Lansingh VC, Carter MJ, Martens M (2007) Global cost effectiveness of cataract surgery. *Ophthalmology* 114:1670–8.

Lewallen S, Courtright P (2002) Gender and use of cataract surgical services in developing countries. *Bull WHO* 80:300–3.

Mathew AA, Turner A, Taylor HR (2009) Strategies to control trachoma. *Drugs* 69:953–70.

Pascolini D, Mariotti SP (2012) Global estimates of visual impairment: 2010. *Br J Ophthalmol* 96:614–18.

Rosenberg T (2013) *The New York Times*, 16 January 2013. A hospital network with a vision. Available at http://opinionator.blogs.nytimes.com/2013/01/16/in-india-leading-a-hospital-franchise-with-vision/

TDR for Research on Diseases of Poverty (2013) Disease Watch Focus: Onchocerciasis. Available at http://www.who.int/tdr/publications/disease_watch/oncho/en/index.html

World Health Organization (2007) A global initiative for the elimination of avoidable blindness: action plan 2006–2011. Available at http://www.who.int/blindness/Vision2020_report.pdf

World Health Organization (2010) Visual impairment and blindness data map. Available at http://www.who.int/blindness/data_maps/en/

World Health Organization (2013a) Prevention of blindness and visual impairment. Global data on visual impairments 2010. Available at http://www.who.int/blindness/en/

World Health Organization (2013b) Prevention of blindness and visual impairment. Priority eye diseases. Available at http://www.who.int/blindness/causes/priority/en/index2.html

World Health Organization (2013c) Prevention of blindness and visual impairment: definition and causes. ICD Update and Revision Platform: Change the Definition of Blindness. Available at http://www.who.int/blindness/en/index.html

Part 6
Other Global
Health Topics

CHAPTER 31

Essential Laboratory Skills

Adam M. Ackerman[1], Peter B. Cooch[2], and Aliyah R. Sohani[3]

[1]Maine Medical Center, Portland, ME, USA
[2]University of California San Francisco, San Francisco, CA, USA
[3]Massachusetts General Hospital and Harvard Medical School, Boston, MA, USA

Key learning objectives

- Gain an appreciation for the role laboratory diagnostics can play in global health.
- Understand principles of basic light microscopy.
- Learn to perform simple laboratory techniques that can be used in a number of settings.
- Understand how to analyze and interpret test results.
- Consider the future of laboratory diagnostics in low-resource settings as technologies improve and advance.

Abstract

Reliance on the results of laboratory tests to help diagnose disease in the developed world has grown to such an extent that healthcare workers would likely be at a loss without easy access to such invaluable data. However, the opposite remains true in many parts of the globe. In low-resource settings, reliance on history, physical examination, and clinical intuition goes extraordinarily far, but some basic knowledge of essential laboratory skills can ensure an accurate diagnosis and appropriate treatment, making a huge difference to a patient's outcome. The purpose of this chapter is to provide the reader with an overview of basic laboratory procedures for use in low-resource settings and to illustrate how familiarity with such skills, as well as ensuring their quality and reliability, play an important role in diagnostic accuracy, ultimately leading to improved patient care and outcome.

Key words: laboratory testing, pathology, infectious disease, low-resource settings, point of care, microscopy, parasitology, diagnostics

Essential Clinical Global Health, First Edition. Edited by Brett D. Nelson.
© 2015 John Wiley & Sons, Ltd. Published 2015 by John Wiley & Sons, Ltd.
Companion website: www.essentialseries.com/globalhealth

Introduction

Laboratory testing is a standard part of diagnosing disease in the developed world. As healthcare students and professionals, we would likely feel at a loss without access to invaluable laboratory data at our fingertips. However, the opposite remains true in many parts of the globe. While reliance on history, physical examination, and clinical intuition goes extraordinarily far in resource-challenged settings, appropriate treatment is predicated on an accurate diagnosis. Therefore, some basic knowledge of essential laboratory skills can make a huge difference to a patient's outcome. The purpose of this chapter is to provide the reader with an overview of basic laboratory procedures for use in low-resource settings and to illustrate how familiarity with such skills, as well as ensuring their quality and reliability, play a key role in making a proper diagnosis, ultimately leading to a better outcome for both the patient and provider.

The most appropriate laboratory assays may vary enormously between regions, depending on resources, availability of trained personnel, and pathologies most likely to be encountered. Local healthcare providers and laboratory professionals represent valuable sources of information when considering which diagnostic tests can best serve a population. In general, laboratory tests should always complement and augment the level of care at local clinics and hospitals. This chapter will focus on tests and concepts that are simple and practical to implement and that provide reliable data that directly impact patient care.

Clinical experience: challenges in providing laboratory services abroad

"We helped write this chapter's introduction while traveling abroad on a project to assess laboratory capabilities at a major clinic serving 15,000 people. Frequent power failures caused us to regularly hunt around for electrical outlets in the hope that one still had electricity flowing. It was an appropriate reminder of the realities of life for many people on the planet, and we wondered how this problem might affect the use of the microscope we just delivered, or the sample in the centrifuge plugged into the wall. Challenges to providing laboratory services while traveling abroad are numerous. A few potential barriers include language, access to clean water, electricity and refrigeration, and availability of equipment, reagents and trained personnel. Flexibility, creativity, patience, and curiosity are the greatest assets you can carry abroad in meeting these challenges."

Adam and Peter, working in the Dominican Republic

Quality and safety in the clinical laboratory

The safety of laboratory personnel is paramount and is closely tied to quality control (QC). Being mindful that each specimen represents vital information about your patient and is potentially infectious will help to ensure the quality of your work and your well-being. Key laboratory safety tips include the following.

- Designated personal protective equipment, such as a lab coat, closed-toe shoes, and protective eyewear, should be worn at all times.
- Protective latex or nitrile gloves must be worn when handling specimens.
- No food or drinks in the laboratory.
- Wash hands after handling specimens and before entering and leaving the laboratory.

In its essence, QC ensures the accuracy, reliability, and reproducibility of laboratory results, helping you to be confident in your diagnosis. Key elements of good QC include the following.

- Label all specimens as soon as possible following collection or receipt.
- Follow the reagent manufacturer's guidelines regarding instrument maintenance and frequency of calibration and running QC samples.
- Take care to prevent cross-contamination between specimens.
- Dispose of expired reagents promptly.
- Ensure that QC is acceptable prior to reporting patient results.

Essential laboratory procedures

Basic light microscopy

Commonplace in most laboratories, the light microscope remains a wonder that can reveal a wealth of information about our patients. Proper use of a light microscope is central to the practice of laboratory medicine across the globe, and most of the techniques described in this chapter rely on it.

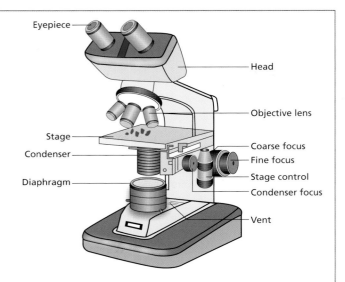

Figure 31.1 Parts of a compound light microscope. Familiarize yourself with your specific microscope. Most models are similar in structure and function, but slight variations exist.

Box 31.1 Microscope maintenance

As with other types of laboratory instrumentation, proper microscope maintenance allows for years of use, even in extreme climates. At the end of each day, wipe down the microscope exterior with a mild soap solution and protect it with a dust cover. Clean the objective lenses with lens paper only when they are noticeably dirty.

If donating a microscope for use in a resource-challenged setting, consider the voltage of the power supply that is generally used in the receiving country. A step-up or step-down transformer may be needed in addition to a power adaptor. Extra microscope bulbs will be invaluable so the laboratory does not have to go far to find one when their light source eventually runs out.

Technique

Figure 31.1 illustrates the major parts of a compound light microscope. Begin by placing the slide on the stage and turning on the light source. Carefully use coarse focus until the specimen becomes visible and then fine focus until the image is clear and sharp. To avoid crushing the slide, always watch the stage when switching objectives or using coarse focus.

As a rule of thumb, start your examination at the lowest power or magnification and sequentially increase to higher-powered objectives. Low power allows assessment of the quality and overall morphology of the preparation. This step is often bypassed at the expense of missing important information. For example, a peripheral blood smear that appears blue on low power may be indicative of leukocytosis.

The high-power 100× objective operates while nearly touching the slide, with a drop of specialized "immersion oil" to bridge the gap. Focus the slide using the highest magnification dry objective (usually 10–40×), then place a small drop of oil on the slide without an objective in place. Pivot the 100× objective into place (the 100× objective should touch the surface of the oil) and use fine focus to sharpen the image.

Most microscopes use a diaphragm to control the amount and angle of light reaching the slide. Use this feature to adjust contrast, in order to make individual objects distinguishable from one another. This is particularly useful when viewing unstained specimens. Box 31.1 describes best how to maintain microscopes.

Fixed slide preparation

Fixed slides are prepared using a common technique from a variety of sources, such as sputum, urine, pus, or cerebrospinal fluid (CSF). Subsequently slides may be stained using various staining methods such as the Gram or acid-fast stains for visualization of infectious organisms. For preparation of peripheral blood smears, refer to the subsequent section on peripheral blood smear evaluation.

Materials

Microscope, glass slides, inoculating loop or sterile swab, clean flame source, 70% methanol, gloves.

Technique

1. If using an inoculating loop, sterilize it in the flame, then let it cool.
2. Collect the desired specimen with the loop or swab. Urine and CSF must be centrifuged to concentrate.
3. Press the loop in the middle of a slide and spread a thin layer of the specimen by moving it in an outward spiral, without reaching the slide edge.
4. Allow to air-dry completely.
5. To fix the sample, pass the slide several times through the flame or add several drops of methanol and let it air-dry.

Gram stain

This simple staining procedure ingeniously allows the visualization and categorization of bacterial species. The process consists of a series of staining and decolorizing steps that give a distinctive purple color for Gram-positive bacteria and pink color for Gram-negative bacteria. Analysis of both the color and morphology can suggest a causative pathogen and guide choice of antibiotic therapy.

Indication

Suspected bacterial infection of most body fluids.

Materials

Microscope, glass slides, Coplin jars, crystal violet stain, Lugol iodine 0.1% solution, 95% ethanol, carbolfuchsin or safranin, clean water, gloves.

Technique

Various methods for applying and washing off stains are illustrated in Figure 31.2(a,b).

1. Smear a sample on a glass slide and fix as described in the previous section on fixed slide preparation.
2. Cover slide with crystal violet stain for 20 s.
3. Wash off the stain with water.
4. Drain the slide and cover the sample with Lugol iodine for 20 s.
5. Wash Lugol iodine off with water.
6. Run 95% ethanol down the slide until it drains clear (approximately 2 s).
7. Cover the sample with safranin or carbolfuchsin for 2 min.
8. Wash off the stain with water and stand the slide upright to air-dry prior to viewing.

Interpretation

Bacteria will only be visible on the highest magnification under immersion oil ($100\times$). Record organism staining, morphology, and grouping. The basic Gram stain interpretive algorithm is illustrated in Figure 31.2(c,d), while common bacterial species and their Gram-staining characteristics are illustrated in Figure 31.3.

Acid-fast stain

The highly pathogenic nature of many acid-fast organisms makes this stain a laboratory essential. The most notable

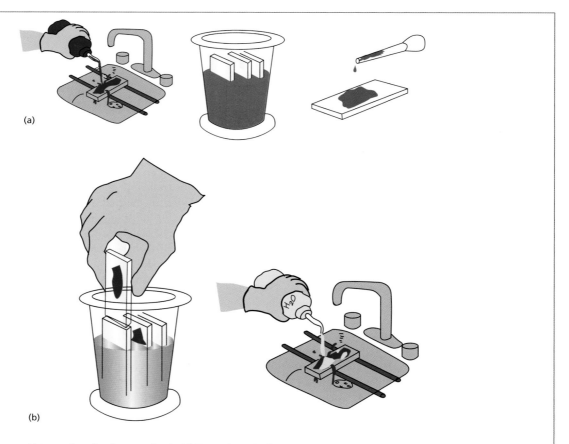

Figure 31.2 Performing and interpreting the Gram stain. (a, b) Examples of different methods of applying (a) and washing off (b) stain.

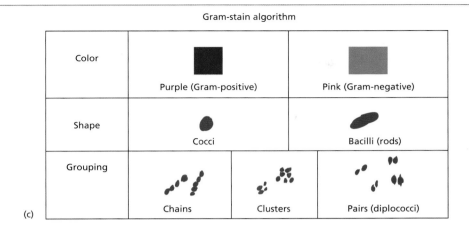

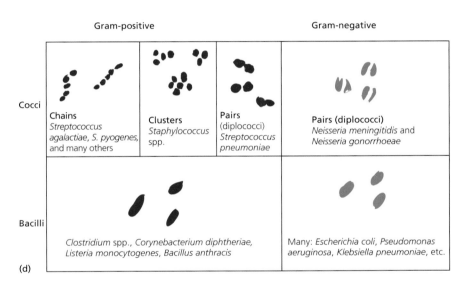

Figure 31.2 (*Continued*) (c, d) The Gram-stain algorithm is used to identify different bacterial species based on their color, shape, and arrangement.

acid-fast pathogen is *Mycobacterium tuberculosis*. This organism, and those like it, contain a large amount of fatty mycolic acid in their cell walls, which makes them resistant to regular Gram staining. However, they retain the carbolfuchsin stain when treated with acid alcohol and are therefore said to be "acid fast." Some pathogens, such as *Nocardia*, *Isospora belli*, and *Cryptosporidium* species, are considered "modified acid fast" as they retain the stain more weakly. The Ziehl–Neelsen technique is described here due to its high sensitivity and specificity (Van Deun *et al.*, 2005). Other techniques are available, including those that do not require the use of heat.

Indications

Suspected infection with *Mycobacterium* or other acid-fast organisms.

Materials

Microscope, glass slides, Coplin jars, Ziehl–Neelsen (carbolfuchsin) stain, acid ethanol, methylene blue, spirit lamp, clean water, gloves. Note that acid-fast staining of suspected *Mycobacterium* should ideally be conducted with a fitted N-95 respirator mask and under a negative-pressure ventilator hood, if available.

Technique

1. Smear a sample on a glass slide and fix as described in the section on fixed slide preparation.
2. Cover slide in Ziehl–Neelsen stain.
3. Gently heat over spirit lamp just until stain begins to evaporate.

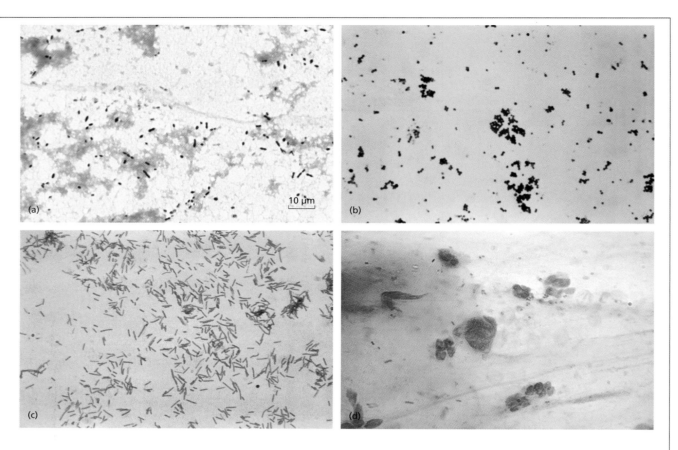

Figure 31.3 Bacterial identification using the Gram stain. (a) *Streptococcus pneumoniae* appears as Gram-positive diplococci. (b) *Staphylococcus aureus* appears as Gram-positive cocci in clusters. (c) *Bacteroides fragilis* appears as Gram-negative rods. (d) *Neisseria gonorrhoeae* appears as Gram-negative diplococci. *Sources*: (a) C. Wojewoda and A. Ross, University of Vermont, Vermont, USA, 2013. Reproduced with permission of C. Wojewoda and A. Ross. (b) CDC Public Health Image Library. (c) CDC Public Health Image Library/Don Stalons. (d) CDC Public Health Image Library/Joe Miller.

4. Allow slide to sit for 5 min.
5. Rinse slide with water.
6. Cover slide with acid ethanol and let sit for 5 min. For *Mycobacterium* species, we recommend 3% HCl acid ethanol. For modified acid-fast organisms, a weaker acid such as 1% H_2SO_4 will give better results.
7. Rinse slide with water.
8. Cover with methylene blue and let sit for 1 min.
9. Rinse slide with water and let dry.

Interpretation

Examine these slides using the same technique as described for Gram-stained slides. Acid-fast organisms will appear red. Cells and non-acid-fast organisms will be counterstained blue.

Fecal wet mounts: laboratory evaluation of gastrointestinal parasites

Stool microscopy is an essential diagnostic technique in laboratories across the developing world, but its sensitivity is very poor for most protozoa, even in professional laboratories. Excellent enzyme-linked immunosorbent assays (ELISAs) and acceptable rapid antigen tests exist for the three most common protozoal pathogens: *Entamoeba histolytica*, *Giardia intestinalis*, and *Cryptosporidium* species (Garcia & Shimizu, 1997; Haque *et al.*, 1998). In contrast, microscopy of fecal wet mounts remains the test of choice for diagnosing helminth infections, as helminth eggs are often easily identified and excreted in high numbers. Stool concentration or filtration, such as the Kato–Katz technique, can increase sensitivity but is not always practical (Knopp *et al.*, 2011). As their name implies, "wet" mounts are unfixed and should be examined as soon as they are made. Wet mounts may also be prepared from vaginal discharge for the evaluation of bacterial vaginosis or *Trichomonas* infection (see Chapter 16 for additional diagnostic criteria).

Indications

- Suspected helminth infestation.
- Diagnosis of selected protozoa.

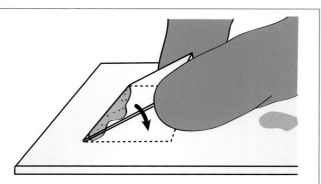

Figure 31.4 Coverslip placement. In order to avoid trapping air bubbles, apply coverslip by holding it at a 45° angle to the slide until liquid completely covers one edge of the coverslip. Then carefully drop the coverslip onto the slide while attempting to maintain as much contact as possible with the liquid portion of the specimen.

Materials

Microscope, glass slides, coverslips, applicator, saline solution, Lugol iodine.

Technique

1. Place one drop of saline solution and one drop of Lugol iodine separated on a slide.
2. Using the applicator, take a small amount of the stool sample and mix separately with each drop.
3. Apply a coverslip to each drop as shown in Figure 31.4. The preparations should be thin enough so that newsprint can be read through it.
4. Examine the saline drop for motile parasites and the Lugol iodine drop for cysts and eggs.

Interpretation

Recognition of characteristic morphologic features of helminth eggs and parasites can allow a species-specific diagnosis (Figures 31.5 and 31.6).

KOH preparations: laboratory evaluation of fungal infection

The potassium hydroxide preparation, or "KOH prep" for short, is used to diagnose fungal infection. It is an important tool to help differentiate cutaneous fungal infection from other causes of dermatitis and to assist in evaluating vaginal discharge for the presence of yeast or *Candida* species (see Chapter 16 for additional diagnostic criteria).

Indications

- Dermatitis of suspected fungal origin.
- Vaginal irritation, itching, or discharge.

Materials

Microscope, glass slides, coverslips, sterile razor, 10% KOH solution, gloves.

Technique

1. For evaluation of dermatitis, hold slide up to skin lesion and brush razor edge lightly over skin to flake off scale onto slide. Use a cotton swab if collecting vaginal discharge.
2. Add one drop of KOH solution to slide surface and apply coverslip (Figure 31.4).

Interpretation

The KOH will dissolve epithelial cells, leaving fungal hyphae and spores or budding yeast forms in the case of candidiasis.

Urinalysis

Urinalysis is a non-invasive technique that can provide insight into a number of genitourinary and systemic processes. Urinalysis strips (also known as urine dipsticks) qualify a spectrum of findings, and the results can help to determine whether additional microscopic examination of centrifuged urine sediment may be needed (see below). Clean-catch, mid-stream urine collection is preferred; use sterile catheterization samples from pediatric patients. Urine dipstick packages typically come with a color guide on the container label for qualitative and semi-quantitative interpretation of the results.

Indications for microscopic analysis of urine sediments

- Clinical: hematuria, suspected renal disease, nephrolithiasis, diabetes, complicated urinary tract infection.
- Laboratory: results of urinalysis strip indicate presence of blood, glucose, ketones, white blood cells, or bacteria.

Materials

Microscope, glass slides, coverslips, centrifuge, centrifuge tube, pipette, gloves.

Technique

1. Add 10 mL of urine to centrifuge tube.
2. Centrifuge at medium speed (approximately 2000 rpm) for 5–10 min. Make sure to balance the centrifuge with a second sample or dummy tube containing the same amount of liquid.
3. Pour off supernatant and resuspend sediment in remaining liquid.
4. Transfer one drop onto a slide with a pipette and apply coverslip (Figure 31.4).

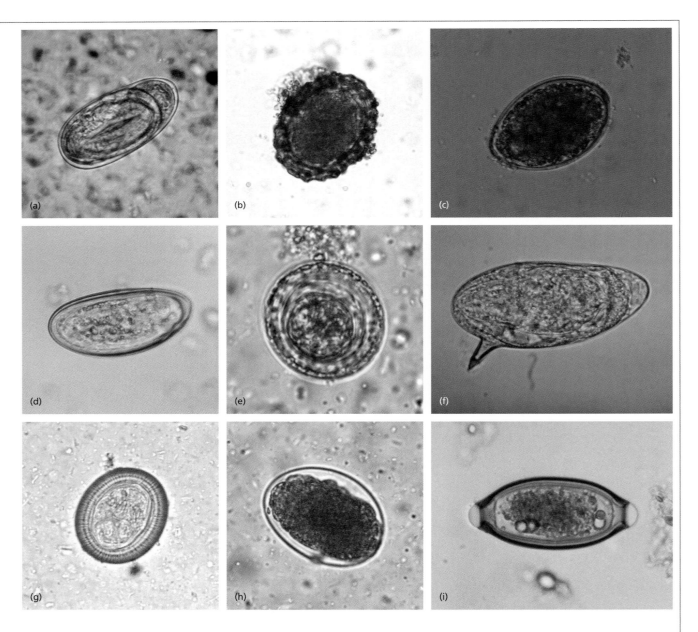

Figure 31.5 Common helminth eggs. (a) The eggs of the two hookworm species *Ancylostoma duodenale* and *Necator americanus* are microscopically indistinguishable. (b) Over a billion humans are believed to be infected with *Ascaris lumbricoides*, whose eggs have a distinctive crenellated appearance. (c) An egg of *Diphyllobothrium latum*, also known as the fish tapeworm, whose infestations may present with Vitamin B$_{12}$ deficiency. (d) The eggs of *Enterobius vermicularis*, or human pinworm, are elongated and flattened on one side. Pinworm eggs and larvae can often be collected from the perianal area using the "Scotch tape/Sellotape test." (e) *Hymenolepis nana*, known as the dwarf tapeworm, is the most common cestode of humans. Unlike *Taenia* species, its eggs are not striated. (f) An egg of *Schistosoma mansoni*, the principal cause of intestinal schistosomiasis. The eggs are visible on low power and have a highly characteristic lateral spine. (g) The eggs of *Taenia solium* (pork tapeworm) and *Taenia saginata* (beef tapeworm) cannot be microscopically distinguished from one another. (h) *Strongyloides stercoralis* is one of the few helminth species capable of autoinfection, i.e., its eggs hatch within the host and restart their life cycle without first needing to be shed in stool. As such, it is often microscopically diagnosed by the presence of larvae rather than eggs. (i) A *Trichuris trichiura* egg, from a parasitic nematode known as human whipworm. *Sources*: (a, f) CDC Public Health Image Library. (b, c, e, h) C. Wojewoda and A. Ross, University of Vermont, Vermont, USA, 2013. Reproduced with permission of C. Wojewoda and A. Ross. (d) CDC Public Health Image Library/B.G. Partin and Dr Moore. (g) CDC Public Health Image Library/M. Melvin. (i) CDC Public Health Image Library/B.G. Partin.

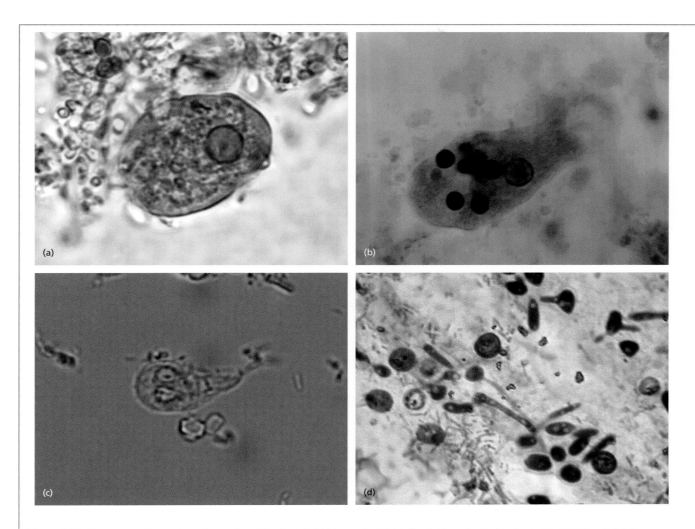

Figure 31.6 Common pathogenic protozoa found in stool. (a) *Entamoeba histolytica* is the principal pathogenic amoeba, but it is morphologically identical to the far more common non-pathogenic organism *Entamoeba dispar*. Analysis by ELISA is usually necessary to differentiate the two species. *Entamoeba dispar* and *E. histolytica* trophozoites have a single nucleus and may be observed to move by pseudopod extension. (b) *Entamoeba histolytica* can rarely be microscopically confirmed by the presence of erythrophagocytosis, as seen in this trichrome stain. (c) The motile trophozoite form of *Giardia intestinalis* has a classic "owl's eyes" appearance and is usually only acquired from liquid stool samples. (d) *Cryptosporidium parvum* and related species are extremely small, ranging from 3 to 5 μm in diameter (about half the size of a red blood cell). They take a red color with modified acid-fast staining. *Sources*: (a) CDC Diagnosis of Parasites of Public Health Concern. Reproduced with permission of CDC Diagnosis of Parasites of Public Health Concern. (b) CDC Public Health Image Library/M. Melvin and Dr Greene. (c) C. Wojewoda and A. Ross, University of Vermont, Vermont, USA, 2013. Reproduced with permission of C. Wojewoda and A. Ross. (d) Ma P, Soave R (1983) Three-step stool examination for cryptosporidiosis in 10 homosexual men with protracted watery diarrhea. *J Infect Dis* 147, figure 2, p. 826. Reproduced with permission of Oxford University Press.

Interpretation

Report the number of visible elements per 40× field. Objects to look for include casts, red blood cells (RBCs), white blood cells (WBCs), bacteria, and epithelial cells. Look for casts under 10× along the edges of the coverslip. If crystals are observed, note the pH to determine their significance. If you are working in a region where urinary schistosomiasis is common, do not forget to look for helminth eggs (Figure 31.7

and Box 31.2). See Table 31.1 for interpretation guide to urine sediment abnormalities.

Peripheral blood smear evaluation

Evaluation of a peripheral blood smear (PBS) is essential to hematology practice in resource-limited settings. It represents a key method for the diagnosis of malaria, and the same technique can be used to help in the evaluation of other etiologies

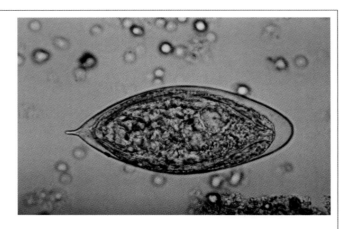

Figure 31.7 *Schistosoma haematobium* egg in a urine sediment sample, easily recognizable by its large size and prominent terminal spine (arrow). *Source*: CDC Public Health Image Library.

Table 31.1 Interpretation guide to urine sediment abnormalities

Abnormality	Interpretation
Squamous epithelial cells	If numerous, suggests a contaminated catch
Erythrocytes/red blood cells	Abnormal if >2 per 40× field. Indicative of microscopic hematuria if urine color is non-bloody on macroscopic assessment. Absence of red blood cells in a sample with gross pink coloring or positive blood on urinalysis may indicate hemoglobinuria.
White blood cells	Bacterial or other urinary tract infection
Red blood cell casts	Suggests renal source of hematuria, such as glomerulonephritis
White blood cell casts	Present in kidney infections, such as pyelonephritis
Bacteria	Consistent with bacterial source of infection. Consider possibility of skin contaminant if urinalysis strip is negative for white blood cells or bacteria.

Box 31.2 Schistosoma haematobium

Chronically high egg burden leads to the symptoms of urinary schistosomiasis, prevalent in the Middle East, South Asia, and Africa. The presence of blood on urinalysis is an effective screening tool for infection, while microscopic analysis of urine sediment is the confirmatory test of choice, with greater than 90% sensitivity for the detection of eggs (see Figure 31.7) (Koukounari *et al.*, 2009).

- For highest egg yield, collect a 10-mL terminal urine sample between 10 AM and 2 PM.
- To concentrate the eggs, centrifuge for 2 min at medium speed (approximately 2000 rpm). Alternatively, commercially available syringes pre-fitted with filters allow egg concentration in the field.
- Examine filter or precipitate at low power, recording total number of eggs. Identifying more than 50 eggs per 10 mL of urine represents a heavy infection.

of anemia. With experience, careful PBS evaluation can even obviate the need for a bedside hemoglobin meter or basic automated cell counter, instrumentation that may not be readily available in many areas.

Indications for preparation of thick and thin peripheral blood smears

- Suspected malarial or other infection (e.g., fevers, chills).
- Signs and symptoms of anemia (e.g., pallor, fatigue, jaundice).

Materials

Two glass slides, Coplin jars or slide racks and plastic containers, methanol, Wright–Giemsa or other suitable stain, clean water, gloves.

Technique

This protocol, as illustrated in Figure 31.8, provides a general guide on how to create thick and thin smears using a widely accepted method and stain (World Health Organization, 2003). Note that a number of different methods, other than Wright–Giemsa, may be used to stain smears. In addition, making a quality PBS may be challenging, and we recommend you practice the technique using the resources of a local laboratory prior to going abroad (see Additional Resources section).

1. For the thick smear, place two small drops of blood on the slide by using a lancet on the patient's third or fourth finger, or by transferring with a pipette a small amount of blood that has already been collected.
2. Use the corner of the second glass slide (spreader slide) to join together the two small drops of blood and create an even thick film.
3. For the thin smear, place one small drop of blood on the glass slide in front of the thick smear.
4. Using the second glass slide as a spreader held at a 45° angle, back into the drop of blood (it will spread along the edge of the spreader slide) and quickly push the spreader along

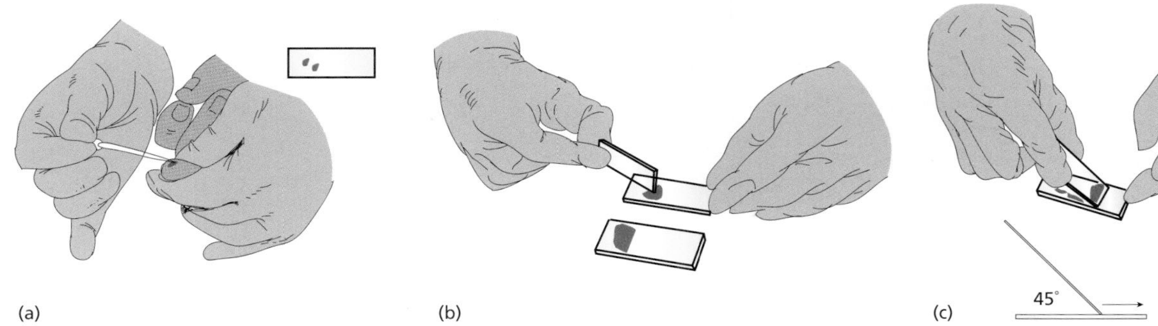

Figure 31.8 Preparation of thick and thin peripheral blood smears. (a) Collect or place drops for thick and thin peripheral blood smears as illustrated. Prepare the thick (b) and thin (c) smears as shown.

the length of the slide. This will create the appearance of a "feathered edge" grossly, which translates to a thin monolayer of cells under the microscope.

5. Allow the smear to air-dry.
6. Immerse the slide(s) in methanol for 5 s and let dry.
7. Transfer the slides to a Coplin jar with Wright–Giemsa stain for approximately 15 min.
8. Wash the slides in three successive Coplin jars or plastic containers filled with clean water to remove excess stain.
9. Allow the slides to dry completely.

Interpretation

Principles of basic microscopy apply to PBS interpretation. Always begin your evaluation on low power and progressively increase to higher magnification for more detailed assessment. Methodical analysis of these samples is important, for example you would not want to miss the presence of schistocytes (a possible clue to sepsis) because you were distracted by a few intracellular parasites. Listed below are key items to assess during low- and high-power PBS evaluation. Examples of specific findings are shown in Figure 31.9. See Chapter 10 for more detailed information related to PBS evaluation for malaria.

Low-power evaluation (10× magnification)
- Observe the overall quality of the PBS. Is the thick smear evenly distributed? Is there a monolayer of RBCs on the thin smear? Are the RBCs intact?
- Is the sample adequately stained? Nuclei of WBCs should appear blue-purple, while RBCs should appear pink-red.

High-power evaluation (100× magnification, oil immersion)
- Concentrate your evaluation in an area of the smear where the RBCs form a monolayer, usually about two 10× fields in from the very edge of the smear. Evaluate the morphology of the RBCs.

- Are they biconcave disks or do they have an abnormal shape (e.g., sickle cells, schistocytes)?
- Are they microcytic, normocytic, or macrocytic? Normal RBCs have a diameter of 7 μm, approximating the diameter of a small lymphocyte nucleus.
- Look at the area of central pallor, which typically occupies about one-third of the cellular diameter. Increased central pallor is indicative of hypochromic anemia, whereas absence of central pallor points to the presence of spherocytes.
- Are there any inclusions (e.g., Howell–Jolly bodies, basophilic stippling) or parasites present inside the cells? Are parasites present between the cells?
- Observe the overall number and distribution of RBCs. Increased empty space between them indicates a decrease in the total RBC count or mass, a sign of anemia.
- To estimate the patient's peripheral counts, examine several 100× fields, count the average number of WBCs and/or platelets per field, and multiply by 15. This provides an approximate WBC or platelet count in units of $\times 10^3/mm^3$.
- If leukocytosis is present, perform a 100-cell manual WBC differential count, noting any abnormalities in morphology and relative number. See Table 31.2 for a guide to interpretation (CAP Hematology and Clinical Microscopy Resource Committee, 1998).
- Observing 8–20 platelets per 100× field corresponds to a normal platelet count. Thrombocytosis is a common finding in iron-deficiency anemia or a variety of infectious or inflammatory states. However, thrombocytopenia in the setting of fever and a characteristic rash can help clinch a diagnosis of dengue fever.

Cerebrospinal fluid analysis

Evaluation of CSF samples can provide diagnostic insight into a variety of conditions affecting the central nervous system (CNS). Since normal CSF is clear and colorless, macroscopic assessment can be done easily at the time of sample collection

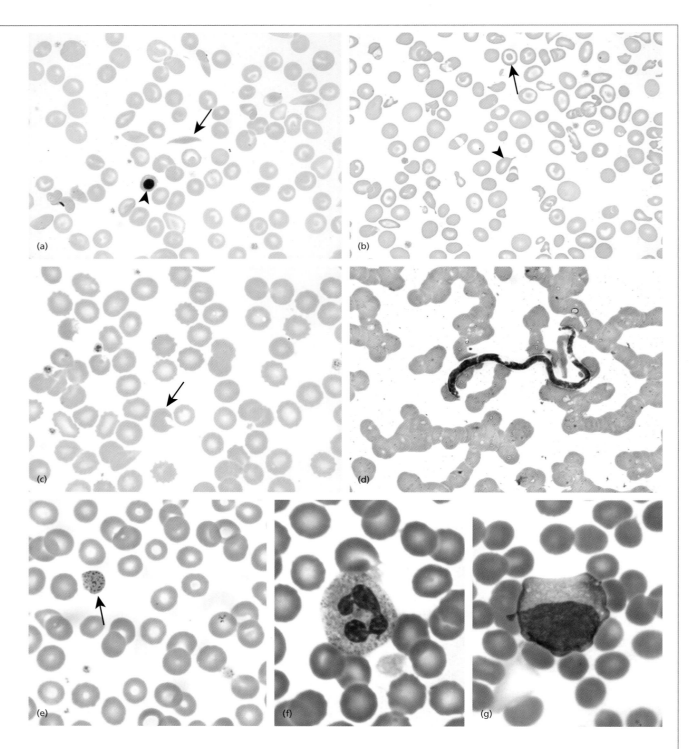

Figure 31.9 Morphologic abnormalities in peripheral blood. (a) Sickle cell disease with drepanocytes or sickled red blood cells (arrow) and a nucleated red blood cell (arrowhead). (b) A case of thalassemia demonstrating marked anisopoikilocytosis (variation in red blood cell shape and size), including numerous microcytes, target cells (arrow), and teardrop cells or dacryocytes (arrowhead). (c) Smear from patient with glucose-6-phosphate dehydrogenase deficiency showing bite cell (arrow). (d) An example of microfilaria infection with elongated cylindrical extracellular form circulating in peripheral blood. (e) Lead poisoning with coarse basophilic stippling (arrow). This finding is not specific to lead intoxication and may be seen in other conditions, including β-thalassemia and bone marrow stress. (f) Segmented neutrophil exhibiting toxic granulation, as evidenced by conspicuous primary granules that are purple in color compared with the pink secondary granules characteristically seen in mature neutrophils. (g) Acute Epstein–Barr virus infection (infectious mononucleosis) characterized by enlarged lymphocytes containing moderate cytoplasm with peripheral basophilic accentuation and adherence to surrounding red blood cells. All images stained with Wright–Giemsa, 1000× magnification. *Sources*: (d) D. Bengo, Mulago Hospital, Kampala, Uganda. Reproduced with permission of D. Bengo. (e) Friedman LS, Simmons LH, Goldman RH, Sohani AR (2014) Case 12-2014: a 59-year-old man with fatigue, abdominal pain, anemia, and abnormal liver function. *N Engl J Med* 370, figure 1a, p. 1544, reproduced with permission from Massachusetts Medical Society.

Table 31.2 Interpretation guide to white blood cell differentials in peripheral blood.

Cell type	Normal range (%)[a]	Increase suggestive of[b]
Neutrophils (segmented and band)	40–70	Bacterial infection. Neutrophils may acquire "toxic" features, with prominent deep pink–red cytoplasmic granules and vacuoles (see Figure 31.9f).
Lymphocytes	22–44	Acute pertussis, typhoid fever, or viral infection; chronic infectious or inflammatory disorders. In acute viral illness (e.g., infectious mononucleosis), lymphocytes are enlarged with a visible nucleolus and abundant cytoplasm showing a peripheral basophilic or bluish accentuation (see Figure 31.9g).
Monocytes	4–11	Chronic viral infection, syphilis, or tuberculosis. Collagen vascular disease, inflammatory bowel disease, sarcoidosis.
Eosinophils	0–8	Invasive parasitic or helminth infections, pernicious anemia, allergic or drug reactions, certain collagen vascular or autoimmune diseases, sarcoidosis, paraneoplastic (certain lymphomas and solid tumors).
Basophils	0–3	Hypersensitivity reaction, tuberculosis, certain types of leukemia
Immature granulocytes (myelocyte, metamyelocyte, promyelocyte)	0–2	Bacterial infection, bone marrow stress, certain types of leukemia
Blasts	0	Severe bone marrow stress due to infection or prematurity, if present in small numbers. Large numbers of blasts (>20% of white blood cells) are worrisome for acute leukemia.

[a] Based on adult normal range at the Massachusetts General Hospital, Boston, USA. Consultation of a standard reference text, such as *Johns Hopkins: The Harriet Lane Handbook*, is recommended for pediatric populations. In addition, regional differences may exist due to variation across race and ethnicity; normal range studies should be conducted as indicated to determine differences in your patient population.
[b] Adapted from CAP Hematology and Clinical Microscopy Resource Committee (1998).

or receipt by the laboratory (Table 31.3). One challenge may lie in discriminating between a traumatic tap versus a true intracranial bleed in visibly bloody samples. However, since lumbar puncture typically involves CSF collection into a series of three to four tubes that are sequentially labeled, assessment of color changes between earlier and later tubes can aid in this discrimination (Table 31.3) (CAP Hematology and Clinical Microscopy Resource Committee, 2006). Microscopic evaluation of CSF, if undertaken, should be performed as soon as possible due to WBC degeneration, which begins within 1–2 hours following collection (Clinical and Laboratory Standards Institute, 2006).

Indications for microscopic CSF analysis

- Clinical: signs and symptoms of suspected meningitis, encephalitis, subarachnoid hemorrhage, or other CNS disease.
- Laboratory: abnormal findings on macroscopic evaluation of CSF (Table 31.3).

To assess for the presence of bacteria, follow the steps outlined in the earlier section on fixed slide preparation and Gram stain-

ing. If tuberculous meningitis is suspected, allow a sample of CSF to sit for 10 min; clot formation is frequently observed (World Health Organization, 2003). Prepare and stain a slide from the sample, using the clot if present, and follow the steps outlined in the earlier section on fixed slide preparation and acid-fast staining.

Materials

Microscope, glass slides, Coplin jars or slide racks and plastic containers, methanol, Wright–Giemsa or other suitable stain, clean water, centrifuge, pipette, gloves. Optional: 22% albumin, Indian ink.

Technique

1. Following macroscopic and Gram-stain evaluation, place the CSF tube in a centrifuge.
2. Centrifuge at low speed (approximately 600 rpm) for 10 min. Make sure to balance the centrifuge with a second sample or dummy tube containing the same amount of liquid.
3. For grossly bloody samples, the supernatant can be assessed for xanthochromia at this step by holding it against a white

Table 31.3 Macroscopic assessment of cerebrospinal fluid.

Abnormal finding	Interpretation
Cloudy or turbid	Increase in white blood cells and protein, suggestive of meningitis. Differential diagnosis: CNS leukemia or metastatic infiltration.
Bloody or blood-tinged	Intracranial hemorrhage, parenchymal infarction, or traumatic tap. A traumatic tap will show streaks and/or large amounts of blood in the first tube with diminishing amounts of blood in later tubes, and the supernatant will appear clear after centrifugation.
Xanthochromia[a] (yellow, orange, or pink tint of supernatant after centrifugation)	Red blood cell breakdown indicative of prior hemorrhage and true intracranial bleed, or hemorrhagic encephalitis such as in HSV. Initial onset at about 2 hours following bleeding event; lasts for up to 4 weeks. Differential diagnosis: hyperbilirubinemia, elevated CSF protein.
Viscous	Cryptococcal infection (increased viscosity due to capsular polysaccharide). Differential diagnosis: metastatic adenocarcinoma (increased viscosity due to mucus).
Clotted	Increased fibrinogen suggestive of bacterial, mycobacterial, or suppurative meningitis; exclude traumatic tap.
Fatty	Fat embolism due to sickle cell disease or surgery.

[a] For grossly bloody samples, evaluate for xanthochromia in supernatant following centrifugation.
Source: adapted from CAP Hematology and Clinical Microscopy Resource Committee (2006), pp. 50–51.

background, using a tube of water for comparison. Aspirate supernatant (it may be utilized if the capability for CSF glucose or protein assays exists) and resuspend precipitate in remaining liquid. If available, add a drop of 22% albumin to make cells more adherent to the glass slide and reduce cellular disintegration (CAP Hematology and Clinical Microscopy Resource Committee, 2006; Clinical and Laboratory Standards Institute, 2006).

4. Transfer one drop of concentrated CSF onto a slide with a pipette.
5. Using a second slide as a spreader slide, make a thin smear of the concentrated CSF and stain with Wright–Giemsa or other appropriate stain. (Follow steps 3–9 for preparation of a thin PBS.)
6. Modification for suspected *Cryptococcus* meningitis: mix one drop of concentrated CSF and one drop of Indian ink on a microscope slide, then place coverslip and examine. Although *Cryptococcus* may be seen on Wright–Giemsa stain (Figure 31.10c), its appearance is enhanced by the Indian ink stain (Figure 31.10d).

Interpretation

Microscopic evaluation of cellular constituents is similar to that of peripheral blood smears. Even after centrifugation, normal CSF is typically paucicellular, containing no RBCs and only a few WBCs, namely lymphocytes (predominate in adults) and monocytes (predominate in neonates). If numerous WBCs are present, count and record at least 100 leukocytes for a differential. See Table 31.4 for an interpretive guide to microscopic CSF analysis. Examples of specific findings are illustrated in Figure 31.10.

Fern test

This test in pregnant women can aid in the diagnosis of active labor or premature rupture of membranes. Urinary leakage is commonly experienced by women during the late stages of pregnancy and may be difficult to distinguish from amniotic fluid based on reported symptoms. However, both the fern and nitrazine tests can identify the presence of amniotic fluid with greater certainty. Since the fern test has a higher specificity and can be performed without reagents, it is described here (Beckmann *et al.*, 2010).

Indications

- Fluid passage during pregnancy.
- Suspected labor or rupture of membranes.

Materials

Microscope, sterile vaginal swab or pipette, glass slide, gloves.

Technique

1. Obtain a sample of vaginal fluid that has been collected without the use of lubricant.
2. Create a thin smear of fluid on the glass slide and allow to air-dry. Do not use heat to speed up drying.
3. Observe under the microscope on low power (10×).

Interpretation

As amniotic fluid dries on a slide, it leaves a distinct pattern reminiscent of a fern leaf due to its sodium chloride content

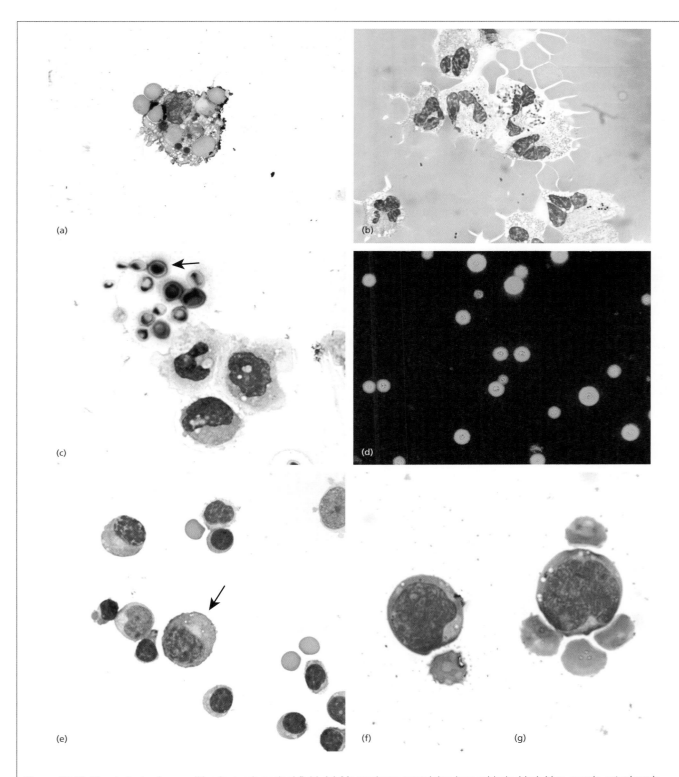

Figure 31.10 Morphologic abnormalities in cerebrospinal fluid. (a) Macrophage containing hemosiderin (dark blue–purple cytoplasmic inclusions) and intact red blood cells (erythrophagocytosis), indicative of true intracranial bleed. (b) Increased numbers of neutrophils, many of which contain phagocytosed bacteria, consistent with bacterial meningitis. Note the large number of red blood cells in the background, suggestive of intracranial hemorrhage or traumatic tap. (c) Cryptococcal meningitis with increased numbers of monocytes and adjacent yeast forms containing a round darkly stained core surrounded by a concentric clear area, representing the mucopolysaccharide capsule (arrow). (d) Indian ink preparation of *Cryptococcus neoformans* fungal meningitis. This staining technique enables better recognition of the organism's clear outer capsule, while the central spore contains grayish granulations. (e) Increased numbers of lymphocytes, as well as a few plasma cells (arrow). Plasma cells are an unusual cell type in CSF and typically reflect meningitis due to syphilis, tuberculosis, or cysticercosis. (f, g) Secondary CSF involvement by Burkitt lymphoma. The neoplastic cells are larger than typical lymphocytes with a high nuclear-to-cytoplasmic ratio, open (rather than condensed) chromatin, small nucleoli and basophilic cytoplasm with small, but conspicuous, vacuoles. Images (a–c) and (e–g) all stained with Wright–Giemsa, 1000× magnification. *Source*: (d) CDC Public Health Image Library.

Table 31.4 Microscopic assessment of cerebrospinal fluid.

Cell type	Increased numbers seen in
Red blood cells	CNS hemorrhage due to stroke. Exclude traumatic tap: look for clearing of fluid color in later tubes, evaluate macroscopically for xanthochromia or microscopically for hemosiderin-laden macrophages or erythrophagocytosis (see Figure 31.10a).
Neutrophils	Bacterial or malarial meningitis (see Figure 31.10b), post-ictal states, infarction, CNS hemorrhage.
Lymphocytes	Viral, mycobacterial, fungal, or parasitic meningitis/encephalitis (i.e., lymphocytic pleocytosis). Other etiologies include Guillain–Barré syndrome and multiple sclerosis (see Figure 31.10e).
Eosinophils	Parasitic infection. Differential diagnosis: drug or foreign body reaction (e.g., ventriculoperitoneal shunt).
Monocytes	Chronic meningitis/encephalitis due to any etiology.
Plasma cells	Meningitis due to syphilis (neurosyphilis), tuberculosis, or cysticercosis. Other causes include Guillain–Barré syndrome, multiple sclerosis, and neurosarcoidosis (see Figure 31.10e).
Macrophages	Various states. Look inside the cytoplasm of these phagocytes for clues: • Organisms: infection • Hemosiderin or intact red blood cells (erythrophagocytosis): prior hemorrhage indicating a true intracranial bleed (see Figure 31.10a) • Fat: parenchymal infarction, vertebral bone infarction due to sickle cell disease, trauma, or traumatic tap.

Source: adapted from CAP Hematology and Clinical Microscopy Resource Committee (2006), pp. 54–55.

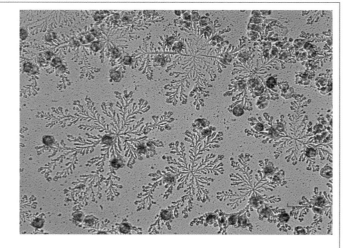

Figure 31.11 Positive fern test. This pattern, reminiscent of a fern leaf, indicates presence of amniotic fluid, as opposed to urine or other vaginal secretions. *Source*: N.J. Garol, University of Vermont, Vermont, USA, 2013. Reproduced with permission of N.J Garol.

Box 31.3 Record maintenance and data collection

Record-keeping and collection of relevant data, including patient-specific identifiers, type of specimen, date and time of sample collection, and results of assays performed on the sample, are an implicit part of the laboratory's function. Findings should be included in the patient's medical record to allow for optimal continuity of care. Although record-keeping is not standardized and you will likely encounter a variety of handwritten and digital methods, the World Health Organization offers several important guidelines related to laboratory records and test report contents (World Health Organization, 2011). Implementation of a simple electronic database may go a long way to help ensure data reliability and retrievability, and electronic records may be easier to incorporate into population-based databases, aiding in public health surveillance and research. Ultimately, the method used for record-keeping must be supported by the resources available at the site and be appropriate to the skill set of local personnel.

(Figure 31.11) (Beckmann *et al.*, 2010). False-positive results may be due to contamination with semen, cervical mucus, or blood.

Box 31.3 describes record maintenance and data collection methods, which apply to the various tests discussed in this chapter.

Additional tests and techniques

Fecal occult blood

Commercial stool guaiac tests for the evaluation of fecal occult blood can be performed anywhere. They typically involve placing a small smear of feces on a testing card. Application of a developer will indicate presence or absence of blood. Keep in mind that an iron-rich diet can lead to a false-positive result.

Point-of-care and rapid antigen tests

Point-of-care testing (POCT) bypasses the need for existing laboratory infrastructure, requires minimal training, and can be performed at the patient's bedside. Many of the tests described in this chapter (e.g., urinalysis strips and stool guaiac cards) utilize principles of POCT, and you may already be familiar with additional examples, such as glucometers, hemoglobin meters, and home pregnancy tests. More recently, rapid antigen tests are a type of point-of-care assay that have become available to aid in the diagnosis of some of the world's most burdensome infections, including malaria and HIV, that have traditionally required more specialized and costly techniques and equipment for diagnosis (Abba *et al.*, 2011; Pant Pai *et al.*, 2012). Effective POCT may also be in the pipeline for active tuberculosis (McNerney & Daley, 2011). While not necessarily the gold standard, many point-of-care and rapid antigen tests are highly sensitive and specific and can be used to screen at-risk populations.

At present, widespread use of POCT is limited by cost and access. Nonetheless, POCT offers an exciting and convenient alternative to traditional assays and is certain to change the practice of global health. Consult with colleagues abroad prior to travel to determine whether select point-of-care assays may be valuable additions to the local diagnostic arsenal.

Dried blood spot cards

Dried blood spot (DBS) cards were initially introduced as a screening tool for detecting metabolic diseases in neonates. As technologies advanced, they found a new role in the diagnosis of viral pathogens, most notably HIV (see Chapter 18, Figure 18.4). DBS cards are a simple, field-friendly method of specimen collection, transport, and storage that can greatly benefit the monitoring of large populations (Bertagnolio *et al.*, 2010). Blood from a finger stick is collected onto three to five circles imprinted on a piece of specialized filter paper and allowed to completely dry (at least 4 hours). Samples should be stored in a plastic bag with silica desiccant to remain viable for up to 2 weeks. Viral RNA, DNA, antibodies, and other proteins remain stable on DBS cards, allowing transport to a central or reference laboratory (Snijdewind *et al.*, 2012). Samples are suitable for a variety of assays, including diagnosis via ELISA and even monitoring viral load and antiretroviral therapy resistance.

Learning laboratory skills prior to your trip

Many of the skills outlined in this chapter can be more easily implemented in the field following some practical exposure and experience. We encourage you to seek the help of laboratory professionals (e.g., laboratory technologists, pathologists) at your home hospital or institution prior to traveling abroad. They are likely to be supportive about organizing some hands-on practical training sessions for you before your departure and may prove to be good contacts to have while traveling abroad.

Additional resources

Guides to advanced testing and additional diagnostic methods

- World Health Organization (2003) *Manual of Basic Techniques for a Health Laboratory*, 2nd edn. Available at http://whqlibdoc.who.int/publications/2003/9241545305.pdf

Atlases and image banks

- CAP Hematology and Clinical Microscopy Resource Committee (1998) *Color Atlas of Hematology: An Illustrated Field Guide Based on Proficiency Testing.* Northfield, IL: College of American Pathologists.
- CAP Hematology and Clinical Microscopy Resource Committee (2006) *Color Atlas of Body Fluids: An Illustrated Field Guide Based on Proficiency Testing.* Northfield, IL: College of American Pathologists.
- CAP Hematology and Clinical Microscopy Resource Committee (2010) *Color Atlas of the Urinary Sediment: An Illustrated Field Guide Based on Proficiency Testing.* Northfield, IL: College of American Pathologists.
- Centers for Disease Control and Prevention (CDC) Public Health Image Bank and Library (PHIL). Available at http://phil.cdc.gov/phil/home.asp
- Partners Infectious Disease Images: eMicrobes Digital Library. Available at http://www.idimages.org/

Laboratory quality assessment and management resources

- World Health Organization (2012) Laboratory assessment tool. Available at http://whqlibdoc.who.int/hq/2012/WHO_HSE_GCR_LYO_2012.2_eng.pdf
- World Health Organization (2011) Laboratory quality management system handbook. Available at http://whqlibdoc.who.int/publications/2011/9789241548274_eng.pdf

REFERENCES

Abba K, Deeks JJ, Olliaro P *et al.* (2011) Rapid diagnostic tests for diagnosing uncomplicated *P. falciparum* malaria in endemic countries. *Cochrane Database Syst Rev* (7):CD008122.

Beckmann CRB, Ling FW, Barzansky BM, Herbert WNP, Laube DW, Smith RP (2010) *Obstetrics and Gynecology*, 6th edn. Baltimore: Lippincott Williams & Wilkins.

Bertagnolio S, Parkin NT, Jordan M, Brooks J, Garcia-Lemma JG (2010) Dried blood spots for HIV-1 drug resistance and viral load testing: a review of current knowledge and WHO efforts for global HIV drug resistance surveillance. *AIDS Rev* 12:195–208.

CAP Hematology and Clinical Microscopy Resource Committee (1998) *Color Atlas of Hematology: An Illustrated Field Guide Based on Proficiency Testing*. Northfield, IL: College of American Pathologists.

CAP Hematology and Clinical Microscopy Resource Committee (2006) *Color Atlas of Body Fluids: An Illustrated Field Guide Based on Proficiency Testing*. Northfield, IL: College of American Pathologists.

Clinical and Laboratory Standards Institute (2006) *H56-A: Body Fluid Analysis for Cellular Composition; Approved Guideline*. Wayne, PA: CLSI.

Garcia L, Shimizu R (1997) Evaluation of nine immunoassay kits (enzyme immunoassay and direct fluorescence) for detection of *Giardia lamblia* and *Cryptosporidium parvum* in human fecal specimens. *J Clin Microbiol* 35:1526–9.

Haque R, Ali IK, Akther S, Petri WA Jr (1998) Comparison of PCR, isoenzyme analysis, and antigen detection for diagnosis of *Entamoeba histolytica* infection. *J Clin Microbiol* 36:449–52.

Knopp S, Speich B, Hattendorf J *et al.* (2011) Diagnostic accuracy of Kato–Katz and FLOTAC for assessing anthelmintic drug efficacy. *PLoS Negl Trop Dis* 5(4):e1036.

Koukounari A, Webster JP, Donnelly CA *et al.* (2009) Sensitivities and specificities of diagnostic tests and infection prevalence of *Schistosoma haematobium* estimated from data on adults in villages northwest of Accra, Ghana. *Am J Trop Med Hyg* 80:435–41.

McNerney R, Daley P (2011) Towards a point-of-care test for active tuberculosis: obstacles and opportunities. *Nat Rev Microbiol* 9:204–13.

Pant Pai N, Balram B, Shivkumar S *et al.* (2012) Head-to-head comparison of accuracy of a rapid point-of-care HIV test with oral versus whole-blood specimens: a systematic review and meta-analysis. *Lancet Infect Dis* 12:373–80.

Snijdewind IJ, van Kampen JJ, Fraaij PL, van der Ende ME, Osterhaus AD, Gruters RA (2012) Current and future applications of dried blood spots in viral disease management. *Antiviral Res* 93:309–21.

Van Deun A, Hamid Salim A, Aung KJ *et al.* (2005) Performance of variations of carbolfuchsin staining of sputum smears for AFB under field conditions. *Int J Tuberc Lung Dis* 9:1127–33.

World Health Organization (2003) *Manual of Basic Techniques for a Health Laboratory*. Geneva: World Health Organization.

World Health Organization (2011) *Laboratory Quality Management System Handbook*. Lyon: World Health Organization.

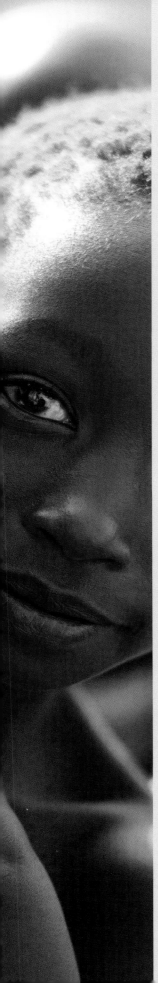

CHAPTER 32
Nursing Care

Patricia A. Daoust[1], Lynda A. Tyer-Viola[2,3], and Kirsti Rinne[4]

[1]Center for Global Health and Massachusetts General Hospital, Boston, MA, USA
[2]Baylor College of Medicine, Houston, TX, USA
[3]Pavilion for Women, Texas Children's Hospital, Houston, TX, USA
[4]University of Utah Medical Center, Salt Lake City, UT, USA

Key learning objectives

■ Understand the role of nursing in global health

■ Discuss the strengths and challenges of nursing care in resource-limited settings.

■ Understand a framework for how the role of the nurse is affected by the environment of care.

■ Identify the fundamental knowledge and skills of nursing care in these settings.

Abstract

In order to provide the most efficient and effective care in the context of global health, it is important for all providers to understand the role of nursing and midwifery. Because of the severe shortage of physicians in the developing world, nurses deliver up to 90% of primary healthcare services, yet the ability to accurately capture the responsibilities and function of nursing is a challenge. Nursing practice varies from country to country and is often determined by the clinical environment, available resources, and the expectations of fellow practitioners. Understanding and optimizing the role of nursing within each healthcare setting improves team effectiveness and maximizes health outcomes.

Key words: nursing, midwifery, global health, resource-limited setting, task-shifting

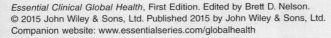

Introduction

The World Health Organization (WHO) estimates there are 35 million nurses and midwives worldwide, comprising 60–80% of the global health workforce (World Health Organization, 2006). In developing countries, where physicians are scarce, nurses deliver up to 90% of all primary healthcare services (Figure 32.1). Despite many challenges, the discipline of nursing is considered in many countries to be the "most trusted profession" (Jones & Saad, 2011). Nurses frequently provide particular care that is as effective as physicians with similar, and in some cases improved, clinical outcomes and increased patient satisfaction (Baldwin *et al.*, 2010). Yet the role of the professional nurse, particularly within the realm of global health, often remains misunderstood.

An in-country government body, such as the Ministry of Health or the Council of Nursing and Midwifery, traditionally defines the scope of nursing practice. However, the defined scope of practice is not always consistent with how nurses actually practice. For example, in many resource-limited settings, nurses frequently provide care for patients beyond their approved scope due to the shortage of physicians. In other settings, however, where nurses may not be recognized for their expertise, they are limited in the care they provide and function more as assistants or ancillary staff.

The goal of this chapter is to provide both non-nursing and nursing providers a better understanding of the profession of nursing and midwifery and the roles and responsibilities that nurses have as important members of the healthcare team in these settings. The chapter will explore the challenges that face the profession, such as severe personnel shortages, limited access to a quality standardized educational system, and cultural barriers that often limit nurses from practicing to the full extent of their training. Also described will be the basic skills and key competencies required for effective global nursing practice and how these can be optimized. Ultimately, the hope is that the information provided will enhance the reader's understanding of nursing, the world's largest cadre of health providers.

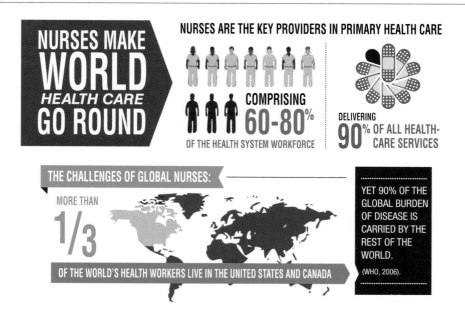

Figure 32.1 Nurses and the delivery of primary care. *Source*: Partners In Health (www.pih.org). Reproduced with permission of Partners In Health.

Box 32.1 ICN definition of nursing

Nursing encompasses autonomous and collaborative care of individuals of all ages, families, groups and communities, sick or well and in all settings. Nursing includes the promotion of health, prevention of illness, and the care of ill, disabled and dying people. Advocacy, promotion of a safe environment, research, participation in shaping health policy and in patient and health systems management, and education are also key nursing roles (International Council of Nurses, 2010).

Table 32.1 Shortages of healthcare workers by region.

WHO region	Number of countries	Number (%) of countries with significant shortages
Africa	46	36 (78%)
Americas	35	5 (14%)
Southeast Asia	11	6 (55%)
Europe	52	0 (0%)
Eastern Mediterranean	21	7 (33%)
Western Pacific	27	3 (11%)
World	192	57 (30%)

Source: data from World Health Organization (2006).

Definition of nursing

The first step to working with nurses is to understand the challenge of accurately defining nursing on a global level. The definition offered by the International Council of Nursing (ICN) is widely accepted by the international nursing community (Box 32.1). Nurses practice in a wide range of environments where roles and responsibilities vary significantly, depending on the clinical setting, the educational background of the nurse, the approved scope of practice, and the nurse's years of experience. Since the role of nurses can vary country to country, it becomes important to ask questions of the local nursing staff to accurately assess clinical knowledge and organizational capacity.

Most nurses in developing countries are *diploma* or *enrolled* nurses; they may or may not have a high-school education but generally receive 2 or 3 years of training in basic nursing skills and can perform simple and, in some cases, more advanced medical procedures. *Auxiliary* or *certified* nurses receive anywhere from a few months to 2 years of training, practice under the direction of a diploma nurse, primarily provide very basic or unskilled care, and have no training in nursing decision-making. Registered nurses have 3 years of post-secondary school education, have a full range of nursing skills, and usually function in supervisory roles (World Health Organization, 2013). Because of a limited number of university-level nursing programs, there are very few baccalaureate-degree nurses in resource-limited settings and even fewer nurses who have master's degrees.

This variation in education, skills set, and role definition creates gaps that affect patient care. For example, in many global settings, the terms "nurse" and "midwife" are frequently used without distinction. Many nursing programs integrate the basic skills related to obstetric care into their curriculum. Trained midwives are usually registered nurses who have practiced for 2 years and then return to school for two additional years of education, based on the International Confederation of Midwives' (ICM) "Essentials competencies for basic midwifery practice" (International Confederation of Midwives, 2013). These defined standards help ensure that, at a minimum, a nurse who calls herself a midwife is competent to perform essential obstetric skills. Therefore, it can be useful to discuss with those providing direct obstetric care their training and competency and not to assume that the nurses in a labor ward are all trained midwives.

Gaps in human resources and current status of nursing

Nurses and midwives are key contributors to improving health outcomes through disease prevention, health promotion, and administering essential life-saving services. They provide care across the lifespan, with treatment aimed at both acute and chronic diseases. Yet the global nurse and midwifery workforce remains understaffed (World Health Organization, 2010). In 2006, the WHO reported a shortage of 2.4 million physicians, nurses, and midwives in 57 countries; 36 (78%) of these countries are in Africa (Table 32.1). In sub-Saharan Africa, 600,000 additional nurses were identified as needed to scale up priority interventions to meet the 2015 Millennium Development Goals (International Council of Nurses, 2004). The results of these efforts remain to be assessed. For comparison, in the United States, there are 937 nurses per 100,000 citizens, while in much of sub-Saharan Africa the average is 90 per 100,000 (World Health Organization, 2006). Sub-Saharan Africa has 11% of the world's population, 24% of the global burden of disease, yet only 3% of the world's qualified healthcare workers (World Health Organization, 2006). The shortage of nurses is devastating in these settings and can greatly exacerbate the health needs of a country (Box 32.2). These gaps in human resources create a challenge for nurses and all clinicians and call for a better understanding of each other's roles and competencies.

Internationally, the professional practice of nursing is guided by a Code of Ethics (International Council of Nurses, 2012). These ethical standards acknowledge nurses and nursing care as a social contract between patients and society

Box 32.2 An example of the consequences of a nursing shortage

A shortage of nurses in Tanzania is undermining the country's efforts to control the spread of malaria, according to Alex Mwita, program manager for the National Malaria Control Program. Mwita reports there are approximately 10,000 nurses working in Tanzania, although the country needs more than 30,000. "With a lack of sufficient nurses, treatment of malaria has become an even bigger problem," Mwita said. At least 2 million people, 70% of whom are pregnant women and children under age 5, die of malaria in Tanzania annually, according to the Ministry of Health (IRIN News, November 29, 2012).

Box 32.3 International Council of Nurses Code of Ethics (2012)

1. Nurses have four fundamental responsibilities: to promote health, to prevent illness, to restore health, and to alleviate suffering.
2. Inherent in nursing is a respect for human rights, including cultural rights, the right to life and choice, to dignity, and to be treated with respect.
3. Nursing care is provided without bias related to age, color, creed, culture, disability or illness, gender, sexual orientation, nationality, politics, race, or social status.
4. Nurses render health services to all members of a community and coordinate services with others.

(Box 32.3). The status of women and the culture of the community affect this contract and how nurses practice, especially in resource-limited settings. Many societies do not view nursing as a desirable profession for women (Hadley & Roques, 2007). Care is impacted by this as well as other contextually bound beliefs because, internationally, the field of nursing generally comprises women. If women are not valued as important members of the healthcare team, it is difficult for patients to see them as competent care providers. Exploring with the staff the role of women in the community will provide a valuable insight into how nurses are valued and practice within the clinical environment.

Importance of working as a clinical team

Caring for people in low-resource settings is complex and requires all clinicians to work as a team. When physicians and nurses support one another and create opportunities to work together, there is a respect for the unique skills and talents that each profession offers. For example, nurses are often not included in daily rounds, even though they are with the patient 24 hours a day. When nurses are part of these patient discussions, they can provide valuable information on the patient's status, answer questions, advocate for the patient, and understand the goals of care and expectations of their role in achieving those goals. It is also an opportunity for physicians to witness what care nurses are prepared to provide and areas where they cannot assume that nurses know specific pathology and treatment regimens. Nurses may need guidance on organizing care and performing specific skills. Conversely, when encouraged to contribute, nurses can provide physicians with the reality and possibilities for care that the environment supports. This is especially useful for visiting physicians adapting to a new setting. Greater collaboration between health professionals, particularly between nurses and physicians, results in greater quality of care, improved patient outcomes, increased overall team competency, and decreased clinical errors (Barr, 2002; Barnsteiner *et al.*, 2007).

Optimizing nursing care

Healthcare professionals may feel frustrated and overwhelmed when working in a developing country. Limited resources and insufficient nursing staff often impede effective patient care. Although staff, infrastructure, and supply shortages need to be addressed, there are creative ways for nursing staff to ensure that all available resources are maximized. These approaches include (i) identifying and focusing on key nursing priorities and (ii) task-shifting care responsibilities or, in other words, designating tasks that require little or no training to less specialized or ancillary staff.

Working with the nursing staff to identify the highest care priorities is critical since nurses are often overwhelmed and distracted with non-clinical activities at the expense of more important patient-related responsibilities. Multiple studies have reported that less than 40% of a nurse's time is spent in providing patient-centered care (Gran-Moravec & Hughes, 2005; Manongi *et al.*, 2009; Al-Kandari & Thomas, 2008). For example, a pediatric ward in Tanzania found that nurses, in an effort to improve their relationship with ancillary staff, would perform housekeeping tasks such as dusting and mopping. Conversely, untrained staff regularly participated in nursing care, such as giving injections. In fact, one nurse reported that there was no distinction between nursing responsibilities and the responsibilities of ancillary staff. This is not a unique finding. Nurses routinely perform tasks that do not require nursing expertise, at the expense of patient care. For this reason, it is important for a collaborative team to define the nursing role and identify ways to optimize nursing practice.

Task-shifting is a collaborative cost-effective method of addressing staffing shortages in resource-limited settings. Much of what is known about the effectiveness of task-shifting was identified through research that focused on the provision of antiretroviral therapy (ART) to HIV-positive patients. A systematic review of the literature found that although more data are needed, task-shifting from doctors to nurses or from nurses to community health workers (CHWs) has potential to maximize already strained resources (Mdege *et al.*, 2012). CHWs are an important component not only of task-shifting but also the implementation of healthcare programs, in collaboration with local healthcare teams (McCord *et al.*, 2012). In all areas of medical treatment, nursing staff can use task-shifting in order to focus on important activities and deliver more effective patient-centered care. In every case, all members of the healthcare team should clearly understand their role and, when appropriate, shift responsibilities. Guidelines on how to implement task-shifting to improve access to care have been developed by the WHO (World Health Organization, 2008). Through prioritization and collaborative task-shifting, the team is not only better able to function efficiently but can also improve overall health outcomes.

Fundamentals of nursing practice in all settings

The specific clinical responsibilities of nurses are not well defined in many clinical settings, especially in resource-limited settings (Kitson *et al.*, 2010). Despite this, all nurses regardless of resources should function with a common purpose to provide "competent, culturally sensitive, and evidence-based nursing and midwifery care" (World Health Organization, 2010). The overall objective in any care setting is to provide collaborative, respectful, and patient-centered care (Kitson *et al.*, 2013). To do this requires basic knowledge and skills, no matter the clinical setting. How individual nurses meet this challenge differs depending on education, resources, support, and the presence of other trained clinicians. There are, however, some recommended competencies that may provide a foundation for success for nurses working in the global health setting, particularly nurses from the developed world (Box 32.4).

Regardless of the system of care or part of the world, several fundamentals of nursing care are universal. Creating a safe environment that promotes healing is a primary goal. Ideally, all patient care tasks should be clearly enumerated so that the clinical team can easily know what each patient needs, which patients require an intervention, and which tasks have been completed. This establishes expectations of the staff and encourages collaboration to achieve patient care goals. Table 32.2 lists basic nursing skills and some innovative ideas on how to accomplish them.

When working with or participating in designing systems of care, consider how nurses can contribute in the following domains of patient care. Specific nursing skills can be modified to the environment, yet the same general principles should apply.

Box 32.4 Key competencies for global nursing practice (Crigger *et al.*, 2006)

1. Open-mindedness and flexibility. Being able to adapt to varying situations while providing healthcare services and remaining open to the values and beliefs of others.
2. Cultural sensitivity and interest. Perceiving the needs of others but not imposing one's own beliefs or moral values or seeing them as a basis of comparison.
3. Optimism, energy, resiliency, and resourcefulness.
4. Honesty and integrity.
5. A stable personal life.
6. Technical and business skills as well as political savvy.
7. Conviction that the work being done is meaningful, and passion for the cause that drives and motivates despite the difficulties encountered along the way (Kim *et al.*, 2006).

Assessment

The nursing assessment incorporates the physiological, psychological, social, and spiritual health of patients. Nurses should be able to perform a basic patient assessment. Collaboration on assessment can also occur by including nurses in patient care rounds. It is essential to define what assessment is required for each patient, the frequency of this assessment, where assessments should be documented, and how changes in the patient's condition are reported.

Caring

The nurse implements interventions that support patient goals and outcomes. Interventions are individualized to the patient's needs, local care setting, and available resources. The nurse collaborates with other members of the team to secure appropriate resources or search for alternative interventions. Explore with the nursing staff what resources are available and how to be creative. For example, staff can build a simple Buck's orthopedic traction device using a 2.3-kg (5-pound) weight/stones, bucket, and rope, or staff can implement a simple system to monitor intravenous fluids using tape and a marker.

Comfort

Nurses provide several interventions that promote patient security and well-being. Comfort and pain management are often lost in a busy clinical environment, and yet these can be the most effective components to achieving patient goals. Comfort can be provided by making pain management a focal point of care, knowing which pain medications are presently available, encouraging a sufficient supply of clean sheets for patients, and helping patients wash daily by providing a bucket and water.

Table 32.2 Knowledge and implementation of skills for basic global nursing.

Vital signs and physical assessment

- Create a system that designates a time of day and documents on a checklist or nursing board that all patients receive, at a minimum, daily vital signs and physical assessments (and more frequently depending on patient acuity).
- Perform and document vital signs. Conduct physical assessments that evaluate (i) cardiac rate and rhythm, (ii) auscultation of lung sounds, and (iii) abdominal assessment, including bowel sounds and the presence and extent of ascites.
- Evaluate for hypoxia and understand the use of oxygen therapy. Oxygen is a therapeutic intervention that requires ongoing assessment, including pulse oximetry. A clipboard at the end of the bed with an oxygen therapy sheet – to document time, mode, amount, and patient oxygen saturation with and without oxygen – can facilitate this increased observation.

Safety and comfort

- Proper organization of a clinical ward, including prioritization of patient needs and safe patient handoff, can dramatically improve care.
- To increase the authority, accountability, and autonomy of the nursing staff, work with the supervisory team to assign nurses to specific patients. This will allow clinicians to interact directly with a nurse to create shared goals for each patient and also allow nurses to more easily focus their attention on each patient's needs.
- To promote a team approach, create a system with the nursing staff to identify when patients have new orders, e.g., flagging a chart with a color marker or using a whiteboard that is visible to staff to communicate a plan of care. Ensure that nurses know how to identify the reason for admission and day-to-day diagnostic needs such as chest X-ray or fasting finger stick (glucose monitoring).
- Ensure the assessment and provision of non-pharmacological aids to promote patient comfort. Identify patients who need frequent turning and skin care, positioning, and toileting. In warm environments, close monitoring of hydration status is imperative.

Infection control

- Although clean running water is often absent in many settings, try to establish the best mode and location for hand hygiene and create a campaign to make this the standard of care at the health facility. Role modeling by clinical supervisors of proper infection control is of the utmost importance. In surgical settings it is vital that all providers understand the process by which something is considered sterile, clean, and soiled
- Identify patients in need of droplet and contact precautions. Especially in settings where tuberculosis is endemic, create a method to identify bed spacing (such as tape on the floor to signify the necessary distance required to prevent cross-contamination), understand the cultural significance of masks and implement a policy on their use, and introduce patient teaching on coughing. Pictures are universal and are good educational tools (Shears, 2013, pp. 217–24; UNAIDS, 2010)

Patient personal care

- In many settings, nurses do not historically provide personal care for patients and instead rely on patients' family members for this important role. Nurses should provide basic care and hygiene to patients, including bathing and oral care. Discuss this need with the nurses and how it can be accomplished in each setting.
- Introduce routine skin assessment and strategies to prevent skin breakdown. Skin and wound care should be a component of the daily nursing physical examination. Identify available resources and materials for wound care. Create a system for wound cleaning and dressing and create a method to ensure appropriate timing and documentation of dressing changes.

Medication administration

- Prior to prescribing in a new setting, review the availability of medications as well as the medication supply and distribution chain. Identifying who is responsible for obtaining and preparing the medications and how the medications are distributed within the facility can help ensure medications are administered correctly.
- Jointly create a system with the nurses in which most medications are provided at the same, limited number of times each day. This can increase compliance and help troubleshoot issues with medication administration.
- Initiation and maintenance of parental medications, including monitoring of intravenous fluids, varies in each setting. Create a system for patients who are nil by mouth for surgery to receive intravenous fluids in hot climates. Proper hydration is important, especially when spinal anesthesia is used.
- Initiate protocols for proper blood transfusion and monitoring for adverse reactions. A system of documentation of vital signs and assessments for transfusion reactions can be created with a bedside form, which includes the transfusion guidelines and a place to document vital signs and patient assessments.

Creating an environment that supports privacy is also imperative and can involve covering patients during examinations and creating privacy dividers with shower curtains between delivery room beds. To increase compliance and to underscore the importance of these clinical approaches, identify a place in the patient chart or on a nursing board to document daily care measures.

Counseling/education

Nurses also provide counseling and education to patients, utilizing active listening that is free of bias and ensures that patients' concerns are addressed. There should ideally be a quiet place in the patient ward wherein nurses can interview and counsel patients in private. Culturally appropriate education materials can also facilitate patient learning and understanding. Establish a system in which, prior to discharge, every patient receives discharge education and a plan for follow-up care.

Conclusion

Global health nursing practice encompasses compassionate care of individuals and communities in collaboration with other clinicians to promote optimal health regardless of resources. Nursing faces many challenges related to preparatory training, status of nurses and women in society, and large gaps in human resources. To work effectively as a team it is important to ask questions of nurses regarding their scope of practice, the level of care they provide, the patients for whom they care, and how to maximize their clinical skills. Optimizing the role of nursing by working as a team to prioritize patient needs will greatly improve the care experience and health outcomes.

Additional resources

- Taylor AL, Hwenda L, Larsen BI, Daulaire N (2011) Stemming the brain drain: a WHO global code of practice on international recruitment of health personnel. *N Engl J Med* 365:2348–51.
- United Nations Programme on HIV/AIDS (UNAIDS). HIV and tuberculosis: ensuring universal access and protection of human rights. Issue paper produced by the UNAIDS Reference Group on HIV and Human Rights, March 2010. Available at http://data.unaids.org/Pub/externaldocument/2010/20100324_unaidsrghrtsissuepapertbhrts_en.pdf
- World Health Organization, African Health Workforce Observatory. Definitions of the 23 health workforce categories. 2007. Available at http://apps.who.int/globalatlas/docs/HRH_HWO/HTML/Dftn.htm

REFERENCES

Al-Kandari F, Thomas D (2008) Factors contributing to nursing tasks incompletion as perceived by nurses working in Kuwait general hospitals. *J Clin Nurs* 18:3430–40.

Baldwin C, Bazarko D, Hancock C, Smith R (2010) Why nurses should be more prominent. Available at http://www.sa-lives.com/entry/13/why-nurses-should-bemoreprominent

Barnsteiner J, Disch J, Hall L, Mayer D, Moore S (2007) Promoting interprofessional education. *Nurs Outlook* 55:144–50.

Barr H (2002) *Interprofessional Education: Today, Yesterday and Tomorrow*. London: Centre for the Advancement of Interprofessional Education.

Crigger N, Brannigan M, Baird M (2006) Compassionate nursing professionals as good citizens of the world. *ANS Adv Nurs Sci* 29:15–26.

Gran-Moravec M, Hughes C (2005) Nursing time allocation and other considerations for staffing. *Nurs Health Sci* 7:126–33.

Hadley M, Roques A (2007) Nursing in Bangladesh: rhetoric and reality. *Soc Sci Med* 64:1153–65.

International Confederation of Midwives (2013) ICM international definition of the midwife. Available at http://www.internationalmidwives.org/who-we-are/policy-and-practice/icm-international-definition-of-the-midwife/

International Council of Nurses (2004) The global nursing shortage: priority areas for intervention. Available at http://www.icn.ch/images/stories/documents/publications/GNRI/The_Global_Nursing_Shortage-Priority_Areas_for_Intervention.pdf

International Council of Nurses (2010) Definition of nursing. Available at http://www.icn.ch/about-icn/icn-definition-of-nursing/

International Council of Nurses (2012) The ICN code of ethics for nurses. Available at http://www.icn.ch/about-icn/code-of-ethics-for-nurses/

Jones J, Saad L (2011) USA Today/Gallup Poll, November 28 to December 1, 2011. Available at http://www.gallup.com/file/poll/151463/Honesty_Ethics_111212.pdf

Kim M, Woith W, Otten K, McElmurry B (2006) Global nurse leaders: lessons from the sages. *Adv Nurs Sci* 29:27–42.

Kitson A, Conroy T, Wengstrom Y, Profetto-McGrath J, Robertson-Malt S (2010) Defining the fundamentals of care. *Int J Nurs Pract* 16:423–34.

Kitson A, Marshall A, Bassett K, Zeitz K (2013) What are the core elements of patient-centred care? A narrative review and synthesis of the literature from health policy, medicine and nursing. *J Adv Nurs* 69:4–15.

Manongi R, Nasuwa F, Mwangi R, Reyburn H, Poulsen A, Chandler C (2009) Conflicting priorities: evaluation of an intervention to improve nurse–parent relationships on a Tanzanian paediatric ward. *Hum Resour Health* 7:50.

McCord G, Liu A, Singh P (2012) Deployment of community health workers across rural Sub-Saharan Africa: financial considerations and operational assumptions. *Bull WHO* 91:244–253B.

Mdege N, Chindove S, Ali S (2012) The effectiveness and cost implications of task-shifting in the delivery of antiretrovial therapy to HIV-infected patients: a systematic review. *Health Policy Plan* 28:223–36.

Shears P (2013) Poverty and infection in the developing world: healthcare-related infections and infection control in the tropics. *J Hosp Infect* 67:217–24.

United Nations Programme on HIV/AIDS (UNAIDS) (2010) HIV and tuberculosis: ensuring universal access and protection of human rights. Issue paper produced by the UNAIDS Reference Group on HIV and Human Rights. http://data.unaids.org/Pub/externaldocument/2010/20100324_unaidsrghrtsissuepapertbhrts_en.pdf

World Health Organization (2006) The global shortage of health workers and its impact. Available at http://www.unep.org/training/programmes/Instructor%20Version/Part_2/Activities/Dimensions_of_Human_Well-Being/Health/Supplemental/Global_Shortage_of_Health_Workers.pdf

World Health Organization (2008) Task shifting: global recommendations and guidelines. Available at http://www.who.int/workforcealliance/knowledge/resources/taskshifting_globalrecommendations/en/

World Health Organization (2010) Strategic directions for strengthening nursing and midwifery services: 2011–2015. Available at http://www.who.int/hrh/resources/nmsd/en/

World Health Organization (2013) WHO Nursing and Midwifery Progress Report 2008–2012, p. 152. Available at http://www.who.int/hrh/nursing_midwifery/NursingMidwiferyProgressReport.pdf

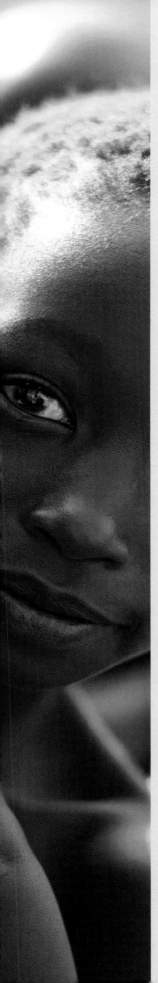

CHAPTER 33
Pharmacy

Diane L. Gal[1], Tana Wuliji[2], Lloyd K. Matowe[3], Marouen Ben Guebila[4], and Radoslaw Mitura[4]

[1]Formerly with the International Pharmaceutical Federation (FIP) Education Initiative, The Hague, Netherlands
[2]University Research Co., LLC (URC), Bethesda, MD, USA
[3]Pharmaceutical Systems Africa, and University of Liberia, Monrovia, Liberia
[4]International Pharmaceutical Students' Federation (IPSF), The Hague, Netherlands

Key learning objectives

- Describe the key barriers to access to medicines in resource-limited settings.
- Understand the management of medicines that are stored and distributed in health facilities.
- Understand how to assess and identify medicine-related problems and needs.
- Learn how to assist the patient on taking their medicines correctly.

Abstract

A healthcare system without medicines seems unthinkable given that they are one of the most important tools we have to prevent illness and improve health. However, a lack of consistent access to medicines, poor quality of medicines, and improper use are common scenarios in many countries around the world. Having an understanding of why these issues happen and how to prevent and manage them is critical. This chapter provides a practical introduction to these complex issues and provides essential guidance on how to reduce barriers to medicine access in resource-limited settings, how to organize medicines that are stored and distributed in health facilities, how to assess medicine-related problems and needs, as well as how to assist the patient in taking their medicines correctly.

Key words: essential medicines, access, availability, pharmacy, pharmaceuticals, pharmaceutical system, pharmaceutical management, supply chain, stock-outs, rational medicine use

Essential Clinical Global Health, First Edition. Edited by Brett D. Nelson.
© 2015 John Wiley & Sons, Ltd. Published 2015 by John Wiley & Sons, Ltd.
Companion website: www.essentialseries.com/globalhealth

Introduction

A healthcare system without medicines seems unthinkable given that they are one of the most important tools we have to prevent illness and improve health. However, a lack of consistent access to medicines, poor quality of medicines, and improper use are common scenarios in many countries around the world. Having an understanding of why these issues happen and how to prevent and manage them is critical.

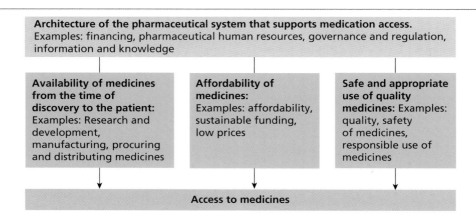

Architecture of the pharmaceutical system that supports medication access.
Examples: financing, pharmaceutical human resources, governance and regulation, information and knowledge

Availability of medicines from the time of discovery to the patient: Examples: Research and development, manufacturing, procuring and distributing medicines

Affordability of medicines: Examples: affordability, sustainable funding, low prices

Safe and appropriate use of quality medicines: Examples: quality, safety of medicines, responsible use of medicines

Access to medicines

Figure 33.1 A framework for access to medicines. *Source:* adapted from Frost & Reich (2008), p. 17.

What are essential medicines?

When health systems have major constraints on resources, the focus must be on providing those medicines that address the priority health needs of the majority of the population, in other words the essential medicines. As the needs in each country can be quite different, countries usually have their own essential medicines list and formularies that describe what should be available and affordable at all times. This may be based on the World Health Organization (WHO) Model List of Essential Medicines (World Health Organization, 2013), which includes the most efficacious and cost-effective evidence-based medicines needed to prevent and manage the acute and chronic diseases that affect populations the most (Kaplan & Mathers, 2011).

What needs to be in place to improve access to medicines?

Access to medicines is defined by the United Nations Millennium Development Goals as having medicines "continuously available and affordable at public or private health facilities or medicine outlets within one hour's walk from each person's home" (United Nations Development Group,

2003). The main objective of the pharmaceutical system is to ensure that quality medicines are accessed and used responsibly by those who need them, when and where they need them, and in a way that is safe, affordable, and equitable. Achieving this is not straightforward and depends on the actions (or processes) of many groups and individuals to come together in a coordinated and well-managed way, as illustrated in Figure 33.1.

The pharmaceutical processes in healthcare systems can be very different between countries, so it is important to be familiar with the local context. Many countries also have critical shortages of pharmaceutical human resources, for instance Zambia, Afghanistan, and Vietnam have five to twenty times more facilities where people can get medicines than the number of trained pharmaceutical human resources (Gal & Bates, 2012). These shortages mean that the roles in pharmaceutical management and the medication-use process (Box 33.1) are often done by those who have not been trained to do these tasks, such as nurses, lay workers, and volunteers. Where pharmacists are available, it is important to coordinate health services with them and involve them in activities to ensure that medicines are accessible and used appropriately (e.g., reviewing prescriptions, identifying medication-related problems, counseling patients on their medicines).

What are the main barriers to access to medicines?

The medication-use process (Figure 33.2) involves a number of steps. These include prescribing, preparation and dispensing, medication administration, and monitoring.

There are many barriers at different levels of the system that can affect the extent to which a patient will benefit from medicines (Table 33.1). Barriers at the individual, household, community, and health service delivery levels can often be addressed and improved by health workers in partnership with patients and the community. Other barriers at the health sector, public policy, and international and regional levels can also affect access to medicines but often require changes to the system that can be beyond the influence of service providers and communities.

An estimated 44 million households experience severe financial hardship and 25 million are pushed into poverty because of healthcare costs every year (Xu *et al.*, 2007). Between 20 and 60% of all health spending in low- and middle-income countries is on medicines (Cameron *et al.*, 2009), and the WHO estimates that around 50–90% of this spending is by patients themselves (also called "out-of-pocket"). Medicines that are not affordable to the health system and/or patient may affect what therapies the patient can access and use. Medicines can be made more affordable by:

- improving the way that medicines are procured and working with manufacturers at the systems level to get better pricing;
- helping patients to access community health insurance schemes; and
- controlling the mark-ups on the price of the medicines sold to patients.

Medicines may not always be available. Only 35% of essential medicines studied were available in the public sector and 66% in the private sector in low- and middle-income countries for various reasons including medicines shortages (Cameron *et al.*, 2009). Even when medicines are available, they may not be quality products or used safely and appropriately. Some have estimated that 15–50% of all medicines in low- and middle-income countries are counterfeited or of substandard quality. Meanwhile, it is estimated that up to half of the medicines prescribed may not be used appropriately by patients (e.g., not taking antibiotics at the right intervals, not completing a course of antibiotics). Medicines have also been estimated to be inappropriately prescribed or dispensed half of the time (e.g., prescribing antibiotics when they are not needed).

If any of these barriers are present, patients may not gain the optimum benefit possible from their medicines and the investments that go into making medicines available may not result in the expected health gains. These issues are very costly to the patient and the health system, with an estimated 8% of global health expenditure or US$500 billion in healthcare costs that could be avoided every year if medicines are used more responsibly (IMS Institute for Healthcare Informatics, 2012).

Box 33.1 Pharmacist and pharmacist-related roles

Pharmacists
Usually 4–6 year degree. Responsible for overseeing and managing medicines supply and use

Pharmacy technicians and assistants
Formal training of up to 2 years. Responsible for stock management and dispensing support

Pharmacy aides
Little or no formal training. Support dispensing and storage of medicines

---

Clinical experience: supporting and collaborating with fellow staff and volunteers

"When we arrived, the cleaning lady was dispensing medicines. We had a hard time telling her that she was not capable of doing the dispensing. Since she wanted to study nursing and enjoyed being in the health clinic, the students supervised her and started building her competencies on dispensing and appropriate medication use."

Luise, pharmacy student working in Tanzania

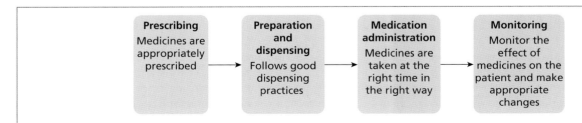

Figure 33.2 Medication-use process.

Table 33.1 Main barriers to access to medicines at individual, household, community, and health service delivery levels.

Level of the health system	Main barriers to access to medicines
Individual, household, and community	Perceptions of the quality of medicines and health services Cost of medicines and health services Demand for and use of medicines Social and cultural barriers (poverty, ethnicity, gender) Medicines not taken or not taken appropriately
Health service delivery	Irregular availability of medicines High medicine prices Medicines not prescribed or dispensed appropriately Low quality of medicines and health services Medicine use not appropriately monitored and therapies not adjusted when needed

Source: adapted from Bigdeli *et al.* (2013).

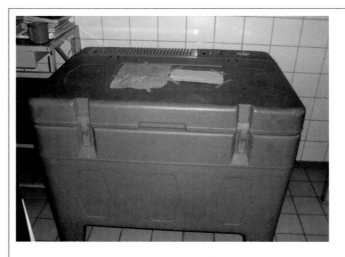

Figure 33.3 Photo of the cooler used in Niger to keep oxytocin cool. Staff in a maternity unit in Niger came up with an innovative idea of using coolers to keep oxytocin in the maternity at the right temperature ready for use when needed as they only had one fridge in the hospital and power was always out. *Source:* USAID Health Care Improvement Project/University Research Co., LLC. Niger Essential Obstetric and Newborn Care Collaborative, USAID Health Care Improvement Portal. Available at https://www.usaidassist.org/resources/niger-essential-obstetric-and-newborn-care-collaborative. Reproduced with permission of University Research Co., LLC.

Managing medicines at health facilities

Good management of medicines and related products at health facilities is critical for ensuring continuous availability of quality medicines. In resource-limited settings, getting medicines to all health facilities may be an obstacle due to:

- a significant proportion of the population living in rural and remote areas;
- difficulty in accessing rural and remote areas, especially areas without roads, during the rainy season, on isolated islands, etc.;
- sporadic distribution of supplies to remote health facilities.

Good management practices are crucial to avoid medicine wastage, deterioration, or undersupply. These include managing the store appropriately, keeping good inventory records, and managing stock levels. Before medicines arrive at the health facility, the supply of medicines that needs to be available must be selected by forecasting what and how many medicines are needed, procuring the medicines, distributing the medicines, and storing them properly (Management Sciences for Health, 2012; World Health Organization, 2004). Once the medicines have arrived at the facility, the management process begins at the store.

Managing the store

If medicines and related supplies are not stored properly and to appropriate standards, they may deteriorate (World Health Organization, 2010a). If they deteriorate, they may lose their potency or have the wrong effect, for example if injectable oxytocin, which is used for prevention and treatment of postpartum hemorrhage, is not kept cold, it will not have the right effect (Figure 33.3). Refrigeration is also needed for many vaccines. If test kits are not stored properly, they produce incorrect results.

A store is a simple way to keep supplies safe. Having all stock in one place also makes it easier to know what is available. A health facility should have a separate room that can serve as the pharmacy store and that can be locked, is in good condition, and is well organized (Figure 33.4). All supplies should be kept in the store and only what is needed daily is taken to the dispensing area. If a health facility does not have a room to use as a pharmacy store, a lockable cupboard should be used.

Extreme temperatures, light, or humidity may cause medicines to deteriorate. Heat affects all medicines, especially liquids, ointments, and suppositories. Some medicines that are light-sensitive, such as injectables, spoil very quickly when exposed to light. Humidity can spoil tablets and capsules because they easily absorb water from the air, making them

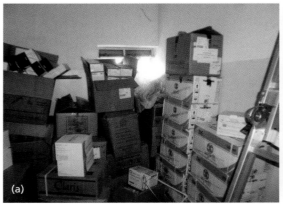 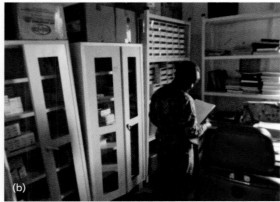

Figure 33.4 Before (a) and after (b) shelving was installed and products organized in a health center in Uganda. Staff also placed thick cardboard in front of the windows to block the sunlight. *Source*: USAID Applying Sciences to Strengthen and Improve Systems Project (ASSIST), Uganda. University Research Co., LLC. Available at http://www.urc-chs.com/project?ProjectID=264. Reproduced with permission of University Research Co., LLC.

> ### Clinical experience: organize the medicines in the store
>
> "I would have liked to have had the time to reorganize the medicines stored at the pharmacy, to at least place the medicines in alphabetical order. We spent so much time just trying to find the right medicine when needed."
>
> Geneviève, pharmacy student working in Kumasi, Ghana

sticky and causing them to deteriorate. Therefore, it is important for all products to be kept in their original packaging, containers, or boxes and in a temperature-controlled, cooled environment as required.

Medicines stored at a health facility should also be arranged by expiration date. The expiration date is useful in storing and managing the stocks of pharmaceuticals. The first-expiration-first-out (FEFO) method of inventory management involves dispensing products with the earliest expiration date first, regardless of the order in which they were received. This method helps prevent expiration of valuable pharmaceuticals.

It is important to identify products that are at risk of theft or abuse, have the potential for addiction, or have legal or regulatory requirements and therefore require storage in controlled access. Medicines such as antiretrovirals or artemisinin-based combination therapies for malaria may need to be kept in secure storage because they are scarce, expensive, and in high demand and short supply. Examples of controlled products requiring secure storage and control include narcotics (e.g., pethidine/meperidine and morphine),

opioids and strong analgesics (e.g., codeine), and psychotropic medicines (e.g., diazepam). This is because these medicines are addictive, used for recreational purposes, and can be sold easily on the streets.

Inventory management and stock control

All medical supplies should be received by at least one staff member at the time of delivery. Sometimes there should be an additional designated person to receive specific items, for controlled substances for example. A record of deliveries should be kept to help staff to find and correct problems that may occur. As supplies are received, the outside of the boxes should be examined for any signs of damage or opening that could indicate theft and the expiration dates of all items should be checked. At a minimum, medicines should have more than 6 months before expiry to be acceptable. Medicine donations can help to save lives by making more medicines available, but only if they are well coordinated and managed, are of quality, and are relevant to the needs. Too often donations of medicines are not carried out in accordance with national and global guidelines for medicine donations as medicines are too close to or past their expiration date (World Health Organization, 2010b).

Maintaining a sufficient stock of items at a health facility has many benefits. Patients receive medicines promptly, and stock-outs can be prevented even when deliveries to the store are delayed. Supplies can be replenished at scheduled intervals. Patients have confidence in the facility and seek help when they are ill. In addition, an effective inventory control system keeps track of and guarantees accountability for supplies.

STOCK CARD

FOLIO NUMBER_____   CARD NUMBER_____

DESRIPTION: **Coartem**				SPECIAL CONDITIONS:		
STRENGTH/ Artemether 20mg+Lumefantrine 120mg SIZE: 24				EXPIRY: January 15, 2014 DATE(S)		
ISSUE UNIT: Blister		AMC		MAXIMUM STOCK		QUNTITY TO ORDER
DATE	TO OR FROM	VOUCHER NUMBER	QUANTITY IN	QUANTITY OUT	BALANCE ON HAND	REMARKS/ BATCH NUMBER
14-May-13					50	
29-May-13	Dispensary	Req #43		5	45	

Figure 33.5 A typical stock card in a primary healthcare facility. *Source*: adapted from the Ministry of Health and Social Welfare, Republic of Liberia. Available at http://www.mohsw.gov.lr/

Stock cards are the inventory management tool used to monitor stock level and consumption of medicines and health supplies. By monitoring the rate of consumption, the staff responsible for managing stocks can forecast future requirements with accuracy. A typical stock card, such as the one illustrated in Figure 33.5, would record valuable stock information. There should be a stock card for each item in the store. In general, stock cards must be kept with the item on the shelf. Use the stock card to track the movement of the item. Record when and how the item is used. This includes all movements, such as when a new item arrives in the store.

When inventory control fails, problems can occur. A patient's condition may worsen because of a delay in treatment, or antimicrobial resistance may develop because a course of treatment was not completed. A patient may even die if life-saving medicines are out of stock. If medicines are not available in rural facilities, patients may have to make long and expensive journeys to obtain treatment. Also, frequent stock-outs may establish or reinforce poor prescribing habits. For example, when a medicine is out of stock, a less suitable alternative may be prescribed.

Successful supply management means that the required items are available for the patients who need them. Supplies are more likely to be available if they are ordered regularly, before the order deadline and in the correct quantities. In general, the amount of supplies to be ordered should be based on the amount that is used or their past consumption. It is also important that ordering is coordinated with the clinicians, in case there have been any changes in services or planned health events so that these can be taken into account (e.g., outreach clinics, vaccination days, increase in number of outpatients, new clinical guidelines). The order forms in many countries include simple calculations to work out the amount of supplies that should be ordered. In some settings, medicines may be redistributed between facilities that have surplus stock and those that need more stock.

Well-maintained stock records contain all the data required for deciding what to order, when to order, and the quantities to order. This helps staff understand the flow of supplies into and out of the healthcare facility. In addition, keeping records serves as the basis for the information needed when ordering new stocks of medicines or when products are recalled.

Using medicines in the treatment and prevention of disease

Assessing and identifying medicine-related needs

Medicinal products are commonly used tools in the prevention, treatment, and cure of disease. Like any tool, their appropriate use requires good understanding of their role, function, effects, and limitations. Selecting and prescribing the most appropriate medicine for a patient first requires an appropriate diagnosis. Take the time to find out what diagnostic facilities and support are available locally and more remotely. Are there rapid diagnostic tests, laboratories for testing, screening and diagnostic checklists and guidelines for common diseases available? One example of this is provided by Camille, a medical student who took part in a rotation at a rural primary healthcare facility in Tanzania:

> It was for me a very interesting experience to discover the medical practice in a different country, in a rural environment, with no diagnostic facilities and very limited resources. The clinic did have laboratory equipment but there was not enough power to run the microscope, so testing blood to properly diagnose malaria was not possible.

Newer rapid diagnostic tests now being made available may help more accurately diagnose malaria (World Health Organization, 2012).

Choosing the best treatment will also depend on the locally available guidelines. Prescribing should follow good prescribing principles and treatment or clinical guidelines, which are often available nationally or within hospitals. Dispensing med-

icines should also follow good pharmacy practice guidelines (International Pharmaceutical Federation & World Health Organization, 2011). General information on the most commonly used medicines may not be available to the medical staff or in the local language. Readily usable and accessible information about medicines, including their appropriate indications for use, dose and duration of treatment, toxicities, major side effects, and contraindications, is of great value to all when choosing the most appropriate medicine. If a facility has internet available, a listing of relevant and freely accessible drug information resources is available online through the International Pharmaceutical Federation Pharmabridge program (International Pharmaceutical Federation Pharmacy Information Section, 2012).

Assessing and identifying medicine-related problems

Since a medicine that is given to a patient is a tool to help that patient achieve a better health outcome, it is important to assess whether the medicine is working. Proper pharmaceutical care implies that "practitioners should assume responsibility for the outcomes of drug therapy in their patients" (Wiedenmayer *et al.*, 2006). This means being able to follow up with patients to assess whether there are any known medicine-related problems. Common types of medicine therapy problems include (Wiedenmayer *et al.*, 2006):

- needing a medicine but not receiving or not taking it;
- taking or receiving the wrong medicine;
- taking a medicine that is not needed;
- taking or receiving too little or too much of the correct medicine;
- experiencing an adverse drug reaction (side effect);
- experiencing a drug–drug or drug–food interaction.

Records of the use of medicines by patients may be established to aid patient care, to reduce medicine-related problems, to monitor medicine use, and to avoid medicine abuse. If available, a simple computer can be an effective option for storing the records (e.g., patient files and stock cards).

Speaking with patients is vital to help identify any potential problems and to ensure patients understand what their medicines should or should not do, so that they can seek further assistance from a health professional if there are any unexpected effects. Patients also need to be counseled and involved in the medication-use process so that they understand the rationale for their therapy, know how to take their medicines, and can adhere to their medicine. Local traditions may play an important role in this process: make sure these are understood so that staff can most effectively educate patients on the prescribed therapy.

In addition, there is also the increased threat in low-resource settings that patients will have greater risk to their safety because of readily available counterfeit or substandard medicines. Educating healthcare professionals and patients on where counterfeits are often sold (e.g., drug sellers, markets, and non-licenced premises) and how to identify substandard products can help to reduce the use of potentially contaminated and harmful medicines. The BE AWARE toolkit offers practical advice on tools and strategies to detect counterfeit medicines and inform patients (http://www.who.int/impact/news/beaware/en/). In certain countries, medicine-tracking systems are being utilized to help reduce the entry of counterfeit products into the markets and healthcare systems (IMS Institute for Healthcare Informatics, 2012).

Clinical experience: local beliefs and counseling and caring for patients

"Appreciating local traditions and beliefs when it comes to healthcare is an important first step to connecting with patients. Many herbal products interact with medicines and need to be discussed with patients. Telling patients what they can and cannot take is unacceptable, and will result in negative patient outcomes. Work *with*, rather than *on*, patients and include their healthcare beliefs. In rural areas, local chemist shops rarely had a pharmacist as there may only be one pharmacist in the entire district. No counseling on proper use of the medicine is performed. We discovered that the route of administration was often being overlooked; many of the local people would crush up antibiotic tablets and sprinkle them into their wounds. Also, many people overdosed on pain medication, not realizing the same active ingredients were found in different preparations."

Cory, pharmacy student working in Ghana

Table 33.2 Assessment of medication use: five prime questions.

Medicine	Question to ask	Explanation
User	"Who is this medicine for?"	If not prescribed by the clinician, always first ask who the medicine is for as the person presenting with the medicines or prescription may not be the person actually using the medicines.
Source	"Where did the medicine come from?"	If a patient comes with a medicine that is not known to staff or the clinic, it is important to find out where the medicine was obtained to identify the product and assess its potential quality and appropriateness.
Purpose	"What is this medicine for?"	It is important that patients understand why they are taking the medicine. This information may also help tailor the information provided to patients.
Directions	New medication: "What were you told about how to take your inhaler?" Refill: "How do you take this medicine?" or "How do you fit this medicine into your day?"	This question is useful for assessing whether the patient understands the medicines (for new medicines) and to assess at refills how patients are taking their medicines.
Monitoring	New medication: "How can you tell whether it is working?" Refill: "How is your pain?" or "What have you noticed since starting this pill?" or "What do you do if you miss taking your medicine?"	These questions will assess patients' understanding of and help in monitoring medicine effectiveness and side effects and assist in detecting any potential quality issues.

Source: adapted from International Pharmaceutical Federation & International Pharmaceutical Students' Federation (2012).

Amoxicillin 500mg

RX# 543   2013/05/14
REF # EC47 7166 9C2D A350

TAKE 1 CAPSULE BY MOUTH IN THE MORNING, AT NOON, AT NIGHT.
Quantity: 30

Figure 33.6 Example of a pictogram medication use label. *Source*: Pictograms Software 2013. Reproduced with permission of the International Pharmaceutical Federation.

Helping the patient understand how to take their medicines

Patients can only remember a limited amount of information, and so the key to helping patients understand their medicines is to prioritize information and focus on key messages.

Techniques are available to check patient understanding, such as asking five prime questions (Table 33.2) and using "teach back" or "show me" techniques, using open questions and patient-friendly educational materials to enhance interaction (International Pharmaceutical Federation & International Pharmaceutical Students' Federation, 2012).

Consider and ask patients if they have any concerns, problems, and questions related to the use of the medicines and provide clear guidance on the best use of the medicine that has been prescribed. When language or health literacy barriers exist between staff and patients, consider using pictograms to help provide the needed information on how to use the medicine (Figure 33.6). Computer software is now freely available in 17 languages to help patients and practitioners communicate through the use of printed pictograms (International Pharmaceutical Federation, 2014).

Health workers have an important responsibility to make sure that life-saving medicines are used in a way that is safe, affordable, and equitable by patients, communities, and the health system. Having the right processes in place can help to ensure that quality medicines are accessible and used responsibly by those who need them, when and where they need them.

REFERENCES

Bigdeli M, Jacobs B, Tomson G *et al.* (2013) Access to medicines from a health system perspective. *Health Policy Plan* 28:692–704.

Cameron A, Ewen M, Ross-Degnan D, Ball D, Laing R (2009) Medicine prices, availability, and affordability in 36 developing and middle-income countries: a secondary analysis. *Lancet* 373:240–9.

Frost LJ, Reich M (2008) *Access: How do Good Health Technologies Get to Poor People in Poor Countries?* Cambridge, MA: Harvard Center for Population and Development Studies. Available at http://www.accessbook.org/

Gal D, Bates I. (2012) Human resources: the 2012 FIP Global Pharmacy Workforce Report. Available at http://www.fip.org/humanresources

IMS Institute for Healthcare Informatics (2012) Advancing the responsible use of medicines. Applying levers for change. Available at http://www.responsibleuseofmedicines.org/wp-content/uploads/2012/09/IIHI-Ministers-Report-170912-Final.pdf

International Pharmaceutical Federation (2014) Pictograms software. Available at http://www.fip.org/pictograms

International Pharmaceutical Federation & International Pharmaceutical Students' Federation (2012) *Counselling, Concordance and Communication: Innovative Education for Pharmacists*, 2nd edn. The Hague, Netherlands: International Pharmaceutical Federation, International

Pharmaceutical Students' Federation. Available at http://www.ipsf.org/pce

International Pharmaceutical Federation Pharmacy Information Section (2012) Open access sources of medicines information. http://www.fip.org/files/fip/Pharmabridge/Open_access_MI_sources_20120120.pdf

International Pharmaceutical Federation & World Health Organization (2011) Good pharmacy practice. Joint FIP/WHO Guidelines on GPP: Standards for quality of pharmacy services. Available at http://www.fip.org/statements

Kaplan W, Mathers C (2011) Global health trends: global burden of disease and pharmaceutical needs. Available at http://apps.who.int/medicinedocs/documents/s20051en/s20051en.pdf

Management Sciences for Health (2012) *MDS-3: Managing Access to Medicines and Health Technologies*. Arlington, VA: Management Sciences for Health, Inc. Available at http://apps.who.int/medicinedocs/documents/s19630en/s19630en.pdf

United Nations Development Group (2003) *Indicators for Monitoring the Millennium Development Goals: Definitions, Rationale, Concepts and Sources*. New York: United Nations. Available at http://mdgs.un.org/unsd/mdg/Resources/Attach/Indicators/HandbookEnglish.pdf

Wiedenmayer K, Summers RS, Mackie CA, Gous AGS, Everard M (2006) *Developing Pharmacy Practice: A*

Focus on Patient Care. World Health Organization and International Pharmaceutical Federation. http://www.fip.org/files/fip/publications/Developing PharmacyPractice/DevelopingPharmacyPracticeEN.pdf

World Health Organization (2004) Management of drugs at health centre level: training manual. Available at http://apps.who.int/medicinedocs/en/d/Js7919e/

World Health Organization (2010a) WHO good distribution practices for pharmaceutical products. Available at http://www.who.int/medicines/areas/quality_safety/quality_assurance/GoodDistributionPracticesTRS957Annex5.pdf

World Health Organization (2010b) International guidelines for medicines donations. Available at http://www.who.int/medicines/publications/med_donationsguide2011/en/index.html

World Health Organization (2012) The pursuit of responsible use of medicines: sharing and learning from country experiences. Available at http://www.who.int/medicines/publications/responsible_use/en/index.html

World Health Organization (2013) WHO model lists of essential medicines. Available at http://www.who.int/medicines/publications/essentialmedicines/en/

Xu K, Evans DB, Carrin G, Aguilar-Rivera AM, Musgrove P, Evans T (2007) Protecting households from catastrophic health spending. *Health Aff (Millwood)* 26:972–83.

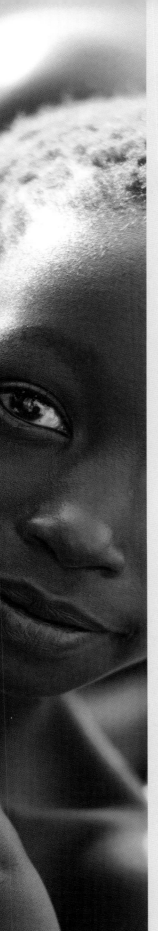

CHAPTER 34

Humanitarian Assistance

Karen Olness, Lauren C. Riney, and Caroline S. Hesko

Case Western Reserve University, Rainbow Babies and Children's Hospital, Cleveland, OH, USA

Key learning objectives

- Describe the acute and chronic effects of disasters on displaced persons.
- List the major organizations involved with global disaster relief and their role in assisting countries.
- Describe problems related to food security and how to address them.
- Describe common obstacles to sanitation and simple interventions to overcome these obstacles.

Abstract

Disaster-producing events occur frequently throughout the world. Regardless of where they occur, there are common problems that require assistance. In 1997, a group of humanitarian non-governmental organizations and the Red Cross and Red Crescent movement framed a Humanitarian Charter related to disaster assistance. The Charter identified standards in five key sectors, including water and sanitation, nutrition, food aid, shelter, and health services. Given the frequency of disasters, it is important that professionals with skills related to these sectors learn about disaster preparedness. This learning should range from international human rights to technical information about food and shelter. This chapter includes information about the effects of disasters on adults and children, about the roles of agencies in disasters, and evidence-based approaches to problems of disease prevention, sanitation, and unclean water. Finally, it includes resources for those who wish to study these issues further.

Key words: disaster, relief, malnutrition, humanitarian, aid, internal displacement, refugee, immunizations, sanitation, mental health

Essential Clinical Global Health, First Edition. Edited by Brett D. Nelson.
© 2015 John Wiley & Sons, Ltd. Published 2015 by John Wiley & Sons, Ltd.
Companion website: www.essentialseries.com/globalhealth

Introduction and epidemiology

Disasters come in many forms, sizes, and geographical locations and can affect a large number of people. Simply, a disaster is any event that causes destruction, affects many lives, and requires assistance from both within and outside the affected community.

The most common disasters that require relief are environmental or natural disasters. These are most often related to extreme weather events such as floods, droughts, tornadoes, blizzards, and hurricanes. Disasters related to geology, such as earthquakes or volcanoes, are less common. Other disasters that require relief are man-made disasters and include biological, chemical, and radioactive disasters as well as governmental collapse, wars, and terrorism (Centre for Research on the Epidemiology of Disasters, 2011).

According to the Annual Disaster Statistical Review, each year close to 300,000 people are killed by natural disasters (Figure 34.1) (CBC News, 2011). Furthermore, disasters displace millions of people throughout the world, with over 30 million people displaced in 2012 alone (Centre for Research on the Epidemiology of Disasters, 2012). Figure 34.2 shows the number of natural disasters reported since 1900. Although the number of reported disasters has greatly increased over the last several decades, the number of persons killed as a result of natural disasters has trended downwards (Figure 34.3). This decrease in casualties is likely the result of the increase in spending on disaster prevention, mitigation, and relief as well as the development of more efficient disaster and healthcare management.

Conflicts also continue to have a deadly public health impact, with the number of deaths among civilians far outnumbering those among combatants. In fact, up to 80–90% of casualties of modern-day wars are civilians, the majority of whom are women and children (UNICEF, 2000). While many of these deaths are directly violence-related, many more deaths during conflict are a result of indirect consequences such as population displacement, disruption of social structure and protections, and limited access to healthcare and essential services. Throughout history, Africa, Asia, and the Middle East have been and continue to be the most affected by these man-made disasters (Figure 34.4).

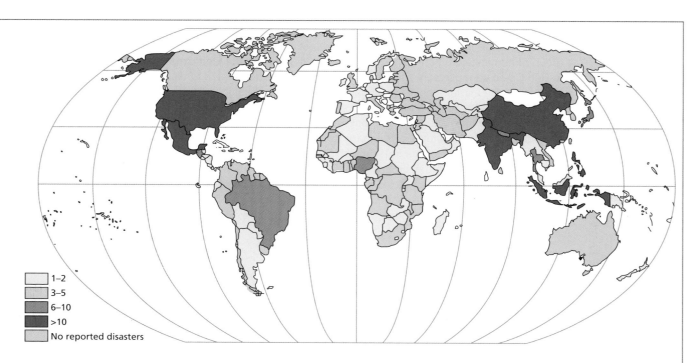

1–2
3–5
6–10
>10
No reported disasters

Figure 34.1 Natural disaster occurrence in 2011. *Source*: EM-DAT, The International Disaster Database. Reproduced with permission of the Centre for Research on the Epidemiology of Disasters.

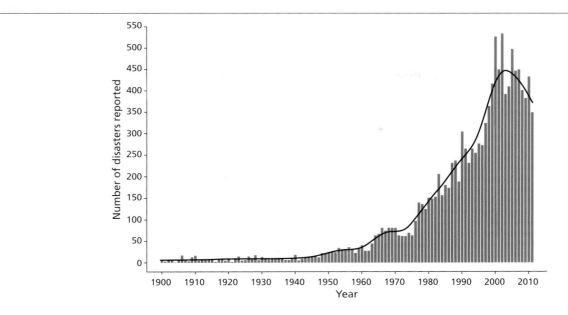

Figure 34.2 Number of disasters reported 1900–2011. *Source*: EM-DAT, The International Disaster Database. Reproduced with permission of the Centre for Research on the Epidemiology of Disasters.

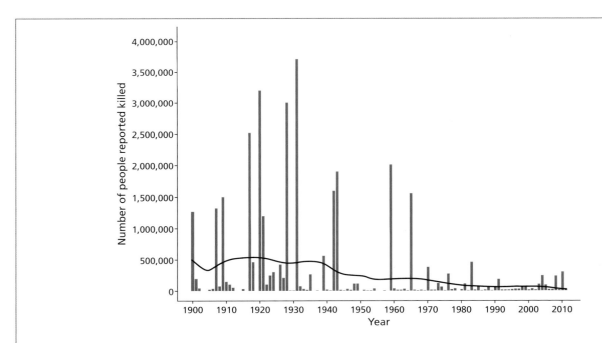

Figure 34.3 Number of people reported killed by natural disasters 1900–2011. *Source*: EM-DAT, The International Disaster Database. Reproduced with permission of the Centre for Research on the Epidemiology of Disasters.

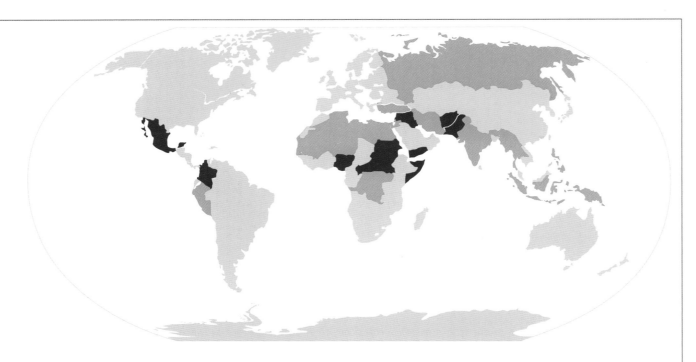

Figure 34.4 Map of ongoing conflicts in the world, as of October 2012. Dark red indicates major wars and civil unrest, with >1000 deaths/year. Orange indicates smaller skirmishes and conflicts, with <1000 deaths/year. *Source*: Wikimedia © Futuretrillionaire. Reproduced under the Creative Commons license.

Red flag

The Centre for Research on the Epidemiology of Disasters (CRED) in Brussels, Belgium defines a disaster as "a situation or event which overwhelms local capacity, necessitating a request to national or international level for external assistance."

Red flag

Internally displaced persons, as defined by the United Nations, are "persons or groups of persons who have been forced or obliged to flee or to leave their homes or places of habitual residence, in particular as a result of or in order to avoid the effects of armed conflict, situations of generalized violence, violations of human rights or natural or human-made disasters, and who have not crossed an internationally recognized state border" (Kälin, 2000).

Refugees and internally displaced persons

As a result of natural and man-made disasters, millions of individuals are displaced from their homes each year. An internally displaced person (IDP) is an individual who has been involuntarily forced to leave his or her home but remains within the borders of his or her country. Refugees are persons who are displaced and relocate into another country.

Currently, over 26 million people are considered IDPs. Most reported IDPs have been uprooted as a result of human rights violations or conflict, so this figure may actually be higher because of others displaced by different reasons (Mooney, 2005). The United Nations High Commissioner for Refugees (2014) reports that, in 2013, 10.4 million persons were refugees under the supervision of UNHCR and about half of these were children.

The countries with the largest populations of IDPs include Colombia, Sudan, Iraq, the Democratic Republic of Congo (DRC), and Azerbaijan with each containing more than 1 million IDPs (Norwegian Refugee Council's Internal Displacement Monitoring Centre, 2012). The United Nation's 1951 Refugee Convention and its amending 1967 Protocol promise refugees protection by UN member states and the international community. However, because IDPs do not cross international borders, they are not provided the same protections. Therefore, national governments have the sole responsibility to provide assistance and to protect their IDPs. This becomes a serious problem as many IDPs are forced to flee and are displaced in the first place because of failing governments or internal conflict.

Red flag

It is estimated that more than 5 million IDPs in 11 countries receive little assistance from their governments, and 70% of these IDPs are women and children (Norwegian Refugee Council's Internal Displacement Monitoring Centre, 2012).

Overview of organizations involved in disaster management

With the increasing number of disasters over the last few decades, an intricate assembly of international, governmental, and non-governmental organizations (NGOs) has come together to provide and assist with humanitarian relief (Table 34.1).

Multiple initiatives have been implemented over the last few decades to foster collaborative partnerships among the major players involved in disaster relief. In the 1990s, there was a tremendous increase in activities among international organizations to assist with global disaster relief. In 1997, agencies came together to improve humanitarian relief and create standards that became known as the Sphere Project (Sphere Project, 2011) (Figure 34.5). The disaster response handbook of standards developed by the Sphere Project members is frequently updated and widely used. Another project to increase efficiency among relief agencies was developed by the UN Humanitarian Reform process and known as the Cluster Approach. The Cluster Approach was created to form successful alliances between Red Cross, UN, and NGO agencies to best prepare and use resources effectively after disasters occur. Agencies with shared objectives are organized into collaborative sectors or clusters, such as clusters for medical care, shelter, nutrition, and water/sanitation. This approach was first put to use after the Pakistan earthquake in 2005 where nine clusters

were established in less than 24 hours (Olness et al., 2014) (Box 34.1).

Acute and chronic effects of displacement

Displacement can have serious effects on adults and children. Most notably, displacement causes a decline in the quality of life of people with regard to health-related conditions. Poor sanitation and unclean water increase the incidence of infectious diseases. People who have been displaced are often unable to access adequate healthcare, so that easily treated diseases linger and cause significant morbidity and mortality. Displacement can also cause separation of families and the breakdown of community structure. This causes psychosocial effects such as anxiety, depression, personality changes, and post-traumatic stress disorder. In the worst cases, increases in suicidal and homicidal thoughts are seen due to increased stressors. In addition, the education of children and adolescents ceases. Lastly, physical, sexual, or emotional abuse is commonly seen in displaced persons. Abusers may be government forces or other parties and can include family members.

The most vulnerable among displaced or refugee populations are women and children. For women, gender-based violence has been a huge issue during times of governmental conflict and other disasters. In Colombia, Sudan, and the DRC, rape has been used to punish communities for political disloyalty, for displacement purposes, and to accomplish ethnic cleansing. In 2006, an estimated 4000 displaced women were raped in the DRC. Additionally, in Uganda, sexual violence and exploitation against women and girls in displacement camps became a large problem (Norwegian Refugee Council's Internal Displacement Monitoring Centre, 2012), Meanwhile, displaced or refugee children are at increased risk of violence, poverty, sexual abuse, forced labor, separation from family, and

Clinical experience

"During several weeks in Haiti after the 2010 earthquake hit, I was based in Port-au-Prince working for a locally owned NGO alongside Haitian colleagues and clinicians. Our immediate goal was to scale up preexisting procurement supply chain to effectively manage the vast influx of medicines and supplies being sent to support the relief effort. On the most fundamental level, what ensured the success of our response was that it was authentically rooted in Haitian leadership. Based on a model of local ownership, rather than one of charity, our partnerships with local leaders within the refugee tent settlements and with the Haitian government allowed the response effort to transcend traditional acute phase paradigms to create more lasting change."

Elisabeth, medical student working in Haiti

Table 34.1 International disaster relief organizations and agencies.

United Nations	Established in 1945 at the end of World War II Protects human rights and promotes equal rights for all nations Provides immediate disaster relief and supports development programs in community development, construction, and agriculture
UN Office for Coordination of Humanitarian Affairs (OCHA)	Coordinates UN assistance in humanitarian crises, provides support for international policy development, advocates humanitarian issues, mobilizes funds quickly Also coordinates relief with non-UN organizations and NGOs
UN High Commissioner for Refugees (UNHCR)	Assists with protecting refugee populations and supports local communities to prevent refugee movements
World Food Program (WFP)	Established in 1961 Provides food aid to populations in need, specifically in non-industrialized countries
World Health Organization (WHO)	Established in 1946 Leader in managing and directing international health as well as assisting in disease control and prevention
United Nations Children's Fund (UNICEF)	Established in 1946 Provides disaster relief to children Supports programs in sanitation, nutrition, and water supply Promotes training, education, and immunizations to improve child healthcare Can provide assistance without permission of existing governments
Inter-Agency Standing Committee (IASC)	Coordinates relief activities for disaster victims involving UN and non-UN humanitarian agencies
International Committee of the Red Cross (ICRC)	Established in 1863, world's oldest relief organization Makes recommendations and creates proposals for humanitarian conventions A neutral independent humanitarian provider offering assistance and protection to victims
International Federation of Red Cross and Red Crescent Societies	Established in 1919 as a consortium of national societies In 1994, joined with six of the world's largest NGOs to create a Code of Conduct to outline how to work in disaster relief
National Red Cross and Red Crescent Societies	Assist with health education and natural disaster relief Provide assistance to victims of armed conflicts
Non-governmental organizations (NGOs)	95% of disaster relief is achieved through about 30 NGOs More than 20,000 organizations worldwide Some receive government funding while others are independently funded through charities and donors Examples: CARE, World Vision, Save the Children

forced recruitment into armed groups. In addition, malnutrition, infectious diseases, and acute and chronic psychological distress are very common in displaced children.

Acute needs and interventions

During a disaster, whether natural or caused by humans, assessing the acute needs of the affected population is critical. Four major areas in which to concentrate interventions during the acute response include nutrition, water and sanitation, housing, and medical care. These areas are of course interdependent. For example, treating a child with a foot laceration with sutures and antibiotics will not suffice if the child lacks shoes or if wound healing is compromised by severe malnutrition.

The devastation caused by disasters is made much worse when it occurs in places already struggling to meet the basic needs of the population. It is important, prior to interventions, that the relief worker be aware of the problems that the community faced before the disaster, such as poor access to safe drinking water (Box 34.2).

Food security

The level of food security in an area will depend largely on pre-disaster levels of food, whether food production means

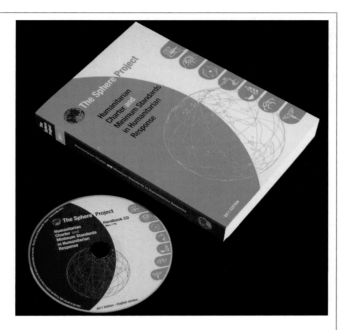

Figure 34.5 The *Sphere Handbook* contains the principles and standards for the provision of humanitarian assistance. *Source*: Sphere Project (2011).

Box 34.2 Understanding the local context: Haiti before the 2010 earthquake (World Health Organization, 2010)

Haiti is the poorest country in the western hemisphere. This was true even before the 2010 earthquake that devastated the already fragile population. As a population:

- 45% lacked access to safe water
- 83% had no access to sufficient sanitation
- 9.1% of children under 5 years of age suffered from acute malnutrition.

Box 34.3 Case example 1

A food aid distribution area has been set up at the hospital after a flood destroyed most of the agricultural land in a village. Each family receives a ration for every member of the household. Prior to leaving the area, you make sure that the two underweight children you are seeing get their food aid, including supplemental ready-to-use therapeutic food (RUTF). A few days later while visiting homebound patients, you notice that multiple families have not eaten their food aid. On further inquiry, you discover that all families were given dry rations to be cooked at home. However, when the river flooded, it swept most of the community's cooking equipment away because the pots were kept next to the river for ease of use.

Box 34.1 Case study: how do you assess a disaster situation in the acute stage?
(World Health Organization, 2005)

1. Leadership: Who is in charge? Is the local government able to help? What organizations are involved and available to help? For example, UN, Red Cross, CDC, FEMA.
2. Demographics: In which geographic area did the disaster occur? Among what population did the disaster occur, and how many people have been affected or displaced?
3. Healthcare: What are the acute healthcare needs? Are there local health workers available to help with the needs?
4. Finance: What resources are needed and what resources are available? Who will be funding the disaster relief work?
5. Medications: Is there any need to mass vaccinate the population to prevent infectious diseases? What medications will most likely be needed at the disaster site and who will supply them?
6. Living conditions: What shelter is available and what is needed? Is there food available? Are sanitation systems in place, and is safe drinking water available?

---

such as farming equipment were destroyed, the feasibility of providing food to affected areas, and the availability of food preparation supplies such as firewood, oil, and cookware (Box 34.3).

Based on the nature and stage of the disaster, who receives food aid and how much they receive will vary. In the acute phase, in the setting of widespread food insecurity, food aid is distributed throughout the community. However, if the disaster occurs in a localized area, a targeted approach is more appropriate. Children (especially those 2–59 months old), pregnant women, and women who are lactating should receive supplemental food in addition to the general ration. Aid can be given as food, vouchers to buy certain commodities, or cash. For example, if local markets are still able to provide certain items, a voucher would be preferable since it supports not only the recipient but also the local merchant.

Dry food aid, or food that is cooked at home, is usually used in areas where patients can safely and easily return home and have the needed equipment to cook. Wet food aid, or food cooked at a site and consumed there, is recommended in refugee camps, at school to help supplement children, and in disasters where navigating home is too unsafe (Sphere Project, 2011). Continued evaluation of food supply distribution is necessary to ensure that it is reaching its intended target. It is essential to determine who in the community should assist with food delivery and allocation. Transparency of ration distribution and having women involved have been shown to be critical to the success of a food aid program and in ensuring empowerment and protection of women (Taylor *et al.*, 2004).

Water and sanitation

Potable water is defined as water that contains less than 10 fecal coliform organisms per 100 mL. It is imperative that potable water is made available as early as possible in a disaster. In areas with commercial water treatment facilities, determining their functionality and capacity as well as protecting them from damage is vital.

> **Red flag**
>
> The minimum amount of water required for each person is 7 L/day.

The average amount of water required per person is summarized in Table 34.2. When setting up a camp, if there will not be access to the minimal required amount of water per person, the location must be changed or water must be trucked in, which can be prohibitively expensive.

Table 34.2 Average water requirements per person per day.

Need	Amount (L/day)	Notes
Total per person	7.5–15	
Survival (food and drink)	2.5–3	Varies depending on climate and health status of the person
Hygiene	2–6	Varies depending on cultural norms
Cooking	3–6	Varies depending on food type and food staples of a community
Health center patient	40–60	Varies depending on disease and acuity
Feeding center patient	20–30	Varies depending on age and food types

Source: data from Sphere Project (2011).

There are four general ways of treating water to make it safe for drinking (Table 34.3). Proper community education about what is considered safe drinking water and explanations that clear water does not mean safe water can help reduce consumption of non-potable water.

The quality of sanitation during an emergency has a major impact on the health and disease burden of the affected community. Potable drinking water and proper sanitation are closely linked. During the acute phase of a disaster, defecation areas should be established. Establishing proper sanitation requires community input on local toileting norms, educating the community on proper sanitation methods, and identifying possible barriers to success (UNICEF, 2005). If there is a body of water or a river near the area of a disaster or within a displacement camp, there should be signs in the local language that explain to the population that they should not defecate or dump waste there (Box 34.4). Because many people will see the water source as an ideal place for relieving themselves, setting up a boundary such as a fence early and engaging the community will help avoid contamination of the water source. It is preferable to emphasize where people can urinate and defecate rather than emphasizing areas where they cannot.

> **Red flag**
>
> Removal of human stool should take priority over removal of animal stool because the amount of diseases affecting humans is greater in human stool (UNICEF, 2005).

Family pit latrines are the most common sanitation method used during emergencies. These are composed of a squatting plate (Figure 34.6) around a hole that should be 1–2 m deep with a privacy screen surrounding the hole. Ideally, one latrine should be constructed for every 20 people (UNICEF, 2005). If communal latrines must be used, it is imperative to have separation among the sexes and adequate privacy measures to ensure compliance and safety. Helping children feel comfortable with the latrine can relieve their fears of falling (Olness *et al.*, 2014).

Housing

Depending on the disaster, the amount and type of shelters available will vary. For example, in a tsunami, entire villages and towns can be swept into the ocean, leaving nothing behind, while an earthquake will result in loss or damage but building materials will still be present. In human conflicts, homes may be burned or destroyed by opposing forces. Young children are particularly vulnerable to increased morbidity and mortality if they do not have proper shelter. To aid in warmth, children should sleep together or with their parents. Kangaroo or skin-to-skin care has been shown to be effective

Table 34.3 Water treatment methods.

Treatment	Method	Notes	Possible pitfalls	Solutions to prevent pitfalls
Storage	Keep water stored and covered for 12–48 hours; longer is preferred	Most pathogens will die in that time Allows sediment to settle (sedimentation) Requires disinfection after storage	Waiting 12–24 hours Water being uncovered or swam in by children	Allow sedimentation overnight. Place in fenced area with guards if needed.
Filtration	Use sand to filter out large debris; an active plankton and algae layer breaks down organic matter	Requires water to flow slowly	Filtration rate based on surface area of sand	Have a two-drum system; stacking drums vertically. use the top drum for sand filtration and allow the water to pass into the bottom drum where it can be stored. A faucet can be attached to the storage drum for access to the water while new untreated water can be poured into the top drum for filtration.
Chemical disinfection	Use chloride or iodine to kill pathogens Calcium hypochlorite is more common	Need to wait 30 min and for free chlorine to be 0.2–0.5 mg/L If water is turbid, requires sedimentation and disinfection	Chlorine taste	Make sure water is not being overtreated since taste is usually unpalatable if levels of free chloride are higher than 0.5 mg/L.
Solar disinfection	Uses the effects of electricity, thermal, or ultraviolet water disinfection	UV-A and cumulative solar energy destroys cell structures of bacteria, creates free oxygen radicals and heats the water	The water bottles must be left in the sun for a lengthy amount of time. Bottles may be harder to obtain and ship than disinfecting tablets.	Bags of water can be packed tighter and shipment becomes less costly than bottles.
Boiling	Bring water to a boil	Boil for an extra minute for every 300 m (1000 feet) above sea level	Boiling requires 1 kg wood per liter of water	Remind people that the water only needs to be brought to a boil, not a vigorous boil.

Source: United Nations High Commissioner for Refugees (2007) *Handbook for Emergencies*, 3rd edn. Geneva: UNHCR.

Box 34.4 Case example 2

A family of five arrives at a new displaced person camp after their village was destroyed by a mudslide. As they move throughout camp, they see numerous signs telling them where they cannot defecate. The father quickly finds an area for toileting that has minimal privacy barriers. Uncomfortable with the amount of openness, the mom and oldest daughter find a more isolated field to relieve themselves. Terrified that they might fall down into the latrine hole, the two young children wander around finding a place to defecate.

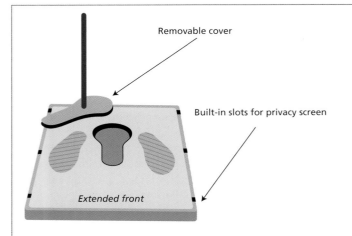

Figure 34.6 Example of a squatting plate.

Table 34.4 Types of housing during a disaster: advantages and disadvantages.

Type	Information	Advantages	Disadvantages
Dispersed settlement	Having those affected by the disaster stay with families in the area	Available in acute phase Builds community Low cost and low administration burden Less environmental impact than a camp	Host families may also be affected by disaster Strain on host families Difficulty distinguishing between hosts and disaster victims can affect need estimates
Mass shelter	Public buildings and community facilities such as schools, hotels, courthouses	Available immediately Water and sanitation facilities are in place No need for new construction	Unable to use buildings for original purpose Can quickly get overcrowded and exceed sanitation and water abilities Buildings can be damaged
Camps	Shelters built specifically for disaster victims	Economies of scale Target population is centrally located Identification and communication is easier	High cost and high administrative burden Can have large local environmental impact Need to construct all required services such as sanitation Increased risk of infection spreading quickly to large numbers Security within the camp and surrounding area may be limited

Source: United Nations High Commissioner for Refugees (2007) *Handbook for Emergencies*, 3rd edn. Geneva: UNHCR.

in providing warmth even to premature infants (Olness *et al.*, 2014). There are three main approaches to housing that can be used during a disaster: dispersed settlement, mass shelter, and camps (Table 34.4).

Medical care

During the acute phase of a disaster, proper triage of healthcare needs is critical in order to decrease morbidity and mortality. Understanding the pre-disaster health system capacity and functionality and the pre-disaster health issues of the community will help with planning and implementation of post-disaster medical care.

During the acute phase of an emergency, medical care can be divided into two main categories.

- Treatment: management of acute injuries, life-threatening infections, and severe malnutrition.
- Prevention: vaccinations, nutritional support, and infection control (malaria bednets, clean water, hand hygiene).

In the acute phase of emergencies, efforts should be made to streamline care, reduce duplication of services, and establish an early warning system for disease outbreaks. Depending on the type of disaster and the infrastructure available, the ability to create field hospitals, clinics, and mobile health centers will vary. When setting up medical care, key questions that need to be answered include the following.

- Location of those affected: urban, rural, isolated due to armed forces or natural barriers.

- Mobility of those affected: road infrastructure, access to vehicles and fuel, physical impairments that decrease mobility, social standing that may impact ability to seek care.
- Resources for the diagnosis and treatment of prevalent diseases and health conditions: laboratory supplies, imaging modalities (e.g., X-ray, ultrasound, ECG), medications that will be needed to treat acute and chronic disease (e.g., antibiotics, HIV medications, tuberculosis medications, pain medications, antimalarial medications).
- Level of training of local practitioners and training of medical volunteers.
- Community attitudes toward medical care, especially care provided by international healthcare workers.

Immunizations

Vaccinations are a cornerstone of public health and are key in helping to reduce morbidity and mortality due to communicable diseases (Table 34.5). Fundamental questions to answer prior to the start of any vaccination campaign include the following.

- What is the baseline level of immunizations in the community?
- What vaccine-preventable diseases (VPD) are present in the community?
- What part of the population is at greatest risk of infection?
- What is the morbidity and mortality associated with a certain VPD?
- What are the community consensus attitudes on use of vaccines among the community?

Table 34.5 Immunizations during a disaster.

Vaccine	When to administer	Who should receive	Storage	Contraindications	Notes
Measles (live)	Highest priority; give during emergency phase	9 months to 5 years are priority 9 months to 14 years In emergency phase, can give as young as 6 months but need to repeat at 9 months with 30-day interval between.	Heat-sensitive Store at 0–8°C	Pregnancy (HIV-positive children *can* and *should* get vaccine)	Must give with Vitamin A 6–12 months of age: 100,000 IU 12–59 months of age: 200,000 IU. Continue supplements every 4–6 months.
Meningococcal Serogroup A and C Inactive	If outbreak, give during emergency phase If no outbreak, give during rehabilitation phase	2–10 year olds are priority	Do not allow to freeze Store at 2–8°C	Should not be given with other vaccines in children with sickle cell disease or asplenia.	Outbreak defined as doubling of cases over 3-week period
Polio OPV (oral polio vaccine, live-attenuated) IPV (inactive polio vaccine)	If endemic within community, give during emergency phase If not endemic within community, give during rehabilitation phase	Children under 5	OPV: −20°C IPV: 2–8°C	OPV should not be used in HIV-positive children. If immediate protection is needed, IPV should be used if pregnant.	OPV is recommended in areas with endemic polio due to increased protection and contact immunity.
Diphtheria, pertussis and tetanus (DPT) (inactive)	Emergency phase	All children under 5	Freezer-sensitive Store at 0–8°C		Tetanus should be given to all females of childbearing age due to risk of neonatal tetanus from contaminated instruments during delivery.
Bacille Calmette–Guérin (BCG) (attenuated live bacteria)	Emergency phase	All children under age 1	Light-sensitive Store at 2–8°C	HIV-positive, even if asymptomatic	

Source: UNICEF (2005), Centers for Disease Control and Prevention (2012), World Health Organization (2012), American Academy of Pediatrics (2012).

- Who within the community (e.g., political leaders, religious leaders, tribal leaders) will be a stakeholder in the process and who may be a cause of resistance to immunizations?
- How and where will vaccines be stored and administered?
- Who will administer the vaccines?

Red flag

Malnutrition is **not** a contraindication to immunization.

Generally, cholera, typhoid, rotavirus, *Haemophilus influenzae* type B, hepatitis A, and varicella vaccinations are not recommended during the early stages of an emergency. Once the situation has stabilized, it is recommended that the World Health Organization (WHO) Expanded Program of Immunization schedule be followed. However, this recommendation can vary slightly depending on the prevalence of certain diseases within a country.

> **Red flag**
>
> Giving Vitamin A with measles vaccine decreases severity of disease if contracted and decreases mortality by 50% in patients with active disease.

Mental health

Man-made disasters are more likely than natural disasters to cause acute and chronic developmental and psychological trauma. This is partly due to the fact that the amount and level of violence a person may witness or experience during a war is greater than in a natural event such as a flood. The response to the disaster by the local, national, and international community also varies greatly depending on the disaster. The rapidity and type of help will have a direct impact on how a person experiences a disaster and how they will react to it in the short and long term (Olness *et al.*, 2014).

In general, women and children are more vulnerable to disasters. Depending on the type of disaster, specific age groups will be at greatest risk for mental health issues. For example, during armed conflicts, adolescent females are vulnerable to being raped and forced into prostitution. Adolescent boys may face forced inscription as child soldiers. Infants and young children are vulnerable due to their inability to care for themselves (Table 34.6). Older children and teenagers are at high risk of psychological sequelae from a disaster due to ability to remember and understand the events they have experienced. How young children respond to disasters depends on their intrinsic personality, how their parents respond, and what early interventions are available to help them.

> **Box 34.5 Case example 3**
>
> You are working in a field clinic in an area destroyed by a recent hurricane. A mother brings in her 4-year-old daughter because she is concerned she may have a urinary tract infection. She explains that her daughter has been toilet trained since the age of 2 but, over the past week, has had multiple episodes of both night and day wetting.

> **Red flag**
>
> Play is critical to healthy development. Create safe opportunities for play, using paper and local materials in creative ways to make toys. Establishing community-level play opportunities helps children recover from disaster trauma.

Regression in development, skills, and behaviors is common after a child experiences a trauma (Table 34.6, Box 34.5). For example, a 5 year old may have temper tantrums similar to a 2 year old as a way to express anxiety and stress. Changes in behavior such as shyness in a normally outgoing child can also be a reflection of stress.

> **Red flag**
>
> PsySTART is a mental health triage system that uses 20 yes–no questions to determine the risk of psychological problems for a person involved in a disaster. Two simple examples of these yes–no questions are "Unaccompanied minor?" and "Saw or heard death or serious injury of others?" (www.psystart.org).

> **Red flag**
>
> Programs used in emergencies include UNICEF's Early Childhood Development Kit, UNICEF's Return to Happiness Program, and the International Resilience Project (Grotberg, 1995).

Chapter 27 offers additional information on the general diagnosis and management of mental health concerns.

Additional resources

General

- United Nations High Commissioner for Refugees (2007) *Handbook for Emergencies*, 3rd edn. Geneva: UNHCR. Available at http://www.unhcr.org/472af2972.html
- UNICEF (2005) *Emergency Field Handbook: A Guide for UNICEF Staff.* Available at http://www.unicef.org/publications/files/UNICEF_EFH_2005.pdf
- Olness K, Mandalakas A, Torjesen K (2014) *How to Help the Children in Humanitarian Disasters*, 3rd edn. Kenyon, MN: Health Frontiers. Available at http://www.ipa-world.org/uploadedbyfck/How%20to%20Help%20Children March16.pdf

Table 34.6 Reaction to a disaster based on age and development.

Age	Response to disaster	Interventions
Toddlers	Regression in learned skills (e.g., toilet training), muteness	Avoid punishment for episodes of incontinence
	Decreased appetite	Reestablish simple routines such as mealtimes and eating as a family
	Model parents' reaction to situation	Encourage parents to seek medical care including mental health services as a way of helping improve their child's health
	Exaggerated startle response, hypersensitivity to noise or weather, irritability	Normalize environment, create calm quiet environment when possible, provide physical contact for reassurance and comfort, frequent feedings (four to five times a day)
School-age children	Somatic complaints (headache and stomach ache)	Affirm that they are experiencing these symptoms, rule out any medical etiology, discuss stress reduction techniques that are used in that culture (e.g., traditional healers, dance, meditation)
	Re-enactment through play	Allow expression of experiences including re-enactment (unless it is destructive or dangerous) as a way for the child to work through and share feelings
	Sleep disorders	Maintain routines: bedtime, waking up, going to school when possible. Try to recreate the sleeping arrangement prior to the disaster
Adolescents	Change in physical activity (increase or decrease)	Encourage regular physical activity, work with community to create safe locations for play
	Rebellion and behavioral problems	Maintain pre-disaster rules for behavior and provide consistent discipline
	Decreased interest in social activities, friends, school, and hobbies	Restart school and community activities as soon as possible, continue to talk about the future to ensure commitment to previous studies and sports

Source: Olness *et al.* (2014).

- World Health Organization (2013) *Pocket Book for Hospitalized Care for Children*, 2nd edn. Available at http://www.who.int/maternal_child_adolescent/documents/child_hospital_care/en/
- Sphere Project (2011) *The Sphere Handbook. Humanitarian Charter and Minimum Standards in Humanitarian Response*. Available at http://www.sphereproject.org/resources/download-publications/?search=1&keywords=&language=English&category=22
- CMO/CIMC Reference Library for the Civilian and Military Practitioner. Center for Disaster Management and Humanitarian Assistance (in CD format), 2004.
- United Nations Universal Declaration of Human Rights: http://www.un.org/en/documents/udhr/
- Eade D, Williams S (2000) *The Oxfam Handbook of Development and Relief*, Vols 1–3. Oxford: Oxfam.
- UNICEF, WHO, UNESCO, UNFPA, UNDP, UNAIDS, WFP, World Bank (2010) *Facts for Life*, 4th edn. http://www.who.int/maternal_child_adolescent/documents/9789280644661/en/
- EM-DAT: The International Disaster Database. Centre for Research on the Epidemiology of Disasters. Available at http://www.emdat.be
- ReliefWeb. Humanitarian news and analysis. Available at http://www.reliefweb.int/

Infectious disease

- Heymann DL (ed.) (2008) *Control of Communicable Diseases Manual*, 19th edn. Washington, DC: American Public Health Association.
- American Academy of Pediatrics, Infectious Diseases Committee (2012) *Red Book*, 29th edn. Elk Grove Village, IL: AAP.
- World Health Organization (2005) *Communicable Disease Control in Emergencies: A Field Manual*. Geneva: World Health Organization. Available at http://www.who.int/diseasecontrol_emergencies/publications/9241546166/en/

Nutrition

- King FS, Burgess A (1993) *Nutrition for Developing Countries*, 2nd edn. Oxford: Oxford University.
- UNICEF. Nutrition in emergencies: basic concepts online lessons. Available at http://www.unicef.org/nutrition/training/

- UNHCR (2009) Guidelines for selective feeding: the management of malnutrition in emergencies. Available at http://www.unhcr.org/4b7421fd20.html
- World Vision (2012) Supporting breastfeeding in emergencies: the use of baby tents. Available at http://www.wvi.org/nutrition/publication/supporting-breastfeeding-emergencies
- UNHCR, UNICEF, WHO, WFP (2009) Food and nutrition needs in emergencies. Available at http://whqlibdoc.who.int/hq/2004/a83743.pdf
- Taylor A, Seaman J, Save the Children UK (2004) Targeting food aid in emergencies. Emergency Nutrition Network Special Supplement Series No. 1, July 2004. Available at http://www.ennonline.net/pool/files/ife/supplement22.pdf

Behavior, mental health, and development

- UNHCR/WHO (1996) Mental health of refugees. http://www.unhcr.org/publ/PUBL/3bc6eac74.pdf
- United Nations (1996) The impact of armed conflict on children. Available at http://www.unicef.org/graca/a51-306_en.pdf
- World Health Organization (2005) The World Health Report: make every mother and child count. Available at http://www.who.int/whr/2005/whr2005_en.pdf

REFERENCES

American Academy of Pediatrics, Infectious Diseases Committee (2012) Poliovirus infections. In: *Red Book*, 29th edn. Elk Grove Village, IL: American Academy of Pediatrics, pp. 588–92.

CBC News (2011) Global disaster impact in 2010, May 10, 2011. Available at http://www.cbc.ca/news/world/story/2011/05/10/disaster-report.html

Centers for Disease Control and Prevention (2012) Vaccine storage and handling toolkit. Available at http://www.cdc.gov/vaccines/recs/storage/toolkit/storage-handling-toolkit.pdf

Centre for Research on the Epidemiology of Disasters (2011) Natural disasters occurrence in 2011 and number of persons reported affected by natural disasters. EM-DAT: The International Disaster Database. Available at http://www.emdat.be/maps-2011

Centre for Research on the Epidemiology of Disasters (2012) Natural disasters trends: Natural disaster occurrence in 2011, number of persons reported affected by natural disasters in 2012, number of disasters reported in 1900–2011, estimated damages in US$ billions caused by reported natural disasters 1900–2011. EM-DAT: The International Disaster Database. Available at http://www.emdat.be/natural-disasters-trends

Grotberg E (1995) *A Guide to Promoting Resilience in Children: Strengthening the Human Spirit.* The Hague: The Bernard van Leer Foundation.

Kälin W (2000) Guiding principles on internal displacement: annotations. Studies in Transnational Legal Policy, No. 32. American Society of International Law and The Brookings Institution Project on Internal Displacement. Available at http://www.law.georgetown.edu/idp/english/Legal_Annotations_32.pdf

Mooney E (2005) The concept of internal displacement and the case for internally displaced persons as a category of concern. *Refug Sur Q* 24(3):9–26.

Norwegian Refugee Council's Internal Displacement Monitoring Centre (2012) IDP definition, guiding principles, and internally displaced women and children. Available at http://www.internal-displacement.org/8025708F004D404D/(httpSectionHomepages)/$first?OpenDocument&count=1000

Olness K, Mandalakas A, Torjesen K (2014) *How to Help the Children in Humanitarian Disasters*, 3rd edn. Kenyon, MN: Health Frontiers, pp. 13–15, 23–33.

Sphere Project (2011) *The Sphere Handbook. Humanitarian Charter and Minimum Standards in Humanitarian Response*, pp. 143–231. Available at http://www.sphereproject.org/resources/download-publications/?search=1&keywords=&language=English&category=22

Taylor A, Seaman J, Save the Children UK (2004) Targeting food aid in emergencies. Emergency Nutrition Network Special Supplement Series No. 1, July 2004. Available at http://www.ennonline.net/pool/files/ife/supplement22.pdf

UNICEF (2000) Patterns in conflict: civilians are now the target. Available at http://www.unicef.org/graca/patterns.htm

UNICEF (2005) *Emergency Field Handbook: A Guide for UNICEF Staff.* Available at http://www.unicef.org/publications/files/UNICEF_EFH_2005.pdf

United Nations High Commissioner for Refugees (2014) Refugee figures. Available at http://www.unhcr.org/pages/49c3646c1d.html

World Health Organization (2005) Communicable disease control in emergencies: a field manual. Available at http://www.who.int/diseasecontrol_emergencies/publications/9241546166/en/

World Health Organization (2010) Public health risk assessment and interventions: Earthquake – Haiti. Available at http://www.who.int/diseasecontrol_emergencies/publications/who_hse_gar_dce_2010_1/en/

World Health Organization (2012) Vaccination in acute humanitarian emergencies: a framework for decision-making. Available at http://www.who.int/immunization/sage/meetings/2012/november/FinalFraft_FrmwrkDocument_SWGVHE_23OctFullWEBVERSION.pdf

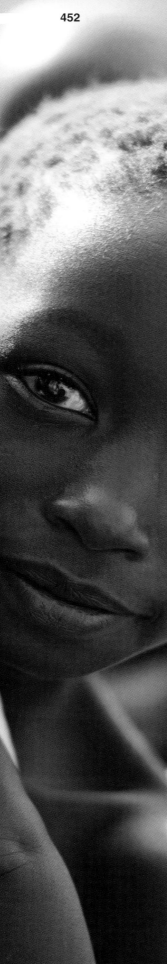

CHAPTER 35
Technologies in Global Health

Roy Ahn[1,2], Nadi Kaonga[1,3], Faiza Yasin[1,4], and Thomas F. Burke[1,2]

[1]Massachusetts General Hospital, Boston, MA, USA
[2]Harvard Medical School, Boston, MA, USA
[3]Tufts University School of Medicine, Boston, MA, USA
[4]Boston University School of Medicine, Boston, MA, USA

Key learning objectives

- Understand the role of various types of technology in improving health in resource-limited settings.
- Identify examples of affordable existing technologies for health, plus emerging technologies.
- Learn about the importance of contextually appropriate technologies for health in resource-limited settings.

Abstract

The role of technologies in advancing global health is evolving. Affordable technology solutions have the potential to transform health systems in resource-limited settings (e.g., microfluidics for rapid diagnostic testing, smartphones for health data collection, insecticide-treated nets for malaria prevention). This chapter describes the myriad types of technology that can improve health in these settings. The chapter also focuses on the technical capability of technologies (i.e., how well the technology works) and on the appropriateness of introducing technologies into these resource-limited environments.

Key words: global health, technology, innovation, resource-poor setting, implementation, uptake, diffusion, microfluidics, diagnostic testing, treatment

Essential Clinical Global Health, First Edition. Edited by Brett D. Nelson.
© 2015 John Wiley & Sons, Ltd. Published 2015 by John Wiley & Sons, Ltd.
Companion website: www.essentialseries.com/globalhealth

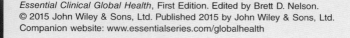

Introduction

From smartphones for health data collection to insecticide-treated bednets for malaria prevention, the role of technology in advancing global public health is expanding and evolving. The World Health Assembly defines health technologies as "the application of organized knowledge and skills in the form of devices, medicines, vaccines, procedures, and systems developed to solve a health problem and improve quality of lives" (World Health Organization, 2013). This definition underscores a major shift in the field, from an early constrained focus on the availability of medicines in developing countries – the World Health Organization (WHO) published its first Model List of Essential Medicines in the late 1970s (Haupt & Guerrant, 2008) – to a much broader contemporary conception of health-promoting technologies.

Despite the ubiquity of health technologies in the world today, a major disparity in access exists between the most developed countries and low- to middle-income countries (LMICs). For instance, the WHO notes the existence of "an estimated 1.5 million different medical devices," while also noting that "[t]he majority of the world's population is denied adequate access to safe and appropriate medical devices within their health systems" (World Health Organization, 2010a).

While the topic of technology and global health is not new, the past decade has witnessed a surge of interest among global health stakeholders. Private and public funders have undertaken efforts to accelerate the diffusion of health-related technologies. The Bill and Melinda Gates Foundation has disbursed more than $450 million since 2003 through its technology-focused Grand Challenges in Global Health program. Similarly, the federal United States Agency for International Development (USAID) started the Development Innovation Ventures program in 2010 to fund and catalyze innovations in health and development (USAID and Development Innovation Ventures, 2013).

The proliferation of technologies has also led to discourse on the need for the appropriate and sustainable design of technologies for LMICs. The introduction of high-tech medical technologies, without careful attention to the health system infrastructure into which it is introduced, may be ineffective at best, and even harmful (Howitt *et al.*, 2012). For example, donated medical equipment may burden recipient health facilities if the equipment is outdated, broken, requires electricity in settings where electricity is sparse, or needs highly technical training to operate. By contrast, a so-called low-tech innovation, such as oral rehydration solution (ORS) for pediatric rehydration, can be extremely effective and impactful in resource-limited settings.

Therefore, prior to its introduction into any community, it is important to consider the following aspects of a technology:

- technical properties;
- safety;
- efficacy and/or effectiveness;
- economic attributes or impacts;
- social, legal, ethical and/or political impacts (Goodman & Ahn, 1999).

The goal of this chapter is to highlight existing and emerging technologies for global health, arranged into three general categories: (i) diagnostics and disease monitoring, (ii) therapeutics and preventive treatments, and (iii) medical and surgical procedures (Howitt *et al.*, 2012). While describing the entire breadth of health technologies is not possible in a single chapter, we provide here illustrative examples of technologies for each of these three categories.

Diagnostics and disease monitoring

Advances in technology have made many diagnostic tests and disease monitoring tools available and affordable for LMICs. For example, point-of-care or rapid diagnostic tests (RDTs) can now be found for various clinical conditions, ranging from malaria to HIV. Hundreds of different RDTs are available on the market, although most use the same general process: the device detects the presence of microbial antigens in a small blood sample. The results, which are available within a few minutes, are easily interpreted from markings on the device. The concept is similar to the over-the-counter pregnancy tests readily found in supermarkets and pharmacies in high-income countries (World Health Organization, 2005; Centers for Disease Control and Prevention, 2010).

A rapidly emerging field within RDTs involves a relatively new technology known as microfluidics. Microfluidics is revolutionizing diagnostic testing for LMICs by developing

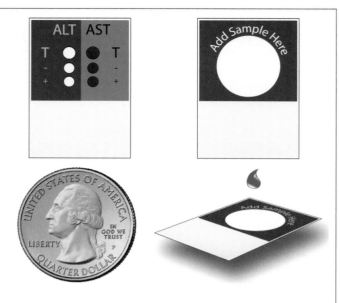

Figure 35.1 Example of point-of-care testing using Diagnostics for All's patterned paper technology. *Source*: Diagnostics For All, Cambridge, MA, USA. Reproduced with permission of Diagnostics For All.

miniaturized tests that obviate the need for expensive testing laboratories or highly skilled laboratory technicians (Yager *et al.*, 2006). For example, biomedical engineers at Columbia University recently developed an affordable, highly sensitive "lab on a chip" for detection of HIV and syphilis. This team has successfully field-tested the point-of-care diagnostic test among volunteers in Rwanda (Chin *et al.*, 2011). The non-profit Diagnostics for All (DFA), based in Cambridge, Massachusetts, has developed paper-based, rapid point-of-care diagnostic tests that require no additional laboratory equipment. The paper tests are compact (the size of a postage stamp), ultra-low cost, require very little blood, and can be disposed of by incineration (Figure 35.1). Finally, researchers at Nationwide Children's Hospital are developing a first-of-its-kind, low-cost, paper-based diagnostic test for preeclampsia. The diagnostic test is based on evidence that women with preeclampsia have misfolded proteins that can be detected by a dye known as Congo Red (Buhimschi *et al.*, 2009).

Information and communication technologies are also emerging as low-cost alternatives for diagnostics, among other uses. Opportunities for the use of mobile phones in global health are diverse: see Table 35.1 for the wide range of mobile health (mHealth) applications in global health. Given that mobile phone use in LMICs is widespread, even in rural areas, various organizations have developed mHealth products that can increase the availability of point-of-care testing and/or connect healthcare providers from developed countries to those in LMICs for the purpose of providing tele-consultation. CellScope, borne out of a laboratory at the University of

California Berkeley, has produced a line of diagnostic scopes (e.g., otoscope, retinal scope) that attach to standard smartphones. MobiSante (Figure 35.2) has developed both a point-of-care smartphone ultrasound device as well as tablet ultrasound device that can be used in LMICs (Mobisante, http://www.mobisante.com/product-overview/).

In addition to diagnostic testing, mobile phones are being used for disease monitoring and to help patients adhere to drug treatment regimens. A 2011 randomized trial in Kenya found that patients who were sent short-message-service (SMS) reminders were more likely than control group patients to adhere to antiretroviral therapy (Pop-Eleches *et al.*, 2011).

Therapeutics and preventive treatments

The use of technology in therapeutics and therapeutic delivery systems is wide-ranging in LMICs and comprise both high-tech and low-tech innovations. These advances include improved vaccine delivery mechanisms, vector control strategies for malaria, and the use of ORS to prevent dehydration.

Disposable syringe jet injections (DSJIs) have emerged as an alternative to the traditional vaccine needle and syringe injection. Rather than a needle, jet injectors (e.g., those made by PATH, http://www.path.org/projects/jet_injector.php) use a high-pressure flow of fluid to break through the skin barrier to deliver the vaccine (Hickling & Jones, 2009). DSJIs minimize the harm associated with the handling of sharps. The incremental cost of using DSJIs per vaccinated individual is $0.57 in Brazil, $0.65 in India, and $1.24 in South Africa (Griffiths *et al.*, 2011). Despite the higher cost, the needle-free design makes it a safe option that can be considered for vaccine delivery. Aerosol vaccine formulations have also been developed and found success in inducing an immune response

Table 35.1 mHealth Applications in Global Health. The application of mobile phones within the health sector is known as mHealth. With increasing mobile phone ownership and decreasing costs of more advanced mobile phones, there are several global health initiatives that have taken advantage of these trends.

Disease reporting/ surveillance	In Zambia, UNICEF's Project Mwana used mobile phones to report test results from the laboratory to the clinic in "real time" via SMS text (Seidenberg et al., 2012).
Microscopy	In Cameroon, India, Thailand, and Vietnam, pilot studies of CellScope, a mobile phone-based digital microscopy tool, are underway. CellScope takes advantage of a mobile phone's camera, turning the mobile phone into a diagnostic device. The device is designed to bring clinical microscopy to remote and/or limited-resource settings (Cook, 2011).
Ultrasound	Mobisante has designed a smartphone attachment that turns the phone into a point-of-care ultrasound machine. It is reportedly less expensive than portable ultrasound machines (Cook, 2011; Seidenberg et al., 2012).
Telemedicine	Cameras and multimedia messages on cell phones have been used for tele-consultations. An image of interest can be sent to a dermatologist or radiologist for diagnosis and treatment advice. Images can also be sent over secure email networks to be read and interpreted on a computer. These forms of telemedicine are in use in countries around the world[a].
Disease management	In South Africa, Cell-Life has implemented a medication reminder system for persons living with HIV/AIDS. Users receive the notifications via text message (de Tolly & Alexander, 2009).
Health provider training	Such information as training guides, checklists, or treatment protocols can be stored on the phone as an application. In India, a pregnancy checklist application has been built for use for Accredited Social Health Activists (ASHAS). CommCare, a mobile phone-based platform, is able to use text, images, and voice to guide literate and non-literate healthcare workers through various health guides and protocols. The WHO and D-Tree International have adapted the Integrated Management of Childhood Illnesses (IMCI) into an electronic format for use on mobile devices, including mobile phones (eIMCI) (Chatfield et al., 2013).[b] Clinicians can carry large collections of reference materials and manuals on hand-held tablets and e-readers for quick access.
Electronic medical record	Existing electronic medical record (EMR) platforms used on computers now have the ability to interface with more mobile information and communication technologies, such as tablets and smartphones. Open-source EMR platforms, such as OpenMRS, have data entry portals through both computers and mobile phones.[c] Similarly, District Health Information System 2 (DHIS2), an electronic platform for data collection, analysis, and visualization, can be updated using their Web portal or a mobile phone.[d] In Malawi, the local NGO Baobab Health has implemented an electronic clinical guide and medical record system that assists clinicians, stores medical record data, and has reduced costs (Driessen et al., 2013).

[a] American Telemedicine Association, http://www.americantelemed.org/learn; Novartis Foundation, telemedicine project in Ghana, http://www.novartisfoundation.org/page/content/index.asp?MenuID=652&ID=1980&Menu=3&Item=44.2
[b] Africa Aid, http://www.africaaid.org/programs/mdnet; Mobile World Live, http://www.mobileworldlive.com/mhealth-tracker
[c] OpenMRS, https://wiki.openmrs.org/display/docs/Mobile
[d] DHIS2, http://www.dhis2.org/mobile

against measles, but further research is needed (Higginson et al., 2011).

Despite innovations in vaccine delivery, cold chain requirements to store and transport refrigerated vaccines remain a significant barrier to successful vaccine delivery in developing countries. Improving the stability of vaccines in the elevated temperatures of many developing nations remains a priority. Vaxess, a start-up based in the United States, has demonstrated the efficacy of using silk polymers to create a heat-stable vaccine that may resist damage when the cold chain is broken (Zhang et al., 2012).

Advances in preventive treatments extend beyond vaccines. Insecticide-treated nets (ITNs) and indoor residual spraying (IRS), as vector control strategies to prevent malaria transmission, have been efficacious and cost-effective in many settings (Centers for Disease Control and Prevention, 2014). Pyrethroid insecticides, effective at low doses and minimally toxic to humans, are currently the only insecticides used to treat bednets (Lengeler, 2004). Five randomized controlled trials in Africa found ITN use alone (without residual spraying) can have very high impact, reducing malaria mortality in children under the age of 5 years by 20% (Lengeler, 2004; Centers for

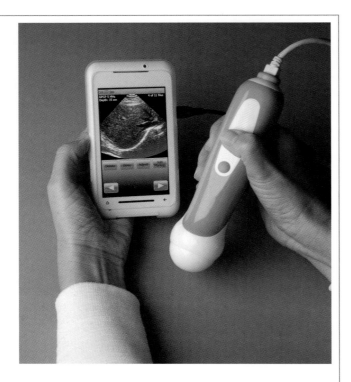

Figure 35.2 MobiSante smartphone ultrasound. *Source*: MobiSante, Inc., Redmond, WA, USA. Reproduced with permission of MobiSante, Inc.

Disease Control and Prevention, 2014). However, as a result of pyrethroids being the only class of insecticide approved for ITN use in the past three decades, pyrethroid resistance is becoming problematic. Therefore, a combination has been suggested of a pyrethroid-treated bednet together with non-pyrethroid IRS. However, this dual-arm approach is more expensive, and the results of its effectiveness have been inconclusive (Yukich *et al.*, 2008).

While the burden of infectious diseases in developing countries remains high, chronic diseases are becoming increasingly prevalent. Consequently, treatment costs and pill burden become significant barriers to effective disease management. Polypills, a single pill combination of multiple drugs, have emerged as a way to mitigate some of these issues. The Single Pill to Avert Cardiovascular Events (SPACE) collaboration designed the Use of Multidrug Pill in Reducing cardiovascular Events (UMPIRE) randomized controlled trial in 2009 to determine the efficacy of a preventative polypill (Thom *et al.*, 2014). The polypill includes 75 mg aspirin, 40 mg simvastatin, 10 mg lisinopril, and 50 mg atenolol. Another version of the polypill used 12.5 mg hydrochlorothiazide in place of the 50-mg atenolol. Preliminary results as presented at the 2012 American Heart Association meeting found a 33% increase in adherence and significant reduction in LDL-cholesterol and systolic blood pressure over 15 months compared with usual care (O'Riordan, 2013).

While not a pill, ORS has successfully been administered to treat diarrheal dehydration. Diarrhea is one of the leading causes of death in children under 5 years of age in developing countries. ORS was first developed in 1969 and has been used since the 1970s as a low-cost alternative to intravenous fluids to treat diarrheal dehydration (World Health Organization, 2006). ORS formulations containing citrate are recommended in tropical countries because the combination allows the formulation to remain stable for up to 2–3 years, increasing shelf-life in that context. ORS is straightforward and can be used for at-home treatment of dehydration (Munos *et al.*, 2010).

Medical and surgical procedures

Health technologies for medical and surgical procedures in LMICs are rapidly emerging and helping providers perform their jobs more effectively, with greater safety, and at lower cost.

Checklists and job aids are great examples of low-cost innovations that hold significant promise for resource-limited settings. The WHO, in conjunction with researchers at Brigham and Women's Hospital in Boston, have pioneered a surgical safety checklist called the Safe Surgery Checklist (Figure 35.3). The checklist has a series of essential steps that the surgical team follows to help avoid preventable (and possibly fatal) mistakes. The checklist has been adapted for use in over 3000 hospitals around the world, including hospitals in Rwanda (World Health Organization, 2008, 2009; Haynes *et al.*, 2009; Edwards, 2013; Safe Surgery 2015 Team, 2013). Another checklist that has gained traction is the safe childbirth checklist (Figure 35.4). Also established by the WHO, the checklist was developed to help avoid preventable deaths related to childbirth in limited-resource settings. A randomized controlled trial is underway to test the effectiveness of this checklist (World Health Organization, 2010b).

A team at Massachusetts General Hospital (MGH) has incorporated checklists and job aids into a novel low-cost uterine balloon tamponade (UBT) system to treat postpartum hemorrhage in LMICs (see Chapter 17, Box 17.4). The system consists of a condom tied by string to a urinary catheter and inflated with clean water through a syringe and one-way stopcock (Figure 35.5). Each kit includes a laminated visual checklist to remind health workers how to use the device. The MGH team has trained health workers in South Sudan and Kenya on UBT, and demonstrated that these providers can safely and effectively place the UBT, thereby saving mother's lives (Nelson *et al.*, 2013).

In the area of newborn health, two low-cost innovations have been developed to combat hypothermia in low-birthweight and premature babies. Embrace's infant warmer uses a sleeping bag design with phase-change materials that are able to help regulate temperature, without the aid of electricity, for up to 6 hours (Stanford University, 2012; Embrace, 2013a). The infant warmer was designed to complement another low-cost innovation, kangaroo mother care (see Chapter 6, Panel 6.2) (Embrace, 2013b). Kangaroo mother care encourages skin-to-skin contact of the mother with the newborn to help keep the newborn warm (World Health Organization, 2003). The practice was first developed and documented in Colombia, where there was a lack of incubators for preterm babies. Evidence on the effectiveness of kangaroo mother care has led to its recommended use in health facilities and at home, under proper guidance.

Several organizations are working to provide people in LMICs with affordable prosthetic limbs. The D-Lab at the Massachusetts Institute of Technology offers a course called Developing World Prosthetics that is solely devoted to the design of affordable prosthetic limbs (e.g., knees, hands) (see http://d-lab.mit.edu). The India-based NGO Bhagwan Mahavir Viklang Sahyata Samiti (BMVSS) distributes the Jaipur Foot, an artificial prosthesis that was designed and developed in the late 1960s. The prosthesis costs $45, which is several orders of magnitude less expensive than similar prostheses on the market. Over the last several decades, the organization has expanded to provide other prostheses and services in 27 countries (see http://jaipurfoot.org/).

Clinical experience

"During my time in Botswana working on an mHealth project, I was able to work alongside healthcare practitioners, government officials, software developers, telecommunication companies, researchers, and funders, and it taught me that clear and constant communication is invaluable to creating a technology product that will best meet the needs of a nation's healthcare system. No single partner can address all the challenges impeding individuals' access to high-quality care, yet each had something crucial to bring to the table – from design, to development, to implementation, and to enhancement of the different mHealth initiatives on which we worked together. Facilitating multidisciplinary collaboration, which requires more than just bringing people together in a physical or virtual space, is something for which I gained a deep appreciation."

Martha, medical student working in Botswana

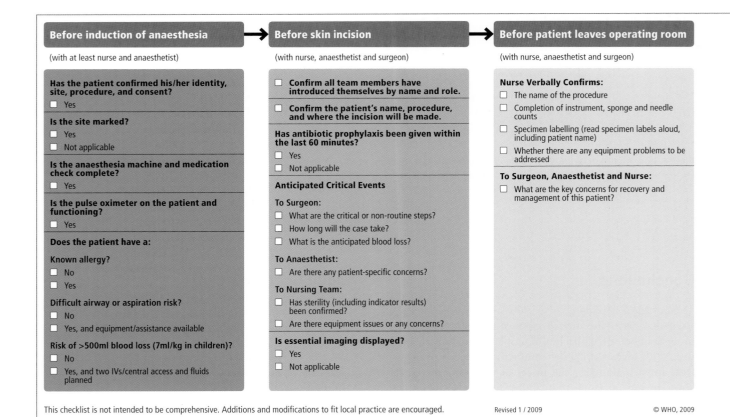

Figure 35.3 The WHO surgical safety checklist. *Source*: World Health Organization (2008). Reproduced with permission of the World Health Organization.

Checklist Item	Qualifying Caption
Does mother need referral? ☐ No ☐ Yes, organized	According to facility's criteria
Partograph started? ☐ Yes ☐ No, will start when ≥ 4 cm	Start plotting when cervix ≥ 4 cm Then cervix should dilate ≥ 1 cm/hour • Every 30 min: plot heart rate, contractions, fetal heart rate • Every 2 hours: plot temperature • Every 4 hours: plot blood pressure
Does mother need to be started on antibiotics? ☐ No ☐ Yes, given	Give antibiotics to mother if any of: • Mother's temperature ≥ 38°C • History of foul-smelling vaginal discharge • Rupture of membranes >18 hours
Does mother need to be started on magnesium sulfate? ☐ No ☐ Yes, given	Give magnesium sulfate to mother if any of: • Diastolic blood pressure ≥ 110 mmHg and 3+ proteinuria • Diastolic blood pressure ≥ 90 mmHg, 2+ proteinuria, and any: severe headache, visual disturbances, epigastric pain
Does mother need to be started on antiretrovirals? ☐ No, confirmed HIV negative ☐ Yes, given *If status unknown, HIV test ordered*	Mothers with CD4 ≤ 350 or clinical diagnosis require treatment Mothers with CD4 >350 require prophylaxis
Confirm supplies are available to clean hands and wear gloves for each vaginal exam	
Encourage birth companion to be present at birth	
Confirm that mother or companion will call for help during labor if mother has any one of the following: bleeding, severe abdominal pain, severe headache or visual disturbance, unable to urinate, or urge to push	

Figure 35.4 A portion of the WHO safe childbirth checklist (Spector *et al.*, 2013). *Source*: World Health Organization (2010b). Reproduced with permission of the World Health Organization.

Conclusions

Technological development in global health is occurring at a staggering pace. The myriad types of technology that can be brought to bear on global health problems are similarly impressive. With increased market competition and an emphasis on wide impact/adoption, the prices of these technologies will lower to the point of affordability for LMICs and thereby dramatically increase access to improved healthcare for poor populations throughout the world.

Additional resources

- World Health Organization. Partnership for maternal, newborn, and child health. Available at http://www.who.int/pmnch/en/
- Maternova: Tools and ideas that save mothers and newborns. Available at http://www.maternova.net
- Innovations for Maternal, Newborn, and Child Health. Available at http://www.innovationsformnch.org
- Grand Challenges in Global Health. Available at http://www.grandchallenges.org
- Grand Challenges Canada. Available at http://www.grandchallenges.ca

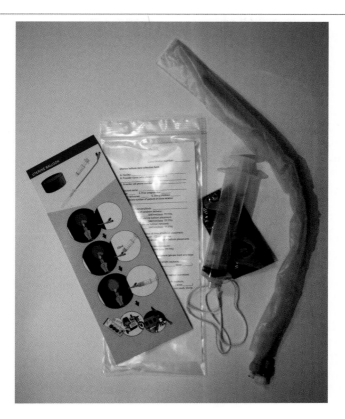

Figure 35.5 MGH's Every Second Matters for Mothers and Babies – Uterine Balloon Tamponade™ package. *Source*: Massachusetts General Hospital Division of Global Health and Human Rights, Department of Emergency Medicine, 2013. Reproduced with permission of Massachusetts General Hospital.

REFERENCES

Buhimschi I, Funai E, Zhao G *et al.* (2009) Assessment of global protein misfolding load by urine "Congo Red Dot" test for diagnosis and prediction of outcome in women with preeclampsia (PE). *Am J Obstet Gynecol* 201:S12–13.

Centers for Disease Control and Prevention (2010) Malaria diagnostics (U.S.): rapid diagnostic test. Available at http://www.cdc.gov/malaria/diagnosis _treatment/rdt.html

Centers for Disease Control and Prevention (2014) Insecticide-treated bed nets. Available at http://www .cdc.gov/malaria/malaria_worldwide/reduction/itn.html

Chatfield A, Javetski G, Lesh N (2013) CommCare evidence base, Dimagi.. Available at https://confluence .dimagi.com/download/attachments/12226140/ CommCare%20Evidence%20Base%20June%202013 .pdf?version=1&modificationDate=1370548380786 &api=v2le.com/webhp?hl=en&tab=ww

Chin CD, Laksanasopin T, Cheung YK *et al.* (2011) Microfluidics-based diagnostics of infectious diseases in the developing world. *Nat Med* 17:1015–19.

Cook J (2011) Ultrasound on the go? Smartphone-based imagine system released by Mobisante. Available at http://www.geekwire.com/2011/mobisante-release -smartphonebased-ultrasound-system/

Driessen J, Cioffi M, Alide N *et al.* (2013) Modeling return on investment for an electronic medical record system in Lilongwe, Malawi. *J Am Med Inform Assoc* 20:743–8.

Edwards C (2013) BBC Health Check: Six questions that could save your life. Available at http://www.bbc.co.uk/ news/health-23252784

Embrace (2013a) The Embrace infant warmers is a product with a mission. Available at http:// embraceglobal.org/main/product

Embrace (2013b) Embrace and kangaroo mother care. Available at http://embraceglobal.org/main/product?section=KMC

Goodman C, Ahn R (1999) Methodological approaches of health technology assessment. *Int J Med Inform* 56:97–105.

Griffiths U, Santos A, Nundy N, Jacoby E, Matthias D (2011) Incremental costs of introducing jet injection technology for delivery of routine childhood vaccinations: comparative analysis from Brazil, India, and South Africa. *Vaccine* 29:969–75.

Haupt E, Guerrant R (2008) Technology in global health: the need for essential diagnostics. *Lancet* 372:873–4.

Haynes A, Weiser T, Berry W *et al.* (2009) A surgical safety checklist to reduce morbidity and mortality in a global population. *N Engl J Med* 260:491–9.

Hickling J, Jones R (2009) Intradermal delivery of vaccines: a review of the literature and the potential for development for use in low- and middle-income countries. Available at http://www.path.org/publications/files/TS_opt_idd_review.pdf

Higginson D, Theodoratou E, Nair H *et al.* (2011) An evaluation of respiratory admin of measles vaccine for prevention of acute lower respiratory infections in children. *BMC Public Health* 11(Suppl. 3):S31.

Howitt P, Darzi A, Yang GZ *et al.* (2012) Technologies for global health. *Lancet* 380:507–35.

Lengeler C (2004) Insecticide-treated bed nets and curtains for preventing malaria. *Cochrane Database Syst Rev* (2):CD000363.

Munos M, Walker C, Black R (2010) The effect of oral rehydration solution and recommended home fluids on diarrhea mortality. *Int J Epidemiol* 39(Suppl. 1):i75–87.

Nelson BD, Stoklosa H, Ahn R, Eckardt M, Walton E, Burke T (2013) Uterine balloon tamponade for postpartum hemorrhage control among community-based health providers in South Sudan. *Int J Gynaecol Obstet* 122:27–32.

O'Riordan M (2013) UMPIRE polypill at AHA. Available at http://www.theheart.org/article/1469635.do

Pop-Eleches C, Thirumurthy H, Habyarimana J (2011) Mobile phone technologies improve adherence to antiretroviral treatment in a resource-limited setting: a randomized controlled trial of text message reminders. *AIDS* 25:825–34.

Safe Surgery 2015 Team (2013) Safe Surgery 2015. The Harvard School of Public Health. Available at http://www.safesurgery2015.org/about-us.html

Seidenberg P, Nicholson S, Schaefer M 2012) Early infant diagnosis of HIV infection in Zambia through mobile phone texting of blood test results. *Bull WHO* 90:348–56.

Spector J, Lashoher A, Agrawal P *et al.* (2013) Designing the WHO Safe Childbirth Checklist program to improve quality of care at childbirth. *Int J Gynaecol Obstet* 122:164–8.

Stanford University (2012) EXTREME design for extreme affordability: Embrace. Available at http://extreme.stanford.edu/projects/embrace

Thom S, Field J, Poulter N *et al.* (2014) Use of a Multidrug Pill In Reducing cardiovascular Events (UMPIRE): rationale and design of a randomized controlled trial of a cardiovascular polypill-based strategy in India and Europe. *Eur J Prev Cardiol* 21:252–61.

de Tolly K, Alexander H (2009) Innovative use of cellphone technology for HIV/AIDS behaviour change communications: three pilot projects. *Cellphones4HIV* March 2009. Available at http://www.w3.org/2008/10/MW4D_WS/papers/kdetolly.pdf

USAID and Development Innovation Ventures (2013) What we do. Available at http://www.usaid.gov/div/about

World Health Organization (2003) Kangaroo mother care: practical guide. Available at http://www.who.int/maternal_child_adolescent/documents/9241590351/en/

World Health Organization (2005) Mechanism of action of malaria rapid diagnostic tests. Available at http://www.wpro.who.int/malaria/sites/rdt/whatis/mechanism.html

World Health Organization (2006) Oral rehydration salts: production of the new ORS. Available at http://whqlibdoc.who.int/hq/2006/WHO_FCH_CAH_06.1.pdf

World Health Organization (2008) World Alliance for Patient Safety. WHO surgical safety checklist and implementation manual. Available at http://www.who.int/patientsafety/safesurgery/ss_checklist/en/

World Health Organization (2009) Safe surgery saves lives: WHO Surgical Safety Checklist. Available at http://www.who.int/patientsafety/safesurgery/en/

World Health Organization (2010a) Medical devices. Fact Sheet No. 346. Available at http://www.who.int/mediacentre/factsheets/fs346/en/index.html

World Health Organization (2010b) Patient safety: safe childbirth checklist. Available at http://www.who.int/patientsafety/implementation/checklists/childbirth/en/

World Health Organization (2013) Technology, Health. Available at http://www.who.int/topics/technology_medical/en/

Yager P, Edwards T, Fu E *et al.* (2006) Microfluidic diagnostic technologies for global public health. *Nature* 442:412–8.

Yukich J, Lengeler C, Tediosi F *et al.* (2008) Costs and consequences of large-scale vector control for malaria. *Malar J* 17:258.

Zhang J, Pritchard E, Hu X *et al.* (2012) Stabilization of vaccines and antibiotics in silk and eliminating the cold chain. *Proc Natl Acad Sci USA* 109:11981–6.

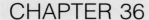

CHAPTER 36
Illness in the Returning Traveler

Christopher Sanford[1] and Claire W. Fung[1,2]
[1]University of Washington, Seattle, WA, USA
[2]The Everett Clinic, Snohomish, WA, USA

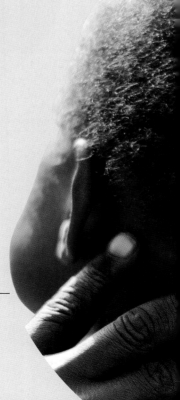

Key learning objectives

- Learn the appropriate work-up for the returned international traveler with gastrointestinal symptoms, fever, and dermatologic disorders.

- Identify potential etiologies of persistent traveler's diarrhea based on clinical presentation and laboratory testing.

- Understand the most common causes of fever in the returned international traveler.

- Become familiar with the most common dermatologic disorders in returned international travelers.

Abstract

A growing number of people travel internationally each year, and among returning international travelers, illness is common. Diarrhea, fever, and rash are the most common complaints. Persistent or protracted diarrhea is diarrhea lasting over 14 days and may require work-up by a physician. Travel-associated fever is a marker of a potentially significant illness and requires prompt evaluation. A common cause of travel-associated fever is malaria. Travel-associated dermatoses include cutaneous larva migrans, localized cutaneous leishmaniasis, and myiasis.

Key words: international travel, post-travel illness, fever, traveler's diarrhea, dermatologic disorders, returned international traveler

Essential Clinical Global Health, First Edition. Edited by Brett D. Nelson.
© 2015 John Wiley & Sons, Ltd. Published 2015 by John Wiley & Sons, Ltd.
Companion website: www.essentialseries.com/globalhealth

Introduction

A growing number of people travel internationally each year. Between 1950 and 2012, the number of international travelers worldwide increased from 25 million to 1 billion annually. This number is anticipated to increase to 1.8 billion by 2030 (United Nations World Tourism Organization, 2011). Among returning international travelers, illness is common. Studies indicate that 20–70% of people who travel from high-income nations to low-income nations report illness associated with their travel (Steffen *et al.*, 1987; Ryan & Kain, 2000), and 1–5% of travelers become sufficiently ill as to seek medical attention during or following travel. Furthermore, between 1 in 1000 and 1 in 10,000 require medical evacuation, and 1 in 100,000 dies (Steffen *et al.*, 1987).

Medical practitioners are increasingly likely to see travelers seeking advice prior to their trips and travelers returning from abroad with illness. For both pre-travel counseling and post-travel care, medical practitioners should be aware of the likelihood of specific travel-associated illnesses depending on the itinerary, activities, and exposures of travelers (Freedman *et al.*, 2006).

Gastrointestinal disorders, fever, and dermatologic disorders are the most common medical problems in ill returned international travelers. In a study of over 40,000 ill returned international travelers, 34.0% were seen for gastrointestinal disease, 23.3% for fever, and 19.5% for a dermatologic disorder (Figure 36.1). These three categories accounted for three-quarters of travel-related diseases (Leder *et al.*, 2013).

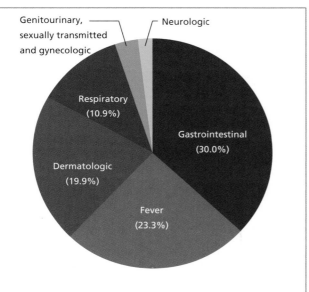

Figure 36.1 Causes of illness in returned international travelers.

Diarrhea

Gastrointestinal infections are the most common illnesses reported in returned travelers (Leder *et al.*, 2013). Traveler's diarrhea (TD) is defined as three or more unformed stools per day plus other gastrointestinal symptoms such as abdominal pain associated with travel. Attack rates of TD range from 30 to 70% of travelers, depending on destination (Centers for Disease Control and Prevention, 2012).

Risk factors for TD include:

- young age;
- adventurous travel (trekking, camping, safaris, tours);
- travel to tropical climates;
- higher socioeconomic status, higher-end hotels;
- medical conditions resulting in immunocompromised state or decreased gastric activity (Steffen, 2005).

TD can be separated into two categories: classical and persistent/protracted. Classical TD has both an incubation period and a mean duration of 3–4 days, and the majority of cases occur within the first week of travel (Von Sonnenburg *et al.*, 2000). Classical TD is brief in duration, usually responds to empiric self-treatment by the traveler, and is most commonly caused by enterotoxic strains of *Escherichia coli* (Centers for Disease Control and Prevention, 2012). Classical TD is not typically evaluated in the physician's office. Persistent/protracted traveler's diarrhea (PTD) is travel-acquired diarrhea that lasts longer in duration (>14 days) after returning from travel and may require evaluation by a physician (International Working Group on Persistent Diarrhea, 1996). PTD can be caused by invasive pathogens (e.g., *Salmonella*, *Shigella*, *Campylobacter*, *E. coli* 0157:H7, *Entamoeba histolytica*) or by non-invasive agents such as *Giardia lamblia*, norovirus (formerly referred to as Norwalk virus), *Vibrio* species, and enterotoxic *E. coli*.

Severity of symptoms and presence or absence of blood or mucus in the stool may be suggestive of certain pathogens over others. However, it is important to note that concurrent infections with more than one enteric pathogen can occur, as well as exacerbations of other chronic gastrointestinal disorders such as irritable bowel syndrome and inflammatory bowel disease.

Clinical presentation

The average case of classical TD is mild, with an average of 4.6 stools daily and complaints of nausea and abdominal pain. Classical TD is self-limited; typically diarrhea resolves within 3–5 days with or without empiric antibiotic treatment (Steffen *et al.*, 1983). Severe disease, however, may lead to orthostatic hemodynamic instability from inability to maintain oral rehydration. In determining the etiology of TD, a detailed history of present illness, including onset, associated symptoms, and duration, is important (Taylor *et al.*, 1999). In classical TD, the abdominal examination typically reveals a soft, non-tender or minimally diffusely tender abdomen with hyperactive bowel sounds. On the other hand, clinical findings in PTD can often include fever, bloody diarrhea, and abdominal pain. Rectal examination may be useful to rule out diarrhea around impacted stool from use of antimotility agents and dehydration, or to exclude other non-infectious causes of gross blood in the stool such as rectal hemorrhoids or fissure.

Laboratory studies and diagnosis

Laboratory studies in the returned traveler with diarrhea may be indicated depending on the duration and severity of illness. The most commonly identified pathogens causing TD are enterotoxic *E. coli*, *Salmonella*, *Shigella*, and *Campylobacter*, accounting for 45–50% of cases. Viruses and protozoa account for 5–10% of cases, and in 30% of cases no pathogen is identified (Black, 1990). Table 36.1 lists diagnostic stool tests that may be useful in identifying the etiology of diarrhea in returned travelers.

Collection of stool for diagnostic testing and handling of specimens requires strict adherence to instructions. Stool specimens should not be contaminated by urine or toilet bowl water. The specimen should be submitted to the laboratory and examined within 1–2 hours of collection. At least three separate specimens (collected no more often than one per day) are needed for optimal identification of parasites (DuPont & Capsuto, 1996). While stool studies are very helpful when positive, they also tend to lack sensitivity.

Some limited blood testing may be helpful in the work-up of PTD. A complete blood count with differential may show leukocytosis with neutrophilia, which can be suggestive of bacterial infection. Marked leukocytosis (>20,000 cells/dL) should raise concern for *Clostridium difficile* infection. Eosinophilia is suggestive of parasitic or invasive helminthic infection. Other blood tests can be used to explore the possibility of hyperthyroidism, systemic inflammation, iron deficiency, or nutritional deficiencies causing malabsorption (de Saussure, 2009).

Treatment

Management of TD should always begin with rehydration. Treatment of TD should then be based on etiology of the disease. Table 36.2 lists treatments for specific etiologies of

Table 36.1 Diagnostic stool tests for returned travelers with diarrhea.

Diagnostic procedure	Indication
Direct examination of stool	Blood in stool suggests inflammatory process Greasy/frothy stool suggests malabsorption
Stool white blood cells	Presence of multiple stool white blood cells suggests bacterial infection
Stool ova and parasites	Detects helminth eggs and larvae Detects protozoan cysts and trophozoites
Stool Gram stain	Comma-shaped organisms suggest *Campylobacter*
Stool wet preparation	Detects live actively mobile protozoan trophozoites
Stool bacterial culture	Detects bacterial enteric pathogens including *Salmonella*, *Shigella*, *Campylobacter*
Stool acid-fast stain	Detects *Cryptosporidium*
Stool trichrome blue stain	Detects microsporidia
Stool safranin stain	Detects *Cyclospora*
Enzyme-linked immunoassay	Separate assays specifically used for detection of *Giardia*, *Cryptosporidium*, *E. coli* 0157:H7, *E. histolytica*, *C. difficile*

Source: adapted from Jong & Sanford (2008).

TD. As discussed, classical TD is self-limited. Empiric self-treatment with antimicrobials (a fluoroquinolone, such as ciprofloxacin, for travelers returning from Africa or Latin America; a macrolide, such as azithromycin, for those returning from Southeast or South Asia) will typically shorten the course of classical TD to 1 day, as compared with 3–5 days if left untreated, as well as reduce associated symptoms like abdominal cramping (De Bruyn *et al.*, 2000).

In the management of PTD, empiric treatment with antimicrobials can be used as both a diagnostic and therapeutic tool. Most bacterial causes of PTD will respond to treatment with an appropriate antibiotic. A fluoroquinolone (e.g., ciprofloxacin) is usually effective for travelers returning from Africa or Latin America; a macrolide (e.g., azithromycin) is preferred for travelers returning from Southeast Asia and the Indian subcontinent due to the high prevalence of fluoroquinolone-resistant *Campylobacter* in those regions. Similarly, a treatment dose of tinidazole (2 g once by mouth) may be used if giardiasis is suspected.

Table 36.2 Common causes of diarrhea in returned travelers.

Etiologic agent	Incubation period	Signs and symptoms	Duration of illness	Possible exposures	Laboratory testing	Treatment/management
Bacteria						
Campylobacter jejuni	2–5 days	Diarrhea (± blood), cramps, fever, vomiting	2–10 days	Uncooked poultry, unpasteurized milk, contaminated water	Stool culture	Supportive care. Erythromycin and quinolones may be indicated early in diarrheal disease
Clostridium difficile	3–7 days	Diarrhea, fever, cramps	Days or several weeks	Antibiotics	*C. difficile* toxin stool culture	Metronidazole or oral vancomycin
Enterohemorrhagic *E. coli* (EHEC) including *E. coli* O157:H7	1–8 days	Severe (often bloody) diarrhea, abdominal pain, vomiting	5–10 days	Uncooked beef, unpasteurized milk/ juice, raw fruits and vegetables, contaminated water	Stool culture (if *E. coli* O157:H7 is suspected, specific testing must be requested)	Supportive care. Monitor renal function, hemoglobin, platelets. Associated with hemolytic–uremic syndrome
Enterotoxigenic *E. coli* (ETEC)	1–3 days	Watery diarrhea, cramps, some vomiting	3–7 days	Fecal–oral	Stool culture (if suspected, must request specific testing)	Supportive care. Antibiotics (TMP-SMX or quinolones) in severe cases
Salmonella species	1–3 days	Diarrhea, fever, cramps, vomiting	4–7 days	Contaminated eggs, poultry, unpasteurized milk/juice/cheese, contaminated raw fruits and vegetables	Stool culture	Supportive care. Antibiotics (TMP-SMX, ampicillin, gentamicin, or quinolones) only indicated for extraintestinal spread
Shigella species	1–2 days	Diarrhea (± blood or mucus), cramps, fever	4–7 days	Fecal–oral	Stool culture	Quinolones
Vibrio cholerae (toxin)	1–3 days	Profuse watery diarrhea and vomiting; severe dehydration	3–7 days	Contaminated water, fish, shellfish, street-vended food typically from Latin America or Asia	Stool culture (if suspected, must request specific testing)	Supportive care with aggressive oral and intravenous rehydration. If confirmed, tetracycline or doxycycline for adults, TMP-SMX for children <8 years old
Vibrio parahaemolyticus	2 hours to 2 days	Watery diarrhea, cramps, nausea/vomiting	2–5 days	Uncooked fish/ shellfish	Stool culture (if suspected, must request specific testing)	Supportive care. Antibiotics (tetracycline, doxycycline, gentamicin, and cefotaxime) if severe
Vibrio vulnificus	1–7 days	Diarrhea, vomiting, abdominal pain, bacteremia, and wound infections. More common in immunocompromised or patients with chronic liver disease	2–8 days	Uncooked shellfish, especially oysters, and open wounds exposed to sea water	Stool, wound, or blood cultures (if suspected, must request specific testing)	Supportive care and antibiotics (ceftazidime and tetracycline or doxycycline)

	Incubation	Symptoms	Duration	Source/transmission	Diagnosis	Treatment
Yersinia enterocolitica	1–2 days	Diarrhea, vomiting, fever, abdominal pain. More common in older children and young adults	1–3 weeks	Uncooked pork, unpasteurized milk/tofu, contaminated water	Stool/vomitus/blood culture (if suspected, must request specific testing). Serology available in research reference labs	Supportive care. Antibiotics (gentamicin or cefotaxime) if septicemia occurs
Virus						
Norovirus	0.5–2 days	Diarrhea (more common in adults), nausea, vomiting, cramps, fever, myalgia	0.5–2.5 days	Shellfish, fecal–oral	Clinical diagnosis, absence of white blood cells in stool, PCR and electron microscopy on fresh unpreserved stool	Supportive care
Parasites						
Cryptosporidium	2–10 days	Diarrhea (usually watery), cramps, low-grade fever	May be relapsing and remitting over weeks to months	Uncooked food or contaminated food by an ill food handler	Specific examination of stool for *Cryptosporidium*	Supportive care, self-limited. If severe, consider paromomycin for 7 days for adults or nitazoxanide for 3 days for children 1–11 years
Cyclospora cayetanensis	1–14 days	Diarrhea (usually watery), loss of appetite, substantial weight loss, cramps, nausea, vomiting, fatigue	May be relapsing and remitting over weeks to months	Various types of fresh produce	Specific examination of stool for *Cyclospora*	TMP-SMX for 7 days
Entamoeba histolytica	2 days to 4 weeks	Diarrhea (often bloody), lower abdominal pain	May last several weeks to several months	Uncooked food or food contaminated by an ill food handler	Stool examination for cysts and parasites (may need at least three samples), serology for long-term infections	Metronidazole and iodoquinol or paromomycin
Giardia lamblia	1–2 weeks	Diarrhea, cramps, gas, bloating	Days to weeks	Uncooked food or food contaminated by an ill food handler	Stool examination for ova and parasites (may need at least three samples)	Metronidazole
Trichinella spiralis	1–2 days for initial symptoms, others begin 2–8 weeks after infection	Diarrhea, nausea, vomiting, fatigue, fever, abdominal discomfort, followed by myalgia, weakness, and occasional cardiac and neurologic complications	Months	Uncooked contaminated meat (usually pork or wild game)	Serology	Mebendazole or albendazole

PCR, polymerase chain reaction; TMP-SMX, trimethoprim/sulfamethoxazole.
Source: adapted from Centers for Disease Control and Prevention (2004).

In some cases, self-treatment of TD among adults may also include antimotility agents in addition to empiric antibiotics and oral rehydration. Loperamide remains the antimotility agent of choice due to the combined effects of antiperistalsis and increased intestinal absorption of fluid and electrolytes (Johnson *et al.*, 1986). However, antimotility agents are contraindicated in children under 3 years of age and should also be avoided if there is evidence of dysentery (high fever, bloody diarrhea) (Bowie *et al.*, 1995; Li *et al.*, 2007). There are mixed data on the effectiveness of diet restriction (avoidance of dairy, fruit juices, concentrated sweets, and high-fat foods) in symptomatic treatment of TD (Huang *et al.*, 2004).

Fever

Fever is reported in 2–3% of North American and European travelers who visit developing nations (Hill, 2000; Wilson & Pearson, 1999). A key source of information on illness in travelers is provided by GeoSentinel, a network of 54 travel clinics around the globe that collects data on ill returned travelers (Leder *et al.*, 2013). According to GeoSentinel data, the most common cause of fever is malaria (29%), followed by dengue fever (15%) (Figure 36.2). Malaria is more disproportionately diagnosed in those returning from Africa, while dengue fever is more common in those returning from Southeast Asia, Latin America, and the Caribbean. Other

common causes of fever include enteric fever (typhoid and paratyphoid), chikungunya fever, rickettsial diseases, viral hepatitis, leptospirosis, tuberculosis, and acute HIV. Typhoid, also known as enteric fever, is more common in those returning from South–Central Asia. Spotted fever rickettsiosis has been found in 6% of those returning with fever from sub-Saharan Africa (most commonly South Africa). In almost 40% of returned febrile travelers, no cause for the fever is identified. Etiologies of fever from three published series are listed in Table 36.3.

Fever in the returned international traveler is a marker of potentially life-threatening illness. Among a large study of over 80,000 ill returned travelers, 4.4% had acute and potentially life-threatening tropical illnesses. Significantly, 91% of those with acute and potentially life-threatening tropical illnesses had fever. The most common diagnoses were *Plasmodium falciparum* malaria (76.9%), typhoid (18.1%), and leptospirosis (2.4%); 13 patients (0.4%) died, 10 as a result of falciparum malaria. Those with elevated risk of falciparum malaria in this large study were males, those visiting relatives and friends, and those visiting West Africa (Jensenius *et al.*, 2013).

Since fever can be a marker for potentially life-threatening illness, medical work-up of the febrile returned international traveler must be conducted promptly. The initial diagnostic work-up should focus on diseases that are life-threatening, treatable, or transmissible (Doherty *et al.*, 1995). During this evaluation and until the patient is well, physicians should have a low threshold for hospitalizing febrile returned travelers.

Obtaining a detailed history of the returned international traveler with fever is mandatory. Important topics to address include where a person has traveled, dates of travel, duration since return, activities during travel, exposure to new sexual partners, exposure to needles and blood, exposure to bodies of fresh water, animal and arthropod bites, pre-travel vaccinations, compliance with malaria prophylaxis, and any treatments to date. Febrile conditions associated with specific exposures are listed in Table 36.4.

The timing of fever onset relative to travel can be useful information in generating a differential diagnosis. With many causes of fever, there is a characteristic amount of time before fever begins (Table 36.5). For example, dengue fever has a relatively brief incubation period, usually 4–7 days (range 3–14 days). Hence, fever appearing in a traveler who returned from the tropics over 14 days prior is unlikely to be due to dengue fever.

Laboratory studies and diagnosis

The work-up of the febrile returned traveler should include complete blood count with differential, hepatic transaminases, renal function tests (e.g., creatinine, blood urea nitrogen), urinalysis, chest X-ray, and, in those with a history of exposure to malaria, thick and thin smears in addition to malaria rapid

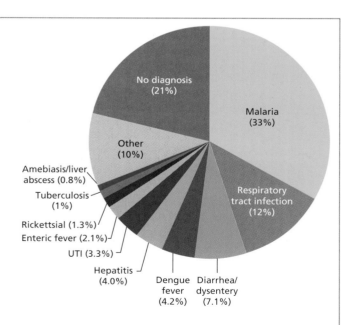

Figure 36.2 Causes of fever in returned international travelers. Data in this figure represent the weight-adjusted averages from studies in Table 36.3.

Table 36.3 Causes of fever from published series (UK, Canada, Australia).

	Doherty *et al.* (1995) (no. of patients 195)	MacLean *et al.* (1994) (no. of patients 587)	O'Brien *et al.* (2001) (no. of patients 232)
Malaria	42%	32%	27%
Respiratory tract infection (i.e., upper respiratory tract infection, pneumonia, and bronchitis)	2.6%	11%	24%
Diarrhea/dysentery	6.6%	4.5%	14%
Dengue	6.2%	2%	8%
Hepatitis	3% (Hepatitis A only)	6%	3% (Hepatitis A only)
Enteric fever	1.5%	2%	3%
Urinary tract infection/pyelonephritis	2.6%	4%	2%
Rickettsial	1.6%	1%	2%
Tuberculosis	1.6%	1%	0.4%
Amebiasis/liver abscess	0	1%	1%
No diagnosis	24.6%	25%	9%

Source: Wilson & Schwartz (2004).

Table 36.4 Febrile conditions associated with specific exposures.

Exposure	Condition
Food and water	
Unsanitary water or food	Hepatitis A or E Enteric fever (typhoid, paratyphoid) Bacterial gastroenteritis Amebiasis
Undercooked meat or fish	Hepatitis A Toxoplasmosis Trichinella
Unpasteurized milk products	*Brucella* Enteric fever *Salmonella* gastroenteritis Tuberculosis (bovis)
Arthropods	
Mosquitoes	Malaria Dengue fever Filariasis *Loa loa* Yellow fever Other arboviruses

(*Continued*)

Table 36.4 Febrile conditions associated with specific exposures. (*Continued*)

Exposure	Condition
Ticks	Tick typhus (Mediterranean or African) Rocky Mountain spotted fever Crimean–Congo hemorrhagic fever Lyme disease Relapsing fever Tularemia Babesiosis *Ehrlichia*
Sandflies	Leishmaniasis Sandfly fever Bartonellosis (Oroya fever)
Blackflies	Onchocerciasis
Tsetse flies	African trypanosomiasis
Reduvid bugs	American trypanosomiasis (Chagas disease)
Chiggers	Scrub typhus
Caves	Rabies Histoplasmosis
Western hemisphere desert area (particularly construction or archeological sites)	Coccidioidomycosis
Animal exposures	Brucellosis Rabies Tularemia Q fever Anthrax Plague Viral hemorrhagic fevers
Sexual contact	HIV Hepatitis B Herpes simplex virus, gonorrhea, syphilis, others
Crowded living conditions; group travel; exposure to ill persons	Meningococcal disease Influenza Tuberculosis Hepatitis A Lassa, Marburg, Ebola virus
Fresh water (swimming, wading)	Schistosomiasis Leptospirosis Hepatitis A

Source: adapted from Sanford (2002).

Table 36.5 Incubation periods.

Short (<10 days)

Malaria
Influenza
Dengue fever
Yellow fever
Enteric bacterial infection
African tick bite fever
Plague
Spotted fever group, including Rocky Mountain spotted fever

Intermediate (10–21 days)

Malaria
Typhoid fever
Leptospirosis
Brucellosis
African trypanosomiasis
Viral hemorrhagic fevers
Q fever
Tick-borne relapsing fever

Long (>21 days)

Malaria
Hepatitis A, B, C, E
Schistosomiasis (Katayama fever)
Leishmaniasis
Amebic liver abscess
Tuberculosis
Filariasis
HIV

Source: adapted from Leggatt (2007).

diagnostic tests (e.g., Binax Now and Paracheck antibody tests). In long-duration travelers, consideration should be given to testing for tuberculosis either by PPD or interferon-gamma release assay (e.g., QuantiFERON-TB Gold) (see Chapter 19). Clinicians should search for malaria even in those with a history of compliance with an efficacious malaria prophylaxis regimen. It is often prudent to save a tube of serum to be used as an acute-phase serum for tests on which clinicians may later decide. Other laboratory tests to consider include specific serologies (e.g., to dengue fever, rickettsial diseases, fungal diseases, *Brucella*, Lyme disease, arboviruses, leptospirosis, filariasis, schistosomiasis), blood cultures, and stool studies including ova and parasite (×3), culture and sensitivity, *Giardia* antigen, and fecal leukocytes.

The presence of an elevated eosinophil count can also guide diagnosis. The most common causes of eosinophilia in high-income nations are allergic and atopic diseases. However, eosinophilia in the returned international traveler suggests possible infection with a tissue-invasive helminth. Infection with *Ascaris*

(roundworm), *Trichinella*, and *Strongyloides* elevate the eosinophil count. Other parasitic infections causing eosinophilia include cysticercosis (caused by *Taenia solium*), echinococcosis, filariasis, hookworm infection, paragonimiasis, schistosomiasis, and visceral larva migrans (Wolfe, 2008; Merck Manual for Health Care Professionals, 2014). Malaria does not elevate the eosinophil count. See Table 36.6 regarding eosinophil count and specific infectious illnesses.

Mild elevation of hepatic transaminases (two to three times upper range of normal) is non-specific, while marked elevation suggests acute viral hepatitis. The presence of fecal leukocytes may indicate infection with an invasive gastrointestinal organism, such as *Salmonella* or *Shigella*.

In the presence of abdominal pain, clinicians should have a low threshold for obtaining imaging (ultrasound or CT, if available) of the abdomen to look for, among other causes of fever, amebic liver abscess.

In stable patients, treatment for malaria should be initiated only after the diagnosis of malaria is confirmed by laboratory testing. In an unstable patient, presumptive treatment of a patient with a clinical scenario consistent with malaria can be initiated prior to laboratory confirmation after consultation with an infectious disease specialist.

Dermatoses

Common causes of dermatologic symptoms in returned international travelers include cutaneous larva migrans, pyodermas, arthropod-related pruritic dermatitis, myiasis, tungiasis, cutaneous leishmaniasis, scabies, and cutaneous fungal infections. In a cohort of 784 American travelers worldwide, 8% (63) experienced dermatoses; 14 were related to insect bites or stings, 10 to sun exposure, seven to dermatophytes (e.g., tinea), seven to contact allergy, and five to infectious cellulitis (Hill, 2000). In a study of 269 patients who presented to a tropical disease clinic in Paris with travel-associated dermatoses, 53% involved an imported tropical disease (Table 36.7) (Caumes *et al.*, 1995).

Cutaneous larva migrans

Cutaneous larva migrans (CLM) (also known as creeping eruption, clam digger's itch, and sand worm eruption) (Figure 36.3) is the most frequent travel-associated skin disease of tropical origin. Most often caused by the larvae of hookworms (*Ancyclostoma* spp.) of dogs, cats, and other mammals, this condition has a worldwide distribution in tropical and subtropical countries. It is transmitted by skin contact with infective larvae in beach sand or soil, usually while walking barefoot, sitting, or lying on beaches.

The incubation period is usually 1–5 days but rarely can be as long as a month or longer. CLM typically presents as a serpiginous erythematous track associated with intense pruritis

Table 36.6 Typical levels of eosinophilia among parasitic infections in travelers. The degree of eosinophilia may differ in individual patients. Non-parasitic causes of eosinophilia include allergic disorders (including asthma), HIV, tuberculosis, leprosy, some fungal infections, some forms of lymphoma and leukemia, etc.

Absent (<400/mm³)

- Amebiasis
- *Ascaris lumbricoides* (adult worm stage)
- Giardiasis
- Leishmaniasis
- Malaria
- Tapeworm
- Toxoplasmosis

Absent to mild (<1000/mm³)

- Clonorchiasis, opisthorchiasis (liver flukes) (chronic)
- Cysticercosis (*Taenia solium*, larval stage)
- *Dientamoeba fragilis*
- Echinococcosis (hydatid disease)
- Enterobiasis (commonly called pinworm in United States and threadworm in UK and Australia)
- Hookworm
- Isosporiasis
- Paragonimiasis (lung fluke)
- Schistosomiasis (chronic)
- Sparganosis tapeworm
- Trichuriasis (whipworm)

Mild to moderate (400–3000/mm³)

- *Ascaris lumbricoides* (larval stage)
- Angiostrongyliasis

Moderate to marked (1000 to >3000/mm³)

- Clonorchiasis, opisthorchiasis (liver flukes) (acute)
- Cysticercosis (if leaking or ruptured cysts)
- Echinococcosis (if leaking or ruptured cysts)
- Hookworm (during larval migration)
- Loiasis (*Loa loa*)
- Paragonimiasis (lung fluke) (during larval migration)
- Schistosomiasis (acute infection, called Katayama fever)
- Toxocariasis
- Trichinosis (acute)
- Tropical pulmonary eosinophilia (occult lymphatic filariasis)

Variable

- Fascioliasis (liver fluke)
- Gnathostomiasis
- Lymphatic filariasis
- Onchocerciasis
- Strongyloidiasis

Source: adapted from Ryan *et al.* (2002).

and mild swelling. Typical locations are the bottom or top of feet, buttocks and, more rarely, trunk or other locations (Malhotra *et al.*, 2006). The track advances from a few millimeters to a few centimeters per day as the larvae advance.

Spontaneous resolution is the rule, usually within weeks to months. Treatment of choice is albendazole 400 mg orally daily for 3 days. Cryotherapy may be ineffective as the larva may be up to 2 cm ahead of the visible burrow. Risk of acquiring CLM is reduced by wearing protective footwear while walking on beaches or soil.

Localized cutaneous leishmaniasis

Leishmaniasis is infection with protozoan *Leishmania* species, for which the vectors are phlebotomine sandflies. Travelers may not notice sandfly bites, as sandflies are silent, small (about one-third the size of mosquitoes or smaller), and bites may be painless. In addition to cutaneous leishmaniasis, the parasite can also cause visceral leishmaniasis, which affects spleen, liver, and bone marrow.

Localized cutaneous leishmaniasis (LCL) is transmitted in over 90 tropical and warm temperate countries. New World LCL is transmitted in forested regions of Latin America and is usually caused by species of *L. braziliensis* and *L. mexicana* complexes. Old World LCL, most commonly caused by *L. major* and *L. tropica*, occurs in sub-Saharan and North Africa, the Mediterranean basin, and the Middle East.

Tourists most commonly acquire this infection in Latin America. Meanwhile, military personnel deployed in the Middle East saw relatively high rates of infection with, for example, over 600 cases of leishmaniasis among US military personnel deployed to Iraq in 2003 alone. Since that time, however, there has been a marked decline in the rate of cases, likely due to improvements in housing for military personnel, control of sandflies, and increased use of personal protection measures (Armed Forces Health Surveillance Center, 2007; Anon., 2012).

Clinical forms of LCL include papule, nodule, plaque, ulcer, and nodular lymphangitis. Cutaneous ulcer is the most frequent clinical presentation of New World LCL, although spread to the mucous membranes can lead to the less common, but severely disfiguring, mucocutaneous form of leishmaniasis. Cutaneous ulcers usually have a well-circumscribed border, a

Table 36.7 Travel-associated dermatoses diagnosed in 269 French travelers presenting to a tropical medicine clinic in Paris.

Diagnosis	Percent
Cutaneous larva migrans	24.9%
Pyodermas	17.8%
Arthropod-related pruritic dermatitis	9.7%
Myiasis	9.3%
Tungiasis	6.3%
Urticaria	5.9%
Rash with fever	4.1%
Cutaneous leishmaniasis	3.0%
Scabies	2.2%
Injuries	1.9%
Cutaneous fungal infections	1.9%
Exacerbation of preexisting illness	1.9%
Sexually transmitted infection	1.5%
Cutaneous herpes simplex	1.1%
Septicemia	1.1%
Acute venous thrombosis	0.7%
Pityriasis rosea	0.7%
Mycobacterium marinum infection	0.7%
Acute lymphatic filariasis	0.4%
Traumatic abrasion	0.4%
Miscellaneous[a]	1.1%
Undetermined	3.3%

[a] Miscellaneous diagnoses were lichen planus, erythema nodosum (manifesting infection with *Salmonella enteritidis*), and Reiter syndrome (of unknown etiology).

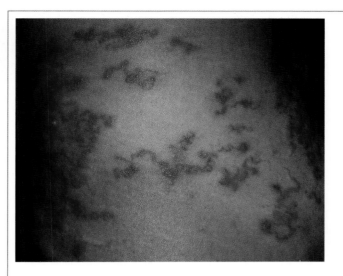

Figure 36.3 Cutaneous larva migrans after hookworm infection. *Source*: Wikimedia © WeisSagung. Reproduced under the Creative Commons license.

crusted base, and are painless (Figure 36.4). Diagnosis is most commonly made with skin biopsy from the ulcer edge. The resulting slit-skin smears are grown on various media, stained with Giemsa, and examined under light microscopy for characteristic amastigotes, or the intracellular form of the parasite (Herwaldt, 1999).

The mainstay of treatment are the pentavalent antimonial agents, sodium stibogluconate and meglumine antimoniate. These two agents have similar efficacy.

Myiasis

Cutaneous myiasis is skin infestation with fly larvae. Myiasis is most frequently caused by the tumbu fly (*Cordylobia anthropophaga*) in sub-Saharan Africa and by the bot fly (*Dermatobia hominis*) in Central and South America. Tumbu fly larvae penetrate the skin after hatching from eggs on clothing and linens that have usually been dried on clothing lines. Lesions typically appear on body parts covered by clothing. On the other hand, bot fly larvae are deposited on the skin by mosquitoes and therefore the lesions are more commonly on uncovered areas of skin. The incubation period for the tumbu fly is 7–10 days, and for the bot fly is 15–45 days.

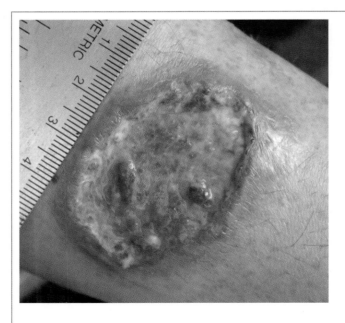

Figure 36.4 Cutaneous leishmaniasis. Additional photos of cutaneous leishmaniasis, including the mucocutaneous form, can be seen in Chapter 20. *Source*: Wikimedia © Layne Harris. Reproduced under the Creative Commons license.

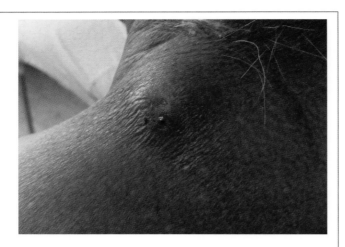

Figure 36.5 Cutaneous myiasis lesion. *Source*: Wikimedia © Petruss. Reproduced under the Creative Commons license.

The skin lesion from either of these flies consists of a 1- to 2-cm furuncular swelling with a minor central punctum that discharges a small amount of serosanguineous or purulent fluid (Figure 36.5). The patient often complains of a sense of movement within the lesion. The number of lesions is typically higher for those with tumbu fly myiasis than with bot fly myiasis. In one study of travelers with myiasis, patients with tumbu fly myiasis had, on average, five lesions compared with 1.7 lesions among those with bot fly myiasis (Jelinek *et al.*, 1995).

Treatment is removal of the larvae. The extraction method is different for the two species. Tumbu fly larvae can be expressed from skin by lateral pressure to either side of the lesion. Bot fly larvae can be extracted after first placing an occlusive substance (e.g., petroleum jelly, bacon fat) over the lesion. Over the course of ensuing hours, the bot fly larvae will migrate toward the surface of the skin, facilitating removal (Brewer *et al.*, 1993). While most travelers are fundamentally unsettled by having wriggling larvae in their skin, significant morbidity, aside from local cellulitis, is rare.

Tumbu fly myiasis can be prevented by ironing clothing and linens after they are dried. Risk of bot fly myiasis can be reduced by covering skin while outdoors, applying DEET or picaridin to exposed skin, applying permethrin to clothing, and sleeping under a permethrin-treated bednet.

Other common etiologies of dermatologic disorders in international travelers include tungiasis (sand flea infestation, most commonly presenting on the feet, often adjacent to a toenail), pyodermas (bacterial skin infections, often secondary to insect bites), dermatophytoses (ringworm, which is more common in the tropics and subtropics), and arthropod-related dermatoses. Chapter 28 provides additional discussion of tropical dermatology.

Other illnesses

Following gastrointestinal disorders, fever, and dermatologic disorders, the three most common remaining categories of illness in returned travelers are respiratory or pharyngeal disorders (10.9%); genitourinary, sexually transmitted infections (Chapter 16), and gynecologic disorders (2.9%); and neurologic disorders (1.7%). The most common respiratory illnesses are non-specific upper respiratory infections, influenza and influenza-like illness, bronchitis, and pneumonia. The most common neurologic disorders include:

- ciguatera intoxication, which results from the consumption of contaminated reef fish and is associated with a syndrome of paresthesia, nerve palsy, and hot–cold temperature reversal that can persist for weeks;
- neurocysticercosis following incidental consumption of the eggs of *Taenia solium* (pork tapeworm);
- tuberculosis meningitis or tuberculoma;
- scombroid poisoning from eating spoiled fish;
- neurotoxic or paralytic shellfish poisoning (Leder *et al.*, 2013).

An important caveat for those caring for returned international travelers is that a significant proportion of illness in the post-travel period is unrelated to travel. Hence, when generating a differential diagnosis for any given symptoms, clinicians should include both travel-related and domestic etiologies.

Additional resources

- Brunette GW (ed.) (2012) *CDC Health Information for International Travel 2012.* New York: Oxfrod University Press.
- Cook GC, Zumla AI (eds) (2008) *Manson's Tropical Diseases*, 22nd edn. Philadelphia: WB Saunders.
- Steffen R, DuPont HL, Wilder-Smith A (eds) (2007) *Manual of Travel Medicine and Health*, 3rd edn. Hamilton, Ontario: BC Decker.
- Guerrant RL, Walker DH, Weller PF (eds) (2011) *Tropical Infectious Diseases: Principles, Pathogens, and Practice*, 3rd edn. Philadelphia: Saunders Elsevier.
- Jong EC, Sanford C (eds) (2008) *The Travel and Tropical Medicine Manual*, 4th edn. Philadelphia: Saunders Elsevier.
- Keystone JS, Kozarsky PE, Freedman DO, Connor BA, Nothdurft HD (eds) (2013) *Travel Medicine*, 3rd edn. Philadelphia: Elsevier Saunders.
- Sanford C (2008) *The Adventurous Traveler's Guide to Health.* Seattle, WA: University of Washington Press.
- Magill AJ, Ryan ET, Solomon T, Hill DR (eds) (2012) *Hunter's Tropical Medicine and Emerging Infectious Disease*, 9th edn. Philadelphia: Saunders Elsevier.

REFERENCES

Anon. (2012) Reported vectorborne and zoonotic diseases, U.S. Army and U.S. Navy, 2000–2011. *MSMR* 19(10):15–6.

Armed Forces Health Surveillance Center (2007) Leishmaniasis in relation to service in Iraq/Afghanistan, U.S. Armed Forces, 2001–2006. *MSMR* 14(1):2–5.

Black RE (1990) Epidemiology of travelers' diarrhea and relative importance of various pathogens. *Rev Infect Dis* 12:S73–9.

Bowie MD, Hill ID, Mann MD (1995) Loperamide for treatment of acute diarrhoea in infants and young children. A double-blind placebo-controlled trial. *S Afr Med J* 85:885–7.

Brewer TF, Wilson ME, Gonzalez E, Felsenstein D (1993) Bacon therapy and furuncular myiasis. *JAMA* 270:2087–8.

Caumes E, Carriére J, Guermonprez G, Bricaire F, Danis M, Gentilini M (1995) Dermatoses associated with travel to tropical countries: a prospective study of the diagnosis and management of 269 patients presenting to a tropical disease unit. *Clin Infect Dis* 20:542–8.

Centers for Disease Control and Prevention (2004) Diagnosis and management of foodborne illnesses: a primer for physicians and other health care professionals. *MMWR Recomm Rep* 53(RR-4):7–12.

Centers for Disease Control and Prevention (2012) Traveler's diarrhea. In: Brunette GW (ed.) *CDC Health Information for International Travel 2012*. New York: Oxford University Press, pp. 56–9.

De Bruyn G, Hahn S, Borwick A (2000) Antibiotic treatment for travellers' diarrhoea. *Cochrane Database Syst Rev* (3):CD002242.

Doherty JF, Grant AD, Bryceson AD (1995) Fever as the presenting complaint of travellers returning from the tropics. *Q J Med* 88:277–81.

DuPont HL, Capsuto EG (1996) Persistent diarrhea in travelers. *Clin Infect Dis* 22:124–8.

Freedman DO, Weld LH, Kozarsky PE *et al.* (2006) Spectrum of disease and relation to place of exposure among ill returned travelers. *N Engl J Med* 354:119–30.

Herwaldt BL (1999) Leishmaniasis. *Lancet* 354:1191–9.

Hill D (2000) Health problems in a large cohort of Americans traveling to developing countries. *J Travel Med* 7:259–66.

Huang DB, Awasthi M, Binh-Minh Le *et al.* (2004) The role of diet in the treatment of travelers' diarrhea: a pilot study. *Clin Infect Dis* 39:468–71.

International Working Group on Persistent Diarrhea (1996) Evaluation of an algorithm for the treatment of persistent diarrhea: a multicenter study. *Bull WHO* 74:478.

Jelinek T, Nothdurft HD, Rieder N, Loscher T (1995) Cutaneous myiasis: review of 13 cases in travelers returning from tropical countries. *Int J Dermatol* 34:624–6.

Jensenius M, Han PV, Schlagenhauf P *et al.* (2013) Acute and potentially life-threatening tropical diseases in western travelers: a GeoSentinel multicenter study, 1996–2011. *Am J Trop Med Hyg* 88:397–404.

Johnson PC, Ericsson CD, DuPont HL, Morgan DR, Bitsura JA, Wood LV (1986) Comparison of loperamide with bismuth subsalicylate for the treatment of acute travelers' diarrhea. *JAMA* 255:757–60.

Jong E, Sanford C (eds) (2008) *The Travel and Tropical Medicine Manual*, 4th edn. Philadelphia: Saunders Elsevier, chapter 27.

Leder K, Torresi J, Libman MD *et al.* (2013) GeoSentinel surveillance of illness in returned travelers, 2007–2011. *Ann Intern Med* 158:456–68.

Leggatt PA (2007) Assessment of febrile illness in the returned traveller. *Aust Fam Physician* 36:328–32.

Li ST, Grossman DC, Cummings P (2007) Loperamide therapy for acute diarrhea in children: systematic review and meta-analysis. *PLoS Med* 4(3):e98.

MacLean J, Lalondi R, Ward B (1994) Fever from the tropics. *Travel Med Advis* 5:27.2–27.14.

Malhotra SK, Raj RT, Pal M (2006) Cutaneous larva migrans in an unusual site. *Dermatol Online J* 12(2):11.

Merck Manual for Health Care Professionals (2014) Eosinophilia. Available at http://www.merckmanuals.com/professional/hematology_and_oncology/eosinophilic_disorders/eosinophilia.html

O'Brien D, Tobin S, Brown GV, Torresi J (2001) Fever in returned travelers: review of hospital admissions for a 3-year period. *Clin Infect Dis* 33:603–9.

Ryan ET, Kain KC (2000) Health advice and immunizations for travelers. *N Engl J Med* 342:1716–25.

Ryan ET, Wilson ME, Kain KC (2002) Illness after international travel. *N Engl J Med* 347:505–16.

Sanford C (2002) Pre-travel advice: an overview. *Prim Care* 29:767–85.

de Saussure PPH (2009) Management of the returning traveler with diarrhea. *Therap Adv Gastroenterol* 2:367–75.

Steffen RF (2005) Epidemiology of traveler's diarrhea. *Clin Infect Dis* 41(Suppl. 8):S536–40.

Steffen RF, van der Linde F, Gyr K, Schar M (1983) Epidemiology of diarrhea in travelers. *JAMA* 249:1176–80.

Steffen RF, Rickenbach M, Wilhelm U, Helminger A, Schar M (1987) Health problems after travel to developing countries. *J Infect Dis* 156:84–91.

Taylor DN, Connor BA, Shlim DR (1999) Chronic diarrhea in the returned traveler. *Med Clin North Am* 83:1033–52.

United Nations World Tourism Organization (2011) Tourism market trends. Available at http://dtxtq4w60xqpw.cloudfront.net/sites/all/files/docpdf/markettrends.pdf

Von Sonnenburg F, Tornieporth N, Waiyaki P *et al.* (2000) Risk and aetiology of diarrhoea at various tourist destinations. *Lancet* 356:133–4.

Wilson MD, Pearson R (1999) Fever and systemic symptoms. In: Guerrant FL, Walker DH, Weller PF (eds) *Tropical Infectious Diseases: Principles, Pathogens, and Practice*. Philadelphia: Churchill Livingston, pp. 1381–99.

Wilson ME, Schwartz E (2004) Fever. In: Keystone JS, Kozarsky PE, Freedman DO *et al.* (eds) *Travel Medicine*. Edinburgh: Mosby.

Wolfe MS (2008) The eosinophilic patient with suspected parasitic infection. In: Jong, EC, Sanford C (eds) *The Travel and Tropical Medicine Manual*, 4th edn. London: Saunders Elsevier.

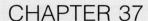

CHAPTER 37
Developing a Career in Global Health

Brett D. Nelson[1,2] and Michael B. Hadley[2]
[1]Massachusetts General Hospital, Boston, MA, USA
[2]Harvard Medical School, Boston, MA, USA

Key learning objectives

■ Review global health opportunities available during each stage of medical training.
■ Discuss potential career paths and employers in global health.
■ Reflect on personal considerations when pursuing careers in global health.

Abstract

Interest in global health among students, clinical trainees, and healthcare providers has reached unprecedented levels. A growing number of individuals are pursuing global health as a specific career choice. Meanwhile, clinical training programs are working to provide students and trainees with needed mentorship and opportunities to gain the experience necessary for this career pursuit. This chapter strives to provide some general guidance about developing a career in global health. We discuss frequent career questions, potential opportunities available during each stage of clinical training, and various global health career models. Lastly, we provide a compilation of resources to help trainees identify career opportunities that align with their global health interests and goals.

Key words: global health, career planning, career development, medical school, residency, fellowship, program delivery, policy, research, mentorship

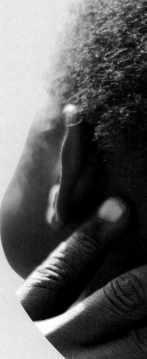

Essential Clinical Global Health, First Edition. Edited by Brett D. Nelson.
© 2015 John Wiley & Sons, Ltd. Published 2015 by John Wiley & Sons, Ltd.
Companion website: www.essentialseries.com/globalhealth

Introduction

A career in global health is one dedicated to addressing health disparities and reducing the burden of disease and mortality in resource-limited settings. Practitioners help secure for those they serve the right to the highest attainable standards of health. Unprecedented numbers of students, clinical trainees, and healthcare providers are participating in global health work today, and while a majority of those participating are periodically involved, a growing number of individuals are also pursuing global health as a specific career choice (Chase & Evert, 2011; Nelson *et al.*, 2012a).

This chapter attempts to provide some guidance to those interested in establishing global health as a significant part of their careers. First, we discuss frequently asked questions regarding the development global health careers. We then review the various global health opportunities available to students and trainees throughout their medical training. Next, we explore different career models and potential employment opportunities. Finally, recognizing that this chapter cannot nearly be comprehensive, we provide a compilation of helpful resources for further reading.

When considering a career in global health, one can begin by considering the questions listed in the self-assessment questionnaire (Box 37.1). Additional discussion of many of these issues is provided throughout the rest of the chapter.

Box 37.1 Self-assessment questionnaire

- **Satisfaction:** What matters most to you and why? What kind of impact do you want to have? What makes up a good day for you? What activities do you enjoy? Are there specific populations you wish to serve? Do you prefer structure or flexibility, desk or fieldwork?
- **Career:** What are your areas of expertise? Do you prefer clinical work, research, policy, management? What other experience or advanced degrees will you need?
- **Family:** How will you maintain your most important relationships? Do you and your partner share the same goals? Can you both find fulfillment in a global health context? Do you have or plan to have children? Would you be comfortable raising them overseas or being away from them for short periods of time?
- **Location:** Where would you like to work? With which languages and cultures are you most comfortable? Would you prefer to work domestically, abroad, or both?
- **Finances:** How much funding will you need? How much debt do you have? How will you finance a career in global health?

Considerations when planning a career in global health

Interests and passions

Individuals are rewarded by careers focused on the issues and populations about which they care most. Therefore, clinicians considering careers in global health should take time to reflect on their goals and whether these goals can be best achieved by working in global health.

Choice of medical specialty

Global health training programs and employment opportunities are regularly filled by clinical generalists (Nelson *et al.*, 2012a). Common specialties include emergency medicine, internal medicine, pediatrics, family medicine, and obstetrics/gynecology. Specialties like emergency medicine and family medicine have often been among the most versatile, empowering clinicians to treat a wide variety of the patients in global health contexts (Hall, 2006).

However, opportunities are growing in other specialties and subspecialties as well. General surgery, ophthalmology, otolaryngology, orthopedics, plastic surgery, and anesthesiology can also be valuable, especially in the form of targeted trips or local skills-training missions (Hall, 2006). Also, with the growing global burden of chronic disease, there are increasing needs for radiologists, oncologists, cardiologists, pulmonologists, endocrinologists, neurologists, dermatologists, pathologists, and other subspecialists.

As you make your decision of which medical specialty to pursue, consider differences in versatility and flexibility among specialties. Explore different residency, fellowship, and funding opportunities (see Additional resources section). And, most importantly, consider your own interests and find a clinical field rewarding in its own right. Regardless of the specialty you select, you can always find ways to be involved globally.

Spouses or partners

When considering global health work, clinicians and their partners should openly discuss each other's goals, hopes, and concerns. If electing to move abroad, both individuals in a couple should first feel confident that they can find fulfillment in a context with different languages, cultures, race/gender/sexual inequalities, job opportunities and earnings, work permits and visas, personal safety and health risks, childcare and education challenges, and separation from friends and family.

Children

Some global health professionals with families are based domestically and are regularly separated from their families as they travel abroad. Others are based abroad and choose to raise their children overseas. If raising children abroad, it is sometimes easiest when children are young and may easily acquire a second language, develop fluency with other cultures, and have tighter relationships with their parents (Hall, 2006). However, teenagers may suffer more from deficient schools, social maladjustment, and parting with friends back home. Health and safety are also concerns for children of all ages. Clinicians considering raising a family abroad should first investigate the perspectives of other parents working in the region regarding safety, costs, schools, community, etc. Alternatively, clinicians sometimes wait until their children have left home for college before beginning an in-country position.

Taking a trial run

Clinicians and their partners may benefit from a trial run of their envisioned global health career. When exploring the idea of a career in global health, it is usually beneficial to try linking with an existing project with a reputable organization, rather than starting with an entirely independent project that may not reflect local needs or the true flavor of global health work. Information on some of the many organizations providing meaningful experiences can be found in the Additional resources section.

Domestic versus international

A career spent abroad is for many clinicians a wonderful blend of meaningful service, humbling challenges, and new experiences. Clinicians should target locations where they can be productive and feel personally comfortable. This requires consideration of local languages, cultures, living conditions, dietary restrictions, personal safety, visas, and access to health services.

Still, life spent abroad may strain relationships with family and friends. Therefore, some clinicians set up a domestic base and make trips abroad, often financing their international work with their part-time domestic work. Although this lifestyle allows partner and children to be based domestically, these clinicians can at times feel stretched between their multiple commitments and geographies.

Alternatively, some global health practitioners work full-time domestically, often in high-level research, management, or consultancy positions. Although this track offers greater stability, these clinicians may miss the privilege of working day to day alongside the international communities they serve. Clinicians desiring both to serve marginalized populations and to work full-time domestically may work among underserved communities in their own country.

Clinical experience

"Global health is my passion and, after 20 years, maintaining a balance between personal and professional life is still a challenge. My work involves extensive international travel for at least 6 months a year. Being self-employed allows me to choose projects that fit my career goals while doing justice to personal commitments. I have been able to set priorities and more or less stick to them, and I am blessed with an extremely understanding and supportive life partner! When working out of home, the line between personal and professional life gets blurred. My strategy is to go completely offline every evening at a specific time, returning the next morning. It is also crucial to set aside some time for exercise and personal endeavors. It's easier said than done but not impossible; the mantra is to judiciously distribute energy between these spaces. The best aspect of global health is interacting with wonderful people and cultures across the world. No profession is without stress but very few satisfy your heart, mind, and soul as a career in global health does."

Kiran, physician and public health professional

Financing a global health career

Clinicians pursuing careers in global health often feel financially pressured. In the United States, for example, 85.5% of medical school graduates carry outstanding loans, with an average educational debt of nearly US$150,000 (Association of American Medical Colleges, 2013). The lack of funding for global health activities means clinicians often self-finance additional training (Nelson *et al.*, 2012a). Also, salaries for positions overseas may be a fraction of their domestic counterparts.

Nevertheless, a career in global health can be financially viable. Part-time employment at home can finance short-term activities abroad. Long-term full-time positions abroad usually provide a salary package sufficient for any reduced cost of living overseas. Additionally, federal loan forgiveness programs may help reduce debt for clinicians employed in certain non-profit organizations. Some clinicians also supplement their income through global health consulting and business ventures. Well-established program- and research-focused individuals may earn salary support through competitive grants from funders like the Bill and Melinda Gates Foundation or the National Institutes of Health (NIH).

Regardless, global health is not considered a path to riches; practitioners must feel fulfilled by their work itself. Over their careers, these practitioners strike a balance between the work they enjoy and the income they need to achieve their personal and familial goals.

Opportunities during medical training

Interest in global health among medical students and residents has reached unprecedented levels (Chase & Evert, 2011). Currently, over 30% of US medical students, for example, participate in global health experiences each year, compared with only 6% in 1984. Similar trends are seen in other Western countries (Association of American Medical Colleges, 1984, 2013; Drain *et al.*, 2007). Likewise, a growing number of physicians-in-training are completing global health electives (Torjesen *et al.*, 1999; Nelson *et al.*, 2008a). Studies demonstrate that these experiences improve trainees' skills as clinicians; global health experiences improve physical examination and language skills, decrease reliance on technology, increase awareness of cultures and costs, and boost physician empathy, flexibility, openness, and confidence (Federico *et al.*, 2006; Drain *et al.*, 2007; Chase & Evert, 2011; Nelson *et al.*, 2012a).

However, medical schools and clinical training programs are struggling to keep up with demands for global health funding, training, mentorship, and experiences overseas (Chase & Evert, 2011; Nelson *et al.*, 2012a). Trainees struggle to find free time, gain worthwhile experience while still developing their skills, and balance family, career, and finances (Drain *et al.*, 2007). Given these barriers interested trainees must be proactive about identifying global health opportunities and building core skills. These skills include communication, advocacy, interpersonal skills, diagnosis and management of endemic diseases, epidemiologic skills for needs-based research, leadership, and an understanding of public health and population-based approaches to health (Evert *et al.*, 2008; Nelson *et al.*, 2008b). Here we discuss some strategies for maximizing one's global health education during clinical training.

Medical school

Many students pursue global health opportunities during medical school. Because of their initially limited clinical training, however, medical students may be at risk of burdening already stretched in-country healthcare programs (Nelson *et al.*, 2012a). Medical students should contribute within their current skills and should not perform clinical duties for which they have not been trained or would not yet be allowed to do in their home country. Therefore, medical students interested in global health should focus first on non-clinical opportunities or on learning in the clinical setting in a largely observer capacity. Within the classroom back home, students can explore different medical specialties, pursue domestically based global health electives (Figure 37.1), or enroll in an advanced-degree program. Extracurricularly, students can learn a new language, attend conferences and student events, identify mentors and role models, and assist with global health research in their areas of interest. However, in all cases, it is imperative that students

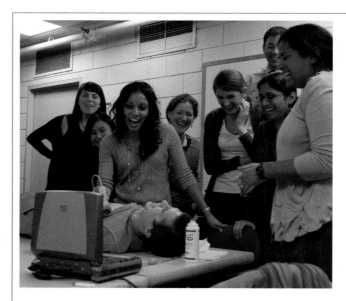

Figure 37.1 Medical students are introduced to various practical skills, including basic bedside ultrasound, during a global health course in Boston. *Source:* B.D. Nelson, Harvard Medical School, Boston, Massachusetts, USA. Reproduced with permission of B.D. Nelson.

not lose focus on mastering the medical school curriculum and becoming a well-trained clinician; without a strong foundation of clinical skills, one cannot be an effective global health clinician.

Residency

Each year, a large number of residents pursue global health experiences, either through international electives and tracks within traditional training programs or, increasingly, as part of dedicated global health residency programs. Currently, there are many 3-year residences with global health curricula, mentorship, and electives abroad (Nelson *et al.*, 2008a). Additionally, there are a growing number of formal global health residency programs, often with an integrated year dedicated to global health research and delivery (Furin *et al.*, 2006; Vinci *et al.*, 2009).

Residents not in a formal global health program can often still use call-free elective time and vacation to pursue international experiences, participate in global health projects, work on dataset analysis, or perform literature reviews (Nelson *et al.*, 2012a). Whenever working abroad, residents deserve and require mentorship and close supervision, even to a greater degree than at home due to novel disease profiles, disease acuity, resource levels, languages, culture, and other variables.

Table 37.1 Examples of post-residency training opportunities. Please note that this list is by no means intended to be comprehensive but simply illustrative of opportunities.

Short-duration global health courses	University of Arizona Global Health Clinical and Community Care Course (3 weeks) Johns Hopkins Summer Institute in Tropical Medicine and Public Health (6 weeks) Harvard Humanitarian Initiative's Humanitarian Studies Course (2 weeks) ICRC's Health Emergencies in Large Populations (HELP) Course (2 weeks)
Diploma or certificate in tropical medicine	London School of Hygiene and Tropical Medicine (3 months) Liverpool School of Tropical Medicine (3 months) Gorgas Course in Clinical Tropical Medicine (Peru) (2 months) Various programs offering the Certificate of Knowledge in Clinical Tropical Medicine and Travelers' Health (CTropMed) from the American Society of Tropical Medicine and Hygiene (2 months) Courses offered through the tropEd network of European and other international institutions
Traditional clinical subspecialty fellowships, with research time focusing on a global health topic	Many traditional subspecialty fellowships have relevance to global health and include research time that can focus on a global health topic (e.g., neonatology, critical care) (2–3 years)
Global health-specific clinical fellowships	Dozens of examples in all major specialties: emergency medicine, family medicine, internal medicine, pediatrics, women's health (1–2 years) (Nelson *et al.*, 2012b)
Research fellowships	Burroughs Wellcome Fund/American Society of Tropical Medicine and Hygiene Postdoctoral Fellowship in Tropical Infectious Diseases (2 years) NIH/Fogarty Global Health Program for Fellows and Scholars Robert Wood Johnson Foundation Clinical Scholars (2 years) Institute of Health Metrics and Evaluation Post-Graduate Fellowship (1–2 years)
Field-based epidemiologic training	Centers for Disease Control and Prevention Epidemic Intelligence Service (EIS) (2 years)
Field- and service-based training programs	US Global Health Service Partnership (a joint program of the US Peace Corps, PEPFAR, and Seed Global Health) (1–2 years) Texas Children's Global Health Service Corps (1 year) Yale/Stanford Johnson & Johnson Global Health Scholars Program (6 weeks) Afya Bora Fellowship in Global Health Leadership (1 year)
Missions with non-governmental organizations	Médecins Sans Frontières (MSF) (Doctors Without Borders) (6–9 months) Médecins du Monde (Doctors of the World)
Internships with international organizations	World Health Organization United Nations

Post-residency training opportunities

Following residency training, there exists a large and growing number of opportunities that can provide additional training and experience in global health. These post-residency opportunities include global health-related didactic courses, diplomas, fellowships, and other field-based experiences (Table 37.1). In recent years, for example, there has been a particularly rapid increase in the availability of clinical global health fellowships, which are available within the fields of emergency medicine, family medicine, internal medicine, pediatrics, surgery, women's health, and others (Figure 37.2) (Nelson *et al.*, 2012b). These global health-specific clinical fellowships are typically 19–24 months and involve clinical service provision abroad, global health research, and some form of didactics,

such as an advanced degree or diploma (Figure 37.3) (Nelson *et al.*, 2012b). Alternatively, a non-clinical fellowship that provides excellent field-based epidemiologic training is the highly regarded Centers for Disease Control and Prevention (CDC) Epidemic Intelligence Service (EIS) program, which may often lead to an entry-level position with, for example, the CDC, USAID, and others.

Making the most of mentorship

A good mentor will provide valuable insight, inspiration, and guidance in career development (Chase & Evert, 2011). As early as possible, a trainee should identify a mentor who understands her goals, knows about her areas of interest, and is enthusiastic, generous, reliable, admirable, and supportive (Sambunjak *et al.*,

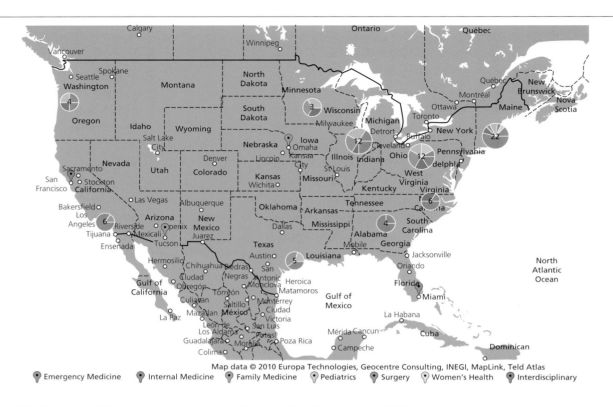

Figure 37.2 Database of US-based clinical global health fellowships (Nelson *et al.*, 2012b).

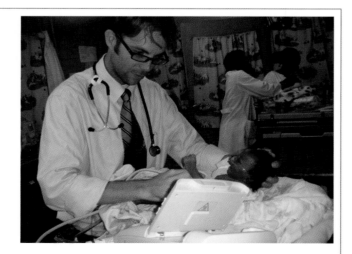

Figure 37.3 A pediatric global health fellow – in this case, a younger version of the editor working in Liberia – conducts a bedside cardiac echocardiogram on a newborn with a suspected congenital heart defect. *Source*: M. Niescierenko, Harvard Medical School, Boston, Massachusetts, USA. Reproduced with permission of M. Niescierenko.

2010; Cho *et al.*, 2011). The trainee should take the lead in cultivating the relationship by creating a plan with high standards and deadlines and by working with the mentor on concrete activities like a research project, manuscript, or presentation (Straus *et al.*, 2009; Cho *et al.*, 2011). If necessary, the trainee should also seek out additional mentors to meet her needs. For example, a trainee could connect with a relatively young mentor to think through immediate next steps in the trainee's career and with a more experienced mentor to provide expertise and in-country contacts for a particular project.

Advanced-degree training

Advanced-degree training may enhance a trainee's impact, employability, and career progression. Trainees often pursue advanced degrees either between third and fourth year of medical school or during a post-residency fellowship. By earning an advanced degree in medical school, the trainee can explore different interests early in one's career pathway. On the other hand, by earning an advanced degree during fellowship, the trainee may more likely immediately apply the knowledge gained. In what follows, we review several advanced training programs relevant to global health careers.

Clinical experience

"Developing a career in global health requires enthusiasm, flexibility, and a bit of perseverance – like most things! Personally, the keys to developing my career have been finding great mentors, flexibility, and, of course, incredibly supportive friends and family. When I am home, I prioritize seeing those closest to me, and then I stay connected via Skype and phone when I travel. Mentorship, both locally and globally, has helped me craft and refine my career. In the end, my best advice is to find something you love doing – if you are passionate about and happy with your work, the positives far outweigh the challenges of a career in global health. I feel very fortunate to have a career that is challenging, rewarding, and ultimately makes me quite happy."

Regan, physician and public health professional

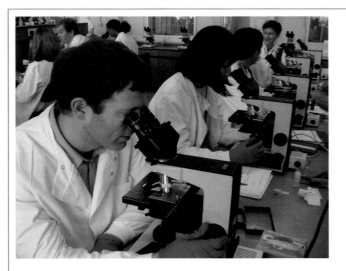

Figure 37.4 Within a Diploma in Tropical Medicine and Hygiene (DTM&H) course from the Royal College of Physicians, clinicians study tropical microscopy and management of tropical diseases. *Source*: B.D. Nelson, Harvard Medical School, Boston, Massachusetts, USA. Reproduced with permission of B.D. Nelson.

MPH

The Master of Public Health (MPH) degree, sometimes offered as a Master of Science (e.g., in International Health), imparts knowledge and skills around population health. During the 1- or 2-year program, students learn epidemiology, biostatistics, demography, health policy, program evaluation, and other skills. Additionally, students can take a diverse selection of electives in areas of interest. The MPH degree is particularly useful and versatile for clinicians interested in long-term involvement in global health service delivery, research, or policy.

MBA, MPP, and MPA

Programs for the degrees of Master of Business Administration (MBA), Master of Public Policy (MPP), and Master of Public Administration (MPA) offer training in management, macroeconomics, finance, and other topics that emphasize effective program administration. Clinicians interested in social entrepreneurship or organizational management might consider the MBA or MPA. Clinicians interested in government administration and policy may consider the MPP or MPA. Additionally, there are combined MBA/MPP programs that cover both domains.

Diploma/certificate in tropical medicine

These shorter programs (2–6 months) train clinicians in the diagnosis and management of tropical diseases found in many developing countries, while providing a basic understanding of related public health interventions. There are over a dozen programs that lead to either a Diploma in Tropical Medicine and Hygiene (DTM&H) from, for example, the Royal College of Physicians (Figure 37.4), or a Certificate of Knowledge in Clinical Tropical Medicine and Travelers' Health (CTropMed) from the American Society of Tropical Medicine and Hygiene.

Language programs

Foreign language proficiency is nearly essential for many long-term in-country global health positions. If you are unsure of your eventual region(s) of interest but are interested in pursuing language training, you could consider one of the more common official UN languages: French, Spanish, or Arabic, in addition to English (United Nations, 2014). There are numerous language programs available, both domestically and internationally, in-person, by multimedia, and online.

Other paths

Clinicians with advanced training in other fields outside of medicine often foster innovation by bringing their unique perspective to global health problems. Examples of some popular and useful paths include anthropology, economics, education, engineering, technology, design, development studies, informatics, law, media studies, and sociology (Hall, 2006).

Career models

Global health is not simply a discipline but rather a set of issues requiring multiple disciplines to solve (Farmer, 2011). Accordingly, there are many ways to get involved. Here, we explore three common global health career models for clinicians

(Nelson *et al.*, 2012a). Each model is open to considerations of full-time versus part-time, domestic versus international, and emergency relief versus long-term development. Many global health careers incorporate facets of each.

Service and program delivery

Clinicians working in the service and program delivery sector design, implement, and evaluate programs that deliver health services to vulnerable populations and those in need (Nelson *et al.*, 2012a). Short-term positions may involve direct clinical service provision or, more sustainably, training local staff. For example, a clinician might spend several weeks with a non-governmental organization (NGO) training local providers in essential newborn care. Alternatively, clinicians can help local service delivery organizations improve quality and efficiency through consulting or monitoring and evaluation.

Longer-term positions are also available in healthcare service and program delivery. In fact, many of the historical examples of global health careers involved clinicians living and working for decades among the populations they served. Albert Schweitzer, a German–French physician and medical missionary, is a well-known example of this model and spent his life providing clinical care in West–Central Africa. Whether with faith-based or non-faith-based organizations, there are countless clinicians who pursue long-term service and program delivery abroad. Although such immersion can come with significant sacrifices, arguably there may be few ways one can have a more rewarding and directly impactful career.

Perhaps even more frequently than providing direct clinical care, clinicians are involved in health program delivery. For instance, a clinician with public health training may lead an in-country team in the design, implementation, and evaluation of a new childhood nutrition program. Clinicians with extensive experience in program delivery, public health, and management may serve as in-country program directors or administrators. These administrators work closely with policy-makers, government, funders, and partner organizations to decide program priorities, allocate resources accordingly, and oversee program implementation.

Research

Global health researchers develop an evidence-based understanding of health issues and how best to address them (Nelson *et al.*, 2012a). Their research covers a variety of topics, including the social determinants of health, healthcare delivery systems, and strategies for preventing and treating disease. Findings from these studies can significantly impact global health delivery, from the level of individual patient care all the way to global guidelines and priorities.

Research careers can also be intellectually rewarding. They often require additional non-clinical skills, such as epidemiology and biostatistics, which can be acquired through advanced-degree programs or fellowships, as discussed above. Researchers may either live abroad or manage ongoing projects through regular short-term visits. They must communicate regularly with local partners, government officials, and ethics boards to ensure their research is feasible and acceptable.

Trainees interested in staying in academic medicine may consider an academic position in global health research. These positions can offer a mix of teaching, research, consultation, and clinical medicine (Hall, 2006). However, careers in academia may include the need for grants, added pressure to publish, and the challenge of balancing various teaching, clinical, administrative, and research responsibilities. Non-academic positions in global health research include program evaluation, data analysis, and consultancy.

Health and social policy

Policy-makers decide how best to allocate resources at the level of populations. Often, they act to redress issues of health inequality as well as guide the operations of health delivery organizations (Nelson *et al.*, 2012a). Examples of such policies include the Millennium Development Goals and the Covenant on Economic, Social, and Cultural Rights, which guarantees the right to the highest attainable standard of health. Clinicians may elect to become involved in policy after fruitful careers in other areas, such as program management, service delivery, or research. As policy-makers, they can have the opportunity to enact far-reaching, meaningful change in health policy.

Types of organizations involved in global health

Finding the right organization with which to work is important, as a career may be shaped as much by an organization as by the particular project. In what follows, we review several general categories of global health organization. Each category offers opportunities in the career tracks discussed above: service and program delivery, research, and policy. Please refer to Chapter 2 for additional information on the roles these organizations play in the global healthcare system.

Multinational organizations

These include United Nations organizations and affiliates such as the World Health Organization (WHO), United Nations Development Program (UNDP), United Nations Children's Fund (UNICEF), United Nations Population Fund (UNFPA), Joint United Nations Programme on HIV/AIDS (UNAIDS), Global Fund, and World Bank. These organizations provide global normative standards and channel extensive multinational funding into worldwide programming and research. Clinicians employed by multinational organizations typically hold non-clinical positions and travel regularly to assist in program design and evaluation. They typically enjoy more stable salaries and benefits but may need to feel comfortable working within large administrative organizations (Hall, 2006). National quotas on the number of positions available for applicants from various member states can make UN positions competitive.

Bilateral and government organizations

These are state-operated agencies, such as the US Agency for International Development (USAID), the UK's Department for International Development (DFID), French Development Agency (AFD), Australian Agency for International Development (AusAid), European Commission, NIH, and CDC. These organizations typically fund and provide technical support for the work of foreign governments and large NGOs operating in developing countries (Drain *et al.*, 2008). Their priorities may be linked with foreign policy and, as a result, can potentially be politicized.

Non-governmental and relief organizations

Included in this category are organizations such as the International Committee of the Red Cross (ICRC), Médecins Sans Frontières/Doctors without Borders (MSF), Oxfam, Project Hope, BRAC, Partners in Health (PIH), International Rescue Committee (IRC), Catholic Relief Services (CRS), CARE, World Vision, Save the Children, local organizations, and many, many others. These organizations often benefit from a highly committed staff, grassroots orientation, and relatively less bureaucracy and political entanglement (Drain *et al.*, 2008). However, they can struggle with financing, coordination, and sustainability (Drain *et al.*, 2008). Long-term salaried positions often require multiple years of global health experience, public health training, and some fluency in the local language. Short-term and volunteer positions have fewer requirements and can be an entry point into the organization and into global health.

Foundations

These non-profit organizations provide funds or support to other organizations. These include the Bill and Melinda Gates Foundation, Wellcome Trust, Clinton Foundation, Carter Center, Children's Investment Fund Foundation, Rockefeller Foundation, and Kaiser Family Foundation, among others. Foundations decide on their respective agendas and may operate in research, advocacy, policy-making, innovation, program design, implementation, and evaluation. Positions within foundations usually require significant experience and are often competitive.

Academic institutions

Universities and affiliated institutions regularly collaborate with funders, benefactors, ministries of health, and in-country partners to improve health in developing countries (Nelson *et al.*, 2012a). Increasingly, these academic medical centers are opening centers and divisions of global health at their institutions. Consequently, full-time and part-time positions within academic institutions may be available for global health educators, researchers, and clinicians. Typically, however, these global health activities are largely supported by applying for grants and other outside funding.

Consultancies and contracting agencies

These agencies frequently complete large contract work for governments and foundations. They include John Snow Inc. (JSI), Management Sciences for Health, Family Health International, and the University Research Corporation, among others. Although most staff are experienced full-time professionals, these organizations may also offer shorter-term assignments for individuals with specific expertise (Hall, 2006).

Conclusion

Trainee and clinician interest in global health continues to grow, and many individuals are seeking to make global health an integral and longitudinal component of their careers. In this chapter, we have reviewed career models, potential employers, frequently asked questions, opportunities available to trainees throughout their training, as well as a compilation of additional readings. We hope these resources can help readers identify potential career opportunities that align with their personal and professional interests and goals in global health.

Clinical experience

"Since graduating from my public health program, I've remained in touch with many of my fellow MPH peers from graduate school. Throughout the course of our training, we frequently discussed our idealistic ideas on the type of work we would be doing once we graduated. We also discussed our fears of being nomadic and missing out on establishing families. Since we all wanted to travel the world, we were afraid we would never meet the right person or be able to balance the lifestyle with our current partners. I have learned through the diverse experiences of my colleagues that, because there isn't a straight path towards 'success,' whether as a global health professional or starting a family as a global health practitioner, there isn't anything to be concerned about. It's kind of like being an entrepreneur. You can create the life you want by finding the piece of global health that works for you."

Brandi, public health professional

Additional resources

- Healthtraining.org: postgraduate training programs in international health. Available at http://www.healthtraining.org
- Consortium of Universities for Global Health online resources. Available at http://www.cugh.org/resources
- Chase MD, Evert J (2011) *Global Health Training in Graduate Medical Education: A Guidebook*, 2nd edn. Bloomington, IN: iUniverse. Available at http://globalhealthimmersion programs.org/rotations/global-health-training-guidebook-2nd-edition/
- Association of Schools of Public Health. Available at http://www.asph.org
- Evert J, Stewart C, Chan K, Rosenberg M, Hall T (2008) *Developing Residency Training in Global Health: A Guidebook*. San Francisco, CA: Global Health Education Consortium.
- Nelson BD. Global health fellowships listing. Available at http://www.globalhealthfellowships.org
- Nelson BD, Izadnegahdar R, Hall L, Lee PT (2012) Global health fellowships: a national, cross-disciplinary survey of US training opportunities. *J Grad Med Educ* 4:184–9.
- Funding and fellowships sponsored by the American Society of Tropical Medicine and Hygiene. Available at http://www.astmh.org/ASTMH_Sponsored_Fellowships/4277.htm
- University of Michigan Center for Global Health. Student Handbook for Global Engagement, 2012. Available at http://open.umich.edu/education/sph/resources/student-handbook-global-engagement/2011
- Global Health Council. Available at http://www.globalhealth.org
- Osborn G, Ohmans P (2005) *Finding Work in Global Health. A Practical Guide for Job-seekers or Anyone Who Wants to Make the World a Healthier Place*. Health Advocates Press.
- American Society of Hygiene and Tropical Medicine. Approved prerequisite courses for certificate of knowledge examination in clinical tropical medicine and travelers' health. Available at http://www.astmh.org/AM/Template.cfm?Section=Approved_Diploma_Courses&Template=/CM/ContentDisplay.cfm&ContentID=2083

REFERENCES

Association of American Medical Colleges (1984) Medical School Graduation Questionnaire: All Schools Report. Washington, DC: Association of American Medical Colleges.

Association of American Medical Colleges (2013) Medical School Graduation Questionnaire: All Schools Summary Report. Washington, DC: Association of American Medical Colleges.

Chase MD, Evert J (2011) *Global Health Training in Graduate Medical Education: A Guidebook*, 2nd edn. Bloomington, IN: iUniverse.

Cho CS, Ramanan RA, Feldman MD (2011) Defining the ideal qualities of mentorship: a qualitative analysis of the characteristics of outstanding mentors. *Am J Med* 124:453–8.

Drain PK, Primack A, Hunt D, Fawzi W, Holmes K, Gardner P (2007) Global health in medical education: a call for more training and opportunities. *Acad Med* 82:226–30.

Drain PK, Huffman SA, Pirtle S, Chan K (2008) *Caring for the World: A Guidebook to Global Health Opportunities*. Toronto, Ontario: University of Toronto Press.

Evert J, Stewart C, Chan K, Rosenberg M, Hall T (2008) *Developing Residency Training in Global Health: A Guidebook*. San Francisco, CA: Global Health Education Consortium.

Farmer PE (2011) More than just a hobby: what Harvard can do to advance global health. *Harvard Crimson*, May 26.

Federico S, Zachar P, Oravec C, Mandler T, Goldson E, Brown J (2006) A successful international child health elective: the University of Colorado Department of Pediatrics' experience. *Arch Pediatr Adolesc Med* 160:191–6.

Furin J, Farmer P, Wolf M et al. (2006) A novel training model to address health problems in poor and underserved populations. *J Health Care Poor Underserved* 17:17–24.

Hall TL (2006) Global health: career options and specialization. Prepared for the American Public Health Association by the Global Health Education Consortium. Available at http://www.cugh.org/sites/default/files/content/resources/modules/To%20Post%20Trainees/Master%20in%20GH%20career%20options%20and%20specialization%20FINAL_JM.pdf

Nelson BD, Lee AC, Newby PK, Chamberlin MR, Huang CC (2008a) Global health training in pediatric residency programs. *Pediatrics* 122:28–33.

Nelson BD, Herlihy J, Burke TF (2008b) A proposal for fellowship training in pediatric global health. *Pediatrics* 121:1261–2.

Nelson BD, Kasper J, Hibberd PL, Thea DM, Herlihy JM (2012a) Developing a career in global health:

considerations for physicians-in-training and academic mentors. *J Grad Med Educ* 4:301–6.

Nelson BD, Izadnegahdar R, Hall L, Lee PT (2012b) Global health fellowships: a national, cross-disciplinary survey of U.S. training opportunities. *J Grad Med Educ* 4:184–9.

Sambunjak D, Straus S, Marusic A (2010) A systematic review of qualitative research on the meaning and characteristics of mentoring in academic medicine. *J Gen Intern Med* 25:72–8.

Straus S, Chatur F, Taylor M (2009) Issues in the mentor–mentee relationship in academic medicine: a qualitative study. *Acad Med* 84:135–9.

Torjesen K, Mandalakas A, Kahn R, Duncan B (1999) International child health electives for pediatric residents. *Arch Pediatr Adolesc Med* 153:1297–302.

United Nations (2014) UN official languages. Available at http://www.un.org/en/aboutun/languages.shtml

Vinci RJ, Bauchner H, Finkelstein J *et al.* (2009) Research during pediatric residency training: outcome of a senior resident block rotation. *Pediatrics* 124:1126–34.

Index

Page numbers in *italic* refer to figures.
Page numbers in **bold** refer to tables.
Page numbers followed by "b" refer to boxes.
Page numbers followed by "p" refer to panels.
In sorting, spaces are ignored so that, for example, "T lymphocytes" comes after "tiredness".